刘士豪论文选集

主审　夏维波　赵维纲　蒋澄宇

主编　李乃适

中国协和医科大学出版社

北　京

图书在版编目（CIP）数据

刘士豪论文选集／李乃适主编 . —北京：中国协和医科大学出版社，2020. 12
ISBN 978－7－5679－1658－6

Ⅰ. ①刘…　Ⅱ. ①李…　Ⅲ. ①内分泌病－文集 ②肾疾病－文集　Ⅳ. ①R58－53 ②R692－53

中国版本图书馆 CIP 数据核字（2020）第 213976 号

刘士豪论文选集

主　　编：李乃适
主　　审：夏维波　赵维纲　蒋澄宇
策　　划：杨　帆
封面题签：李乃适
责任编辑：顾良军

出版发行：中国协和医科大学出版社
　　　　　（北京市东城区东单三条 9 号　邮编 100730　电话 010－65260431）
网　　址：www. pumcp. com
经　　销：新华书店总店北京发行所
印　　刷：中煤（北京）印务有限公司

开　　本：710×1000　　1/16
印　　张：31
字　　数：470 千字
版　　次：2020 年 12 月第 1 版
印　　次：2020 年 12 月第 1 次印刷
定　　价：165.00 元

ISBN 978－7－5679－1658－6

（凡购本书，如有缺页、倒页、脱页及其他质量问题，由本社发行部调换）

序 一

　　北京协和医院在中国现代医学发展的历史长河中有着非常显著的地位。刘士豪教授作为北京协和医院培养出的佼佼者，不仅是我国内分泌学的奠基人和开拓者，而且在事实上成为了转化医学的先行者。20世纪50年代，他的力作《生物化学与临床医学的联系》一经问世，就在学术界产生了巨大的影响。而其中精华，正是他几十年医教研过程中对如何在临床医学中研究生物化学、又如何将生物化学运用到临床医学实践中去的深刻体会和体系建构。在该书的序言中，他写道："如果能引起生物化学工作者深入临床，临床工作者深入生化，使二者更密切地结合起来向医学进军，则本书抛砖引玉的目的即已达到。"这一句话，实际上和当前转化医学的思想不谋而合，也非常完美地解释了刘士豪教授取得巨大学术成就的深层次原因。这一思想目前已经成为当今学术界的主流思想，而我院也必将顺应学术潮流，按照这一行之有效的体系进一步提高，以期获得更为瞩目的进展。

　　《刘士豪论文选集》的出版是我院百年协和系列纪念活动中浓墨重彩的一笔。这本书的出版，不仅让大家能够一窥刘士豪教授如何实践他的学术思想，也必将给我们的医教研活动带来重要启发。因此这本书的出版，不但是内分泌科的一件盛事，更是我们北京协和医院学术经典的完美重现。希望协和的年轻人和广大医务工作者从中得到更大的收获！

中国医学科学院北京协和医院名誉院长

中国科学院院士

2020 年 11 月

序 二

刘士豪教授是我国内分泌学的奠基人之一，学术成就有目共睹。刘士豪教授、朱宪彝教授和邝安堃教授对于我国内分泌学的开创性贡献是特别值得我们敬仰的。也正是基于此，我在担任中华医学会内分泌学分会主任委员期间特地设立了 3 位前辈的冠名讲座，迄今已是第 12 年。曾正陪教授和夏维波教授也分别在 2010 年和今年的刘士豪冠名讲座上做了精彩的学术报告。刘士豪教授和朱宪彝教授提出"肾性骨营养不良"的疾病命名已是我国现代医学史上的一座丰碑。两位教授的贡献在当时已经站在了国际前沿，也正是我国在现阶段真正特别需要的原创性科研。当前内分泌疾病的管理与相关研究已越来越成为国家关注的重点之一，我们从事内分泌学的医生比过去任一年代都更为幸运，理应做出更多更好的研究。

《刘士豪论文选集》即将付梓，这不仅对了解刘士豪教授的学术成长历程至关重要，对全国内分泌学界如何进行原创性科研工作也大有裨益。原创性科研不仅需要扎实的工作基础和实事求是的科研作风，而且需要善于总结、勤于思考的"有准备的头脑"；而多学科合作等一系列符合科研规律的科研体系建设也是不可或缺的。我们全国内分泌学界的同仁，无论是协和还是瑞金，抑或是其他医院的内分泌代谢科医生，都应将前辈的严谨学风和创新精神传承下来，推动我国内分泌代谢病学科的不断进展，争取在世界内分泌代谢病学界再创辉煌！

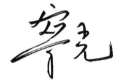

上海交通大学医学院附属瑞金医院院长

中国工程院院士

中华医学会内分泌学分会第八届委员会主任委员

2020 年 12 月

序 三

中华医学会内分泌学分会成立于 1980 年底，40 年来有力地促进了全国内分泌事业的发展。而在此之前，从中华医学会自 1915 年成立开始，有关内分泌专业的学术研讨实际上从未间断。刘士豪教授在内分泌学界崭露头角后即一直参与中华医学会以及《中华医学杂志》（英文版）的学术活动。他的处女作，也即这部论文集所收录的第一篇论文，就是发表于《中华医学杂志》（英文版）的前身之一《博医会报》。1932 年中华医学会和博医会合并以后，刘士豪教授作为北京协和医院内科学系内分泌代谢与肾脏病专业的团队核心，对学会和杂志的支持力度更为突出。以"骨软化症的钙磷代谢"为题的 13 篇系列论文中，有 4 篇发表于《中华医学杂志》（英文版）。他的许多论文都是先在学会会议上交流再发表于《中华医学杂志》（英文版）；这一批国际前沿水平的研究成果在中华医学会会议上得以分享，对国内学术界的推动作用可想而知。他还曾兼任北京医师会副会长，对北京地区的整个现代医学发展都起过一定的作用。新中国成立后，他也始终不遗余力地推动学术活动，并且于 1964 年中华医学会在广州举办的内分泌、代谢及肾脏病学学术会议上作了主旨报告，题为"内分泌研究发展的方向"，亦即这本论文集收入的最后 1 篇论文，其观点高屋建瓴，许多论断即使现在读来也不觉过时。可以说，刘士豪教授的一生，不仅是在世界内分泌学界发出"中国声音"的一生，同时也是推动我国内分泌事业发展的一生。

值此刘士豪教授诞辰 120 周年之际，《刘士豪论文选集》的出版是我们内分泌学界的一件非常值得纪念的大事。我们内分泌学分会也必将以刘士豪教授等学界前辈为榜样，推动全国的内分泌事业不断发展和进步。

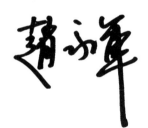

山东省立医院院长

中华医学会内分泌学分会第十一届委员会主任委员

2020 年 11 月

序 四

2020 年是不寻常的一年，而对于我国内分泌学界来说，刘士豪教授诞辰 120 周年也同样是今年的一件大事。临近岁末，又获悉《刘士豪论文选集》即将出版，很是高兴。北京协和医院内分泌团队于 20 世纪三四十年代在钙磷代谢领域取得了丰硕成果，为世界内分泌学界所瞩目；加拿大钙磷代谢专家帕菲特（Parfitt）认为那一时期的协和资料"构成了人类关于维生素 D 缺乏症及其处理的全部知识宝库"。刘士豪教授长期是这一团队的核心人物，他的论文集基本代表了那一时期协和内分泌及肾脏病学领域的研究成果。因此，这本论文选集的出版，不仅对医学史研究者来说是一大喜讯，对我们内分泌学工作者领略那一时代的协和研究风貌也大有裨益。

刘士豪教授在全国内分泌学界有着非常高的影响力，为全国内分泌学科的发展作出了重要贡献。他在上世纪 60 年代早期开办了内分泌高级研修班，当时名额很少，获得进修机会的医生，回到当地以后对当地的内分泌事业的发展都起到了相当大的推动作用。我们辽宁内分泌的前辈（也是中国医大附一院内分泌科的奠基人）、我的导师富朴云教授经过严格选拔后获得了在协和进修的机会。在上世纪的 90 年代，我的学术研究的起步阶段也受益于协和老师的热情指教。特别是史轶蘩教授严谨的治学态度成为我终生的楷模。更早的时期，朱宪彝教授、周寿恺教授也都是协和内分泌团队的重要成员，他们后来分别去了天津和广州，对推动两地的内分泌临床与科研水平发挥了非常重要的作用。

今天，全国内分泌学界的学术水平已经大为提高，这一切来自几代内分泌学者不辞辛苦的努力。刘士豪教授作为早期协和团队的核心，这方面贡献尤为突出。《刘士豪论文选集》的出版，也让我们能够更好地纪念这位中国内分泌事业的奠基人和开拓者。我衷心地祝愿夏维波教授领导的团队继承和弘扬刘士豪教授的治学精神，为我国的内分泌事业作出更大更多的贡献。

中国医科大学附属第一医院教授

中华医学会内分泌学分会第九届委员会主任委员

2020 年 11 月

序　五

　　今年是刘士豪教授诞辰 120 周年，在这样一个双甲子的纪念年出版《刘士豪论文选集》是一件特别有意义的事。刘士豪教授是北京协和医院著名内科学教授，是我国的内分泌学家和医学教育家，迄今他的学术贡献仍能得到世界公认。他和北京医学界的关系极其紧密。自1925 年毕业以来，除了出国学习的 3 年余时间，几乎所有的行医生涯他都在北京度过，可谓名副其实的"京城名医"。而成立于1922 年的北京医学会，一直致力医学学术交流，刘士豪教授自然是北京医学会的重要成员。1940 年，当全国形势一片混乱、日美关系濒临破裂的前夜，尽管协和医院仍然能够运行依旧，但大量的英美著名教授已经纷纷撤离，而北京亦有诸多名医也早早奔赴大西南。而刘士豪教授在这危难之际选择了留守北京，并且出任了北京医学会副会长，为北京医学界始终维持高水平医疗和北京地区的医学学术交流作出了突出贡献。

　　《刘士豪论文选集》的出版，既是北京协和医院的一大盛事，同样也是我们北京医学会的一件大事！刘士豪教授的学术成就大量体现于他所发表的论文，因此，《刘士豪论文选集》的出版，对我们全面认识他当年的学术成就有着不可替代的意义。

封国生

北京医学会会长

2020 年 11 月

序 六

第一次见到刘士豪教授的字迹和照片是在 10 多年前的一次偶然机会，在北京协和医院的学术会堂出席学术活动我偶然看到了协和医院院史展览。这位久负盛名但从未谋面的中国现代内分泌学奠基人的照片和他亲自撰写的医疗文书第一次跃入我的眼帘。刘教授辉煌的人生和卓越的才华深刻地印在我的脑海里，难以磨灭。为纪念为我国内分泌事业作出巨大贡献的先驱，中华医学会内分泌学分会在 2009 年年会上由宁光教授提议，首次设立了刘士豪、朱宪彝和邝安堃教授冠名讲座。在撰写冠名讲座短片的内容时，我冥思苦想，努力在脑海中复现刘教授当时的工作情景，写出了"至今，我们仍然能从他呕心沥血完成的巨著中看到他那治学严谨、和蔼可亲的身影"，以表达我们虽未谋面、但曾相识并受益于刘教授渊博知识的感觉。

2012 年和 2018 年我有幸两次被中华医学会内分泌学分会推选做刘士豪教授冠名讲座。通过北京协和医院李乃适教授和其他同仁提供的宝贵资料，我更加全面地了解了这位迄今中国最伟大的内分泌代谢病专家。刘教授不仅天资聪颖、才华出众，学术成就更是无人能及。

他创立的多个"第一"至今仍是我国内分泌学领域之最：

刘士豪于 1936 年报道了中国第一例胰岛素瘤并成功治愈。

刘士豪是协和毕业生中第一位临床学系教授，1941 年成为协和医院内科学教授。

刘士豪在国际上第一个命名"肾性骨营养不良"疾病，他也是迄今唯一命名了一个被国际上广泛认可的内分泌代谢疾病的中国学者。1942 年 4 月，刘士豪和朱宪彝于《科学》(Science) 共同撰文提出了"肾性骨营养不良"的命名，并于国际上首次提出用双氢速变固醇治疗有效。他提出的"肾脏是使维生素 D 活性不能发挥作用的根源，可能肾衰时产生一种特殊因子，抑制了维生素 D 的活性但不能抑制 A.T.10. 的活性"的预言，30 年后这一设想得到了科学证实。

刘士豪带领团队自 20 世纪 40 年代起首先开展了多种内分泌疾病临床和基础研究，在糖尿病、原发性醛固酮增多症、肾性尿崩症等方面均卓有建树。

刘士豪于 1957 年建立了 24 小时尿 17 羟皮质类固醇的测定法。同年出版了《生物化学与临床医学的联系》一书。

20 世纪 50 年代末创建了我国第一个内分泌科——北京协和医院内分泌科并任科主任。

刘士豪于 1965 年成功建立了放射免疫法测定胰岛素。

……

这一个个"第一次"彰显出刘教授与生俱来的超人天赋，也让我们更加体会到了他呕心沥血、不懈努力、奋发进取的科学精神。刘士豪教授是我国现代内分泌代谢学的先驱，数以百计千计内分泌学后来者的领路人。他于 20 世纪 60 年代开办的多期学习班，为全国最早萌芽的临床内分泌学科培养了一大批骨干师资和科研队伍，为后来全国范围相继成立的内分泌专科奠定了基础。刘教授为我国内分泌代谢事业作出的巨大贡献和他留给我们的宝贵财富不仅在过去和现在激励了一批又一批内分泌人，而他也必将当之无愧地成为我们一代又一代内分泌人为之骄傲的楷模。

值此刘士豪教授诞辰 120 周年之际，我们全体内分泌同仁缅怀我们的先驱，学习和传承刘教授终身为我国内分泌事业奉献的精神，团结奋战，再创辉煌。

中国人民解放军总医院教授

中华医学会内分泌学分会第十届委员会主任委员

2020 年 12 月

序 七

在 1936 年经典国际期刊《临床研究杂志》(*Journal of Clinical Investigation*) 的第 3 期，署名刘士豪、娄克斯、周寿恺和陈国桢的一篇论文赫然在列。这是世界上发表的第 17 例胰岛素瘤，也是我国第 1 例胰岛素瘤。这篇论文，不仅在当时是罕见病研究的典范之作，即使以当前的视角，也能给我们许多启发。胰岛素瘤在今天仍然可被认为是一种罕见病，更不必说在 20 世纪 30 年代的中国了。"老协和"的内分泌代谢与肾脏病学研究团队，是一个极为出色的临床与研究团队：他们既从临床上推测出了胰岛素瘤的诊断，又在手术后对肿瘤标本做了极为出色的动物研究，从而使临床诊断得到了进一步的证实。这几乎是在当时的条件下能够做的最完备的研究。几乎文献中探讨的可能有效的方法，在协和的代谢病房都进行了探讨和必要的实践，用协和的数据为探讨这些方法是否有效提供了有力的证据。这篇论文收录在本论文集的第三编，为我们对"老协和"如何研究罕见病提供了一个绝佳的范例，也促使我们思考当前如何更好地进行罕见病研究。

除了科研以外，这篇论文所体现出来的病历书写，也已经达到了几近完美的水平，从对症状的一层层详细描述，到查体的细致入微，都可以代表老协和的病历书写标准，值得我们精读并有针对性地学习。

十年树木，百年树人。协和要想长盛不衰，则前辈们在论文中、在病历中、在言传身教中体现的协和精神是必须得到传承和发扬的。《刘士豪论文选集》在百年协和即将到来之际出版，对于协和精神的传承，有着非凡的意义。

中国医学科学院北京协和医院院长

2020 年 12 月

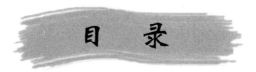

目　录

第一编　风华正茂

第二编　赴美求学

第三编　胰瘤研辨

第四编　骨病深耕

第五编　名世之作

第六编　英伦进阶

第七编　贫血探秘

第八编　一代宗师

附　录

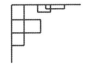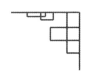

第一编　风华正茂

　　第一编收录了刘士豪教授担任实习医师、住院医师和总住院医师期间的论文。1924 年 10 月，刘士豪尚未毕业时即发表了第 1 篇学术论文《The influence of cod-liver oil on the calcium and phosphorus metabolism in tetany》，探讨了鱼肝油对 2 例搐搦症患者钙磷代谢的影响。这是他学术生涯的开端，也是他研究钙磷代谢的开端。这篇论文特地致谢了 G.A. Harrop 教授。Harrop 教授是当时北京协和医院的内科客座教授，也是张孝骞教授赴美进修时的导师；由此也可初步了解刘士豪的学术师承。本编第 2 篇论文《The partition of serum calcium into diffusible and non-diffusible portions（透析血清钙质之研究）》发表于当年创刊的我国著名学术期刊《中国生理学杂志》，探讨了发挥生理作用的血清钙到底是"非渗透性钙"还是"渗透性钙"，以翔实的数据为这一关键问题提供了重要证据。第 3 篇《Plasma acid-base equilibrium in malaria》和第 4 篇《Studies on plasma lipoids. 1. Fatty acids of blood plasma in diabetes and nephrosis》同样发表于《中国生理学杂志》。《Plasma acid-base equilibrium in malaria》研究了疟疾的酸碱平衡问题，得出了阴性结果，但结论同样非常重要，以客观数据否定了原先的错误结论。《Studies on plasma lipoids. 1. Fatty acids of blood plasma in diabetes and nephrosis》探讨糖尿病和肾病患者的血清脂肪酸水平，是林树模与刘士豪合作所著，也是生物化学方法在内分泌学的应用。实际上刘士豪在这一时期发表了 15 篇学术论文，涉及内分泌代谢的诸多方面，因篇幅所限不得不忍痛割爱，可参看附录一。

𝔗𝔥𝔢
𝕮𝔥𝔦𝔫𝔞 𝕸𝔢𝔡𝔦𝔠𝔞𝔩 𝕵𝔬𝔲𝔯𝔫𝔞𝔩.

VOL. XXXVIII.   OCTOBER, 1924.   NO. 10

THE INFLUENCE OF COD-LIVER OIL ON THE CALCIUM AND PHOSPHORUS METABOLISM IN TETANY.*

LIU SHIH-HAO, M.D., Peking.

The close association between rickets and infantile tetany is a clinical observation of long standing. The relationship has been further verified by chemical studies which have indicated a disturbance in the balance between calcium and phosphorus in both conditions. In infantile tetany[1] there is a diminution of the calcium content of the blood, the inorganic phosphorus remaining normal or slightly above normal in the majority of the cases. It has been shown that the calcium content of the blood rises with the disappearance of the symptoms of tetany. In rickets[2], however, the blood calcium is usually normal or nearly so, while the phosphorus is reduced 40 per cent to 60 per cent or even more. When a cure results from the use of cod liver oil, ultra-violet radiation, exposure to sunlight, or the use of proper dietary regime, the phosphorus of the serum rises to normal limits, and there is a deposition of tricalcium phosphate in the bone. When rickets is complicated by tetany, certain cases may show only a low concentration of calcium, while still others may present a diminution of both calcium and phosphorus.

According to the available evidence, it seems that the defective calcification in rickets[3] may be accounted for by the fact that the bone-forming elements, calcium and phosphorus, are present in the blood in such low concentrations that the precipitation of tricalcium phosphate is impossible. Similarly it is believed that the symptoms of tetany are attributable to the low calcium concentration in the blood and tissues, because numerous researches

---

*From the Department of Medicine, Peking Union Medical College, Peking.

have demonstrated the important relation of calcium salts to irritability of the central nervous system. Their withdrawal, as by applying oxalate to the cortex, leaves the latter in a state of hyperirritability, which can be made to disappear by supplying a solution of calcium salts. Furthermore, the addition of calcium to a solution of sodium salts allays the stimulating effect of the latter on the isolated frog muscle.

It is believed [5] that calcium salts in blood exist in three forms, namely, (a) as highly dissociable compounds with protein; (b) as undissociated crystalloid molecules; and (c) as free ions. Presumably, calcium salts exert their physiological effect only to such extent as physico-chemical conditions permit their presence as calcium ions. Any condition that decreases the dissociation of calcium in the blood would tend to produce symptoms of tetany even though the total calcium in the blood were normal. When the concentration of the ionized calcium is lowered, hyperirritability of the neuro-muscular system results. Rona and Takahashi [6] have shown that increase in the bicarbonate content of the blood diminishes the ionized calcium, whereas increase in the hydrogen ion concentration permits a larger concentration of calcium ions. For this reason symptoms of tetany appear as a result of the administration of alkalies,[7] gastric operations,[8] or hyperpnœa,[9] where a definite increase of bicarbonate or a decrease of hydrogen ion concentration has been demonstrated. Recently Gamble and Ross [10] have found following the administration of calcium chloride, ammonium chloride, and hydrochloric acid, to infants with tetany, that the plasma bicarbonate is decreased, and the hydrogen ion concentration of the plasma is increased, while the tetanoid symptoms disappear. The first two factors increase the ionization of calcium so that enough ions are present to allow normal irritability of the nerves.

In addition to the bicarbonate content and the hydrogen ion concentration, another factor that influences the ionization of calcium is its total concentration in the plasma. Of the total calcium about one-third is bound by protein and may be left out of consideration, because, as shown by Salversen and Linder,[11] the lowered calcium in tetany is not due to a primary decrease in the protein-bound calcium, but is caused by a decrease in the diffusible fraction. This fraction comprises the free calcium ions and the

Influence of Cod-liver Oil on Metabolism in Tetany.　795

undissociated crystalloid molecules of calcium salts. Using the formula of Rona and Takahashi[6] the calcium ion concentration is found to be about 3. mg. per 100 c.c. of blood, a value experimentally confirmed by Brinkman and Van Dam.* The remaining third is said to be present as undissociated calcium carbonate in supersaturated solution. These two fractions are present in a constant ratio as expressed in the following equation[7]:

$$\frac{(Ca++)\,(CO_3--)}{(Ca\,CO_3)} = K$$

In order to maintain this constant, any decrease in the diffusible calcium would involve the undissociated molecules as well. When the calcium ions are sufficiently decreased, tetany occurs. In the majority of cases of tetany, where there is no increase of plasma bicarbonate nor decrease of hydrogen ion concentration, one may conclude that the low total calcium in the blood is responsible for the diffusible calcium concentration, the immediate cause of tetany.

But the question arises : "What causes the low total calcium in the blood of infants with tetany?" In rickets the low phosphorus content of the blood, which mainly accounts for the failure of calcification of the bones, has been shown to be due to defective absorption of this element through the gastrointestinal tract by the metabolism experiments of Schabad and Schloss. [9] [10] Normally, 70 per cent or more of the phosphorus excreted by breast fed infants appears in the urine, and with children on cow's milk about 60 per cent is thus excreted. In rickets the conditions are quite reversed : much the larger part may be eliminated through the bowel. When recovery takes place following the administration of cod liver oil a return to normal occurs; the phosphorus may be quite unchanged in amount but that in the feces is greatly reduced. Retention occurs at the expense of the fecal phosphorus. Recent work by Orr, Holt, Wilkins, and Boone [12] has further shown that ultra-violet radiation, like cod liver oil, causes large amounts of calcium and phosphorus to be retained in the body, and the increased calcium and phosphorus are found in the urine after the radiation, indicating an increased absorption from the intestines. They conclude that the defective absorption from the intestine found in active rickets is the cause of the

---

*Referred to under Reference 10. Original article is not available.

low concentrations of calcium and phosphorus found in the serum and is the ultimate cause of the defective calcification of the bones of the rachitic infants. The condition of affairs in tetany, however, remains obscure, although this latter disease has been extensively treated with cod liver oil[13], and ultra-violet radiation[14]. It has been the purpose of this study to determine, in the first place, whether or not the low serum calcium in tetany is due to the defective absorption of this substance through the intestine; and in the second place, whether or not the efficacy of cod liver oil in the treatment of tetany lies in its ability to promote the absorption of calcium from the intestinal canal.

METHODS OF INVESTIGATION.

The subjects were two girls, each of whom showed on admission to the hospital marked carpopedal spasm, Chvostek's sign, Trousseau's sign, and the typical electrical reactions characteristic of tetany. They came from an orphanage in Peking containing about fifty girls and seventy boys, varying from 10 to 18 years in age. About ten of the girls complained of stiffness of the fingers during the winter months, and showed on examination varying degrees of the facial phenomenon. In all of the cases this was the first symptom complained of, although several later had difficulty in walking. None of the boys were affected similarly. Investigation into the living conditions showed that the girls stayed indoors practically all the time in the colder months, studying two hours and working on embroidery eight hours daily. The boys were employed in rug weaving, so that their hands were employed approximately to the same extent. They had better facilities for getting out into the open air and running about in the sunlight, which were denied the girls.

The diet in the orphanage is practically constant throughout the year. It consists of the following foodstuffs : for breakfast, millet gruel, corn bread, salted turnip; for lunch, wheat bread, vegetable; For supper, corn bread, vegetable. A portion of meat is served once a month, and the vegetables are varied according to the season. Bean sprouts are obtainable in January and February; onions and bean curd in February and March; spinach in April; egg-plant and gourds, May to July; pearl melons in August and September; and cabbage, October to January. During the period of study the patients were

Influence of Cod-liver Oil on Metabolism in Tetany. 797

kept on a uniform diet resembling the orphanage diet as closely as possible, and both the intake and the composition of this diet were accurately known.

The patients remained in the hospital for about ten weeks. The period during which they were studied is divisible into two parts, namely, a control period of five weeks without treatment, and a second period of equal length during which they received cod liver oil, 15 c.c. three times daily. Toward the end of each of these periods four consecutive days were set apart as metabolism periods. During each of these the total 24-hr. urine was collected and the creatinin was determined to insure the obtaining of complete specimens. Stools were collected and marked off to correspond to the 4-day period with charcoal. From the specimens of stool and urine, the output of calcium and phosphorus of each period was determined; and from the amount and composition of the food taken, the intake of calcium and phosphorus was calculated. Values for milk were taken from Babcock [15] while those for other foods were taken from Shermann and Gettler [16]. During the two periods determinations of the calcium and phosphorus of the blood serum and of cerebro-spinal fluid were made. The electrical reactions were also obtained, and in order to determine whether a condition of alkalosis existed, the carbon-dioxide combining power was estimated both before and after treatment. The pH of the gastric contents during the two periods was also determined to see whether a decreased gastric acidity might be present as a factor in the causation of tetany in these cases [29].*

---

* The methods employed in this study were the following : calcium in urine was determined by McCrudden's gravimetric method [17] with brom-crysol purple as the indicator. For the determination of phosphorus in urine, the Briggs' modification of Bell and Doisy's method [18] was used.

The total stools of each period were put together, thoroughly mixed and evaporated to dryness on a steam bath. Alcohol (95 per cent) was added and the mixture evaporated to dryness again. The process was repeated once more, making two additions of alcohol in all. The residue was ground up, put in a dessicator overnight, and weighed. Exactly 2 gm. of the air-dried stool were ashed by Stolte's method [19]. Calcium was determined by McCrudden's procedure [18] and phosphorus by the molybdic acid method [20].

For blood serum and cerebro-spinal fluid, the method of estimation employed for calcium was that of Kramer and Tisdall [21]; for phosphorus, that of Briggs [18]; and for carbon-dioxide combining power, that of Van Slyke and Cullen [22].

The pH of gastric contents was estimated by the method of Shohl and King [23].

REPORT OF CASES

Case 1. Hospital No. 4319.

Li Fu-chen, aged 16, was admitted to the Peking Union Medical College Hospital on January 18, 1924, complaining of rigidity of hands for two months. Discharged well on April 3, 1924. A year ago (February 20, 1923), patient had an attack of tetany, promptly relieved by calcium therapy. Two months before admission she began to have spastic attacks in both hands. These gradually increased in severity and frequency. A week prior to admission both of her feet became involved, and she became practically incapacitated. Menstruation commenced in November, 1923.

On admission, patient was fairly well developed and nourished. Height 142.5 cm. Weight 37.3 kg. Her hands and feet intermittently assumed the typical positions of carpopedal spasm. Chvostek's and Trousseau's signs were present. X-ray of the long bones showed no evidence of rickets. During the first period, when no medication was given, her symptoms persisted without any marked change. With the commencement of cod liver oil therapy, however, her symptoms began to clear up, until about ten days after the treatment was commenced no clinical signs of tetany could be detected. The electrical reactions typical of tetany, before treatment, returned to normal after treatment. Chemical examination of the blood and cerebro-spinal fluid both before and during treatment gave the results shown in Table 1. Table 3 shows the calcium and phosphorus excretion in stool and urine during the 4-day periods before and after medication.

Case 2. Hospital No. 655.

Pai Jui-fang, aged 15, admitted to the Peking Union Medical College Hospital on January 9, 1924 with the complaint of spasms in both hands and feet for 16 days prior to admission. Discharged well on April 3, 1924. The patient had had chronic tuberculous lymphadenitis of the neck operated on here two years ago, and had phlyctenular ophthalmia a year ago.

TABLE I.—CALCIUM, PHOSPHORUS, AND CARBON-DIOXIDE COMBINING POWER OF BLOOD SERUM AND CEREBRO-SPINAL FLUID BEFORE AND AFTER TREATMENT. (CASE I.)

	Before Treatment			After Treatment		
	Mg. per 100 c.c. Calcium	Mg. per 100 c.c. Phosphorus	Vol. % CO_2	Mg. per 100 c.c. Calcium	Mg. per 100 c.c. Phosphorus	Vol. % CO_2
Blood serum	5.8	2.38	53%	10.5	4.80	59%
Cerebro-spinal fluid	3.3	1.41	55%	5.9	1.35	58%

Influence of Cod-liver Oil on Metabolism in Tetany.　799

TABLE 3.—THE CALCIUM AND PHOSPHORUS INTAKE AND OUTPUT BEFORE AND AFTER COD LIVER OIL TREATMENT. (CASE 1).

CALCIUM.

	Intake	Excretion				
		Urine	Stool	Total	Percentage in Urine	Percentage in Stool
Before Treatment	0.458	9.033	0.367	0.400	8.25%	91.75%
After Treatment	0.687	0.130	0.450	0.580	22.32%	77.68%

PHOSPHORUS.

	Intake	Urine	Stool	Total	Percentage in Urine	Percentage in Stool
Before Treatment	2.573	0.609	0.674	1.282	47.47%	52.53%
After Treatment	3.859	2.178	1.296	3.474	62.69%	37.31%

About two weeks before admission, she began to notice numbness and spasticity, first of the hands, then of the feet. The spasms were at first intermittent, but were continuous for the two days prior to admission, and caused considerable muscular pain. Physical examination showed a poorly developed and moderately emaciated girl with hands and feet in severe carpopedal spasm, complaining of pain in the extremities. There were marked facial phenomenon and Trousseau's sign. Height 128.7 cm. Weight 24.2 kg.

On admission patient was given calcium lactate and full diet. Her symptoms were relieved somewhat under this treatment. After January 20, however, calcium lactate was discontinued, the patient put on the orphanage diet, and the symptoms quickly returned. The same procedure was followed in this case as in Case 1, except that from February 21 she was given 1,000 c.c. of fresh cow's milk in addition to the diet described on account of her poor nutrition. Shortly after commencing treatment with cod liver oil her spasms were relieved and the facial phenomenon and Trousseau's sign disappeared.

The electrical reactions during the control period showed the hyper-excitability characteristic of tetany. They became normal again after treatment.

Chemical studies of blood and cerebro-spinal fluid yielded very low values for calcium and phosphorus which were raised to normal by the cod liver oil treatment as illustrated in Table 2. Results of the metabolic studies of calcium and phosphorus before and after treatment are tabulated in Table 4.

TABLE 2.—CALCIUM AND PHOSPHORUS CONTENT OF BLOOD
AND CEREBRO-SPINAL FLUID BEFORE AND AFTER
TREATMENT. (CASE 2).

	Before Treatment		After Treatment	
	Mg. per 100 c.c. Calcium	Mg. per 100 c.c. Phosphorus	Mg. per 100 c.c. Calcium	Mg. per 100 c.c. Phosphorus
Blood serum	5.4	2.63	10.3	5.44
Cerebro-spinal fluid...	3.8	1.44	5.9	3.80

TABLE 4.—THE CALCIUM AND PHOSPHORUS INTAKE AND OUTPUT
BEFORE AND AFTER COD LIVER OIL TREATMENT. (CASE 2).

CALCIUM.

	Intake	Excretion				
		Urine	Stool	Total	Percentage in Urine	Percentage in Stool
Before Treatment	0.458	0.049	0.398	0.447	11.02%	88.98%
After Treatment	4.687	0.138	0.107	0.245	56.26%	43.74%

PHOSPHORUS.

Before Treatment	2.573	0.082	0.100	1.081	7.55%	92.45%
After Treatment	6.819	0.547	0.130	0.677	80.81%	19.19%

DISCUSSION

These two cases presented all of the clinical evidence and
laboratory findings of idiopathic tetany. No parathyroid
deficiency [24] was present; no symptoms pointed to the gastric form
of tetany; and they had never had intravenous injection of
alkalis.

The recent paper of Pincus and Kramer [25] states that normally
the blood serum calcium averages 9.6 mg. per 100 c.c.; and

phosphorus, 2.9 mg. per 100 c.c. The values for cerebro-spinal
fluid are just half as much as those for serum, namely calcium 4.8
and phosphorus 1.3. In these two cases in the active stage of
tetany the calcium concentration in blood serum was 5.8 and 5.4
respectively, which were very low values. Cerebro-spinal fluid
showed still lower results, namely 3.3 in the first case and 3.8 in
the second, emphasizing further the importance of low calcium
concentration as the cause of the hyperirritability of the nervous
system. As has been mentioned before, the concentration of
calcium ions in blood necessary to maintain the normal irritability
of the nervous system is about 3 mg. In the cerebro-spinal fluid a
greater proportion of the total calcium is probably present in ionic
form so that about 3 mg. of free calcium ions may still be available.
Since the protein concentration of the cerebro-spinal fluid is very
low (0.02 per cent) in comparison with that of plasma (7-9 per cent)
the protein bound calcium must be negligible in quantity. Any
decrease of cerebro-spinal fluid calcium may be regarded as a
clearer and more direct evidence of tetany than a decrease of the
blood calcium.

After treatment with cod liver oil, the calcium and phosphorus
contents of blood and cerebro-spinal fluid were raised to normal.
This together with the disappearance of the clinical signs of tetany
and the decreased irritability to electrical stimuli is taken as
evidence that the cure of the tetany was brought about by cod liver
oil alone, an observation which agrees with that of Brown,
Maclachlan, and Simpson [13].

The action of cod liver oil in the cure of tetany may
be better understood by analyzing the metabolism data on
calcium and phosphorus. In the first case, calcium retention
before the cod liver oil treatment was 12.62 per cent, and this
became 15.58 per cent after the treatment. A comparison of the
urinary and stool excretion of calcium before and after cod liver oil
therapy reveals that as a result of the treatment there was a
marked increase in the proportion of the total calcium output
excreted through the urine with a correspondingly decreased
excretion through the stool, showing that there was actually more
calcium absorbed through the gastro-intestinal tract, metabolized
in the body, and then excreted through the kidneys.

Phosphorus retention in this case, contrary to what was expected, was less after the treatment than before. However, there was a distinct increase in the urinary excretion of phosphorus at the expense of the stool excretion.

Figures for the second case are more clear cut. Calcium and phosphorus showed parallel results. In spite of the large increase in the intake of calcium and phosphorus during the period of treatment, the total excretion of both of these elements was much less than that before the treatment. The relatively high output and low intake in the active stage of the disease resulted in a low retention, especially of calcium. On the other hand, during the treatment period the retention of both calcium and phosphorus was tremendously increased. The urinary excretion of both calcium and phosphorus was greatly increased during the second period, indicating that a much greater proportion of the intake was absorbed into the system and the excess eliminated through the urine.

From this evidence we conclude that the low calcium in these cases was associated with defective absorption through the intestine, and that cod liver oil exerts its beneficial effect on tetany by promoting the absorption from the intestinal canal.

While it is assumed that cod liver oil increases the absorption of calcium and phosphorus from the intestine, it is perfectly possible that it may act by diminishing their re-excretion through the gastro-intestinal tract. Birk[26] injected calcium intravenously into a rachitic child and found that it was largely excreted through the intestine. When phosphates were thus injected, very little was eliminated with the stool. Sjellema[27] showed that rabbits on a low calcium diet might excrete three times as much calcium as that present in the food, and still give feces with about the same percentage of calcium as in periods of positive calcium balance. This was interpreted by the author as pointing to a physiological rôle for calcium in the production of feces. Cod liver oil acted by decreasing the amount of calcium necessary for this purpose. How far the results on rabbits under normal conditions are applicable to human cases of tetany cannot be stated. It seems altogether probable that calcium and phosphorus are absorbed together and that cod liver oil promotes that absorption of these substances rather than that it limits their re-excretion through the intestines.

Influence of Cod-liver Oil on Metabolism in Tetany.　803

We may conclude that in these cases of tetany the intestinal absorption of calcium was decreased with a resulting low concentration of calcinm in the serum and cerebro-spinal fluid. Under the influence of cod liver oil, the absorption of calcium from the limited intake was increased so that the level of calcium concentration in blood and cerebro-spinal fluid necessary to maintain the normal irritability of the nervous system was restored and the tetany disappeared.

The mechanism whereby cod liver oil increases the absorption is influenced by two factors, namely, the reaction of the gastro-intestinal tract and the amount of fat intake. Holt and his colleagues[28] have shown that in infants and children calcium absorption depends not only upon the intake of calcium salts, but also upon the amount of fat ingested. The optimal absorption of calcium occurs when the intake of fat exceeds 3.0 to 4.0 gm. per kilo body weight. The fat present in the cod liver oil may be a contributing factor to the increased absorption.

With regard to the reaction of the gastro-intestinal canal, alkalies diminish mineral absorption, while acids increase it. Babbott and his co-workers[29] have recently shown that the normal pH of the gastric contents of infants is 4.2 and in infantile tetany this is increased to 5.3. With the disappearance of symptoms of tetany, the pH returns to normal. The gastric acidity in our cases of tetany was normal and seems to have had no bearing on the symptoms.

CONCLUSION

1. In certain cases of tetany, the low calcium content of blood and cerebro-spinal fluid is probably due to deficient absorption of this element through the intestines. Low calcium content means low calcium ion concentration, which is directly responsible for the symptoms.

2. Cod liver oil, when administered to such cases, increases the retention of calcium and, to a lesser extent, of phosphorus as well. The urinary excretion of these elements is at the same time increased, indicating an increased absorption from the intestines.

Note.—The writer wishes to express his thanks to Dr. G. A. Harrop, of Peking, for his encouragement and help in the preparation of this paper.

BIBLIOGRAPHY

1. Kramer, B., Tisdall, F. F., and Howland, J., Am. J. Dis. Child., 1921, xxii, 560 and 431.

2. Kramer, B., and Howland, J., Am. J. Dis. Child., 1921, xxii, 105.

3. Howland, J., Medicine, 1923, ii, 347.

4. McCollum, E. V., and Voegtlin, C., J. Exp. Med., 1909, xi, 118.

5. Howland, J., and Kramer, B., Monatschrift f. Kinderheilkunde, 1923, xxv, 279.

6. Rona B., and Takahashi, D., Biochem. Zeitschr., 1913, xlix, 370.

7. Howland, J., and Marriott, W. McK., Quart. J. Med., 1918, xi, 289. Harrop, G. A., Johns Hop. Hosp. Bul., 1919, xxx, 62.

8. McCann, W. S., J. Biol. Chem., 1918, xxxv, 553.

9. Collip, J. B., and Backus, A., Am. J. Physiol., 1920, li, 568.

10. Gamble, L., and Ross, G. S., Am. J. Dis. Child., 1923, xxv, 455, and 471.

11. Salversen, H. A., and Linder, G. C., J. Biol. Chem., 1923, lviii, 635.

12. Orr, W. J., Holt, L. E., Wilkins, L., and Brown, F. H., Am. J. Dis. Child., 1923, xxvi, 362.

13. Brown, A., MacLachlan, I. F., and Simpson, R., Am. J. Dis. Child., 1920, xix, 413 ; Canad. Med. Ass. J., 1921, xi, 522.

14. Huldschinsky, K., Ztschr. f. Kinderh., 1920, xxvi, 207 ; Casparis, H., and Kramer, B., Johns Hop. Hosp. Bul., 1923, xxxiv, 219 ; Hoag, L. A., Am. J. Dis. Child., 1923, xxvi, 186.

15. Leach, A. E., Food Inspection and Analysis, Third Edition, 1914, John Wiley and Sons, New York.

16. Shermann, H. C., and Gettler, A. O., J. Biol. Chem., 1912, xi, 323.

17. McCrudden, F. H., J. Biol. Chem., 1911-1912, x, 197.

18. Briggs, A. P., J. Biol. Chem., 1922, liii, 13.

19. Tisdall, F. F., and Kramer, B., J. Biol. Chem., 1921, xlviii, 1.

20. Hawk, P. B., Practical Physiological Chemistry, Seventh Edition, 570.

21. Tisdall, F. F., J. Biol. Chem., 1923, lvi, 439.

22. Van Slyke, D. D., and Cullen, G. E., J. Biol. Chem., 1917, xxx, 289.

23. Shohl, A. T., and King, J. H., Johns Hop. Hosp. Bul., 1920, xxxi, 152.

24. Salversen, H. A., J. Biol. Chem., 1923, lvi, 443.

25. Pincus, J. B., and Kramer, B., J. Biol. Chem., 1923, lvii, 463.

26. Birk, W., Monatschr. f. Kinderh., 1908, vii, 450 ; Birk, W., and Orgler, Monatschr. f. Kinderh, 1910, ix, 544.

27. Sjollema, B., J. Biol. Chem., 1923, lvii, 271.

28. Holt, L. E., Courtney, A. M., and Fales, H. L., Am. J. Dis. Child., 1920, xix, 97, and 204.

29. Babbott, F. L., Johnston, J. A., Haskins, C. H., and Shohl, A. T., Am. J. Dis. Child., 1923, xxvi, 475 ; Babbott, F. L., Johnston, J. A., Haskins, C. H., ibid., 1923, xxvi, 486.

Chinese Journal of Physiology, 1927, Vol. I, No. 3, pp. 331—344

THE PARTITION OF SERUM CALCIUM INTO DIFFUSIBLE AND NON-DIFFUSIBLE PORTIONS*

SHIH-HAO LIU

(From the Department of Medicine, Peking Union Medical College, Peking)

Received for publication May 18, 1927

In view of the consistent finding of a decreased blood calcium in infantile and parathyreoprive tetany, this has generally been held as directly responsible for the increased irritability of the neuromuscular system. But difficulty arises when it is occasionally found that the level of blood calcium does not parallel the severity of symptoms of tetany. Moreover, in other types of tetany, namely, gastric tetany, tetany following sodium bicarbonate administration, and following hyperpnoea, the blood calcium usually does not change. Conversely, in certain varieties of nephritis as reported by Salvesen and Linder (18), and in kala-azar, as will be shown presently, there is a distinct lowering of blood calcium without any evidence of tetany. These discordant observations, among others, have led to the recent tendency to study the state of calcium as it exists in the blood.

With no method available for directly measuring calcium ions in the blood, attempts have been made to separate serum calcium into diffusible and non-diffusible portions, thus indirectly, perhaps incompletely, gaining an idea of the state of calcium in the blood. Three types of methods have been employed, namely, compensation dialysis by Rona and Takahashi (16), von Meysenbug and his co-workers (11), and Cruickshank (5); ultra-filtration by Cushny (7), and Neuhausen and Pincus (14); and simultaneous determination of the calcium contents of blood and cerebro-spinal fluid, assuming that the latter is a protein-free filtrate of blood by Cameron and Moorhouse (1).

---

*An abstract of this paper is being published in the Proceedings of the Society for Experimental Biology and Medicine, June, 1927.

On account of the divergent results obtained with different methods, the important question whether the diffusible or the non-diffusible calcium is reduced in tetany has not been satisfactory answered. The general impression, without much experimental basis, has been that the diffusible calcium is reduced in tetany. Cruickshank (5), and Cameron and Moorhouse (1), however, conclude that in tetany parathyreopriva the reduction is mainly in the non-diffusible fraction. On the other hand, von Meysenbug and McCann (10), and Moritz (12) found that both the diffusible and non-diffusible calcium were reduced in the same ratio.

Similarly the question as to what binds the non-diffusible calcium is in an unsettled state. Rona and Takahashi (16) were the first to suggest that the non-diffusible calcium might be bound to protein. Loeb (9) by *in vitro* experiments demonstrated that the amount of clacium that diffuses through a collodion membrane at pH 7.4 varies directly with the protein concentration. Cameron and Moorhouse (1), however, rejected this hypothesis, and suggested instead that the non-diffusible calcium is bound to some organic substance which may be the parathyroid hormone. Greenwald (8) has proposed that some of the calcium may be combined with an organic substance intimately associated with parathyroid function and probably diffusible.

In the hope of throwing light on some of these questions and of studying the manner of increase of blood calcium under the influence of parathyroid hormone and cod liver oil, the following observations were undertaken.

METHOD

For the separation of diffusible and non-diffusible clacium, the method of combined ultra-filtration and dialysis of Moritz (12) and Updegraff, Greenberg, and Clark (19) was employed with a few modifications. The arrangement of apparatus is shown in fig. 1. Collodion sacs (C) were cast from Pyrex test tubes of an internal diameter of 12 mm. These were kept in normal saline containing a few drops of chloroform in the ice chest. The outer tube (G) is simply a Pyrex test tube 140 mm long and of an internal diameter of 18 mm. Negative pressure is applied between the sac and the outer tube by means of a suction pump at S. A bottle (W) is arranged between the suction pump and the filtration apparatus so as to prevent back flow of water into the

PARTITION OF SERUM CALCIUM

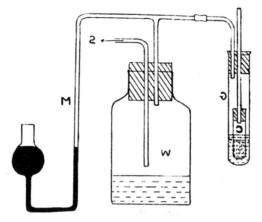

Fig. 1.　Arrangement of apparatus.

tube (G) incident to variation of water flow through the suction pump. A mercury manometer (M) is also interposed to register the pressure maintained.

For ultra-filtration and dialysis, 2 cc of serum were placed in a freshly prepared collodion sac carefully tested for leaks; and 2 cc of distilled water, in the outer tube. Of ascitic and pleural fluids, 4 cc were employed on account their low calcium content. Filtration with the sac in contact with the water in the outer tube was allowed to proceed for 5 hours under a negative pressure maintained at 150 mm of mercury. At the end of the period, the fluid remaining in the sac was measured and transferred to a 15 cc centrifuge tube of the Tisdall type, and the sac carefully washed and the washings added to the centri-fuge tube. The fluid in the outer tube was treated in the same way. Both the inner and outer fluids were analysed for calcium by the method of Tisdall as modified by Clark and Collip (2). Total calcium was estimated in a separate portion as a check. The albumin and globulin contents of plasma and other body fluids were determined by Wu and Ling's method (20).

RESULTS

Control cases.

The calcium partition and proteins of blood were determined in nine hospital patients with conditions unassociated with disturbances in calcium metabolism, with a total serum calcium ranging from 9.2 to

10.6 mg per 10.0 cc. The results are given in table 1. The diffusible calcium varied from 4.5 mg or 42.5 per cent to 5.8 mg or 58.0 per cent, the non-diffusible calcium from 4.1 mg or 42.3 per cent to 6.1 mg or 57.5 per cent. The average figures of 5.0 mg or 51.2 per cent for the diffusible and 4.8 mg or 48.8 per cent for the non-diffusible calcium agree very well with the results of those who have used the same method for normal cases.

TABLE 1.

Blood calcium distribution and proteins in 9 patients with conditions unassociated with disturbances in calcium metaoblism

Case No.	Condition	Non-diffusible serum calcium		Diffusible serum calcium		Total serum calcium	Plasma albumin	Plasma globulin
		mg per 100 cc	percent	mg per 100 cc	percent	mg per 100 cc	percent	percent
7843	Obesity	6.1	57.5	4.5	42.5	10.6	4.6	2.0
16621	Neurasthenia	5.8	56.3	4.5	43.7	10.2	4.3	1.3
15237	Tuberculous peritonitis	5.0	50.5	4.9	49.5	10.4	3.6	1.2
15549	Hemolytic jaundice	4.9	50.5	4.8	49.5	9.8	3.9	1.1
15194	Pulmonary tuberculosis	4.5	48.9	4.7	51.1	9.2	3.2	1.9
4937	Auricular fibrillation	4.4	46.8	5.0	53.2	9.6	3.2	2.2
16556	Chronic arthritis	4.2	42.0	5.8	58.0	10.0	3.6	2.0
16264	Leprosy	4.1	44.6	5.1	55.4	9.2	3.5	1.6
16041	Banti's disease	4.1	42.3	5.6	57.7	9.7	3.6	1.0
	Mean	4.8	48.8	5.0	51.2	9.9	3.7	1.6

The plasma albumin in these cases ranged from 3.2 to 4.6 per cent with an average of 3.7 per cent, and globulin from 1.0 to 2.2 per cent with an average of 1.6 per cent.

Conditions associated with low total serum calcium.

In the two cases of tetany studied (table 2), both the diffusible and non-diffusible calcium were reduced with a relatively greater reduction in the diffusible fraction. Protein figures were approximately normal.

In three cases of nephrosis with a total calcium ranging from 7.7 to 8.6 mg, the distribution of serum calcium showed a normal, or even slightly higher than normal diffusible portion, and a markedly reduced non-diffusible portion. Similar striking results were obtained in four cases of kala-azar having a total serum calcium varying from 6.6 to 7.6 mg while their diffusible calcium remained normal, their non-diffusible calcium suffered a great reduction. None of these cases of nephrosis and kala-azar showed any clinical signs of tetany, and their electrical reactions were normal.

TABLE 2.

Blood calcium distribution and proteins in conditions with low blood calcium

Case No.	Condition	Non-diffusible serum calcium		Diffusible serum calcium		Total serum calcium	Plasma albumin	Plasma globulin
		mg per 190 cc	percent	mg per 100 cc	percent	mg per 100 cc	percent	percent
15846	Tetany	4.3	53.7	3.7	46.3	8.0	3.4	1.7
15810	„	3.8	59.4	2.6	40.6	6.5	4.2	1.8
13769	Nephrosis	3.3	38.4	5.3	61.6	8.6	1.8	1.2
13896	„	2.3	29.1	5.6	70.9	7.9	1.9	1.2
14418	„	2.0	25.9	5.7	74.1	7.7	1.8	1.5
16440	Kala-azar	3.0	39.5	4.6	60.5	7.6	2.3	3.4
16501	„	2.7	36.0	4.8	64.0	7.7	2.6	2.0
16182	„	1.8	26.1	5.1	73.9	6.9	1.9	1.4
16239	„	1.7	25.4	5.0	74.6	6.6	1.2	0.6

In these cases, there was a marked decrease of plasma proteins. The reduction of albumin was pronounced and uniform, while globulin was distinctly low in three and high in one out of the seven cases.

Pleural and ascitic fluids.

In table 3, the data of eight pleural and ascitic fluids are given. The calcium contents of these fluids were distinctly low, and the reduc-

TABLE 3.

Calcium distribution and proteins in pleural (P) and ascitic (A) fluids

Case No.	Condition	Fluid	Non-diffusible calcium		Diffusible calcium		Total calcium	Albumin	Globulin
			mg per 100 cc	percent	mg per 100 cc	percent	mg per 100 cc	percent	percent
12338	Pleurisy	P.	2.0	29.8	4.7	70.2	6.7	0.2	0.05
16429	„	P.	1.6	21.9	5.7	78.1	7.2	0.1	0.07
16290	„	P.	1.0	18.5	4.4	81.5	5.5	0.1	0.09
16392	Cirrhosis of Liver	A.	0.9	14.5	5.3	85.5	6.2	0.11	0.7
16102	Banti's disease	A.	0.8	13.3	5.2	86.7	5.9	0.4	0.2
14418	Nephrosis	P.	0.8	12.9	5.4	87.1	5.8	0.3	0.1
16249	Cardiac failure	P.	0.3	6.0	5.7	94.0	5.3	0.06	0.04
16249	Cardiac failure	A.	0.2	3.8	5.1	96.2	5.4	0.07	0.04

tion was chiefly in the non-diffusible fraction which was almost negligible in amount in the last two cases. The diffusible calcium, however, remained about 5 mg, corresponding to the normal value obtained for serum. Going along with the decrease of non-diffusible calcium, the protein contents of these fluids were extremely low.

The effect of cod liver oil.

The efficacy of cod liver oil in the treatment of infantile tetany and its ability in raising blood calcium have been repeatedly observed by various authors. It would be interesting to see which portion of the calcium is raised. One case of tetany in a girl of 16, apparently of the infantile type (table 4, case I) was given cod liver oil 15 cc twice daily for 12 days. The elevation of calcium was reflected in both the diffusible and non-diffusible calcium, but the rise was very much greater in the diffusible than in the non-diffusible portion (fig. 2). Case II, a case of nephrosis with a total calcium of 7.7 mg, was given 45 cc of cod liver oil daily for 12 days. The rise of total calcium was not marked in this case. The slight increase of serum calcium obtained seemed to be

TABLE 4.

The effect of cod liver oil on blood calcium distribution and proteins

Cod Liver Oil	Date	Non-diffusible serum calcium		Diffusible serum calcium		Total serum calcium	Plasma albumin	Plasma globulin
		mg per 100 cc	percent	mg per 100 cc	percent	mg per 100 cc	percent	percent
Case I. Hospital No. 15846. Tetany.								
Control 15 cc b.i.d.	Mar. 25	4.3	53.7	3.7	46.3	8.0	3.4	1.7
from Mar. 30	Apr. 4	4.5	46.4	5.2	53.6	9.8	4.2	1.6
to April 10	11	4.7	42.9	6.1	57.1	9.8	4.7	1.7
Case II. Hospital No. 14418. Nephrosis.								
Control 15 cc t.i.d.	Mar. 24	2.4	25.9	5.7	74.1	7.7	1.8	1.5
from Mar. 27	31	2.4	27.3	6.4	72.7	8.2	1.9	1.6
to April 7	Apr. 7	2.0	25.0	6.0	75.0	8.0	2.1	1.5

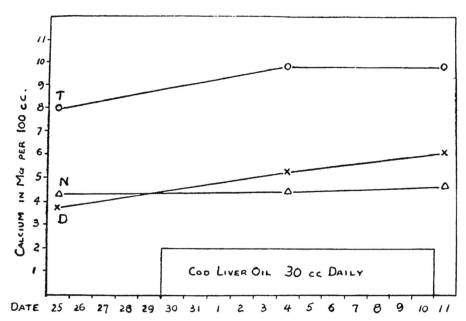

Fig. 2. Case I. Effect of cod liver oil on total (T), diffusible (D), and non-diffusible (N) calcium.

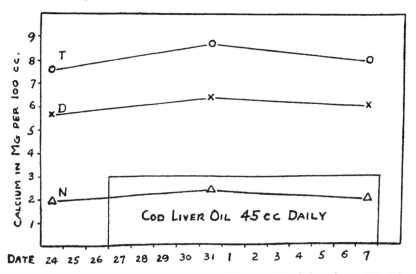

Fig. 3. Case II. Effect of cod liver oil on total (T), diffusible (D), and non-diffusible (N) calcium.

mainly in the diffusible fraction (fig. 3). Simultaneous determinations of plasma proteins showed no striking change, although there was a tendency for the albumin to increase somewhat.

The effect of parathyroid hormone.

Since the discovery of an active parathyroid extract by Collip and his colleagues (3,4), we have a potent agent for raising blood calcium as well as in the treatment of tetany. The manner of increase of calcium in the blood was studied in two cases (table 5). The first case, following other lines of treatment, was already convalescent with an almost normal total serum calcium in normal partition. Under the influence of parathyroid extract, the blood calcium showed a further rise to a maximum of 10.4 mg, and the rise was again chiefly in the diffusible fraction (fig. 4). The second case is a man of 46 having chronic tetany of 4 years duration, probably associated with a parathyroid deficiency. He had a total serum calcium of 6.5 mg with a proportionate decrease

TABLE 5.

The effect of parathyroid hormone on blood calcium distribution and proteins

Collip's Parathyroid Extract	Date	Non-diffusible serum calcium		Diffusible serum calcium		Total serum calcium	Plasma albumin	Plasma globulin
		mg per 100 cc	percent	mg per 100 cc	percent	mg per 100 cc	percent	percent
Case I. Hospital No. 12947. Tetany.								
Control 230 U from	Apr. 1	4.2	45.7	5.2	54.3	9.2	3.6	2.0
April 6-8 300 U from	8	4.2	41.2	6.0	58.5	10.2	4.9	2.1
April 8-11 200 U from	11	4.6	44.2	5.8	55.8	10.4	4.8	1.7
April 11-13	13	4.0	40.4	5.9	59.6	9.9	3.6	1.2
Case II. Hospital No. 15810. Tetany.								
Control 200 U from	Apr. 13	3.1	46.3	3.6	53.7	6.5	5.0	1.7
April 13-15 180 U from	15	3.1	31.3	6.8	68.7	9.6	4.2	2.1
April 15-18 150 U from	18	4.1	36.9	7.0	63.1	11.1	3.8	1.8
April 18-20	20	4.6	41.1	6.6	58.9	11.1	3.7	1.3

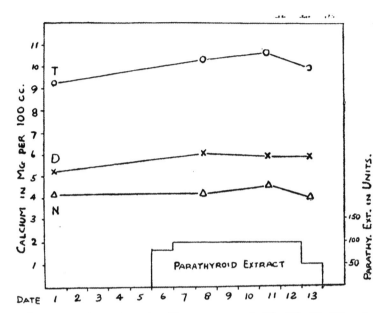

Fig. 4. Case I. Effect of parathyroid extract on total (T), diffusible (D), and non-diffusible (N) calcium.

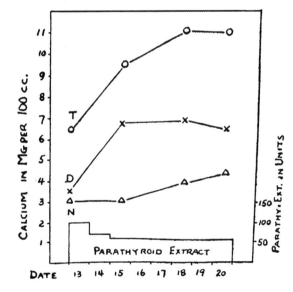

Fig. 5. Case II. Effect of darathyroid extract on total (T), diffusible (D), and non-diffusible (N) calcium.

of both the diffusible and the non-diffusible fractions. After the injection of parathyroid extract, his serum calcium rose to 11.1 mg. Both the diffusible and non-diffusible calcium showed a rise, but the rise in the diffusible portion was distinctly greater than that of the non-diffusible portion, an effect similar to that of cod liver oil (fig. 5). There was no consistent change in the blood proteins, although the albumin tended to decrease, especially in case II.

DISCUSSION

From the foregoing data, it is clear that in "normal" individuals, the partition of serum calcium into diffusible and non-diffusible fractions is fairly constant. In certain diseased conditions, either the diffusible or the non-diffusible calcium or both may be decreased with a resulting low total calcium. When the non-diffusible calcium is decreased without any decrease in the diffusible calcium as in nephrosis and kala-azar, no signs of tetany appear, even though the total serum calcium may be at a level as low as that ordinarily considered associated with tetany (17). A decrease of diffusible calcium in certain types of nephritis without evidence of tetany has been reported by Salvesen and Linder (18), and Pincus, Peterson and Kramer (15), but the similar results obtained in kala-azar seem to be a new finding adding further evidence in support of the view that the non-diffusible calcium plays a relatively unimportant rôle in the maintenance of normal nervous irritability.

Furthermore, from the results on the cases of tetany reported here, the decrease of calcium seems to be chiefly in the diffusible fraction. Pincus and others (15), using the method of ultra-filtration found that in infantile tetany and in post-operative tetany of dogs, the filtrable calcium was greatly reduced, while the non-filtrable calcium remained normal. This is in agreement with the results presented, and emphasises the importance of the diffusible calcium in the control of neuro-muscular irritability.

Under the influence of either cod liver oil or parathyroid hormone, the total serum calcium rises, but with a greater rise in the diffusible than in the non-diffusible portion so that the former reaches the normal level with a resulting disappearance of tetany. Moritz (13) who studied the effect of injecting parathyroid extract on the serum calcium of rabbits, found that both the diffusible and non-diffusible calcium were increased, but that usually the diffusible calcium was increased more than the non-diffusible calcium, in agreement with the present observations on human cases.

It seems that there is overwhelming evidence in favor of the view that it is the diffusible calcium that is physiologically active in the control of neuro-muscular irritability, whatever the diffusible calcium actually consists of.

In regard to the state of non-diffusible calcium, it seems that definite evidence has been brought forward in this communication to show that it is associated with serum protein. In nephrosis and kala-azar where the proteins, especially albumin, are low, the non-diffusible calcium is correspondingly low. In ascitic and pleural fluids, with an extremely low protein content, the non-diffusible calcium is present only in small amounts. This agrees in general with the work of Salvesen and Linder (18) who found that the decrease of total serum calcium, in non-uremic cases of Brights' disease paralleled the decrease in plasma protein and thought that the reduction of calcium was probably in the non-diffusible fraction, although this was not actually estimated.

Csapó and Faubl (6) fractionated the serum proteins and found that each fraction carried down with it a certain amount of calcium which was held quite tenaciously. Of the serum proteins, albumin seemed to carry down the most calcium. The fact that in the cases of nephrosis and kala-azar presented here, the decrease of non-diffusible calcium parallels the decrease of albumin more closely than globulin would lend support to the view that albumin is more important in holding calcium in the non-diffusible form.

From the foregoing discussion, althogh it is quite proboble that the non-diffusible calcium (associated with the plasma proteins), is unimportant in the control of nervous irritability, the slight decrease of non-diffusible calcium in tetany without any decrease of protein remains yet unexplained, unless it be assumed as did Salvesen and Linder (18) that with a primary decrease of diffusible calcium, some of the non-diffusible form becomes diffusible tending to maintain any possible equilibrium between the two. Further work, however, seems necessary along this line.

SUMMARY

1. Using a method of combined ultra-filtration and dialysis for the partition of calcium into diffsuible and non-diffufible fractions, the decrease of serum calcium in tetany is found chiefly in the diffusible form, while that in nephrosis and kala-azar with no evidence of tetany is exclusively in the non-diffusible form. This indicates that it is the disffusible rather than the non-diffusible calcium that is physiologically active in the control of neuro-musclar irritability.

2. Under the influence of both parathyroid hormone and cod liver oil, the rise of serum calcium is mainly in the diffusible portion, further emphasising the importance of the diffusible calcium in maintaining normal neuro-musclar irritability.

3. Definite evidence has been brought forward that the non-diffusible is calcium in some way bound to serum proteins especially albumin.

LITERATURE

1. CAMERON, A. T. AND MOOR-   J. Biol. Chem., 1925, **63**, 687-720.
   HOUSE, V. H. K.
2. CLARK, E. P. AND COLLIP, J. B.   J. Biol. Chem., 1925, **63**, 461-464.
3. COLLIP, J. B.   J. Biol. Chem., 1925, **63**, 395-438.
4. COLLIP, J. B., CLARK, E.P. AND   J. Biol. Chem., 1925, **63**, 439-460.
   SCOTT, J. W.
5. CRUICKSHANK, E. W. H.   Brit. J. Exper. Path., 1923, **4**, 213-223.
6. CSAPÓ, J. UND FAUBL, J.   Biochem. Ztschr., 1924, **150**, 508-514.
7. CUSHNY, A. R.   J. Physiol., 1919-20, **53**, 391-398.
8. GREENWALD, I.   J. Biol. Chem., 1926, **67**, 1-28
9. LOEB, R. F.   J. Gen. Physiol., 1926, **8**, 451-461.
10. MEYSENBUG, L. V. AND Mc-   J, Biol. Chem., 1921, **47**, 541-545.
    CANN, G. F.
11. MEYSENBUG, L. V., PAPPEN-   J. Biol. Chem., 1921, **47**, 529-539.
    HEIMER, A. M., ZUCKER, T. F.
    AND MURRAY, M. F.
12. MORITZ, A. R.   J. Biol. Chem., 1925, **64**, 81-89.
13. MORITZ, A. R.   J. Biol. Chem., 1925, **66**, 343-351.
14. NEUHAUSEN, B. S. AND PINCUS,   J. Biol. Chem., 1923, **57**, 99-106.
    J. B.
15. PINCUS, J. B., PETERSON, H. A.   J. Biol. Chem., 1926, **68**, 610-609.
    AND KRAMER, B.
16. RONA, P. AND TAKAHSHI, D.   Biochem. Ztschr., 1911, **31**, 336-344.
17. SALVESEN, H. A.   J. Biol. Chem., 1923, **56**, 443-456.

18. SALVESEN, H. A. AND LINDER,　　J. Biol. Chem., 1923-24, **58**, 617-634.
    G. C.
19. UPDEGRAFF, H., GREENBURG,　　J. Biol. Chem., 1926-27, **71**, 86-126.
    D. M. AND CLARK, G. W.
20. WU, H. AND LING, S. M.　　Chinese J. Physiol., 1927, **1**, 161-168.

透析血清鈣質之研究

劉士豪

北京協和醫學校內科系

　　血清中之無機成分，鈣質比較他種原質，居特殊地位。如用火棉膠製成小囊，盛以血清，置此囊於蒸餾水中，加以副壓力過濾，其他成分，均可滲透此囊而入水中，惟鈣質則不然，一半入水，一半仍留囊中。故正常血清100CC含鈣質10mg者，約半數爲「有滲透性」，半數爲「無滲透性」。病症中如手足搐搦症，呈神經過敏現象，其血清鈣質較平常爲少。用火棉膠囊過濾法檢察，乃知「無滲透性」之鈣質并不減少，而「有滲透性」之鈣質，異常減少。患黑熱症及患腎炎症者，其血清鈣質亦異常低減，而并不發現神經過敏之病狀。用上法試驗，結果爲「無滲透性」之鈣質減少，而「有滲透性」之鈣質之多寡與平常無異。由此可見「有滲透性」之鈣質，對于神經之敏感有莫大關係，至於「無滲透性」之鈣質，則爲比較的不重要。

　　手足搐搦症治療法，用魚肝油或甲狀旁腺內分泌液，効力甚力，并可增長血清鈣質。其增長之鈣質，大半爲「有滲透性」者，更可證明神經之敏感性，全賴「有滲透性」之鈣質以爲約束。

「無滲透性」之鈣質，其不能透析火棉膠囊之原因，據多半研究家之設想，均以其與血清蛋白質結合，故不能自由彌散，但此說并無確實證據．此篇試驗結果：凡患黑熱症或腎炎症者，其血清「無滲透性」之鈣質減少時，其血清蛋白質亦必同等的減少，二者相依而行．分析腹水及胸水鈣質，亦能證明此點，蓋腹水及胸水所含之蛋白質極少，其「無滲透性」之鈣質爲量亦極少．由此觀之，「無滲透性」之鈣質，確與蛋白質有關，似無疑義．

Chinese Journal of Physiology, 1928, Vol. II, No. 2, pp. 151—156.

PLASMA ACID-BASE EQUILIBRIUM IN MALARIA*

SHIH-HAO LIU

(From the Department of Medicine, Peking Union Medical College, Peking)

Received for publication January 31, 1928

Indian workers on malaria have long thought that there is a condition of "acidosis" in the blood of patients with malaria. This is based largely upon the apparent close resemblance between the malarial paroxysm and the anaphylactoid phenomenon produced by the injection of a foreign protein into the body, and the presence of acidosis in the latter condition. Sinton (7), employing the bicarbonate tolerance test of Sellards (5), showed that patients with malaria required approximately twice as much sodium bicarbonate as normal persons in order to render the urine alkaline to litmus. He concluded that there was a moderate degree of acidosis in malaria, and obtained a reduction in the incidence of relapses in the series of cases of malaria treated with quinine combined with alkali (6).

Direct evidence of the existence of acidosis in the blood in malaria, however, has been lacking. The present paper has for its purpose a study of the acid-base equilibrium of the blood in malaria by direct measurements of the reaction and electrolyte distribution of the plasma.

EXPERIMENTAL

Thirteen cases of malaria were available for study. One case was aestivo-autumnal malaria and the remaining cases tertian malaria. Venous blood was obtained both during the paroxysm at the height of the fever (39.5-40.5°C), and during the remission with normal temperature. The study of the acid-base equilibrium consisted of measurements of pH, total base, CO_2 capacity, chloride and protein content.

The bicolorimetric method of Hastings and Sendroy (1) was employed for the determination of pH. Blood was taken from the vein without

*Read before the Chinese Physiological Society, Peking, January, 1928.

stasis or contact with air, and colorimetric comparisons were made of the plasma at 38°C.

For total base, the method of Stadie and Ross (9) was used. The benzidine solution was standardized once every two weeks. Determinations were made from serum.

Total CO_2 capacity was determined by the method of Van Slyke and Cullen (11). The bicarbonate (HCO_3) combined with base was calculated from the following formula devised by Peters et al. (3):

$$HCO_3 = \frac{CO_2 - 2.85}{2.24}$$

in which CO_2 = total CO_2 capacity in volumes percent as determined, 2.85 = volumes percent of CO_2 dissolved in plasma at 40 mm of CO_2 tension at 38° C, and 2.24 = gas constant. The HCO_3 is expressed as milli-equivalents per liter.

Chloride was determined as sodium chloride by the method of Meyer and Short (2). Plasma was used. Sodium chloride in mg per 100 cc was reduced to milli-equivalents by the following equation:

$$Cl = \frac{NaCl \times 10}{58.06}$$

in which NaCl = sodium chloride in mg per 100 cc, 58.06 = the molecular weight of sodium chloride and Cl = chloride in milli-equivalents per liter.

Proteins were estimated by Wu and Ling's (13) method. Only the plasma albumin and globulin were determined. The determination of fibrinogen was not made, as it is of relatively small magnitude and its omission probably does not invalidate our conclusions for comparative purposes. The base bound by protein was calculated by the equation $P = 2.03$ Pr, where P = milli-equivalent of base bound by protein, Pr = protein in percent, and 2.03 = the base combining power of protein for human blood obtained by Van Slyke (12).

Total acid (A) is calculated as the sum:

$$A = HCO_3 + Cl + P$$

in which HCO_3, Cl and P represent respective milli-equivalents of bicarbonate, chloride and protein combined with base, and A therefore represents the total base-combining power of the inorganic acids and proteins of the plasma or serum. The difference between this and total base represents the inorganic phosphates, sulphates and salts of organic acids. The failure to determine the inorganic phosphorus and sulphur makes the sum total of the acids incomplete. Under ordinary circumstances inorganic phosphates amount to 1.5 to 2.0 milli-equivalents and inorganic sulphates are negligible in amount. Therefore, for comparative purposes, a study of the total base in relation to HCO_3, Cl and P is sufficient.

RESULTS AND DISCUSSION

The results obtained in 13 cases of malaria are presented in table 1, and the average values of the various constituents in these cases while afebrile and during fever are given in table 2. From table 1, it can be seen that all the values obtained are within normal limits with the methods employed.

Plasma pH remained constant; the greatest variation did not exceed 0.05 which is within the experimental error. As the variations were slight and they occurred both ways, identical results were obtained when the readings during remissions and those in paroxysms were averaged.

Although the values of HCO_3, the amount of bicarbonate combined with base, were all within normal limits, the values during the febrile periods were consistently lower than those during the afebrile periods. The decrease on the average amounts to 2.2 milli-equivalents. It remains to be determined whether this slight depletion of HCO_3 is characteristic of malarial paroxysm or dependent on the effect of the fever alone. Stadie, Austin and Robinson (8) in studying the effect of temperature on the acid-base equilibrium of blood and serum, demonstrated that at constant pH, HCO_3 decreases with increase of temperature. The decrease amounts to 0.48 milli-equivalents per degree of increase of temperature. In infections of various kinds with fever, Peters and his co-workers (4) showed a similar decrease of bicarbonate. In typhoid fever*, there is also a tendency for the bicarbonate to decrease during the febrile periods. Thus the slight decrease of HCO_3 during malarial paroxysm may well represent the result of fever rather than the specific effect of malaria.

Regarding chloride, all except two cases showed a decrease during fever as compared with the values during afebrile periods. The average decrease of chloride is 3.3 milli-equivalents, which is somewhat more

*Unpublished results.

S. H. LIU

TABLE 1.

Plasma acid-base equilibrium in malaria

Case	Condition	pH	Total base (B) m-eq. per liter	HCO₃ m-eq. per liter	Cl m-eq. per liter	Protein m-eq. per liter	Total acid (A) m-eq. per liter	Residual base (B - A) m-eq. per liter
9356	Afebrile	7.34	159.0	28.5	95.4	13.0	126.9	32.1
	Fever	7.34	152.2	22.1	94.0	14.0	130.1	22.1
15621	Afebrile	7.40	170.4	30.9	93.5	7.9	132.3	38.1
	Fever	7.40	170.4	26.3	90.5	11.6	128.4	42.0
15810	Afebrile	7.38	156.8	27.7	97.8	13.6	139.1	17.7
	Fever	7.40	158.8	26.1	97.3	12.2	135.6	23.2
16899	Afebrile	7.33	160.2	29.3	97.8	13.4	140.5	19.7
	Fever	7.38	168.0	27.6	96.8	12.4	136.8	31.2
17743	Afebrile	7.40	157.2	26.5	101.5	11.6	139.6	17.6
	Fever	7.40	175.8	25.0	96.3	9.1	130.4	45.4
17756	Afebrile	7.35	147.0	23.3	102.5	12.6	138.4	8.6
	Fever	7.35	170.8	22.9	103.6	12.2	138.7	32.1
17878	Afebrile	7.38	160.2	29.2	117.0	11.4	157.6	2.6
	Fever	7.40	162.0	26.8	97.2	11.4	134.4	27.6
17880	Afebrile	7.34	157.8	25.3	102.2	12.4	139.9	17.9
	Fever	7.35	154.4	23.0	100.5	11.4	134.9	19.5
17953	Afebrile	7.34	164.6	24.7	103.6	11.4	139.7	24.9
	Fever	7.30	167.8	20.9	106.8	11.4	139.1	28.7
18085	Afebrile	7.40	159.0	24.5	102.5	10.8	137.8	21.2
	Fever	7.37	169.4	24.5	100.5	13.4	138.4	31.0
18192	Afebrile	7.48	164.6	22.4	98.8	12.0	133.2	31.4
	Fever	7.43	150.0	21.3	87.7	11.4	120.4	29.6
18266	Afebrile	7.45	157.8	26.4	99.4	11.4	137.2	20.6
	Fever	7.48	170.4	24.4	95.6	9.1	129.1	41.3
18530	Afebrile	7.38	139.5	28.5	97.3	9.3	135.1	4.4
	Fever	7.33	132.7	27.3	94.0	9.1	130.4	2.3

TABLE 2.

Average values from table 1

	Afebrile	Fever	Difference
pH	7.38	7.38	0
Total base (B), m-eq. per liter	158.0	161.7	+ 3.7
HCO₃, m-eq. per liter	26.7	24.5	− 2.2
Cl, m-eq. per liter	100.7	97.0	− 3.7
Protein, m-eq. per liter	11.6	11.4	− 0.2
Total acid (A), m-eq. per liter	139.0	132.9	− 6.1
Residual base (B-A), m-eq. per liter	19.0	28.8	+ 9.8

marked than the decrease of HCO_3. Although hypochloremia has long been recognized as characteristic of pneumonia (10), it may also be found in other infectious fevers (4). Unpublished observations of the author on typhoid fever also indicate that during the febrile periods the plasma chloride is lowered, tending to return to normal during convalescence.

Protein variations were rather irregular and occurred both ways, and as a result the difference between the average values during fever and remission is negligible.

Total base, A, represents the total base-combining power of bicarbonate, chloride and proteins and the difference in total acid between the two periods is the summation of the differences in the individual constituents. In this series of cases there is an average total decrease of 6.1 milli-equivalents of acids (HCO_3, Cl, P) during the febrile paroxysm.

This decrease in total acid plus the slight increase in total base during the febrile periods represents the excess of residual base probably bound by organic acid produced as a result of the paroxysm. In this series of experiments the excess of organic acids on the average amounts to 9.8 milli-equivalents. The nature of the excess of organic acids, however, is not determined.

SUMMARY AND CONCLUSIONS

The results of a study of the acid-base equilibrium of the plasma in 13 cases of malaria are presented. The measurements include pH, total base, CO_2 content, chloride and proteins. All the values obtained are within normal limits. During the febrile paroxysm, the pH remains unchanged, but there is a slight increase of total base with a slight decrease of bicarbonate and chloride. All these changes tend to increase the residual base and the excess of residual base during fever is probably bound by organic acids of undetermined nature. All these variations, though uniform, are considered to be the result of fever, and not due to the specific effects of malarial infection.

156　　　　　　　　　　S. H. LIU

LITERATURE

1. HASTINGS, A. B. AND SENDROY,　J. Biol. Chem., 1924, **61**, 695-710.
    J., JR.
2. MYERS, V. C. AND SHORT, J. J.　J. Biol. Chem., 1920, **44**, 47-53.
3. PETERS, J. P., BULGER, H. A.,　J. Biol. Chem., 1926, **67**, 141-158.
    EISENMAN, A. J. AND LEE, C.
4. PETERS, J. P., BULGER, H. A.,　J. Biol. Chem., 1926, **67**, 219-235.
    EISENMAN, A. J. AND LEE, C.
5. SELLARDS, A. W.　　　　　　The principles of acidosis and clinical me-
    　　　　　　　　　　　　　thods for its study, Cambridge, U.S.A. 1917.
6. SINTON, J. A.　　　　　　　Indian Med. Gaz., 1923, **58**, 406-415.
7. SINTON, J. A.　　　　　　　Indian J. Med. Res., 1923-24, **11**, 1051-1056.
8. STADIE, W. C., AUSTIN, J. H.　J. Biol. Chem., 1925, **66**, 910-920.
    AND ROBINSON, H. W.
9. STADIE, W. C. AND ROSS, E. C.　J. Biol. Chem., 1925, **65**, 735-754.
10. SUNDERMAN, F. W., AUSTIN,　J. Clin. Invest., 1926, **3**, 37-64.
    J. H. AND CAMAC, J. G.
11. VAN SLYKE, D. D. AND CULLEN,　J. Biol. Chem., 1917, **30**, 347-368.
    G. E.
12. VAN SLYKE, D. D.　　　　　Quoted by Atchley, D. W. and Benedict,
    　　　　　　　　　　　　　E. M., J. Biol. Chem., 1927, **73**, 1-14.
13. WU, H. AND LING, S. M.　　Chinese J. Physiol., 1927, **1**, 161-168.

瘧疾血清中之酸鹼性之平衡

劉士豪

北京協和醫學校內科學系

辛氏 (Sinton) 云，患瘧病者常有血酸症；但此說并無直接之證據．著者於十三例之瘧疾，直接檢查其血清中之「氫遊子之濃度」(pH)，「鹽基總數」(total base)，「重炭酸鹽」(bicarbonate)，「氯化物」(chloride)，及「蛋白質」(protein)．結果以上各質均合正常之量度，并無血清過酸之表示．在瘧熱發作時，「鹽基總數」比較熱退時稍多；而「重炭酸鹽」及氯化物則稍減．此種變遷甚微，無論何種熱病，均可發生，非瘧病特然也．由此觀之，瘧疾血清中酸鹼各質，平衡如常，并無特殊之變化．

·Chinese Journal of Physiology, 1928, Vol. II, No. 2, pp. 157—162.

STUDIES ON PLASMA LIPOIDS. I. FATTY ACIDS OF BLOOD PLASMA IN DIABETES AND NEPHROSIS*

SCHMORL M. LING and SHIH-HAO LIU

(From the Chemical Laboratory, Department of Medicine, Peking Union

Medical College, Peking)

Received for publication February 3, 1928

It is a well known fact that in diabetes mellitus of moderate or severe form there is a pronounced tendency for fat and other lipoids of the blood to be abnormally high. A similar change was also observed in nephritis by Müller (7). Epstein (3) considered hypercholesterolemia as one of the outstanding features of nephrosis. To explain this characteristic change several possibilities have been suggested. Diminished ability of the organism to utilize fat is one of the prominent possibilities, but direct evidence of this has been lacking. According to Leathes' hypothesis of fat catabolism (6), desaturation is a necessary preliminary step in the utilization of the comparatively stable fatty acids of the food and stored fat of the body and by desaturation these fatty acids are rendered more susceptible to further oxidation and possibly to other changes. This process is believed to take place mainly in the liver and the desaturated fatty acids are carried from the liver to different organs by the blood. Therefore highly unsaturated fatty acids may be present in the blood. If there is a difference in the degree of unsaturation of the fatty acids of blood plasma in normal and diseased conditions, some light may be thrown on the nature of the disturbance of fat metabolism that occurs in diabetes mellitus and nephrosis.

*Read before the Seventh Biennial Conference of the National Medical Association of China, Peking, January, 1928.

157

METHOD

For analysis 20 to 30 cc of venous blood were obtained from subjects under fasting conditions. It was oxalated and centrifuged at once. For the separation of fatty acids Bloor's method (1) was used. The plasma, 10 to 15 cc, obtained from the blood by centrifuging, was treated with 5 gm of stick potassium hydroxide and digested on a steam bath for 6 hours. The mixture was then carefully neutralized with concentrated hydrochloric acid and extracted with ether in separate portions until the ether was colorless. The ether extract was washed once with water and the ether distilled off. The residue was dissolved in petroleum ether and the fatty acids were separated from the "unsaponifiable matter". For the separation of the solid from the liquid fatty acids the method of Twitchell (9) based on the difference in solubility of the lead salts of the liquid and solid fatty acids in cold alcohol was used. Iodine number determinations were made on the liquid fatty acid fraction, using Wijs' method (10).

Beyond carrying out the various separations and determinations as quickly as possible and protecting the solutions from free access of air by stoppering the containers and by keeping weighing bottles in a vacuum desiccator, no special precaution was taken to avoid oxidation of the unsaturated fatty acids.

RESULTS

Fourteen samples of blood plasma were examined, four of which were obtained from normal healthy individuals, five from hospital patients with diabetes mellitus of moderate severity and five from nephrosis patients. The results of the examinations are shown in table 1.

As may be seen from the table, normally total lipoids vary from 380 to 445 mg per 100 cc of plasma, of which about 45 per cent are unsaponifiable. The liquid fatty acids range from 136 to 210 mg per 100 cc of plasma and constitute 70 to 90 per cent of the total fatty acids, with an average iodine number of 156. 6. In both diabetes mellitus and nephrosis the total lipoids are increased, the increase being more marked in the latter than in the former. Apparently this increase is due to a proportionate accumulation of all the fatty substances, since the percentages of the "unsaponifiable matter" and the liquid fatty acids are practically unchanged. On the other hand the liquid fatty acids are much less unsaturated, as indicated by the iodine number, which varies from 45 to 98 in the case of diabetes mellitus and from 59 to 87 in the case of nephrosis.

TABLE 1.
Fatty acids of blood plasma
mg per 100 cc

Hospital No.	Diagnosis	Total lipoids		"Unsaponifiable"		Total fatty acids		Solid fatty acids	Liquid fatty acids		Iodine number of liquid fatty acids
		By weight A	Sum of C and D B	By weight C	Per cent of total lipoids (B)	By weight D	Sum of F and G E	F	By weight G	Per cent of total fatty acids (E)	
	Normal	445	431	210	49	221	210	71	139	66	160.8
	"	414	368	117	32	251	240	30	210	87	133.7
	"	380	327	177	54	150	150	14	136	90	161.0
	"	386	377	150	40	227	227	20	207	90	171.0
18379	Diabetes mellitus	500	479	179	37	300	267	13	254	95	97.9
18614	"	510	448	246	55	202	154	40	114	74	45.3
18830	"	420	409	218	53	191	186	28	158	85	55.7
18861	"	333	297	111	37	186	184	14	170	92	52.5
18603	"	525	478	161	31	317	317	28	289	91	95.4
18008	Nephrosis	985	917	395	40	522	484	80	404	84	80.0
18767	"	871	856	356	41	500	475	63	412	87	66.1
18492	"	915	902	362	40	540	498	78	420	84	87.4
19083	"	915	892	207	28	685	675	60	615	91	59.4
19106	"	1125	1077	342	32	735	700	60	640	91	62.1

DISCUSSION

The outstanding feature of the results shown in the above table is that the iodine number decreases as the amount of fat in the blood plasma increases. The iodine numbers of the liquid fatty acids in normal plasma are all relatively high, considerably higher than those reported by Csonka (2). But his results are hardly comparable with ours, as his work was done on whole blood. In diabetic lipemia the iodine numbers of various samples of liquid fatty acids vary from 45 to 98. This is of the same order as that reported by Fischer (4), Neisser and Derlin (8), Imrie (5), and Csonka (2) who found that the fatty acids of the blood had an iodine number of 60.6, 54, 73, and 83 to 90 respectively. With regard to the degree of unsaturation of the fatty acids of the blood plasma in nephrosis very little has been reported. The data at hand show beyond question that these fatty acids are less unsaturated, as indicated by their iodine number, than those of normal plasma.

From these results it is clear that the iodine numbers obtained for fatty acids from normal blood plasma in our experiments were higher than that of oleic acid (90). The numbers varied from 134 to 171. This indicates the presence of fatty acid of the linoleic series ($C_n H_{2n-4} O_2$), the iodine number of which is 181. The nature of the fatty acids in the various components of plasma lipoids has yet to be determined.

The fact that with increased fat in the blood plasma the iodine number of the fatty acids became lower, being 45 to 98 in the case of diabetes mellitus and 59 to 87 in the case of nephrosis, suggests an access of a large amount of the stored fat of the body. Before a definite conclusion can be drawn, it is desirable to determine, if this unusual amount of fat with low iodine number is due to accelerated discharge of fat from storage cells, when there is no corresponding acceleration in the rate at which the liver deals with it, so that the unaltered fat is forwarded to the blood stream.

SUMMARY

The fatty acids of normal blood plasma are highly unsaturated with an average iodine value of 156.6, while in diabetes mellitus and nephrosis they are much less unsaturated and their iodine value is lower, being 45 to 98 in the former and 59 to 87 in the latter.

LITERATURE

1.　BLOOR, W. R.　　　　　　　J. Biol. Chem., 1923, 56, 711-724.
2.　CSONKA, F. A.　　　　　　J. Biol. Chem., 1918, 33, 401-409.
3.　EPSTEIN, A. A.　　　　　　Am. J. Med. Sci., 1917, 154, 638-647;
　　　　　　　　　　　　　　　　1922, 163, 167-186.
4.　FISCHER, B.　　　　　　　Virchow's Arch. f. path. Anat. u. Physiol.
　　　　　　　　　　　　　　　　u. klin. Med., 1903, 172, 30-71.
5.　IMRIE, C. G.　　　　　　　J. Biol. Chem., 1915, 20, 87-90.
6.　LEATHES, J. B.　　　　　　The Harvey Lectures, Philadelphia and Lon-
　　　　　　　　　　　　　　　　don, 1908-9, p. 213-239.
7.　MÜLLER, J.　　　　　　　　Ztschr. f. physiol. Chem., 1913, 87, 469-483.
8.　NEISSER, E. UND DERLIN, L.　Ztschr. f. klin. Med., 1904, 51, 428-438.
9.　TWITCHELL, E.　　　　　　J. Indust. Eng. Chem., 1921, 13, 806-807.
10.　WIJS, J. J. A.　　　　　　J. B. Leathes and H. S. Raper's Monograph
　　　　　　　　　　　　　　　　on the fats, London, 1925, 2nd ed., p. 70-73.

血漿中脂質之研究

其一· 糖尿病及腎病人血漿中脂酸,

林樹模　　　劉士豪

北京協和醫學校內科學系

　　康健人血漿中脂酸，其未飽和度(unsaturation)極高，所以脂酸，每百公分平均能吸收碘一五六·六公分．糖尿病及腎病人血漿中脂酸，其未飽和度較低；前者所有脂酸,每百公分祇能吸收碘四五至九八公分；後者所有脂酸,每百公分祇能吸收碘五九至八七公分．

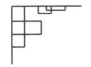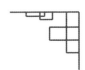

第二编　赴美求学

　　第二编选取了刘士豪教授第一次出国在纽约洛克菲勒医学研究所学习时期的论文。刘士豪在 1928 年赴美进修，师从著名生物化学家范斯莱克（Donald D. Van Slyke）。范斯莱克与福林（O. Folin）同为美国生物化学界两大学术权威，在国际上享有盛名。他在 1922 年曾经被聘为协和的客座教授，在协和生物化学系与吴宪合作，做出了一批重要成果。刘士豪得名师指点，系统进行了生物化学的学习。同时，他在范斯莱克指导下与 Sendroy 合作研究了血气分析中有关二氧化碳张力的问题，发表了 3 篇论文。本编可管窥刘士豪教授在美国学习研究内容之一斑。

GASOMETRIC DETERMINATION OF OXYGEN AND CARBON MONOXIDE IN BLOOD.

By JULIUS SENDROY, Jr., AND S. H. LIU.*

(*From the Hospital of The Rockefeller Institute for Medical Research, New York.*)

(Received for publication, July 21, 1930.)

Van Slyke and Neill (1), in their original description of the manometric blood gas apparatus, described a method for the determination of O_2 and CO which was sufficiently exact for most purposes. However, estimation of the CO was less exact than that of O_2. While O_2 was determined by specific absorption with $Na_2S_2O_4$ solution, the CO had to be estimated by subtracting from the residual CO + N_2 a value of 1.2 or 1.4 volume per cent corresponding to the mean N_2 content of blood. CO could not be determined by absorption, because no suitable absorbing solution was available which did not form an unmanageable clot when mixed with the blood in the extraction chamber. The procedure by which CO is estimated by subtraction of the mean N_2 content of blood from the CO + N_2, is definitely less exact than one in which CO could be determined by direct absorption. Furthermore, the estimation by subtraction of the mean N_2 is not valid for blood saturated under experimental conditions with inert gases other than air at atmospheric pressure.

A technique which made possible the precise determination of CO by direct absorption was later devised by Van Slyke and Rob-scheit-Robbins (2) who used the Harington-Van Slyke (3) modification of the extraction chamber of the manometric apparatus. At the bottom of this extraction chamber there is an added cock, by means of which the chamber and the gases in it can be washed with successive portions of cleaning and absorbing solutions. The blood could be washed out and the CO measured by absorp-

* On leave of absence from the Department of Medicine, Peking Union Medical College, Peiping, China.

133

tion with cuprous chloride solution. The results were highly exact, but the numerous washings made the procedure rather long, 40 to 50 minutes being required for an analysis. Also, an inconvenience was introduced in this analysis, with the necessity for using the special Harington-Van Slyke extraction chamber, while all other analyses described for the manometric apparatus can be carried out with the simpler Van Slyke-Neill chamber.

In the present paper a procedure is described in which determination of CO by absorption is accomplished in analyses made with the Van Slyke-Neill chamber. The mixture of $O_2 + CO + N_2$ extracted from blood is removed to a micro-Hempel pipette, where the O_2 is absorbed, by a technique similar to that employed previously for manometric determination of amino nitrogen (4). The extraction chamber is then washed free of blood, and the gases are returned for completion of the analysis. The procedure equals in accuracy the Van Slyke-Robscheit-Robbins method, is less laborious, and can be carried through in 25 to 30 minutes.

Description of Method.

Reagents.

Acid Ferricyanide Reagent.—This is prepared for use each day by mixing equal parts of the following two solutions; (*a*) 32 gm. of potassium ferricyanide and 8 gm. of saponin dissolved in water to make 1 liter of solution, (*b*) 8 cc. of concentrated lactic acid (sp. gr. 1.20), diluted to 1 liter.

Alkaline Pyrogallate.—15 gm. of pyrogallic acid in 100 cc. of a saturated solution of KOH (sp. gr. about 1.55). This absorbent is kept under paraffin oil in a stoppered bottle and is not used until 3 weeks after preparation. If kept confined under oil in the modified Hempel pipette used for this work, one portion of pyrogallol solution may be used for 30 to 40 analyses.

Air-Free N Sodium Hydroxide.—Approximately 40 gm. of NaOH per liter solution. This is extracted air-free for use daily, and kept under oil in a calcium chloride tube ((1) p. 534).

Glycerol-Salt Solution.—One volume of glycerol is mixed with 3 volumes of saturated NaCl solution.

Winkler's Cuprous Chloride Solution.—200 gm. of CuCl, 250 gm. of NH₄Cl, and 750 cc. of water. The addition of a few gm. of

J. Sendroy, Jr., and S. H. Liu　　135

pure metallic copper serves to keep the CuCl in reduced state. This solution is freed of air, kept under a layer of paraffin oil, and should be used within 4 hours after having been rendered air-free.

Caprylic Alcohol.—This is used to prevent foaming.

Procedure.

The analysis consists of the following steps.

1. The gases, CO_2, O_2, CO, and N_2 are extracted from the blood sample in the chamber of the Van Slyke-Neill apparatus.

2. CO_2 is absorbed by the addition of N NaOH.

3. The mixture of residual gases, O_2, CO, and N_2 is transferred to the Hempel pipette containing alkaline pyrogallate, which absorbs the oxygen.

4. The blood is removed from the extraction chamber and replaced by air-free glycerol-salt solution.

5. The mixture of residual gases, CO and N_2, is returned to the chamber of the apparatus.

6. CO is absorbed by the addition of Winkler's reagent.

The details of the successive steps are given below. Since much of the technique has already been described in papers on other manometric analyses, it would be advantageous for the reader not already familiar with the manometric apparatus to consult previous papers referred to (1–4) for more complete explanations of general details and precautions.

The directions below apply when 2 cc. samples are used. The procedure for 1 cc. samples is given in a later section.

1. Extraction of Gases from Blood Sample.—From the cup of the Van Slyke-Neill apparatus, 2 drops of caprylic alcohol are admitted into the extraction chamber, followed by 8 cc. of the acid ferricyanide reagent. The stop-cock is sealed with mercury, and the chamber is evacuated and shaken for 2 minutes. The extracted air is ejected ((4) p. 428) and 4 cc. of the air-free reagent are allowed to run up into the cup. The blood sample is delivered from a 2 cc. rubber-tipped, stop-cock pipette ((1) p. 531). Traces of blood remaining in the cup are washed into the chamber with 1 cc. of the reagent, and the stop-cock is sealed. The chamber is evacuated and shaken for 3 minutes to extract the blood gases.

2. Absorption of CO_2 with NaOH.—Mercury is readmitted to

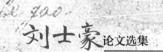

the chamber until the level of the liquid above comes to within a few cc. of the 2.0 cc. mark. 2 cc. of air-free N NaOH are placed in the cup, of which 1 cc. is slowly admitted into the chamber ((1) p. 545). The stop-cock is sealed and p_1, representing the total pressure of the gases O_2, CO, and N_2, is observed with the solution level at the 2.0 cc. mark.[1]

3. Transfer of Gases to Hempel Pipette and Absorption of Oxygen.
—The Hempel pipette ((4) p. 437) contains alkaline pyrogallate protected by a layer of oil in the upper bulb. A little of the solution is run out to clear the stop-cock a (Fig. 1) of any air that may be present, then the capillary limbs, l and r, are filled with mercury from the cup c above. 1 cc. of mercury is poured into the cup k of the Van Slyke-Neill apparatus, and all air is dislodged from the capillary leading down from the cup to the chamber.

The stop-cock of the manometric apparatus which admits mercury from the leveling bulb to the extraction chamber is opened, and the leveling bulb is raised to such a height, (this will have to be determined by the analyst) that the extracted gases will be compressed into a bubble at the top of the chamber at *slight* positive pressure. The stop-cock is closed, and the leveling bulb set at rest in the uppermost ring, above the chamber.

The free end of the Hempel pipette, with mercury flowing through l from the cup c above, is thrust firmly down into the cup k so that the rubber tip fits snugly. Stop-cock a is opened in the position indicated (Fig. 1). Stop-cock b is then opened. At this point, if the internal pressure of the gas bubble has been correctly fixed, a small amount of the gas should run into the capillary limb of the Hempel pipette under its own pressure. The rest of the gas, followed by the blood solution, is forced up into the Hempel pipette by admitting mercury slowly from the leveling bulb into the extraction chamber. As soon as the blood solution has passed slightly beyond the stop-cock a, the latter is turned in a clockwise

---

[1] If the precipitate formed by the interaction of the blood with the acid reagent obscures the meniscus, gentle movement of the chamber by hand will facilitate the solution of the proteins in the added alkali. Reading p_1 may then be taken over a clear solution. When dealing with darkly colored solutions, a source of light placed in back of the chamber has been found to be of great help in the adjustment of the meniscus to the volume mark. The light should only be used momentarily at the time of adjustment, so that no increase in temperature of the jacket and chamber may occur.

direction to the closed position shown in Fig. 1, position *a*, and the Hempel pipette is withdrawn.[2]

The free arm *l* is cleared of blood solution by the admission of mercury from cup *c*, and the capillary *r*, by continued turning of *a* in a clockwise direction, is likewise cleared of blood solution and gas. The pipette is set aside for the absorption of oxygen. Occasional gentle movement of the gas bubble to and fro, or in a horizontal rotatory manner facilitates the absorption, which is complete in 3 to 4 minutes.

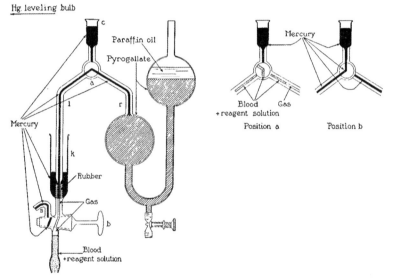

FIG. 1. Arrangement of apparatus for different stages of transfer of gas between extraction chamber and Hempel pipette.

4. Replacement of Blood Solution by Air-Free Glycerol-Salt Solution in Extraction Chamber.—In the meanwhile, the blood solution is removed from the chamber, which is then flushed two or three times with water. 5 cc. of glycerol-salt solution are then admitted into the apparatus and rendered air-free by shaking the evacuated

[2] In order to minimize the contamination of the absorbent by the blood solution, which precipitates in the pyrogallate and may even serve to trap gas, it is important to allow as little blood solution to pass into the capillary limb *r* as possible.

chamber for 2 minutes. The extracted air is expelled, and 1.5 cc. of the glycerol-salt solution are admitted into the cup k, 3.5 cc. remaining in the chamber.

5. Transfer of CO and N₂ from Hempel Pipette to Extraction Chamber.—1 cc. of mercury is poured into the cup k, stop-cock a is turned counter clockwise, and the Hempel pipette is placed in position while mercury is flowing from cup c into cup k (Fig. 1, position b). Stop-cock a is then turned counter clockwise to the position shown in Fig. 1. The mercury leveling bulb is placed in its lower position and stop-cock b is opened. The stop-cock connecting leveling bulb and extraction chamber is carefully opened, and, by withdrawal of mercury from the bottom of the chamber, the gas bubble from the Hempel pipette is slowly drawn into the top of the chamber. The minimum possible amount of pyrogallate solution is allowed to flow past the stop-cock a, which is then again turned back to the position indicated in Fig. 1, position b. By careful manipulation, with alternate opening and closing of the stop-cock a, the last portion of gas (and a slight amount of pyrogallate) is completely driven down, followed by mercury from cup c into the chamber, which is then sealed through stop-cock b.

The glycerol-salt solution level is lowered slightly below, then allowed to come to rest at the 2.0 cc. mark where a reading is taken. Due to the slow drainage of the viscous solution, two or three successive readings may be necessary to obtain the constant final reading, to be denoted as p_2. When CO is not present in too great amount, greater accuracy in its measurement is gained by obtaining a new base line reading, denoted by p'_2, at the 0.5 cc. mark. In this work, most of the CO pressure differences have been read at the 0.5 cc. mark.

6. Absorption of CO by Winkler's Solution.—6 cc. of the air-free Winkler's reagent are placed in cup k. Of this, 5 cc. are slowly admitted into the chamber at slight negative pressure (leveling bulb at height corresponding to the bottom of the chamber ((3) p. 581)). Due to the trace of pyrogallate which has followed the gas from the Hempel pipette into the chamber, the introduction of the first few drops of CO absorbent causes a precipitate to form. This, however, upon further addition of the reagent, drops to the bottom of the liquid, leaving the top with a clear meniscus. Absorption of CO is complete in 2 minutes. The solution is gently lowered to the 0.5 or 2.0 cc. mark, and the pressure p_3 is observed (see Van Slyke and Robscheit-Robbins (2) for precautions).

Determination of Corrections c_1 and c_2.—Before calculating the amounts of oxygen and carbon monoxide from the pressure differences $p_1 - p_2$ and $p'_2 - p_3$ (or $p_2 - p_3$), respectively, it is necessary to apply a correction in each case. Such corrections take into account whatever amounts of air may have been introduced with the reagent and not extracted the first time, and differences in pressure readings which result when either the *vapor tension* or the *volume* of the liquid above the mercury is altered.

To obtain the first correction c_1, the procedure previously outlined is followed. 2 drops of octyl alcohol and 8 cc. of the acidified ferricyanide reagent are extracted for 2 minutes, the extracted air is ejected, and 4 cc. of the solution are admitted into the cup k. 3 cc. are readmitted into the chamber and the extraction is repeated for 3 minutes. 1 cc. of air-free N NaOH is added and the reading p_2 made at the 2.0 cc. mark.

The chamber is cleaned and 5 cc. of glycerol-salt solution are extracted for 2 minutes. Following the ejection of extracted air, 3.5 cc. of the solution are left in the chamber. Reading p_2 is then made at the 2.0 cc. mark.

The difference in pressure $p_1 - p_2 = c_1$ and represents the correction to be applied to the $p_1 - p_2$ difference obtained in the analysis of the blood. In this work, the reading at 2.0 cc., over 3.5 cc. of glycerol-salt solution, has been found to be consistently between 1 and 2 mm. lower than the same reading over 8 cc. of the ferricyanide-NaOH mixture. This correction is largely the algebraic sum of two factors, namely, the *increase* in p_2 over p_1 due to the decrease in volume from 8 cc. to 3.5 cc., and the *decrease* in p_2 from p_1 due to the lower vapor tension of the glycerol-salt solution as compared with the tension of the ferricyanide-NaOH mixture.

To obtain the second correction c_2, a reading p'_2 at the 0.5 cc. mark is taken with the same 3.5 cc. of glycerol-salt solution, immediately after the 2.0 cc. reading. After the addition of 5 cc. of air-free Winkler's reagent, the reading p_3 is taken at the 0.5 cc. mark. When readings for CO are made at the 2.0 cc. mark (which, however, will occur only in analyses of blood of high CO content), the p'_2 reading is omitted, and p_3 is read at 2.0 cc., as in the analysis.

The difference in pressure

$$p'_2 - p_3 \text{ (or } p_2 - p_3) = c_2$$

and represents the correction to be applied to the $p'_2 - p_3$ (or $p_2 - p_3$) difference obtained in the analysis of the blood. At the 0.5 cc. mark the reading over 5 cc. of Winkler's reagent has been found to range from 3 to 5 mg. lower than the same reading over 3.5 cc. of glycerol-salt solution. Here also, the correction is the resultant of two factors; namely, the *decrease* in p_3 from p'_2 due to increase in volume from 3.5 to 5.0 cc., and the *increase* in p_3 over p'_2 due to the higher vapor tension of the glycerol-salt-Winkler's solution mixture as compared with the tension of the glycerol-salt solution alone.

The analyst should determine these two corrections for each day's analyses. If a new lot of any reagent is introduced during a series of analyses, the c corrections are redetermined.

Calculations.

The pressure of O_2 gas from the sample analyzed is calculated as

$$p_{O_2} = p_1 - p_2 - c_1$$

where the O_2 content in terms of volumes per cent or millimols per liter is calculated as

$$O_2 \text{ content} = p_{O_2} \times \text{factor.}$$

The values of the appropriate factor are taken from Column 9, Table II or Table III, of Van Slyke and Neill's paper (1) for a sample of 2 cc., $S = 7$ cc., $a = 2.0$ cc., and $i = 1.0$.

The pressure of CO gas from the sample analyzed is calculated as

$$p_{CO} = p'_2 - p_3 - c_2$$

where the CO content in terms of volumes per cent or millimols per liter is calculated as

$$CO \text{ content} = p_{CO} \times \text{factor.}$$

The values of the appropriate factor are taken from Column 8 of the same tables, Tables II and III (1), for a sample of 2 cc.,

$S = 7$ cc., $a = 0.5$ cc., and $i = 1.0$. In some instances, when CO is present in large amounts, it may be necessary to take these readings (p_2 and p_3) at the 2.0 cc. mark, in which case the factors used will be the same as those for oxygen given above.

Estimation of O_2 and CO with 1 Cc. Blood Sample.

When the blood is about half saturated with O_2 and half with CO, or when it is necessary to economize in the amount of material used, one may obtain accurate results with blood samples of 1 cc. When one or both gases are present in small amount, there is a decrease in the percentage accuracy with which the less abundant gas is determined, since the absolute error (about 0.001 cc. of gas) remains constant. Whether the resultant error is relatively too great to permit use of the 1 cc. sample depends upon the purpose of the analysis. The amounts of reagents required are less than when 2 cc. samples are used, *all* readings are made at 0.5 cc., and the c corrections are different.

Briefly, the changes from the technique described for 2 cc. samples are as follows. Instead of 8 cc. of acid ferricyanide, only 5.5 cc. are rendered air-free. Of this, 4 cc. are run up into the cup k, and the 1 cc. sample is introduced into the chamber. This is then followed by 1 cc. of the reagent, thus making 3.5 cc. of liquid to be shaken. Of the N NaOH used to absorb the CO_2, only 0.5 cc. is introduced into the chamber. Reading p_1 is made at 0.5 cc. After the return of the gas from the Hempel pipette, reading p_2 is taken over 3.5 cc. of air-free glycerol-salt solution at the 0.5 cc. mark. For the CO absorption, 3.5 cc. of air-free Winkler's solution are introduced into the cup, of which 2.5 cc. are used for absorption. Reading p_3 is also taken at the 0.5 cc. mark. The c_1 and c_2 corrections are determined in the manner described in the previous section, the appropriate amounts of reagents being used.

The gas contents are calculated from

$$O_2 \text{ content} = (p_1 - p_2 - c_1) \times \text{factor}$$

and

$$CO \text{ content} = (p_2 - p_3 - c_2) \times \text{factor}$$

where the factor to be applied is obtained from Column 6, Table II of Van Slyke and Neill's tables of factors (1) for sample = 1 cc., $S = 3.5$ cc., $a = 0.5$ cc., and $i = 1.0$.

O₂ and CO in Blood

Determination of Blood O₂ or CO Alone.

Obviously, the procedure described with 1 or 2 cc. blood samples may be used when either O_2 or CO content alone is the aim of the analyst. While this method offers no advantage over the original Van Slyke-Neill technique for blood O_2, for CO it is less subject to the possible errors pointed out by those authors ((1) pp. 563 and 564).

When CO content alone is desired, the use of N NaOH is omitted. The gases liberated by the acid ferricyanide are transferred directly to the Hempel pipette, where CO_2 and O_2 are absorbed by the pyrogallol solution. The base line pressure reading p_1, with 3.5 cc. of air-free glycerol-salt solution, is made at either the 0.5 or 2.0 cc. mark. The final reading p_2, after the CO absorption by Winkler's reagent, is taken at the same volume as that at which p_1 was read. The appropriate c corrections in each of the above cases are determined as before.

EXPERIMENTAL.

The present method has been rigorously tested and compared with four other different techniques for the analysis of oxygen or carbon monoxide or a mixture of both, in blood. The results given in the following serve to indicate both the relative accuracy of the various methods, and the absolute accuracy of the newly modified procedure. The data presented are representative but not selected results. Of all the analyses done in preliminary tests of the method less than 10 per cent would have to be discarded because of inaccuracies outside the limit of experimental error.

Analysis of Blood for O₂ Content Only.

In order to test the accuracy of the gas bubble transfer from the extraction chamber to the Hempel pipette and back again, results of blood oxygen content analyses by the new technique were compared with values obtained by the method of Van Slyke and Neill. Table I is indicative of the good agreement obtained.

Analysis of Blood for CO Content Only.

For the purpose of comparing results with the Van Slyke-Robscheit-Robbins (2) technique, the experiments grouped in Table II were performed. They indicate good agreement. Even

J. Sendroy, Jr., and S. H. Liu 143

when CO is present to the extent of only 4.5 volumes per cent, the comparison of results from 2 cc. samples used in the new technique, with results from 5 cc. samples by the Van Slyke-Rob-

TABLE I.

Results of Analyses of Blood for Oxygen Content Only.

Experiment No.	Volumes per cent O$_2$ by method of:			
	Van Slyke-Neill.		Authors.	
		Average.		Average.
1	20.40	20.40	20.34 20.32	20.33
2	24.40 24.35	24.38	24.28 24.34	24.31
3	20.19 20.28 20.33	20.27	20.25	20.25
4	21.99 21.93	21.96	21.97 21.95	21.96

TABLE II.

Results of Analyses of Blood for CO Content Only.

Experiment No.	Volumes per cent CO by method of:			
	Van Slyke-Robscheit-Robbins.		Authors.	
		Average.		Average.
1	8.12 8.36	8.24	8.07 8.07	8.07
2	11.57 11.61	11.59	11.56 11.56	11.56
3	4.66 4.62	4.64	4.75 4.72	4.73

scheit-Robbins method, shows no appreciable difference between the two sets of determinations.

The reliability of the method for CO absorption was tested in another way. A portion of fresh ox blood was placed in the double tonometer system used in this laboratory (5). The system was evacuated and refilled with hydrogen three times, then equilibrated by rotation for 20 minutes at room temperature. The process of blood reduction and elimination of oxygen was repeated. Following this, a calculated amount of pure CO gas made from formic acid was added to the system. A low tension of 10 or 12 mm. was sufficient to saturate the blood thoroughly with CO while the amount physically dissolved at this pressure was so small (0.02 to 0.03 volume per cent) as to be negligible. The blood and gas phase were again allowed to come to equilibrium, after which the blood was analyzed for CO according to directions given in preceding sections.

Another portion of blood was evacuated and equilibrated the same number of times as the first, except that air was used as the gas phase. The O₂ capacity was finally estimated by analyzing for oxygen according to Van Slyke and Neill (1) and subtracting the physically dissolved O₂ according to the equation

$$(1) \quad \text{Dissolved } O_2 \text{ (vol. per cent)} = \frac{B - W}{760} \times 20.9 \times \alpha_{O_2} \times 0.84$$

where $B - W$ represents the barometric pressure minus the water vapor tension at the temperature of saturation and α_{O_2} is the Bunsen solubility coefficient at the same temperature, for oxygen in water. The numerical constants 20.9 and 0.84 are respectively the percentage of oxygen in air, and the approximate water content of blood.

The combining capacity of the blood for O₂ and CO should be the same. Table III shows the results of two such experiments. In Experiment 1, it may be added, further analyses indicated an oxygen content of 0.25 volume per cent, incomplete reduction of the sample saturated with CO thus accounting for the slightly lower CO results.

Finally, the CO content of a sample of blood thoroughly saturated with that gas was confirmed in still another way. The blood was equilibrated with an atmosphere of almost pure CO, then put aside in a closed vessel over mercury. 2 cc. samples were withdrawn for analysis according to the method described in this paper. After analysis, the amount of CO *unextracted* in the course of the analysis was calculated by multiplying the *total* CO by the appropriate factor for unextracted gas obtained from the equations developed by Van Slyke and Stadie (6). At equilibrium,

TABLE III.

Comparison of O_2 and CO Blood Capacities.

Experiment No.	Volumes per cent gas by method of:			
	Van Slyke-Neill.		Authors.	
	O_2		CO	
		Average.		Average.
1	22.36		22.12	
	22.32	22.34	22.18	22.15
2	19.67			
	19.81	19.74	19.71	19.71

TABLE IV.

Determination of CO Extracted from Blood in Van Slyke-Neill Apparatus.

Volumes per cent CO.					
Total by authors' method.		Calculated.		Extracted, analysis by I_2O_5 method.	
	Average.	Unextracted.	Extracted.		Average.
22.68				22.61	
22.53	22.60	0.09	22.51	22.93	22.77

the ratio of unextracted gas to the total gas present is defined by the equation

$$(2) \qquad \frac{\dfrac{A\,\alpha'}{A - S}}{1 + \dfrac{A\,\alpha'}{A - S}}$$

where A = volume of gas phase, S = volume of liquid phase, and α' = the Ostwald solubility coefficient at the prevailing temperature. To determine the accuracy of the results, several other samples were extracted in the evacuated chamber of the Van Slyke

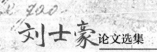

146 O$_2$ and CO in Blood

apparatus. In each case, after extraction, the stop-cock *b* (see Fig. 1) of the chamber was opened to dilute the extracted CO with outside air. The gas in the chamber was then completely transferred through the capillary side arm *S* of the apparatus through stop-cock *b*, by displacement with mercury, into an 800 cc. partially evacuated tonometer. Air was admitted into the tonometer to atmospheric pressure. Following this, the gas was displaced by glycerol-salt solution and passed over hot I$_2$O$_5$. The iodine liberated by the CO was absorbed in KI solution and

TABLE V.

Comparison of Results of Combined Analysis of Blood for Both O$_2$ and CO by Method of Van Slyke and Robscheit-Robbins and by That of the Authors.

Experi-ment No.	Volumes per cent gas by method of:							
	Van Slyke-Robscheit-Robbins.				Authors.			
	O$_2$		CO		O$_2$		CO	
		Average.		Average.		Average.		Average.
1	11.22	11.22	12.14	12.14	11.37		12.02	
					11.27	11.32	11.94	11.98
2	10.78		11.22		10.54		11.42	
	10.74	10.76	11.45	11.34	10.56	10.55	11.32	11.37
3	5.71	5.71	6.21		5.61		6.32	
			6.16	6.19	5.63	5.62	6.36	6.34
4	15.40		5.42		15.56		5.46	
	15.54	15.47	5.46	5.44	15.47	15.51	5.48	5.47
5	5.85		6.05		5.65		6.26	
	5.74	5.80	6.20	6.13	5.56	5.60	6.31	6.29

then titrated with sodium thiosulfate. More complete details as to the procedure employed will be given in a later publication from this laboratory. Table IV shows that CO, thus determined by an entirely independent method of measurement, agrees very well with the results obtained by the manometric technique.

Combined Analysis of Blood for O$_2$ and CO Content.

The accuracy of the procedure having been tested against other methods with respect to one or the other of the two gases, experiments were performed for the purpose of confirming results by the

J. Sendroy, Jr., and S. H. Liu   147

combined technique. The first of several series of such experiments is recorded in Table V, where comparative results with respect to the Van Slyke-Robscheit-Robbins method are given. In view of the fact that the latter method was not designed for oxygen analysis, and its use for that purpose introduces several

TABLE VI.

Comparison of Results of Combined Analyses of Blood for Both O_2 and CO by Several Different Methods.

Experiment No.	Blood sample.	Content.	Van Slyke-Neill. O_2	Van Slyke-Robscheit-Robbins. O_2	CO	Authors. O_2	CO	Calculated.* O_2	CO
1	A	O_2 + CO		0.41	18.98				
				0.32	18.97				
	B	O_2	18.97						
			19.08						
	C	1 A : 1 B†					9.22		
							9.38	9.69	9.49
2	A	O_2 + CO		0.26	22.64				
				0.20	22.69				
	B	O_2	22.64						
			22.50						
	C	1 A : 1 B†				11.37	11.39		
						11.32	11.58	11.40	11.33
3	A	O_2	23.79						
			23.71						
	B	CO							
	C	1 A : 1 B†		11.85	12.54	11.86	12.55		
				11.93	12.55	11.89	12.55	11.88	

* O_2 values calculated from Van Slyke-Neill and Van Slyke-Robscheit-Robbins analyses. CO values calculated from Van Slyke-Robscheit-Robbins analyses.

† 1 part A + 1 part B.

extra steps in the published procedure, the agreement in values is quite satisfactory.[3]

[3] The additional steps involved in analyzing blood for oxygen by the Van Slyke-Robscheit-Robbins method were the following. After the extraction of the blood gases, 2 cc. of air-free N NaOH were added to absorb

Table VI gives comparative results, analyzed and calculated, for experiments with mixtures of ox blood saturated with CO and with O_2, the bloods having been analyzed for CO or O_2 before and after the mixture was prepared. From the preliminary analyses by the Van Slyke-Neill and Van Slyke-Robscheit-Robbins methods, values of O_2 and CO for the mixture were calculated. The agreement of the analytical data with the calculated values is as good as could be expected considering the number of steps involved in preparing the final mixtures.

The most rigorous test of the accuracy of results by the combined method is that based on the principle of the identity of the oxygen- and carbon monoxide-combining power of a given sample of blood. When blood is equilibrated with an atmosphere containing either O_2 or CO at a tension sufficient to have all of the available hemoglobin combined with gas, the amount of O_2 and CO combined in either case will be identical. The amounts of *dissolved* O_2 or CO will depend on the tension of the respective gases, as indicated by Equation 1 where CO may be substituted for O_2. As shown by Sendroy, Liu, and Van Slyke (7) the tension of CO required to saturate blood with that gas will be but $\frac{1}{210}$ part of the tension of O_2 required to combine all the blood hemoglobin with oxygen. In the one case, therefore, one may have the blood fully combined with CO, with a negligible amount of dissolved CO present, while in the other, when the blood is fully combined with O_2, a correction must be made for dissolved gas.

Table VII indicates the results obtained by analysis of mixtures of blood, the amounts of O_2 or CO in which could be calculated from O_2 or CO capacity data. Thus, for instance, in Experiment 1 (Table VII), a certain portion of blood (Sample A) was saturated with air, and analyzed for O_2 as in the regular O_2 capacity method

---

CO_2, and the blood solution was removed from the Harington-Van Slyke chamber through the lower stop-cock. The chamber was washed once with air-free glycerol-salt solution. This was rejected and then replaced by another 5 cc. over which the reading at the 2.0 cc. mark was taken. The difference between this reading and the subsequent one following the absorption of oxygen by pyrogallate gave the pressure due to O_2. A new table of factors similar to that given by Van Slyke and Robscheit-Robbins was calculated for use in oxygen analyses.

J. Sendroy, Jr., and S. H. Liu　　149

TABLE VII.

Comparison of Results of Combined Analyses of Blood for CO and O₂
Compared with Values Calculated from O₂ Capacity Results.

Experiment No.	Blood sample.	Volumes per cent gas by method of:			Calculated.[*]	
		Van Slyke-Neill.	Authors.			
		O_2	O_2	CO	O_2	CO
1	A, saturated with air.	20.36t 19.84c				
	B, saturated with CO at 10 mm.			19.93		19.84
	C = 3 parts A + 1 part B.		15.06	5.05	15.25	4.96
2	A, saturated with air.	20.34t 19.82c				
	B, saturated with CO at 10 mm.			19.85		19.82
	C = 1 part A + 1 part B.		10.19	9.97	10.17	9.92
3	A, saturated with air.	20.65t 20.16c				
	B, saturated with CO at 10 mm.					20.16
	C = 5 parts A + 1 part B.		17.20	3.43	17.21	3.36
	D = 5 parts A + 2 parts B.		14.79	5.75	14.75	5.76
4	A, saturated with air.	21.76t 21.26c				
	B, saturated with CO at 10 mm.					21.26
	C = 15 parts A + 2 parts B.		19.10	2.58	19.20	2.50
	D = 5 parts A + 1 part B.		17.90	3.63	18.13	3.55
5	A, saturated with air.	22.59t 22.09c				
	B, saturated with air containing CO.		0.33	21.69		
	C = 1 part A + 5 parts B.		4.21	17.96	4.05	18.06
6	A, saturated with air.	19.45t 18.98c				
	B, saturated with CO at 10 mm.					18.98
	C = 1 part A + 2 parts B.		6.59	12.57	6.49	12.65
	D = 1 part A + 5 parts B.		3.26	15.59	3.24	15.81

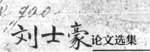

TABLE VII—Concluded.

Experiment No.	Blood sample.	Volumes per cent gas by method of:			Calculated.	
		Van Slyke-Hiller.	Authors.			
		CO	O₂	CO	O₂	CO
7	A, saturated with air.				22.07t 21.57c	
	B, saturated with CO at 10 mm.	21.57t				
	C = 2 parts A + 1 part B.		14.54	7.13	14.71	7.19

t = total gas.   c = combined gas.

*O₂ values calculated from total O₂ according to Van Slyke-Neill method.   CO values calculated from combined O₂ values.

of Van Slyke and Neill.   The total O₂, by analysis, was 20.36 volumes per cent.   The calculated dissolved O₂ was 0.52 volumes per cent, thus making the O₂-combining power of the sample equal to 19.84 volumes per cent.   Hence, the CO-combining power of the same blood, when exposed to an atmosphere containing CO at sufficient tension, should be identical with this value.

Accordingly, a second portion of blood (Sample B, Experiment 1) was saturated with an atmosphere containing enough CO to combine completely with the amount of blood present and to have in excess an amount which would make the CO tension at equilibrium 10 mm. of mercury.   The dissolved CO was therefore negligible.

The saturation of the blood in each case was made at room temperature and repeated to make three saturations in all, according to the technique of Austin et al. (5).   Hence, the concentration of the blood, due to the several evacuations of the tonometers, was the same in each case.

Blood (Sample B, Experiment 1) was analyzed for CO according to the new technique and the results (19.93 volumes per cent) checked well with the calculated value (19.84 volumes per cent) obtained from the Van Slyke-Neill analysis for O₂ capacity.

Definite volumes of blood (Samples A and B) were then accurately measured out and mixed, 3 parts by volume of Sample A to

J. Sendroy, Jr., and S. H. Liu　　　151

one of Sample B, and the analyses carried out by the combined technique. Again the results were compared with the calculated values.

In Table VII, there has been included, for convenience in presentation, an experiment somewhat different from the preceding ones. In Experiment 7 the procedure employed was the reverse of that in the others, in that the *CO capacity*, as estimated by the

TABLE VIII.

Comparison of Combined Analyses of Blood for O₂ and CO with 1 Cc. and 2 Cc. Samples.

Experi-ment No.	Volumes per cent.							
	O₂				CO			
	1 cc. sample.		2 cc. sample.		1 cc. sample.		2 cc. sample.	
		Average.		Average.		Average.		Average.
1	10.03	10.03	10.11	10.11	11.09	11.09	11.01	11.01
2	10.80		11.01		11.77		11.71	
	10.71		10.95	10.98	11.70		11.73	11.72
	10.91	10.81			11.65	11.71		
3	16.05		16.01		6.17		6.18	
	16.16	16.10	15.96	15.99	6.15	6.16	6.19	6.18
4	11.13		10.97		11.56		11.76	
	11.00	11.06	10.92	10.95	11.62	11.59	11.78	11.77
5	19.07		18.89		3.18		3.12	
	18.72		18.87	18.88	3.20		3.15	3.14
	18.88	18.89			3.18	3.19		

method of Van Slyke and Hiller (8), was used as the basis of calculation of O₂ values. Actually, blood Samples A and B were equilibrated as before, with air and with a low tension CO + H₂ mixture. The blood mixture (Sample C) was prepared and kept over mercury. After analysis for O₂ and CO by the combined technique, samples of the same mixture were employed for the estimation of the CO capacity within the apparatus. Experiment 7 thus constitutes another independent confirmation of the values given by the modified technique. The agreement of calculated and analyzed values in this table is within the limit of error to be expected in the preparation by volume of blood mixtures such as these.

Analysis of 1 Cc. Samples.

In order to determine the relative accuracy of results obtained by reducing the size of the blood sample to 1 cc., the results given in Table VIII were obtained. Apparently, for the mixtures here used, 1 cc. and 2 cc. samples give results agreeing within the limit of error of the method.

SUMMARY.

An improved technique is described for the determination of oxygen and carbon monoxide in a single blood sample by the use of the Van Slyke-Neill manometric apparatus.

BIBLIOGRAPHY.

1. Van Slyke, D.D., and Neill, J. M., *J. Biol. Chem.*, **61**, 523 (1924).
2. Van Slyke, D. D., and Robscheit-Robbins, F. S., *J. Biol. Chem.*, **72**, 39 (1927).
3. Harington, C. R., and Van Slyke, D. D., *J. Biol. Chem.*, **61**, 575 (1924).
4. Van Slyke, D. D., *J. Biol. Chem.*, **83**, 425 (1929).
5. Austin, J. H., Cullen, G. E., Hastings, A. B., McLean, F. C., Peters, J. P., and Van Slyke, D. D., *J. Biol. Chem.*, **54**, 121 (1922).
6. Van Slyke, D. D., and Stadie, W. C., *J. Biol. Chem.*, **49**, 1 (1921).
7. Sendroy, J., Jr., Liu, S. H., and Van Slyke, D. D., *Am. J. Physiol.*, **90**, 511 (1929).
8. Van Slyke, D. D., and Hiller, A., *J. Biol. Chem.*, **78**, 807 (1928).

MANOMETRIC ANALYSIS OF GAS MIXTURES

II. CARBON DIOXIDE BY THE ISOLATION METHOD

By DONALD D. VAN SLYKE, JULIUS SENDROY, Jr., AND SHIH HAO LIU*

(From the Hospital of The Rockefeller Institute for Medical Research, New York)

(Received for publication, January 7, 1932)

In this paper there is described a procedure whereby the CO_2 in a gas mixture is first isolated from other gases by absorption with alkali solution in the chamber of the manometric apparatus. The other gases are then ejected, the absorbed CO_2 is set free by acid, and is determined as in blood analyses. By this procedure the CO_2 in any desired volume of gas can be absorbed, and then set free and determined by the pressure it exerts at 2 or 0.5 cc. volume. The error with the usual manometric chamber, is, as in blood gas determination, less than 1 per cent of the amount of CO_2 determined, and could doubtless be further reduced by modifying the manometric chamber. Thus Van Slyke, Hastings, Heidelberger, and Neill (1922), using a chamber of 100 instead of 50 cc. total volume, with measurements of CO_2 pressures at 5 instead of 2 cc. volume, limited the error of blood CO_2 determinations to about 1 part in 500. The analyses published in this paper were obtained with the usual 50 cc. chamber, and therefore do not represent the maximum accuracy that could be obtained by modifying the chamber for that purpose.

A carbon dioxide method in which, as in this, the error in terms of per cent of the total gas mixture diminishes in proportion to the CO_2 content, is especially adapted to analysis of gas mixtures containing small amounts of carbon dioxide. With the isolation method, and the usual 50 cc. manometric chamber, one can readily determine the CO_2 content of atmospheric air to 0.0003 volume

---

* On leave of absence from the Department of Medicine, Peking Union Medical College, Peiping, China.

531

per cent, or 0.01 of the amount present. Such precision with apparatus modeled on the usual principles of gas analysis can be obtained only with most elaborate precautions, because it would involve measurement of total gas volumes with an accuracy of 1 part in 300,000.

The method serves well for determination of carbon dioxide in expired or alveolar air, where the CO_2 content runs from 6 to 2 per cent. The error, with the usual manometric chamber employed, is within 1 per cent of the amounts of CO_2 determined.

In analyses of gases with more than 10 or 15 per cent of CO_2, the simple absorption method, described in the preceding paper (Van Slyke and Sendroy, 1932), is preferable, unless it is desirable to use minimal gas samples. In that case the micro form of the method here described can be used, with samples of only 1 to 1.5 cc.

Reagents

5 N Sodium Hydroxide, Approximate.

1 N Hydrochloric Acid, Approximate—83 cc. of concentrated hydrochloric acid of 1.19 specific gravity diluted to a liter.

0.1 N Sodium Hydroxide, Approximate, of Minimal CO_2 Content—Sodium hydroxide is dissolved in an equal volume of water and the solution is let stand till the nearly insoluble Na_2CO_3 has settled. Of the supernatant solution, 6 cc. are pipetted into 1 liter of water, which has been freed of CO_2 by adding a drop of concentrated hydrochloric acid and boiling. About 1 cc. of 1 per cent alizarin red solution is added. The 0.1 N alkali solution is immediately poured into 50 cc. flasks or bottles closed with paraffined corks or vaselined glass stoppers. After one of these flasks has been opened to use part of the solution, the residue is thrown away. As an alternative method of preservation larger amounts of the alkali may be kept in closed air-free containers over mercury, as shown in Fig. 6 of Van Slyke and Neill (1924).

Apparatus

The only special apparatus besides the manometric is a 25 cc. burette for holding CO_2-free NaOH solution. The tip of the burette is provided with a rubber ring and must be long enough to fit into the cup of the manometric chamber, as shown in Fig. 3 of Van Slyke (1927). The top of the burette is closed by a 1-hole

Van Slyke, Sendroy, and Liu 533

stopper into which is fitted a soda-lime tube to prevent entrance of atmospheric CO_2. When the burette is not in use the outlet is kept immersed in mercury to minimize absorption of atmospheric CO_2 by the alkali at the tip.

METHOD A, FOR GAS SAMPLES NOT EXCEEDING THE VOLUME OF THE MANOMETRIC CHAMBER

In this method the sample is measured in one portion by the pressure it exerts at 50 or 2 cc. volume in the chamber. It is the method of choice when the gas analyzed contains over 1 (and less than 10) per cent of CO_2, or when the CO_2 content is less than 1 per cent and maximal accuracy is not essential. When the CO_2 content is less than 1 per cent, Method B, described later in this paper, is more exact, but it is somewhat less rapid.

It is desirable that the analyst familiarize himself with the introductory sections on general technique in Paper I of this series (Van Slyke and Sendroy, 1932).

Introduction and Measurement of Sample

Macro Samples—Before the gas sample is admitted to the chamber one estimates the approximate pressure in mm. which a sample of desirable size will exert at 50 cc. volume. A desirable sample will contain 0.5 to 1.0 cc. of CO_2, which will give a pressure of 200 to 400 mm. at 2 cc. volume. A simple rule to follow to calculate the pressure which a sample of desired size will exert at 50 cc. is to divide 1200 by the expected percentage of CO_2 in the gas. *E.g.*, if alveolar air, with probably 6 per cent CO_2, is analyzed, a sample is taken which will give a P_S of $\dfrac{1200}{6} = 200$ mm. pressure at 50 cc. The CO_2 in this sample will then exert $0.06 \times 200 = 12$ mm. pressure at 50 cc., and 25 times as much, or 300 mm. at 2 cc. when P_{CO_2} is determined in the final measurement. When expired air from a Tissot spirometer, with a CO_2 content of usually about 4 per cent is analyzed, one takes sufficient sample to give a P_S of about 300 mm. If gas of less than 1.5 per cent CO_2 content is analyzed, as large a sample as possible is taken; enough to give a P_S of 500 mm.

Before the sample is admitted the chamber is washed with acidulated water, which is ejected by slow admission of mercury.

534 II. Manometric CO_2 by Isolation

The p_0 reading is then taken, with the chamber empty of gas and the mercury at the 50 cc. mark. The sample of desired size is then admitted as described for "Admission of sample regulated by pressure" in the preceding paper (Van Slyke and Sendroy, 1932). The p_1 reading is then taken with the mercury meniscus again at the 50 cc. mark.

$$P_S = p_1 - p_0$$

Micro Samples—A sample of about 1.5 cc. volume at atmospheric pressure is admitted as described by Van Slyke and Sendroy (1932) for "Admission of sample regulated by volume." The readings of p_0 and p_1 in this case are taken with the mercury in the chamber at the 2 instead of the 50 cc. mark.

Absorption of CO_2 from Gas Sample

After the gas sample has been measured, 3.0 cc. of the CO_2-free 0.1 N sodium hydroxide solution, measured to 0.1 cc., are admitted into the chamber from the soda-lime guarded burette. The addition of alkali is made in the manner described for "Quantitative transfer of solution to the chamber without washing" in a previous paper (Van Slyke, 1927). Before inserting the burette tip into the cup of the chamber, 0.5 cc. of the solution is wasted, in order to remove from the tip the drop which may have absorbed CO_2 from the air.

After admission of the alkali, the mercury in the chamber is lowered until only the lower third of the chamber is filled with the metal. The chamber is then shaken rather slowly for 2 minutes. This causes complete absorption of the CO_2 by the alkali, which is thrown about on top of the mercury in such a way that it comes into thorough contact with the gas.

The residual gases are then ejected. It is not necessary that the last few c.mm. of gas be ejected, but it is essential that none of the alkali solution rise into the cup. The ejection of gas is therefore stopped when the alkali solution has entered the bore of the stop-cock.

After ejection of unabsorbed gases, 1 cc. of the 1 N hydrochloric acid is placed in the cup, and 0.5 cc. is run into the chamber. The CO_2 is now determined as described for blood analyses (Van Slyke and Neill, 1924). The stop-cock of the chamber is sealed with

Van Slyke, Sendroy, and Liu 535

mercury and the liberated CO_2 is extracted by 2 minutes shaking at the 50 cc. mark. The reading p_2 is then taken, with the precautions for this measurement given by Van Slyke and Neill (1924, p. 533).

The reading of the gas pressure p_2 is taken with 2 cc. of gas volume, unless so little CO_2 is present that the P_{CO_2} at 2 cc. volume is less than 100 mm. In this case the reading is taken with the gas at 0.5 cc. volume.

The stop-cock controlling the mercury in the chamber is opened, and the CO_2 is absorbed with 0.3 cc. of 5 N sodium hydroxide solution, as described on p. 546, of Van Slyke and Neill. Then reading p_3 is taken with the same gas volume as at the p_2 reading. The alizarin indicator serves to show that the entire solution in the chamber turns alkaline.

A *blank analysis* is performed, in which no gas is admitted to the chamber. The pressure fall observed when the 5 N sodium hydroxide is added is the c correction. It should not exceed 4 to 6 mm. with the gas at 2 cc. volume if the 0.1 N alkali solution has been prepared and handled with the above outlined precautions to minimize its CO_2 content.

$$P_{CO_2} = p_2 - p_3 - c$$

Calculation

The CO_2 content of the gas is calculated as:

$$\text{Volumes per cent } CO_2 = \frac{P_{CO_2}}{P_S} \times \text{factor}$$

The values of the factor are given in Table I.

The factors of Table I are calculated as follows: The volume, V_{CO_2}, of CO_2, in cc., reduced to $0°$, 760 mm., present in the sample, is calculated by multiplying P_{CO_2} by the factor, f_1, which is derived from Equation 4 of Van Slyke and Neill (1924).

$$f_1 = \frac{i\,a}{760\,(1 + 0.00384t)} \left(1 + \frac{S\,\alpha'}{A - S}\right)$$

A = total volume of chamber at lower mark = 50 cc. in present chamber; S = volume of solution from which the CO_2 is extracted = 3.5 cc. in this analysis; a = volume at which the pressure of

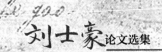

the extracted CO$_2$ gas is measured = 2 or 0.5 cc.; t = temperature centigrade; α' is the distribution coefficient of CO$_2$ between

TABLE I

Factors by Which Ratio, P_{CO_2}:P_S, Is Multiplied in Order to Calculate Volume
Per Cent of CO$_2$

Temperature	Factors when sample pressure is taken at 50 cc. volume		Factors when sample pressure is taken at 2 cc. volume	
	P_{CO_2} measured with gas at 2 cc. volume	P_{CO_2} measured with gas at 0.5 cc. volume	P_{CO_2} measured with gas at 2 cc. volume	P_{CO_2} measured with gas at 0.5 cc. volume
°C.				
10	4.444	1.132	111.1	28.29
11	32	29	110.8	22
12	21	26	0.5	15
13	11	24	0.3	09
14	02	22	0.0	04
15	4.393	20	109.8	27.98
16	83	17	9.6	92
17	73	15	9.3	87
18	65	13	9.1	82
19	58	12	9.0	77
20	51	10	8.8	72
21	44	08	8.6	68
22	37	06	8.4	63
23	30	04	8.3	59
24	24	02	8.1	54
25	18	00	7.9	50
26	12	1.099	7.8	47
27	06	97	7.6	44
28	00	96	7.5	41
29	4.295	95	7.4	38
30	91	94	7.3	34
31	86	93	7.2	31
32	82	92	7.0	27
33	77	91	6.9	24
34	73	90	6.8	20

the gaseous and aqueous phases; i = factor correcting for reabsorption of CO$_2$ while the volume of the extracted gas is being

diminished from $A - S$ to a cc. The values of i used are those found by Van Slyke and Sendroy (1927); viz., 1.017 when P_{CO_2} is measured at 2 cc. volume, and 1.037 when P_{CO_2} is measured at 0.5 cc. volume. (Values of 100 f_1 are given in Table IV.)

The volume, V_S, of the sample, in cc. reduced to 0°, 760 mm., is calculated by multiplying P_S by f_2.

$$f_2 = \frac{a}{760 \ (1 + 0.00384t)}$$

The symbols, a and t, have the same significance as above. The coefficient 0.00384 instead of the usual 0.00367 is used in the denominator in order to correct for expansion of the mercury in the manometer with temperature, as discussed by Van Slyke and Neill (1924) on p. 540 of their paper. The calculation of V_S as $V_S = f_2 \, P_S$ is an application of the general formula used for reductions of gases to standard conditions; viz.,

$$\text{Volume of gas at } 0°, 760 \text{ mm.} = (\text{volume at } t°, P \text{ mm.}) \times \frac{P}{760 \ (1 + 0.00384t)}$$

In the present case, the volume at $t°$, P mm., is a, the volume of the gas in the chamber when the manometer is read.

The volume per cent of CO_2 in the sample is calculated as:

$$\text{Volume per cent } CO_2 = \frac{100 \times V_{CO_2}}{V_S} = \frac{100 \, f_1 \, P_{CO_2}}{f_2 \, P_S} = \frac{P_{CO_2}}{P_S} \times \text{factor}$$

The factor is $\dfrac{100 \, f_1}{f_2}$, values of which are given in Table I.

Table II indicates the results obtained by the macro analysis of gas mixtures of varying CO_2 content (from 0.03 to 10 per cent), by the method of isolation described in this section. The results are compared with those obtained by the usual method of Haldane analysis. In the case of Samples 2 and 3 in Table I, these mixtures, because of their small CO_2 content could not be accurately analyzed in the Haldane apparatus. The values given are those calculated by the addition of CO_2-free air to known, measured volumes of pure CO_2.

TABLE II

Determinations of CO_2 in Air by Method A, in Which Both Sample and Isolated CO_2 Are Measured by Pressure

Macro samples measured by pressure at 50 cc. volume

		Manometric analysis		Haldane analysis for CO_2, 9 to 10 cc. samples
	Sample No.	Approximate size of sample in terms of P_S at 50 cc.	CO_2 content found	
			per cent	*per cent*
Air of 0.03 to 1 per cent CO_2 content. P_S at 50 cc., P_{CO_2} at 0.5 cc.	1	150	0.90	0.88
			0.90	0.90
	2	520	0.031	0.033*
			0.031	
			0.031	
			0.031	
	3	500	0.079	0.076*
			0.077	
			0.078	
			0.080	
Air of 3 to 10 per cent CO_2 content. P_S at 50 cc., P_{CO_2} at 2 cc.	4	160	3.25	3.32
			3.30	3.32
	5	170	5.31	5.21
				5.25
	6	170	10.75	10.70
			10.61	10.71
	7	150	3.89	3.87
			3.92	3.86
			3.89	3.87
	8	140	6.72	6.78
			6.71	6.78
			6.78	6.78
	9	170	9.94	10.00
			10.01	9.99
			9.90	
			9.93	
	10	150	3.12	3.13
				3.13
	11	150	3.05	3.00
			3.05	3.03
	12	150	10.34	10.31
			10.34	10.32
			10.36	
	13	150	6.98	6.98
			7.00	6.97
	14	160	4.91	4.86
			4.87	4.88

* Mixture of known CO_2 content.

538

Table III covers the results of micro analyses with samples of 0.5 to 1.5 cc.

TABLE III

Determinations of CO₂ in Air by Method A, in Which Both Sample and Isolated CO₂ Are Measured by Pressure

Micro samples measured by pressure at 2 cc. volume

Sample No.		Manometric analysis		Haldane analysis for CO₂, approximately 10 cc. samples
		Approximate size of sample in terms of P_S at 2 cc.	CO₂ content found	
			per cent	*per cent*
Air of 17 to 25 per cent CO₂ content. P_S at 2 cc., P_{CO_2} at 0.5 cc.	15	450	25.70	25.58
			25.65	25.64
				25.69
	16	400	17.62	17.56
			17.65	17.63
				17.64
Air of 3 to 10 per cent CO₂ content. P_S at 2 cc., P_{CO_2} at 0.5 cc.	17	360–510	3.27	3.31
			3.28	3.35
			3.34	3.34
			3.34	
	18	370–390	6.63	6.56
			6.54	6.55
			6.60	6.57
			6.67	
			6.69	
			6.52	
	19	360–380	9.43	9.46
			9.38	9.46
			9.36	9.48
			9.41	
	20	370–390	6.44	6.53
			6.46	6.53
			6.45	
	21	370–380	5.89	5.88
			5.92	5.83
			5.91	5.87
	22	430	6.50	6.56
				6.58
	23	500	5.86	5.95
				5.97

Example of Calculation—Analysis of CO₂ in air mixture (Sample 14, Table II) gave the following.

Measured at 23.0° at the 50 cc. mark	Measured at 23.1° at the 2 cc. mark
mm.	mm.
$p_1 = 242.2$	$p_2 = 335.7$
$p_0 = \;\;86.0$	$p_3 = 155.0$
$P_S = 156.2$	$p_2 - p_3 = 180.7$
	$c = \;\;\;5.2$
	$P_{CO_2} = 175.5$

Multiplying $\dfrac{P_{CO_2}}{P_S}$ by the appropriate factor, 4.330, from Table I, we obtain

$$\text{Volume per cent } CO_2 = \frac{175.5}{156.2} \times 4.330 = 4.87$$

Corrections for Calibration Errors of Chamber and for Effect of Measuring P_S Over a Mercury Meniscus—If a, the volume at which P_S is measured, is other than the 50 or 2 cc. assumed in calculating the factors of Table I, the observed P_S will have to be multiplied by the correction factor $\dfrac{a}{2}$ or $\dfrac{a}{50}$ to obtain the exact P_S for use with the factors of Table I. Similarly, if the volume at which P_{CO_2} is measured is other than the assumed 0.5 or 2.0 cc. the observed P_{CO_2} will require multiplication by $\dfrac{a}{0.5}$ or $\dfrac{a}{2}$ in order to obtain the exact P_{CO_2} for use with the factors of Table I.

In a well calibrated chamber the deviations from the assumed volumes will be negligible, except for P_S values, measured in the micro determinations, over a mercury meniscus at the 2 cc. mark. The chambers are calibrated for gas measurements over water menisci, and the gas space over a mercury meniscus at a given mark is greater than over a water meniscus at the same mark. If the bore of the chamber at the 2 cc. mark is 4 mm., as is generally the case, we have found that the gas space over a mercury meniscus at that mark is 0.012 cc. greater than over a water meniscus. The value of P_S measured at a 2 cc. mark exact for a water meniscus will then require multiplication by the correction factor $\dfrac{2.012}{2.000} = 1.006$, when the measurement is made over a mercury meniscus.

In general, if a represents the supposed gas volume (0.5, 2.0, or 50 cc.) held by the chamber over a water meniscus at a given mark, a' the actual volume above a water meniscus found in checking the calibration, and c_a the increase in gas volume measurement that results from changing from a water meniscus to a mercury meniscus, then the observed pressure, P_S, or P_{CO_2}, must be corrected by multiplication by $\dfrac{a'}{a}$ if the pressure is observed with the gas over an aqueous meniscus, and by $\dfrac{a' + c_a}{a}$ when the pressure is observed with the gas over a mercury meniscus. In the CO_2 determinations in gas mixtures above described, $\dfrac{a' + c_a}{a}$ is significant only in the measurement of P_S values at the 2 cc. mark for micro samples. For P_S measured with the gas at 50 cc. volume, as is the case except when larger samples are taken, the difference between mercury and water menisci is only enough to affect P_S by about 1 part per 1000, and may ordinarily be neglected. P_{CO_2} values in this analysis are all measured over water menisci, so that the c_a correction does not apply to P_{CO_2}.

METHOD B, FOR PRECISE DETERMINATION OF SMALL PROPORTIONS OF CO₂ IN AIR

The procedure is the same as the above, except that here a larger sample, 200 or 300 cc. of air, is shaken in successive portions with alkali in the manometric chamber, the absorbed CO_2 being then extracted from solution and measured as above. The 0.03 per cent of CO_2 in ordinary outdoor air can thus be measured with an accuracy of 1 part per 100.

The sample is measured by volume in a container of the type shown on the left in Fig. 1. The container, of, for example, 250 cc. volume, is calibrated by weighing it first empty, except for a film of water on the inner wall, and then with the bulb between the two cocks filled with water. The container, of which the inner walls should be moist, is connected with a mercury leveling bulb, and is completely filled with a sample of the air, the mercury being withdrawn as far as the lower cock. The container is then immersed in a water bath at a temperature about 1° higher than

542   II.   Manometric CO_2 by Isolation

that of the room, and after thermal equilibrium has been reached, the top stop-cock is exposed to the air and opened for a moment to release the internal pressure. The barometric pressure and the temperature of the water bath are recorded.

The container is then connected to the manometric chamber as shown in Fig. 1 by a flexible rubber tube of about 2 mm. bore and just sufficient length to permit the chamber to be shaken without

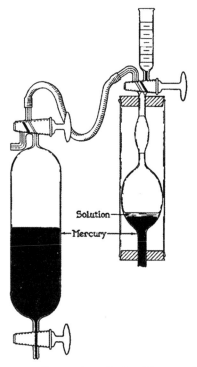

Solution—
—Mercury—

Fig. 1. Method of sampling and analysis of large volumes of gas with the manometric chamber.

disturbing the container. The connecting tube is then filled with mercury from the chamber, and about 35 cc. of the sample are run into the chamber. 3 cc. of the approximately CO_2-free 0.1 N sodium hydroxide are then admitted to the chamber as above described, and the CO_2 in the air is absorbed by shaking slowly for 4 minutes, with 10 or 15 cc. of mercury in the chamber. The unabsorbed gas, except for a small bubble, is then ejected. Then another portion of the sample is admitted and its CO_2 is absorbed in the same manner. This procedure is repeated until all the gas from the calibrated container has passed through the chamber and has been shaken with the alkali. When the last portion of gas is run into the chamber a little mercury from the container is permitted to follow and fill the left-hand bore of the cock of the chamber.

After the CO_2 from the last portion of air has been absorbed, the unabsorbed air is ejected without loss of solution, and 0.5 cc. of 1 N hydrochloric acid is admitted to the chamber. The CO_2 is extracted from the solution, and P_{CO_2} is measured as directed for Method A. Manometer reading p_1 is taken with the CO_2 gas at 0.5 or 2.0 cc. volume, according to the amount present, and p_2 with the residual gas at the same volume after the CO_2 has been absorbed with 5 N alkali. The value of the c correction is determined in a blank analysis, in which no air is run through the chamber.

Calculation

$$P_{CO_2} = p_1 - p_2 - c$$

$$\text{Volume per cent } CO_2 \text{ in air} = \frac{P_{CO_2} \times 100 f_1}{C \times f_2}$$

C is the capacity in cc. of the container in which the gas sample was measured by volume.

$100 f_1$ is the factor from Table IV, by which P_{CO_2} is multiplied in order to obtain 100 times the cc. of CO_2 present, reduced to 0°, at 760 mm.

f_2 is the usual factor, $\dfrac{B - W}{760 (1 + 0.00367t)}$, by which the observed volume of a moist gas is multiplied to obtain the volume reduced to 0°, 760 mm. B = barometric pressure, corrected for temperature, W = vapor tension of water at the temperature, $t°$ centigrade, at which the gas volume is observed. The values of f_2 are not given here, as they are found in any text-book of gas analysis or of physicochemical tables. In place of values of $\dfrac{1}{1 + 0.00367t}$ and values of B corrected for temperature, one may use uncorrected

544   II.   Manometric CO_2 by Isolation

values of B with the factor $\dfrac{1}{1 + 0.00384t}$. The use of the coefficient 0.00384 instead of 0.00367 makes a sufficiently exact correc-

TABLE IV

Values of Factor, 100 f_1, by Which P_{CO_2} Is Multiplied to Obtain 100 V_{CO_2};
for Use in Calculating Results from Method B

Temperature	Factor when P_{CO_2} is measured with gas at 2 cc. volume	Factor when P_{CO_2} is measured with gas at 0.5 cc. volume
°C.		
10	0.2818	0.0718
11	00	14
12	0.2783	09
13	67	05
14	50	01
15	35	0.0697
16	19	93
17	04	89
18	0.2690	86
19	75	82
20	62	78
21	48	75
22	34	71
23	20	68
24	07	65
25	0.2594	61
26	81	58
27	69	55
28	57	52
29	45	49
30	33	46
31	22	43
32	11	40
33	00	37
34	0.2489	34

tion for the expansion of mercury in the barometer, whether the
scale is glass or brass (see Van Slyke and Neill, 1924, p. 540).

Examples of Calculation—The nature of the results obtained in

analysis of atmospheric air, and of the calculations involved, are
indicated by the data in Table V.

TABLE V

*Calculation of CO_2 Determined in Atmospheric Air by Method B, in Which
Sample Is Measured by Volume from Separate Container*

Readings of p_1 and p_2 were made with gas at 0.5 cc. volume

	Analysis I	Analysis II
Measurement of samples		
C, cc..............	291.9	268.6
t, °C..............	24.3	24.2
B, mm............	765.2	765.2
W, "	22.8	22.7
f_2..................	0.897	0.897
Measurement of CO_2 pressures		
Temperature, °C..	23.3	21.8
p_1, mm............	256.0	270.0
p_2, "	107.3	133.9
$p_1 - p_2$, mm......	148.7	136.1
c, mm.............	13.6	13.6
P_{CO_2}, mm.........	135.1	122.5
$100 f_1$.............	0.0667	0.0672
Calculations		
Volume per cent CO_2......	$\dfrac{135.1 \times 0.0667}{291.9 \times 0.897} = 0.0344$	$\dfrac{122.5 \times 0.0672}{268.6 \times 0.897} = 0.0342$

SUMMARY

Carbon dioxide is isolated from other gases by shaking the gas
mixtures in any desired volume with alkali solution in the chamber
of the Van Slyke-Neill manometric apparatus. The other gases
are ejected, and the CO_2 absorbed is set free with acid and determined, as in estimations of plasma CO_2 content.

The method is especially adapted to accurate determination of
CO_2 when the latter is present in minimal proportions, as in atmospheric air, in which the CO_2 content can be estimated easily within
0.0003 volume per cent.   In respired air the method gives results
exact to within $\pm$ 0.05 volume per cent.

546 II. Manometric CO_2 by Isolation

BIBLIOGRAPHY

Van Slyke, D.D., *J. Biol. Chem.*, **73**, 121 (1927).

Van Slyke, D.D., Hastings, A. B., Heidelberger, M., and Neill, J. M., *J. Biol. Chem.*, **54**, 481 (1922).

Van Slyke, D.D., and Neill, J. M., *J. Biol. Chem.*, **61**, 523 (1924).

Van Slyke, D.D., and Sendroy, J., Jr., *J. Biol. Chem.*, **73**, 127 (1927); **95**, 509 (1932).

MANOMETRIC ANALYSIS OF GAS MIXTURES

III. MANOMETRIC DETERMINATION OF CARBON DIOXIDE TENSION AND pH, OF BLOOD

By DONALD D. VAN SLYKE, JULIUS SENDROY, Jr., AND SHIH HAO LIU*

(*From the Hospital of The Rockefeller Institute for Medical Research, New York*)

(Received for publication, January 7, 1932)

Hasselbalch, in 1916, showed that the pH of blood could be calculated by Henderson's mass law equation from the observed CO_2 tension and the CO_2 content. Difficulties attending determination of the CO_2 tension of blood as drawn, however, prevented the immediate application to blood analysis of this simple principle, which promised to obviate the technical difficulties of electrometric methods and the errors of colorimetric ones.

With modern refinements of the technique for CO_2 determinations in plasma, Eisenman (1926–27) solved the problem by determining the CO_2 absorption curve of the separated serum (curve with CO_2 tensions as abscissæ, CO_2 contents as ordinates), and interpolating on the curve the CO_2 content of the serum of the shed blood. The abscissa of the curve at the interpolated point indicates the CO_2 tension.

The present paper offers another procedure, which avoids the necessity of plotting a CO_2 absorption curve, and of depending upon interpolation. The CO_2 tension of blood is determined by equilibrating the blood at body temperature with a relatively small bubble of gas, a principle introduced by Pflüger (1872) and applied by Krogh (1908). Under the conditions used, the gas assumes the CO_2 tension of the blood, which is ascertained by determining the CO_2 content of the equilibrated bubble. In the present method the bubble is analyzed by the micro gas analysis

---

* On leave of absence from the Department of Medicine, Peking Union Medical College, Peiping, China.

THE JOURNAL OF BIOLOGICAL CHEMISTRY, VOL. XCV, NO. 2

described in the preceding paper (Van Slyke, Sendroy, and Liu, 1932).

A portion of the blood is then centrifuged, and the CO_2 content of the plasma is determined by the Van Slyke-Neill (1924) method. Since conditions of equilibration are such that the CO_2 content of the blood is not significantly changed, the blood used for equilibration can afterwards be used to supply the plasma for analysis. Because of the complications which the cells and the degree of oxygenation introduce by varying the value of pK' in the Henderson-Hasselbalch equation (Warburg, 1922; Van Slyke, Wu, and McLean, 1923), the pH calculation is greatly simplified by basing it on the CO_2 content of plasma or serum rather than on that of whole blood.

From the CO_2 tension and the plasma CO_2 content obtained, the plasma pH is calculated by the Henderson-Hasselbalch equation, with values for pK' and the solubility coefficient of CO_2 determined in previous papers from this laboratory (Hastings, Sendroy, and Van Slyke, 1928; Van Slyke, Sendroy, Hastings, and Neill, 1928). The deviation of the plasma pH values thus gasometrically determined, from values determined with the standard hydrogen electrode, has in none of our analyses exceeded 0.04 pH_s and in the majority of analyses has not exceeded 0.02.

The results obtained by the procedure outlined give the acid-base balance of the blood plasma in terms of CO_2 tension, plasma pH, and CO_2 and bicarbonate contents. Sufficient blood remains for oxygen analyses, so that the factors most frequently sought in studies of the acid-base balance are obtained with the one blood portion of 9 cc.

In case conditions render impracticable the anaerobic centrifugation to obtain plasma for CO_2 determination, the CO_2 content and oxygenation may be determined in the whole blood, and from these values and the CO_2 tension the plasma CO_2 may be estimated, with an error not exceeding 2 volumes per cent, by means of the nomogram given in Fig. 2.

One factor of perhaps definite importance is neglected in this, as in all previous methods for routine determination of blood pH. Havard and Kerridge (1929) have reported that shed blood kept at 38° suffers, in a few minutes after drawing, a fall of 0.02 to 0.05 in pH. After this drop they found the pH to remain constant, except for the slow fall that later sets in as the result of lactic acid formation from glucose.   If the blood was cooled to 18° as soon as drawn, the initial pH fall required an hour and a half.   These observations, made with glass electrodes, have been confirmed with hydrogen and quinhydrone electrodes by Laug (1930), who found a fall of 0.02 to 0.04 in the pH of plasma when the blood was kept at 36° for 13 minutes after being drawn.   There is yet no explanation of the chemical cause of the slight but definite acidi-fication.   However, it appears that pH values found in plasma and serum by the techniques commonly applied, and by the one presented in this paper, are about 0.03 lower than the pH in the circulating blood.   Such a limited error does not seriously impair the utility of the pH values in acid-base studies.

Error Involved in Equilibration

If oxygenated blood is equilibrated with air $+$ CO_2, the CO_2 tension in the gas will approach within 0.3 mm. the original CO_2 tension of the blood, even if the original difference between blood and gas is as much as 10 mm. of CO_2 tension.   The degree of approximation is indicated by the following calculation.

If we assume that 1 cc. of gas is equilibrated with 9 cc. of normal blood, and that the initial CO_2 tension of the gas phase is 40 mm., while that of the blood is 50 mm., the gas bubble, in order to raise its CO_2 tension to 50 mm., will take from the blood 0.0126 cc. of CO_2 (calculated at 0°, 760 mm.) and thereby reduce the blood CO_2 content by 0.14 volume per cent.   The fall in CO_2 tension caused by removing the 0.0126 cc. of CO_2 from the blood is about 0.3 mm. (see Fig. 91, p. 897, of Peters and Van Slyke, 1931).

The equilibration must be accomplished also without markedly changing the oxygenation of the hemoglobin in the blood, or the CO_2 tension will be altered.   Oxygenated hemoglobin acts as a stronger acid than reduced hemoglobin, so that increase in the HbO_2 decomposes $BHCO_3$ into H_2CO_3, with corresponding rise in the CO_2 tension, and *vice versa* (for discussion of this phenomenon, see Peters and Van Slyke, p. 900 *et seq.*, 1931).   However, when the gas bubble equilibrated with the blood is only $\frac{1}{9}$ the volume of the latter, and the initial p_{O_2} of the blood is set at 80 mm. for arterial, and 25 mm. for venous blood, the changes in oxygenation of the hemoglobin are too slight to affect seriously the CO_2 tension.[1] This conclusion may be derived from the following calculation.

9 cc. of normal blood combine with about 1.80 cc. of O_2 to completely oxygenate the hemoglobin. To change the p_{O_2} of the 1 cc. gas bubble by 10 mm., 0.0126 cc. of O_2 are required, which is enough to saturate 0.007 of the hemoglobin in the 9 cc. of blood. From Fig. 91, p. 897, of Peters and Van Slyke (1931), one can estimate that, with blood CO_2 content constant at 50 volumes per cent, change from complete oxygenation to complete reduction causes a decrease of 13 mm. in the CO_2 tension of blood. Hence, if the HbO_2 of the blood gives to the gas bubble, or the Hb takes from it, enough O_2 to change the p_{O_2} of the bubble 10 mm., the resultant change in blood CO_2 tension will approximate 0.007×13 mm., or about 0.1 mm.

When the initial O_2 tension of the bubble is set at 80 mm. for arterial blood and 25 mm. for venous, it appears that oxygenation changes will rarely affect the CO_2 tension by more than 0.2 mm. (see Fig. 107, p. 987, of Peters and Van Slyke, 1931). In fact, the effect on p_{CO_2} of measured differences, up to 30 mm., between the initial oxygen tensions of the bubble and the blood has not been experimentally detectable (see Table III).

It appears that equilibration under the conditions used may be depended on to bring the CO_2 tension of the gas bubble within 0.5 mm. of the original CO_2 tension of the blood, and that when greater errors occur in blood p_{CO_2} determined by the present method they are probably attributable to the micro analysis of the equilibrated gas bubble. This analysis is subject to a maximum error of about 0.2 volume per cent of CO_2, equivalent to 1.5 mm. of CO_2 tension. The maximum error to be expected in the p_{CO_2} determination is therefore about $0.5 + 1.5 = 2$ mm. This is in fact nearly the limit of error we have encountered, as seen in Tables I and II.

Calculation of Plasma pH by Henderson-Hasselbalch Equation, and Sources of Error Involved

This equation, its derivation from the law of mass action, and its various forms, have been discussed by Austin *et al.* (1922) and

[1] For brevity we shall use the symbols p_{CO_2} and p_{O_2} to indicate carbon dioxide tension and oxygen tension, respectively.

on p. 874 *et seq.* of Peters and Van Slyke (1931). The form in which it serves to calculate plasma or serum pH from the CO_2 tension and total CO_2 content of the fluid is expressed in Equations 1 and 2.

$$(1) \qquad pH_s = 6.10 + \log \frac{[CO_2]_s - 0.067 p_{CO_2}}{0.067 p_{CO_2}}$$

when $[CO_2]_s$ is expressed in volumes per cent of CO_2 in the plasma or serum.

$$(2) \qquad pH_s = 6.10 + \log \frac{[CO_2]_s - 0.0301 p_{CO_2}}{0.0301 p_{CO_2}}$$

when $[CO_2]_s$ is expressed in millimols of CO_2 per liter of plasma or serum.

$[CO_2]_s$ indicates the total CO_2 content of the serum or plasma, p_{CO_2} the CO_2 tension in mm. of mercury, pH_s the pH of serum or plasma.

These are special forms of the general Henderson-Hasselbalch equation

$$(3) \qquad pH = pK' + \log \frac{[BHCO_3]}{[H_2CO_3]}$$

In Equations 1 and 2 pK' is represented by the constant, 6.10, $BHCO_3$ is calculated as [total CO_2] $-$ [H_2CO_3], and [H_2CO_3] is calculated as

$$(4) \qquad \text{Volume per cent } CO_2 \text{ as } H_2CO_3 = 100 \ \alpha \times \frac{p_{CO_2}}{760}$$

$$= 0.067 p, \text{ when } \alpha = 0.51$$

To calculate [H_2CO_3] in millimols per liter, the volume per cent factor is multiplied by 10, and divided by 22.26, the volume of 1 mol of CO_2 at 0°, 760 mm. The factor 0.0301 is thus obtained.

It is evident that the precision of the gasometric pH_s depends upon the accuracy of four values; the $[CO_2]_s$ and p_{CO_2} determined in the analysis, and the constants, pK' and α. Each of these four values offers a possible source of error to the calculated pH_s. It appears that we may estimate these sources of error as follows:

552 III. Manometric Blood CO_2 Tension and pH

Solubility Coefficient of CO_2—The value of α in normal human serum was found by Van Slyke, Sendroy, Hastings, and Neill (1928) to be 0.510, with variations only in the third decimal place. The presence of much lipoid in pathological serum, such as may occur in nephrosis, was found to increase the solubility, sometimes to as high as 0.54, because of the high solubility of CO_2 in fats and oils. However, even in such serum, it is probable that the value 0.510 represents approximately the solubility of CO_2 in the *water phase*, and that the use of the value, $\alpha = 0.51$, in calculating $[H_2CO_3]$, seldom involves an error of over 1 per cent. An error of 1 part per 100 in $[H_2CO_3]$ would alter the calculated pH_s by 0.004.

Total CO_2 Content of Plasma—In the ordinary 50 cc. form of the Van Slyke-Neill apparatus, plasma CO_2 can be determined with an error not exceeding 1 part in 200. Such an error would affect calculated values of pH_s by 0.002. If the plasma CO_2 content is not determined directly, but estimated from blood CO_2 by Fig. 2, the error in $[CO_2]_s$ is increased to a possible (though unusual) maximum of 1 part in 20, and the resultant error in calculated pH_s is raised to 0.02.

CO_2 Tension—When the blood CO_2 tension is determined by the method described in this paper, the maximum error, indicated by Tables I to III, is about 1 part in 20. Such an error in p_{CO_2} would cause an error of 0.02 in the calculated pH_s.

The Constant, pK'—pK' is not an absolute constant, but diminishes as the total electrolyte content of a solution, expressed in terms of ionic strength, increases. The relationship is indicated by the formula $pK' = 6.33 - 0.5\sqrt{\mu}$ where μ represents ionic strength (Hastings and Sendroy, 1925). The increase in electrolyte content caused by adding oxalate to blood should accordingly depress somewhat the pK' value of plasma below that of serum separated without addition of any electrolyte. The data of Cullen (1922), however, indicate a pK' for normal horse oxalated plasma only 0.003 below that for the serum of the same blood. An increase in the value of pK' may be expected in some pathological conditions (especially in severe nephritis) where the total electrolyte content of the plasma is subnormal, so that the use of a normal average pK' for such sera should give pH_s results slightly too low. The data of Hastings, Sendroy, and Van Slyke (1928) show, in fact, pK' values in two nephritics higher by 0.02 units than the average normal value. It is probable that, for serum and plasmas of abnormal electrolyte content, a correction for pK', estimated from the deviation of total base from its normal value, could be applied. The magnitude of such correction could be estimated from the formula of Hastings and Sendroy quoted above. Its application to serum and plasma would need to be tested, however, before routine application.

Hastings, Sendroy, and Van Slyke (1928) found in sixteen determinations with human sera, of which six were nephritic, a total range of pK' values between 6.097 and 6.122 in normal sera, and between 6.108 and 6.134 in nephritic sera. The average of all the values was 6.105, and this agreed with the mean calculated from data of other authors reported since 1922. Accordingly 6.10 was taken as the value of serum pK'. This value for pK' has since been generally used, and is employed in calculation of gasometric pH values by the present method. From our data in Table IV,B, it can be seen that a pK' value of 6.11 would give gasometric pH values in slightly closer average agreement with the electrometric values, but the difference is not decisive enough to warrant the slight change from the pK' value established by the data quoted above.

According to the above considerations a gasometric pH_s determination by the present method is subject to the following maximum errors from the four values on which the pH_s calculation depends: 0.002 pH from plasma CO_2 content, directly determined; 0.004 from probable variations in the solubility coefficient, α, of CO_2 in plasma; 0.010 from variations in pK'; 0.020 from errors in determining p_{CO_2} by the method described in this paper. The total is a maximum error of 0.036 pH_s, which in fact is about that indicated by the data of Table IV,B. The maximum total error is to be expected only in the rare case that all the errors from the four values on which the calculation is based are maximal, and in the same direction.

Apparatus

The vessel designed for the equilibration of the blood with a prepared gas mixture is shown in B, Fig. 1. The body B is of 10 cc. total capacity, the smaller bulb being marked for 1 cc. gas volume, leaving 9 cc. for the blood. Stop-cock S is bored at a 90°

angle to allow communication between any two adjacent openings. Stop-cocks and all capillaries leading to them are of 1 mm. bore. The bulb G, of 1 cc. capacity, has been introduced so that after blood and gas phase have been brought into equilibrium, the gas may be separated from the blood at 38° before the vessel is removed from the water bath.

PROCEDURE

Preparation of Gas Mixtures

For equilibrating venous blood, a gas mixture having 50 mm. p_{CO_2} and 25 mm. p_{O_2} at 38° is used.   For arterial blood, the initial gas tensions used are 40 mm. p_{CO_2} and 80 mm. p_{O_2}.   The remainder of the gas mixture may be either nitrogen or hydrogen.

The gas mixtures are stored in 300 cc. containers of the type shown as T in Fig. 1.   We have prepared the gas mixtures with the aid of the gas manifold described by Austin *et al.* (1922, p. 129). The modification introduced by Van Slyke, Wu, and McLean (1923, p. 805), in which the gas mixtures are made up by pressure measurements, has been used.   Gas mixtures may thus be rapidly prepared in which the tensions of CO_2 and O_2 are within 1 mm. of those desired.

Introduction of Gas into Tonometer—The larger vessel, T, in Fig. 1, contains the prepared gas mixture. B and the three capillary tubes at its top are filled with mercury. G is filled with mercury from H.   With cock S in position *3*, a drop of caprylic alcohol is drawn from cup C into the capillary below the cup. C is then partially filled with mercury from above, and B and T are connected as shown in Fig. 1.   The connecting capillary X is of 0.5 mm. bore, and has at its tip a tapered rubber ring, R, shown inserted into cup C.   About 3 cc. of mercury are admitted into T from leveling bulb A, then capillary X is cleared of air by connecting it with T and allowing gas from T to waste through X and bubble out through the mercury in C.   The interiors of B and T are connected by turning the proper cocks, then by lowering the leveling bulb D the mercury is withdrawn from B and replaced by gas from T.   Stop-cocks S', S, and F are closed in the order given. S is left closed between positions *2* and *3*.   Clamp K is closed and the rubber tube is disconnected from S'.   Capillary X and the mercury are removed from cup C.

Van Slyke, Sendroy, and Liu 555

Drawing Blood and Introducing It into Tonometer—The blood is drawn into a tube coated with enough dried neutral potassium oxalate and ammonium fluoride to make the final concentrations in the blood 0.2 and 0.1 per cent, respectively. The necessary volume of a *neutral* solution containing 20 gm. of potassium oxalate

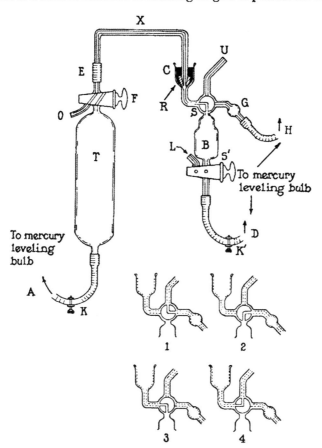

FIG. 1. Apparatus for equilibration of blood. *B* is the tonometer in which the blood is to be equilibrated. *T* is a gas container, from which *B* is about to be filled with a gas mixture approximating the CO_2 and O_2 tensions of ordinary venous or arterial blood.

and 10 gm. of ammonium fluoride per 100 cc. is spread on the inside of the vessel and dried with a current of air. The blood is drawn without contact with air. For this purpose it may be drawn under oil, as described by Van Slyke and Cullen (1917). However, it is preferable to draw it directly into a closed tube over mercury, as described on p. 131 of Austin *et al.* (1922). If first drawn into a tube with oil, the blood is transferred to a closed tube over mercury (tube *J*, Fig. 3, of Austin *et al.*, 1922).

The tonometer, *B*, previously filled with the desired gas mixture, is connected to the blood tube through the lower cock, *S'*. A few drops of blood are run through the outlet *L*. Then stop-cock *S* is opened in position *3* to let out displaced gas, and the vessel is filled through *S'* with blood to the 1 cc. mark. Cock *S* is closed in position midway between positions *3* and *4*. Leveling bulb *D* is again connected to the lower stem of tonometer *B*, and the stem is cleared of blood by mercury from *D* wasted through the outlet *L*.

As an alternative procedure, the blood may be drawn into a syringe containing paraffin oil, and forced directly from the syringe into tonometer *B* through a short rubber tube of 2 mm. bore. In this case the necessary layer of oxalate and fluoride is placed on the inner wall of the syringe. During the delivery of blood from the syringe into *B*, the point of the syringe is held downwards, with the connecting tube to *B* bent into a U, so that no oil may enter *B*.

Equilibration of Blood and Gas at 38°—The tonometer *B* in an upright position is immersed as far as the upper cock in water at $38° \pm 0.1°$. Leveling bulbs *D* and *H*, attached to the tonometer, are suspended outside the bath. A droplet of mercury is placed in cup *C*. The tonometer is held in the bath for 1 or 2 minutes, then *S* is turned to position *3* to allow escape of enough of the warmed air to lower the pressure within the chamber to atmospheric. The escape of gas is indicated by movement of the droplet of mercury in cup *C*. Cock *S* is closed and the tonometer is left in the bath for another minute, after which *S* is again opened. This procedure is repeated until there is no further indication of the escape of gas when the cock is opened.

Cock *S* is turned from position *3* in a clockwise direction to a position midway between positions *1* and *2*. A rubber stopper is inserted into the mouth of cup *C* to keep out water from the bath. The entire tonometer is then immersed in the bath and is rocked in such a manner that the bubble moves from one end of the chamber to the other. An automobile wind-shield wiper, run by compressed air or vacuum may be used for this purpose. 10 minutes suffice for attainment of CO_2 equilibrium. At the end of that period the tonometer, still in the bath, is placed in an upright position for 1 or 2 minutes to permit drainage of blood from the wall of the upper part of the chamber. Then, with leveling bulb H slightly elevated, stop-cock S is turned to position 2 just long enough to permit a droplet of mercury from G to pass into the chamber B. The mercury removes blood from the bore of cock S, from which it might otherwise enter G when the gas is transferred to this bulb.

Separation of Equilibrated Blood and Gas—This operation is preferably performed without removing the tonometer from the bath. If one works quickly, however, the tonometer may be taken out and the gas bubble transferred to bulb G before temperature change has significantly affected the distribution of CO_2 between the gas and blood.

The tonometer is either removed from the bath, or, preferably, placed in an upright position with only the part above cock S above the surface of the bath. The stopper is removed from C. Leveling bulb H is placed slightly below and leveling bulb D slightly above the tonometer. Cock S is then turned to position 2. A portion of the gas from B escapes at once into G. Most of the remaining gas is driven into G by admitting mercury from leveling bulb D into the bottom of chamber B. The admission of mercury is stopped when almost all of the gas has been transferred to G, and before any blood has entered the bore of cock S. Cock S is then turned to position 3 and the small bubble of gas left in B, followed by a little blood, is allowed to escape into cup C.

S is turned to position 4, and cup C and the bore of the cock are cleaned by drawing water, and then acetone in succession through U. The separated gas and blood may now be analyzed at the operator's convenience. If, however, the blood is not analyzed at once, it should be chilled in ice water and kept cold until used. Even then the blood analysis should be made on the same day. Before removal of either the blood or gas for analysis, the tonometer should be brought to room temperature.

Determination of CO_2 Content of Gas Bubble—This analysis is carried out as described in the preceding paper (Van Slyke, Sendroy, and Liu, 1932). The technique described for measuring micro gas samples is followed. To transfer the gas sample from

558 III. Manometric Blood CO₂ Tension and pH

bulb G of Fig. 1 to the Van Slyke-Neill manometric chamber, the arm U is connected glass to glass with the side arm of the chamber. Mercury is then run back and forth between cup C of the tonometer and the Van Slyke-Neill chamber to drive all gas bubbles out of the connections. Manometer reading p_0 is taken, with the meniscus of the mercury at the 2 cc. mark in the gas-free manometric chamber. The mercury leveling bulb attached to H is then placed higher than the leveling bulb of the manometric apparatus, cock S is turned to position 1, and all the gas in G is passed into the manometric chamber followed by a little mercury to seal the cock of the chamber. The mercury meniscus in the chamber is again brought to the 2 cc. mark and manometer reading p_1 is taken. The pressure exerted by the gas sample at 2 cc. volume is calculated as

$$P_S = p_1 - p_0$$

The absorption of CO_2 with NaOH solution and the rest of the analysis are then carried out as described in the preceding paper (Van Slyke, Sendroy, and Liu, 1932).

Centrifugation of Blood and Determination of Plasma CO₂ Content—Tube X of Fig. 1 is replaced by another glass capillary, of which the descending outlet limb is long enough to reach to the bottom of a centrifuge tube. The blood is then passed into a centrifuge tube containing a layer of oil. The oil is at once replaced by a layer of low melting paraffin, and the blood is centrifuged. The paraffin is pierced with a warm cork-borer, and 1 cc. samples of the plasma are withdrawn into pipettes and used for determination of the CO_2 content of the blood, according to Van Slyke and Neill (1924).

Calculation

From the volume per cent CO_2 content of the gas bubble, C, the CO_2 tension is calculated by the usual formula.

$$p_{CO_2} = 0.01\ C\ (B - 49)$$

where B is the barometric pressure in mm. of mercury and 49 is the vapor tension of water at 38°.

From the value of p_{CO_2} and the CO_2 content of the plasma, the plasma pH is calculated by Equation 1 or 2, previously given. Or

Van Slyke, Sendroy, and Liu   559

the calculation may be made graphically by the line-chart given in Fig. 1 of Van Slyke and Sendroy (1928), and reproduced in Fig. 87 of Peters and Van Slyke (1931).

Estimation of Plasma CO_2 Content from Whole Blood CO_2 Content and CO_2 Tension—The chart in Fig. 2 is analogous to that in Fig.

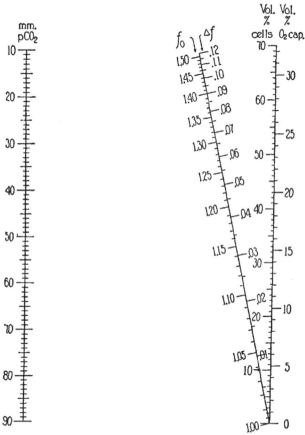

FIG. 2. Line-chart for estimating plasma CO_2 content from whole blood CO_2 content.

3 of Van Slyke and Sendroy (1928) for estimating the CO_2 content of plasma from that of whole blood, with the aid of a factor dependent on the oxygen capacity and pH_s of the blood. In the present chart, Fig. 2, a scale for p_{CO_2} replaces that for pH_s. The

use of the chart is exactly the same as that of the former one, except that p_{CO_2} values are used in place of pH_s.　The CO_2 tension values are more convenient in connection with the determinations outlined above, because the p_{CO_2} is directly determined.　Theoretically, the use of p_{CO_2} is not so precise as the use of pH_s to correct for the effect of reaction changes on the distribution of bicarbonate, in accordance with Donnan's law, between cells and plasma.　In practice, however, we have found little difference between the two charts in the accuracy with which they estimate plasma CO_2 content from whole blood values.　The error in plasma CO_2 estimation is usually less than 1 volume per cent, but may be as great as 2.5 volumes per cent.

Fig. 2 can be used to estimate plasma CO_2 contents from whole blood values when working conditions are not convenient for centrifuging the blood to obtain plasma for direct analysis.　Any such indirect estimation of plasma CO_2 content, however, increases by about 0.02 the possible error in the pH_s calculated, as has been already shown in the discussion of "Calculation of plasma pH by Henderson-Hasselbalch equation, and sources of error involved."

EXPERIMENTAL

Blood CO_2 Tensions Set by Saturation with Known Gas Mixtures Compared with Tensions Subsequently Found in Blood by Present Method

Blood was treated with oxalate and fluoride, as directed for the present method.　Then, in order to set the CO_2 and O_2 tensions of the blood at known levels, it was subjected to preliminary saturation with large volumes of gas, in which CO_2 was mixed with H_2, or with H_2 and O_2, or with air.　The "first saturation method" of Austin *et al.* (1922) was used, in which a tonometer with two chambers is employed, such that, after saturation is finished, the gas phase can be separated for analysis in a large chamber and the blood in a small one.　The composition of the gas, with which the blood had been saturated, was determined in a Haldane air analysis apparatus.　From the analysis of the gas the CO_2 tension of blood present, given in Tables I to III, was calculated, and, in Table III, also the O_2 tension of blood present.　The limit of error of the Haldane air analysis is 0.03 volume per cent of CO_2 or O_2, corresponding to 0.2 mm. tension of these gases. The CO_2 tension of blood present may therefore be considered to be ascertained within 0.2 mm.

Of the blood thus prepared, 9 cc. portions were transferred to tonometer B of Fig. 1, and were equilibrated as described in this paper, with 1 cc. portions of analyzed gas mixtures. A 1 cc. bubble was used, consisting of CO_2 and H_2 for previously reduced blood

TABLE I

Determinations of CO_2 Tension in Reduced Horse and Ox Blood Previously Saturated with Hydrogen Gas Containing Known Tensions of CO_2

Blood No.	Initial CO_2 tension of gas bubble	CO_2 tension of blood		
		Present	Found from final p_{CO_2} of gas bubble	Error
	mm.	*mm.*	*mm.*	*mm.*
1	45.8	41.8	42.5	+0.7
2	45.8	51.6	49.3	−2.3
3	44.1	50.7	51.8	+1.1
4	42.6	38.0	36.3	−1.7
5	42.6	50.2	47.9	−2.3
6	36.8	37.2	37.0	−0.2
7	36.8	44.9	44.3	−0.6
8	44.4	45.6	46.9	+1.3
9	44.4	38.1	38.7	+0.6
10	45.3	50.6	53.0	+2.4
11	45.3	40.8	39.0	−1.8
12	44.7	49.2	48.3	−0.9
13	44.7	40.5	41.5	+1.0
14	45.5	48.6	47.2	−1.4
15	45.5	40.1	41.9	+1.8
16	42.5	35.4	37.1	+1.7
17	42.5	47.6	46.9	−0.7

(Table I), of CO_2 and air for previously oxygenated blood (Table II), and of CO_2, H_2, and O_2 for blood oxygenated in varying degrees (Table III). The 1 cc. portions of gas used were prepared with CO_2 tensions, and, in Table III, O_2 tensions, differing to varying extents from the previously set tensions of the blood, but within such limits of difference as are likely to occur in determinations of the CO_2 tension of drawn venous or arterial blood.

The results indicate that the error of blood CO_2 tensions de-

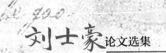

TABLE II

Determinations of CO₂ Tension in Oxygenated Ox Blood Previously Saturated with Air Containing Known Tensions of CO₂

Blood No.	Initial CO_2 tension of gas bubble	CO_2 tension of blood		
		Present	Found from final p_{CO_2} of gas bubble	Error
	mm.	*mm.*	*mm.*	*mm.*
1	37.6	44.7	43.6	−1.1
2	47.8	43.7	43.0	−0.7
3	44.1	41.6	43.1	+1.5
4	34.2	41.6	41.6	0.0
5	38.4	43.3	43.3	0.0
6	38.4	45.0	45.0	0.0
7	38.4	46.1	44.7	−1.4
8	38.4	36.0	38.3	+2.3
9	43.0	45.9	46.7	+0.8
10	43.0	36.3	36.9	+0.6
11	40.7	45.9	46.5	+0.6
12	40.7	36.3	35.5	−0.8
13	43.6	37.0	38.7	+1.7
14	45.7	37.0	37.7	+0.7
15	40.8	37.0	39.4	+2.4
16	41.7	44.4	44.7	+0.3
17	39.4	44.4	42.4	−2.0
18	43.5	49.1	49.8	+0.7
19	38.5	49.1	50.0	+0.9

TABLE III

Determinations of CO₂ Tension in Ox, Horse, and Human Blood of Varying Degrees of Oxygenation

Each blood was previously saturated with a gas mixture containing CO_2, H_2, and O_2 at known tensions.

Blood No.	Initial tensions of gas bubble		Gas tensions present in blood		CO_2 tension found in blood	Error in CO_2 tension found
	CO_2	O_2	CO_2	O_2		
	mm.	*mm.*	*mm.*	*mm.*	*mm.*	*mm.*
1	41.2	140.3	46.6	139.2	46.7	+0.1
2	43.5	52.3	46.6	139.2	43.1	−3.5
3	43.7	73.8	52.3	54.7	51.8	−0.5
4	43.7	73.8	39.9	102.1	39.4	−0.5
5	42.3	68.0	43.9	86.8	45.0	+1.1
6	42.3	68.0	44.3	50.0	43.4	−0.9
7	41.2	66.8	38.9	85.4	38.6	−0.3
8	41.2	66.8	46.8	47.9	46.2	−0.6
9	51.7	30.3	57.5	47.8	57.3	−0.2
10	51.6	41.4	57.5	47.8	59.6	+2.1
11	46.5	61.5	57.5	47.8	59.4	+1.9
12	45.6	70.9	52.8	47.1	51.2	−1.6

562

termined as described in this paper averages approximately 1 mm. Except for Blood 2 of Table III, in which the initial oxygen tension of the equilibrating bubble was intentionally made greatly different from that of the blood, the maximum error is 2.4 mm. of CO_2 tension.

Comparison of Electrometric and Gasometric pH_s Determinations in Human Venous Blood

The blood was obtained partly from hospital patients and partly from normal individuals. It was collected over mercury without contact with air, as described by Austin *et al.* (1922), in tubes provided with potassium oxalate and fluoride to prevent coagulation and lactic acid formation. No particular effort was made to prevent stasis, hence the CO_2 tensions are a little higher and the pH_s values a little lower than usual for blood drawn from the arm vein without stasis. Each sample of blood was divided into two portions.

Portion I was transferred to tonometer *B* of Fig. 1, and was used for determination of the CO_2 tension by the method described in this paper. After the gas bubble had been withdrawn from the tonometer for analysis, the residual blood in *B* was used for determinations of blood CO_2 content, oxygen content, and oxygen capacity by the methods of Van Slyke and Neill (1924). The results of the analyses are given in Table IV, *A*.

Portion II was transferred to a centrifuge tube containing a layer of paraffin oil, which was at once replaced by melted paraffin. The blood was centrifuged under the solidified paraffin. The separated plasma was drawn into a tube over mercury, as described by Austin *et al.* (1922), and was used for electrometric determination of the pH, and, in Bloods 9 to 13, for determination of the plasma CO_2 content.

For the electrometric pH determination at 38° the electrode chamber of Clark (1915) was used, with thermometer added as described by Cullen (1922). The electrode was filled with about equal volumes of plasma and gas. The gas used was hydrogen to which sufficient CO_2 was added to give in each case the p_{CO_2} which the blood was found to have by the writers' method in Portion I.

The H_2-CO_2 gas mixtures used in the electrometric pH_s deter-

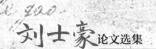

564 III. Manometric Blood CO₂ Tension and pH

TABLE IV
A. Analyses of Venous Human Blood as Drawn

Blood No.	O₂ capacity of blood	O₂ saturation of blood	CO₂ content of whole blood = $[CO_2]_b$	CO₂ content of plasma = $[CO_2]_s$		Determinations of CO₂ tension		
				Determined directly on separated plasma	Estimated from $[CO_2]_b$ by Fig. 2	Initial tensions in gas bubble used in tonometer		Final P_{CO_2} in gas bubble = blood P_{CO_2}
						CO₂	O₂	
	vols. per cent	per cent	vols. per cent	vols. per cent	vols. per cent	mm.	mm.	mm.
1	20.93	77.3	57.88		69.27	45.2	67.7	60.4
			57.91		69.72	58.3	67.1	59.4
2	21.55	58.0	55.74		67.05	45.2	67.7	55.1
			55.52		66.65	58.3	67.1	56.5
3	21.48	61.0	53.61		64.10	48.3	67.1	57.2
			53.87		64.70	45.2	67.7	53.6
4	18.46	69.0	55.18		64.98	60.0	44.6	50.2
			55.16		64.95	45.8	67.8	50.0
5	19.77	61.8	54.03		63.93	60.0	44.6	52.0
6	12.47	39.0	61.42		67.45	60.0	44.6	61.8
			61.53		67.60	45.8	67.8	61.9
7	19.78	60.1	57.70		67.92	60.0	44.6	60.2
			58.01		68.30	45.8	67.8	60.7
8	10.68	41.7	60.55		65.52	60.0	44.6	60.9
9	20.77	84.2	54.14	65.62	65.76	44.8	40.2	48.9
10	16.41	55.4	55.08	62.49	62.77	51.6	41.4	55.0
11	21.04	72.3	52.93	63.22	63.78	51.6	41.4	49.5
12	22.42	61.6	53.80	65.04	65.18	46.5	61.5	54.5
13	19.86	65.2	48.00	57.03	56.23	51.7	30.3	57.3
			48.30	57.03	56.50	51.6	41.4	59.6
			48.09	57.03	56.38	46.5	61.5	59.4
14	21.98	42.0	62.00		74.06	46.3	23.7	65.3
			62.00		73.90	49.1	13.8	65.8
15	20.23	67.0	57.14		68.11	46.3	23.7	54.0
			57.14		67.96	47.5	33.2	55.3
16	23.51	80.1	48.82		60.60	40.3	23.4	47.3
			48.93		60.58	48.7	14.7	47.7
			48.87		60.60	48.4	0.0	47.5
17	19.95	50.8	56.76		66.80	46.3	23.4	56.6
			57.17		67.33	48.7	14.7	56.3
			57.19		67.27	48.4	0.0	58.6
18	21.25	31.4	59.17		69.74	46.0	23.5	65.3
			59.36		69.97	48.6	0.0	65.4

TABLE IV—*Concluded*

B. *pH$_s$ Values Found in Bloods of Table IV, A*

| Blood No. | Gasometric pH$_s$ | | pH$_s$ by H$_2$ electrode | Error of gasometric pH$_s$ if electrometric is exact | |
	From p_{CO_2} and directly determined [CO$_2$]$_s$	From p_{CO_2} and [CO$_2$]$_s$ estimated from whole blood CO$_2$		Gasometric pH$_s$ from direct [CO$_2$]$_s$	Gasometric pH$_s$ from [CO$_2$]$_s$ estimated from [CO$_2$]$_b$
1		7.30	7.32		−0.02
		7.32	7.32		±0.02
2		7.33	7.35		−0.02
		7.32	7.35		−0.03
3		7.30	7.30		0.00
		7.33	7.30		+0.03
4		7.36	7.39		−0.03
		7.36	7.39		−0.03
5		7.34	7.38		−0.04
6		7.28	7.31		−0.03
		7.28	7.31		−0.03
7		7.30	7.32		−0.02
		7.30	7.32		−0.02
8		7.27	7.29		−0.02
9	7.37	7.38	7.39	−0.02	−0.01
10	7.31	7.30	7.33	−0.02	−0.03
11	7.36	7.36	7.40	−0.04	−0.04
12	7.33	7.33	7.33	±0.00	0.00
13	7.24	7.23	7.20	+0.04	+0.03
	7.22	7.22	7.20	+0.02	+0.02
	7.22	7.22	7.20	+0.02	+0.02
14		7.30	7.32		−0.02
		7.30	7.32		−0.02
15		7.34	7.34		0.00
		7.34	7.34		0.00
16		7.31	7.36		0.00
		7.35	7.36		−0.01
		7.36	7.36		0.00
17		7.32	7.31		+0.01
		7.33	7.31		+0.02
		7.30	7.31		−0.01
18		7.27	7.27		0.00
		7.27	7.27		0.00

minations were made up by pressure as described above for "Preparation of gas mixtures."   In this case, however, where exactness was necessary, a correction was required for the change in vapor tension of water between the room temperature, at which the gas mixture was made, and the electrode temperature of 38° to which the plasma and gas were brought for the pH determination.   If one represents barometric pressure by B, room temperature by t, vapor tension of water at 38° by W_{38}, and vapor tension of water at $t°$ by W_t the CO_2 pressure that must be measured at room temperature is calculated as follows:

$$\text{Measured } p_{CO_2} \text{ at } t° = \text{desired } p_{CO_2} \text{ at } 38° \times \frac{B - W_t}{B - W_{38}}$$

Mixtures made by this method and then subjected to gas analysis were found to be within 1 mm. of the desired CO_2 tension, and usually within 0.5 mm.   Any difference in CO_2 tension between plasma and gas put into the electrode chamber would be reduced to less than half by interchange between plasma and gas, so that the final CO_2 tension in the plasma used for electrometric pH estimation can be assumed to be within less than 0.5 mm. of the tension found by our method in blood Portion I.   An error of 0.5 mm. in setting the CO_2 tension in the electrode chamber would affect the determined pH by approximately 0.005.   It appears probable that the total error of the electrometric pH determination may be considered to be within the limit of ±0.01 pH.

The electrodes were standardized with 0.1 N hydrochloric acid, which was assumed to have a pH of 1.08.   The system used and the standardization have been discussed, on pp. 708–709 of a previous paper (Van Slyke, Hastings, Murray, and Sendroy, 1925).

The results in Table IV, B show a maximum deviation of the gasometric pH_s from the electrometric of ±0.04 pH.   In the majority of cases the deviation does not exceed 0.02 pH.

Since the observed deviations represent the sum of errors between the gasometric and electrometric determinations, it appears that the maximum error in the gasometric pH_s does not usually exceed 0.03 pH.

SUMMARY

Gasometric methods are described for determining in blood the carbon dioxide tension and the plasma pH.

Van Slyke, Sendroy, and Liu 567

The CO_2 tension is obtained by equilibrating blood with $\frac{1}{9}$ its volume of a gas mixture which contains CO_2 and O_2 in tensions approximating those of average venous or arterial blood. The gas bubble attains the CO_2 tension of the blood, which is then determined by micro gas analysis of the bubble with the method described in the preceding paper.

The pH of the plasma is calculated by the Henderson-Hasselbalch equation from the CO_2 tension found in the blood and the CO_2 content determined by analysis of subsequently separated plasma.

The maximum errors are ± 2.5 mm. of CO_2 tension and ± 0.04 pH; the usual errors are less.

With one sample of blood and an entirely gasometric technique carried out with the manometric apparatus, these determinations give the acid-base balance of the plasma in terms of pH, CO_2 or bicarbonate content, and CO_2 tension.

The writers are much indebted to Dr. A. Alving and Dr. J. M. Steele for obtaining samples of human blood.

BIBLIOGRAPHY

Austin, J. H., Cullen, G. E., Hastings, A. B., McLean, F. C., Peters, J. P., and Van Slyke, D. D., *J. Biol. Chem.*, **54**, 121 (1922).

Clark, W. M., *J. Biol. Chem.*, **23**, 475 (1915).

Cullen, G. E., *J. Biol. Chem.*, **52**, 521 (1922).

Eisenman, A. J., *J. Biol. Chem.*, **71**, 611 (1926–27).

Hasselbalch, K. A., *Biochem. Z.*, **78**, 112 (1916).

Hastings, A. B., and Sendroy, J., Jr., *J. Biol. Chem.*, **65**, 445 (1925).

Hastings, A. B., Sendroy, J., Jr., and Van Slyke, D. D., *J. Biol. Chem.*, **79**, 183 (1928).

Havard, R. E., and Kerridge, P. T., *Biochem. J.*, **23**, 600 (1929).

Krogh, A., *Skand. Arch. Physiol.*, **20**, 254, 279 (1908).

Laug, E. P., *J. Biol. Chem.*, **88**, 551 (1930).

Peters, J. P., and Van Slyke, D. D., Quantitative clinical chemistry, Baltimore, **1** (1931).

Pflüger, E., *Arch. ges. Physiol.*, **6**, 69 (1872).

Van Slyke, D. D., and Cullen, G. E., *J. Biol. Chem.*, **30**, 289 (1917).

Van Slyke, D. D., Hastings, A. B., Murray, C. D., and Sendroy, J., Jr., *J. Biol. Chem.*, **65**, 701 (1925).

Van Slyke, D. D., and Neill, J. M., *J. Biol. Chem.*, **61**, 523 (1924).

Van Slyke, D. D., and Sendroy, J., Jr., *J. Biol. Chem.*, **79**, 781 (1928).

568 III. Manometric Blood CO_2 Tension and pH

Van Slyke, D. D., Sendroy, J., Jr., Hastings, A. B., and Neill, J. M., *J. Biol. Chem.*, **78**, 765 (1928).

Van Slyke, D. D., Sendroy, J., Jr., and Liu, S. H., *J. Biol. Chem.*, **95**, 531 (1932).

Van Slyke, D. D., Wu, H., and McLean, F. C., *J. Biol. Chem.*, **56**, 765 (1923).

Warburg, E. J., *Biochem. J.*, **16**, 153 (1922).

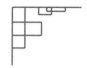
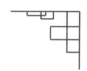

第三编　胰瘤研辨

第3编仅包括1篇论文——《Adenoma of pancreatic islet cells with hypoglycemia and hyperinsulinism: Report of a case with studies on blood sugar and metabolism before and after operative removal of tumor》，但意义重大，为我国首例胰岛素瘤的研究，发表于1936年的《临床研究杂志》（*Journal of Clinical Investigation*）。胰岛素瘤迄今仍然为一种典型的罕见病，在20世纪30年代就更为罕见，因为1924年才有病例报道怀疑胰岛素瘤的诊断，1927年才有经手术证实的第一例胰岛素瘤，1929年才真正出现了首例经手术缓解的胰岛素瘤病例。本篇论文是世界上第17例经手术证实的胰岛素瘤病例。该论文无论是在临床处理还是基础研究均可作为罕见病研究的经典之作。无论是病历书写和临床观察的精细程度，还有刘士豪教授设计的对肿瘤标本提取物进行胰岛素的生物测定，都在这篇论文中体现得淋漓尽致。

ADENOMA OF PANCREATIC ISLET CELLS WITH HYPOGLYCEMIA AND HYPERINSULINISM

REPORT OF A CASE WITH STUDIES ON BLOOD SUGAR AND METABOLISM BEFORE AND AFTER OPERATIVE REMOVAL OF TUMOR

By S. H. Liu, H. H. Loucks, S. K. Chou and K. C. Chen

(*From the Departments of Medicine and Surgery, Peiping Union Medical College, Peiping, China*)

(Received for publication December 16, 1935)

Shortly after Banting and Best's discovery of insulin (1), Harris (10) in 1924, on the basis of cases of hypoglycemia with symptoms similar to those of insulin shock and relievable by feeding, postulated the occurrence of spontaneous "hyperinsulinism" as opposed to the "hypoinsulinism" of diabetes. The first verification of this hypothesis appeared in 1927 in a report by Wilder, Allan, Power and Robertson (26) of a case of intractable hypoglycemia. The patient, on exploration, showed carcinoma of the islet tissue of the pancreas with metastasis to the liver. Insulin was demonstrated in the hepatic metastases. Two years later Howland, Campbell, Maltby and Robinson (12) reported the first case of pancreatic islet adenoma which was diagnosed preoperatively, identified at operation and excised with favorable result.

In the past few years the literature on hyperinsulinism has grown tremendously. A review by Whipple and Frantz (25) of all the published cases of hyperinsulinism and islet tumor has appeared very recently. According to their analysis of the 157 cases reported, 75 cases of hypoglycemia were ascribed to hyperinsulinism without verification at operation or autopsy. Of the 82 remaining cases in which the pancreas was examined, normal tissue was recorded in 13 instances, hypertrophy of the islands in 4 instances and chronic inflammatory change in 3, leaving 62 instances in which a tumor of the pancreatic islands was found. Analyzing further the 62 cases of tumor, exactly 50 per cent were incidental necropsy findings without recorded hypoglycemia. The group of 31 cases of tumor associated with hypoglycemia consists of 10 discovered at autopsy and 21 at operation. Among the last 21 cases, 4 were instances of carcinoma in which death occurred shortly after operation in 2 instances.

There remain 17 patients with adenoma, the excision of which led to eventual recovery. Thus in spite of frequent reports of hypoglycemia and hyperinsulinism, adenoma of the pancreatic islets, verified at operation with favorable outcome after extirpation of the tumor is a relatively rare condition. We are reporting the history of such a case together with the results of blood sugar and metabolism studies and biological assay of the tumor for insulin.

CASE REPORT

A Chinese man, M. T. L., aged 49 years, a mine foreman, was admitted to the Hospital on November 23, 1934, for attacks of unconsciousness and convulsions. He apparently had been well until April 1930 when, on one occasion, his consciousness became clouded after he had been awakened suddenly at night. His normal mental state returned in 3 hours after he had been given food. A similar attack occurred in September of the same year after the omission of breakfast. On that occasion he showed, in addition, haphazard movements of his limbs and profuse perspiration. Feeding again brought him out of coma. In March 1931 a strenuous journey by bicycle was followed by weakness and stiffness of the legs and collapse from which he recovered promptly after taking food. He once went to sleep without supper, and at 4 o'clock the next morning became semicomatose and then delirious, moving his arms violently, running out of his room and shouting loudly. Thereafter the attacks became more frequent, recurring approximately once every one to three months. Involuntary urination occurred during one of the attacks.

In February 1934 generalized clonic convulsions were first noticed, accompanied by coma. Subsequently similar seizures recurred almost every night, usually between 2 and 4 a.m. According to the description given by his wife, the onset of the seizures was marked by a cessation of the snoring which occurred regularly during sleep and the opening of his eyes accompanied by staring and grimacing. Twitching movements first involved the lower limbs and then the upper. In the beginning the movements were slight and then more violent. Occasionally the tongue was bitten. Each series of con-

249

S. H. LIU, H. H. LOUCKS, S. K. CHOU AND K. C. CHEN

vulsions usually lasted a few minutes and would be followed by an interval of relative quietness during which the patient could be induced to swallow some carbohydrate foods which his wife had learned to feed him in order to abolish the attacks.

During the intervals between the attacks the patient apparently was normal except for an impaired memory of recent events. He grew very fat during the two years prior to admission, his appetite being enormously increased. There was no loss of libido or potency. He had abandoned his work in 1932.

In the past history there was a record of smallpox at the age of 12, dysentery at 37, urethral discharge at 38, and an acute febrile illness of unknown nature at 42.

Physical examination. Between attacks the patient appeared perfectly comfortable. Temperature 37.4° C., pulse 80, blood pressure 104/70, height 172 cm., weight 96.7 kgm. The patient was well developed and markedly obese, with fat distributed generally without special predilection for given regions. Distribution of hair was normal except for a tendency toward the feminine type in the pubic region. The ocular fundi showed a slight degree of perivasculitis of the retinal vessels; visual fields normal. Thyroid gland was not enlarged. Lungs were normal. Heart was not enlarged, and the radial arteries were not thickened. Masses or individual organs could not be palpated within the abdomen. External genitalia were normal; prostate gland not enlarged. Neurological examination revealed nothing of significance. Dr. H. I. Chu, who saw the patient first in the Outpatient Clinic, suggested the diagnosis of hypoglycemic syndrome.

Laboratory data. Urinalysis gave normal findings and stools proved negative for ova or parasites. The red blood count was 5.9 million; hemoglobin, 15.3 grams; and white blood cells, 12,100 with 67 per cent neutrophiles. The blood sugar during the postabsorptive period as determined on many occasions was between 40 and 50 mgm. per cent. Icterus index was 6. A bromsulphalein test revealed no retention of the dye after 30 minutes. Roentgenologic examination of the skull showed a normal sella turcica. The basal metabolic rate was 1,977 calories per diem or + 3.0 per cent. Blood Wassermann reaction was negative.

The ordinary three-meal diet was not adequate to prevent convulsive seizures which usually came between 4 and 5 a.m. The patient therefore was given a diet containing 3,000 calories with 473 grams carbohydrates divided into 5 equal portions served at 8 a.m., 12 noon, 5 p.m., 10 p.m. and 3 a.m. This regimen kept him free from symptoms for a few days, but after that mild attacks re-appeared before the 3 a.m. and 8 a.m. feedings, and the diet had to be increased to 3,500 calories with 600 grams carbohydrates.

During the interval between admission and operation various studies on blood sugar and metabolism were made, which are described later.

Operation. On January 2, 1935, with the patient under ether anesthesia a laparotomy was performed (H. H. L.).

The abdomen was opened through a left rectus incision extending from the xiphoid process to a point about 3 cm. below the umbilicus. The subcutaneous and omental fat was large in quantity and a portion of the greater omentum was excised in order to facilitate exposure. The usual exploration revealed the fact that the liver was small with smooth surfaces and a thin, almost knife-like edge. The gallbladder, stomach, duodenum, small intestine, appendix and colon all appeared normal. The spleen was small. It was difficult to palpate the kidneys on account of excessive perirenal fat.

A duodenal tube was passed to deflate the stomach, and the pancreas was approached through the gastrocolic omentum. Along the upper margin of the right half of the body of the pancreas at approximately the point of junction of the head and body lay a tumor 2.5 cm. in diameter which was somewhat firmer in consistency than the rest of the gland. It was dark red in color and was elevated slightly above the surface of the gland. It appeared to be contained within a thin capsule and was enucleated easily from its bed in the pancreas. Numerous large veins ran between the capsule and the substance of the gland and hemostasis presented some difficulty, ligatures and the coagulating current both being employed. An iodoform gauze drain was packed lightly into the denuded area, and two cigarette drains were placed down to the level of the pancreas. The gastrocolic omentum was closed by interrupted sutures of fine silk. The abdominal wall was closed in layers around the drains, the closure being reinforced by three stay sutures of silver wire.

Postoperative course. For some hours prior to and during the operation, as well as for some hours subsequently, the patient was given a 5 per cent solution of glucose in normal saline by means of a continuous intravenous drip (40 drops per minute). The blood sugar at 9 a.m. (before operation) was 59, and at 1 p.m. (shortly after operation) it was 158; later in the day it rose to 264 mgm. per cent and sugar appeared in the urine. Temperature 39.3° C.; pulse 130. Glucose by intravenous drip was discontinued and 400 cc. of citrated blood were given.

On the next day the temperature went higher (40.4° C.), and the respirations increased to 34 per minute. Aside from slight cough and a few râles heard at the bases of both lungs, there was nothing to indicate a pulmonary complication. A moderate bloody discharge drained from the operative wound. One cigarette drain was removed. The white blood cell count was 8,850. The blood sugar was maintained between 175 and 245 mgm. per cent, and the urinary sugar totaled 4 grams in 24 hours. Insulin was started, and given in doses of ten units three times a day.

On the third day the fever began to subside, the general condition improving. The blood sugar was 238 to 300 mgm. per cent; the urine sugar 17 grams. The iodoform gauze drain was removed.

On the fourth day the patient was well enough to take a high caloric diet. The blood sugar was 276 mgm.

per cent and the urinary sugar totaled 22 grams. On the fifth day the temperature became normal. The last drain was removed and some serosanguineous discharge came from the wound. The hyperglycemia and glycosuria tended to diminish. Insulin was discontinued on the 7th day, and the blood sugar became normal and the urine sugar-free on the 9th day, before a calculated diabetic diet was started. From then on convalescence was uncomplicated, the wound closing gradually and the discharge becoming less in amount. The patient was up and about three weeks after the operation and did not experience any of the symptoms which had been present previously. A number of the preoperative observations on blood sugar and metabolism were repeated, and the results are described later. Although the patient showed evidence of a slight diabetic tendency as indicated by a sugar tolerance test, he tolerated a full diet with a normal fasting blood sugar and without glycosuria. He was discharged on February 22, 1935, in good condition except for a small sinus at the upper part of the wound which still drained thin fluid resembling pancreatic juice. His weight was 81.8 kgm., a loss of 14.9 kgm. compared with that on admission.

Examination on May 20, 1935, five months after operation, showed that the patient was well, and was without recurrence of the preoperative symptoms. The sinus had closed shortly after discharge. The fasting blood sugar was 111 mgm. per cent. A 24-hour specimen of urine contained no sugar. The weight was 80.8 kgm.

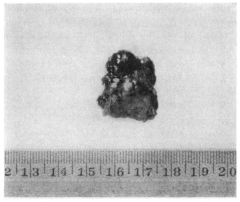

FIG. 1. GROSS APPEARANCE OF THE TUMOR REMOVED FROM THE PANCREAS.

STUDIES OF THE TUMOR

Anatomical observations. The tumor as shown in Figure 1 appeared nodular, dark red in color, and firm in consistency, measuring 2.5 × 2.0 × 1.5 cm. in diameter. It weighed 4.41 grams. The anterior surface was covered by a thin fibrous capsule, while its posterior surface, i.e., that portion of the tumor in contact with the gland, was studded with small areas of pancreatic tissue. The cut surface was grayish, cellular in appearance and showed many congested blood vessels. Microscopically the tumor consisted of a diffuse solid growth of cells which were uniform in size, well differentiated and morphologically identical with those of Langerhans' islands (Figure 2). In some areas the cells were arranged in cords or trabeculae much like the structure of normal islands. Mitotic figures were not seen. The anterior surface was entirely encapsulated, but the posterior surface was cut across irregularly, and in certain areas, immediately beneath the capsule groups of pancreatic acini were present.

Biologic assay for insulin. The method of extraction used was that of Best, Jephcott and Scott (2). A portion of the tumor weighing 1.92 grams was extracted, and the volume of extract made up to 20 cc. The assay was done on two rabbits of comparable weight which had been deprived of food for 24 hours prior to injection. As seen from Table I, the extent and duration of hypo-

TABLE I

Results of assay of extract of the tumor for insulin on rabbits

	Blood sugar		
	Control	2 hours	4 hours
	mgm. per cent	mgm. per cent	mgm. per cent
Rabbit 1			
January 4, weight 1570 grams, 0.5 cc. of *insulin* (0.5 unit).............	141.4	75.7	117.1
January 6, weight 1510 grams, 0.5 cc. of *extract* (0.05 gram)..........	124.2	72.2	101.9
Rabbit 2			
January 4, weight 1820 grams, 0.5 cc. of *extract* (0.05 gram)..........	138.5	83.6	111.1
January 6, weight 1724 grams, 0.5 cc. of *insulin* (0.5 unit).............	117.1	78.2	118.8

glycemia in both rabbits after the injection of tumor extract happened to approximate those after 0.5 unit of insulin. Therefore the tumor tissue was considered to contain approximately 10 units of insulin per gram. According to Best, Jephcott and Scott, beef pancreas yields on the

S. H. LIU, H. H. LOUCKS, S. K. CHOU AND K. C. CHEN

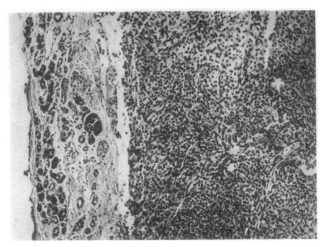

Fig. 2 *A*. Photomicrograph of a Section near the Periphery of the Tumor Showing Acinar Tissue in the Capsule (left) and Tumor Tissue with Trabecula Formation (right).

Magnification 111 times.

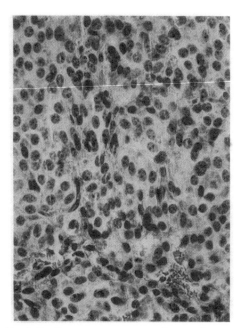

Fig. 2 *B*. Photomicrograph of a Section Showing Cytology of the Tumor in Greater Detail.

Magnification 445 times.

average 3,000 units of insulin per kgm. or 3 units per gram as determined by their method. The high insulin content of the tumor justifies the diagnosis of hyperinsulinism in this patient.

In the literature, there are recorded three successful attempts to extract insulin or an insulin-like substance from a tumor of the pancreas removed at operation (5, 8, 26). It appears that the tumor in our case had a higher insulin content than that of the tumors previously reported.

OBSERVATIONS ON THE BLOOD SUGAR AND RESPIRATORY METABOLISM

Behavior of blood sugar in relation to meals. While the patient was being given a diet of 3,000 calories with 473 grams of carbohydrate distributed evenly among five meals, the capillary blood sugar was determined hourly throughout 24 hours by the Folin-Wu method (7) adapted to 0.1 cc. samples. The results are plotted in Figure 3, from which one notes that the blood sugar rose to a maximum within 1 to 3 hours after each meal. The maxima, which varied from 65 to 115 mgm. per cent, were below normal after meals, although the values were low to start with. The more significant abnormality lies in the failure of the blood sugar to maintain a normal level during the postabsorptive period. Within 4 to 5 hours after each meal when absorption could

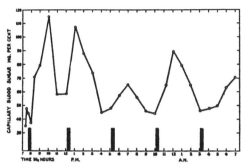

FIG. 3. HOURLY BLOOD SUGAR THROUGHOUT 24 HOURS IN RELATION TO MEALS WHICH ARE INDICATED BY VERTICAL BARS.

hardly be complete it promptly fell to 44 to 58 mgm. per cent. If, therefore, meals had been delayed, it is reasonable to suppose that the level would have continued to fall until symptoms occurred. Therefore, the condition can be characterized as one of pronounced postabsorptive hypoglycemia in which frequent feedings were necessary to prevent the development of symptoms.

Correlation between the level of blood sugar

and the clinical picture. On one morning with breakfast omitted, the patient was observed carefully, and the capillary blood sugar, blood pressure and pulse rate were determined at approximately 10-minute intervals. As seen from Figure 4, the observations were commenced at 8:00 a.m. when the patient was quiet and mentally clear with the blood sugar fluctuating at 45 to 50 mgm. per cent. He remained in this condition for about 25 to 30 minutes, after which without appreciable change in the level of the blood sugar he became slightly drowsy, but easily arousable. The drowsiness gradually deepened so that in another 30 minutes when awakened he again fell asleep and began snoring at once. The blood sugar level remained practically unchanged. The period of profound drowsiness lasted 25 minutes before it passed into a stage of excitement. Then the patient became restless, opened his eyes in a staring manner and yawned repeatedly. The fists were clenched tightly, and the legs were moved about purposelessly. At times, fine twitchings of the muscles of the hands and face were noticed. The patient still seemed to recognize loud calls or commands, but was unable to answer or act upon them. The blood sugar level tended to fall somewhat, slightly below 45 mgm. per cent. This period lasted 10 minutes before active generalized clonic convul-

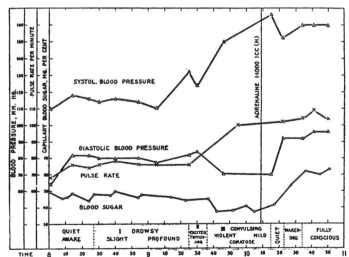

FIG. 4. CORRELATION BETWEEN LEVEL OF BLOOD SUGAR AND MENTAL STATE. BLOOD PRESSURE AND PULSE RATE ALSO INDICATED.

sions began. The convulsions increased gradually in violence, the patient's whole body being thrown about the bed with such force that several men were required to hold him down. Breathing was stertorous, with frothing at the mouth. Violent seizures continued for 15 minutes before they gave place to milder convulsive movements of the limbs. With the onset of convulsions the blood sugar dropped to about 37 to 40 mgm. per cent. The blood pressure began to rise during the excitement and reached 150/70 during the convulsions. The pulse rate also was increased. One cubic centimeter of 1:1,000 solution of adrenalin given subcutaneously was followed in 5 minutes by a subsidence of the convulsions and in 15 minutes, by consciousness.

It seems that the hypoglycemic syndrome in this patient can be divided conveniently into three stages. The first stage was characterized by drowsiness and a gradually deepening depression. The second stage was ushered in by excitement which progressed into the convulsive seizures of the third stage. During the first stage which lasted for an hour there was no significant decrease of blood sugar compared with that of the period of relative well-being. Even when the second stage was reached, the lowering of blood sugar was slight, if any. It was not until after the convulsions had started that definite further lowering of the blood sugar occurred. From these observations it may be inferred that hypoglycemia has to be maintained for a certain length of time, which in this patient amounted to over two hours, before the central nervous system suffers sufficiently to manifest itself by convulsions. It seems that besides the level of the hypoglycemia, the duration is an important determining factor in the symptomatic manifestations. Unfortunately, our observations did not extend over a sufficiently long period prior to the symptoms to enable us to estimate accurately the duration of the critical level of blood sugar necessary to initiate an attack.

The effect of adrenalin. A detailed study of the blood sugar level and its relation to symptomatic manifestations following the administration of adrenalin is given in Figure 5. The efficacy of adrenalin in relieving the hypoglycemic syndrome, a well known phenomenon, was demonstrated clearly in this case. With the patient

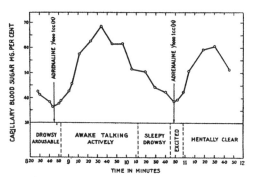

FIG. 5. EFFICACY OF ADRENALIN IN RAISING BLOOD SUGAR AND RELIEVING SYMPTOMS.

mentally drowsy and the blood sugar at the low level of 36 mgm. per cent, 1 cc. of adrenalin injected hypodermically was followed within 10 minutes by a return of consciousness associated with a rise of the blood sugar to 42 mgm. per cent. A maximum level of 68.6 mgm. per cent was reached about 45 minutes after the injection. From then on it commenced to fall, and 85 minutes after the injection it reached a level of approximately 50 mgm. per cent at which time the patient again began to feel drowsy. Two hours after the injection the blood sugar was back to the original low level, and the patient once more was in a semicomatose condition. A second injection of adrenalin at this point brought about a similar reaction, although the maximum level of blood sugar attained was somewhat lower.

It may be noted here that there apparently was a difference in the blood sugar level referable to a given mental state depending on whether the blood sugar was increasing or decreasing. During the ascent of the curve following the injection of adrenalin, consciousness was almost regained at 42 mgm. per cent, while during its descent drowsiness supervened at 50 mgm. per cent. The difference was probably significant, although no attempt was made to determine the true glucose content of blood which might not have shown such discrepancies.

The action of adrenalin was studied further by the simultaneous determination of the venous blood sugar and serum inorganic phosphorus (6) following the administration of this drug both preoperatively and after convalescence from the operation. As shown in Figure 6, the adrenalin hyperglycemia before operation, as in previous observations, reached its peak 40 minutes after injection, and the blood sugar returned to the in-

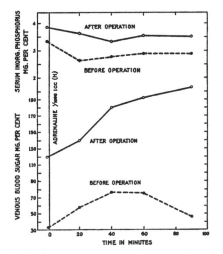

Fig. 6. Comparison of the Effect of Adrenalin on Blood Sugar and Serum Inorganic Phosphorus before and after Operative Removal of the Tumor of Islands of Langerhans.

itial level in 90 minutes. However, after operation, at which the source of excess insulin was removed, adrenalin caused a much more extensive and prolonged rise in the blood sugar; at 90 minutes after injection when the study was terminated, a maximum value of 198 mgm. per cent was obtained. The serum inorganic phosphorus curve before operation was on a lower level and showed a more definite decline following the administration of adrenalin than that obtained by the same procedure after excision of the tumor.

These observations may be summarized by saying that although adrenalin was very promptly effective in combating the hypoglycemic syndrome, thus acting as a true antagonist to insulin, its action was considerably curtailed and shortened in the presence of excess insulin. The fact that adrenalin was repeatedly effective indicated that a considerable store of glycogen in the liver or other tissues was available for conversion into glucose.

Effect of pituitrin, pitressin, and ephedrine. One cubic centimeter of pituitrin (Parke, Davis

and Co.) was given hypodermically on one occasion when the blood sugar was only 38 mgm. per cent and the patient was emerging from drowsiness into excitement; 15 minutes later the blood sugar rose to 42 mgm. per cent, and the patient was somewhat clearer for a short while (10 minutes) before returning to the pre-injection state. One and a half cubic centimeters of pitressin (Parke, Davis and Co.) was then given subcutaneously, and its action was observed to be similarly slight and doubtful. On another occasion ephedrine was used (100 mgm. hypodermically) without the slightest effect on the course of the patient's symptoms or the level of the blood sugar.

Effect of levulose. One morning when the patient was slightly drowsy and the blood sugar was 48 mgm. per cent, he was given, instead of his usual breakfast, 50 grams of levulose dissolved in 250 cc. of water. The drowsiness persisted and gradually deepened and 70 minutes after the ingestion of levulose restlessness set in and progressed to mild convulsive attacks. The blood sugar, however, rose to 55 mgm. per cent in 30 minutes and fell to 44 mgm. per cent in 70 minutes at which time mild convulsions supervened. This ineffectiveness of levulose in combating the hypoglycemic syndrome is in conformity with the results of Cori (3) who showed that levulose cannot be utilized by the tissues until it first has been converted into glycogen by the liver. The slight rise of blood sugar probably represented levulose which was ineffective in counteracting the symptoms.

Comparison of the effect of glucose per rectum and by mouth. Although glucose often has been administered per rectum, doubt still exists as to whether it is absorbed through this route. Our patient afforded an excellent indicator with which to test the efficacy of the absorption of glucose by rectum inasmuch as very slight changes in the level of the blood sugar were manifested by marked changes in his mental state. As indicated in Figure 7, 600 cc. of 10 per cent solution of glucose given per rectum in three installments within a period of one hour did not prevent the gradual lowering of the blood sugar or the progression of drowsiness to the subsequent state of excitement and convulsions. This is a sharp contrast to the efficacy of glucose administered by mouth, by which route even much smaller amounts

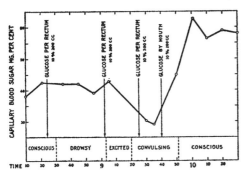

Fig. 7. Ineffectiveness of Glucose per Rectum in Combating the Hypoglycemic Syndrome in Contrast to the Efficacy of Glucose by Mouth.

of glucose brought about immediate amelioration of symptoms and a rise of the blood sugar. This observation indicates that glucose in this concentration per rectum is not absorbed or is absorbed so slowly that physiologic effects are not demonstrable. This conclusion is in agreement with that of Scott and Zweighaft (21).

Effect of glucose on blood sugar, metabolic rate and respiratory quotient before and after operation. The study consisted of half-hourly analyses of the capillary blood sugar, hourly determinations of the metabolic rate and estimations of urinary nitrogen, both before and for 4 hours after the ingestion of 170 grams of glucose. The expiratory gas was collected in a Tissot gasometer for a period of 10 to 15 minutes each time and analyzed for O_2 and CO_2 in a Haldane apparatus. Urinary nitrogen was determined by the Kjeldahl method. The data on blood sugar, respiratory quotient, caloric output, and calculated composition of metabolic mixture during the experimental periods are presented in Figure 8 and Tables II and III.

In Figure 8, the blood sugar curve before operation is seen to deviate from normal in two respects. First, the peak (156 mgm. per cent) was not reached until two hours after the ingestion of glucose. Second, after a normal level had been reached at the end of three hours the curve continued to fall to the level of 51 mgm. per cent at the end of the fourth hour, a low level comparable to that which existed before glucose was administered. It seems that the excess insulin present in the blood stream prevented a more prompt

attainment of the maximal level. As soon as this was reached, more insulin was called forth. The excess insulin together with the diminishing amount of glucose entering the blood stream from

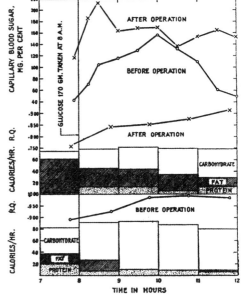

Fig. 8. The Effect of Glucose Ingestion on Blood Sugar, Respiratory Quotient, Metabolic Rate, and Composition of the Metabolic Mixture before and after Operation.

TABLE II

Effect on respiratory quotient and metabolic rate of 170 grams glucose ingested at 8:00 a.m.

Time	Total respiratory quotient		Nonprotein respiratory quotient		Calories per hour		Calories per 24 hours		Metabolic rate		Increase over basal rate	
	A*	P†	A*	P†	A*	P†	A*	P†	A*	P†	A*	P†
a.m.									per cent	per cent	per cent	per cent
7–8	0.883	0.765	0.910	0.763	82.4	74.7	1977	1793	3.0	0.0	0	0.0
8–9	0.925	0.848	0.987	0.855	91.5	77.7	2197	1866	14.4	4.0	11.0	4.0
9–11	0.987	0.856	1.010	0.866	92.1	80.8	2210	1941	15.1	8.2	11.8	8.2
10–11	0.992	0.878	1.014	0.884	86.6	78.6	2079	1885	8.2	5.2	5.1	5.2
11–12	0.972	0.914	0.987	0.931	80.1	78.8	1924	1892	0.1	5.5	−2.8	5.5

* A, before operation, height 172 cm., weight 95.0 kgm., surface area 2.08 square meters, Aub-DuBois standard 80.0 calories per hour.

† P, after operation, height 172 cm., weight 82 kgm., surface area 1.94 square meters, Aub-DuBois standard 74.7 calories per hour.

TABLE III

Combustion of protein (from urinary nitrogen), carbohydrate and fat (from nonprotein respiratory quotient) before and after ingestion of 170 grams glucose at 8 a.m.*

Time	Protein				Carbohydrate				Fat			
	A†		P‡		A†		P‡		A†		P‡	
a.m. 7–8	grams	calories	grams	calories	grams	calories	grams	calories	grams	calories	grams	calories
	4.48	19.0	0.46	2.0	11.0	46.0	3.4	14.1	1.84	17.4	6.19	58.6
8–9	1.76	7.4	2.97	12.6	16.0	65.9	7.9	33.0	1.94	18.2	3.39	32.1
9–10	2.30	9.7	2.79	12.8	19.7	82.4	8.8	37.0	0.0	0.0	3.27	31.0
10–11	1.98	8.4	1.34	5.3	18.7	78.2	11.6	44.4	0.0	0.0	3.06	28.9
11–12	1.37	5.8	3.12	13.2	17.0	71.0	12.0	50.2	0.35	3.3	1.63	15.4
Total for last 4 hours	7.41	31.3	10.22	43.9	71.4	297.5	40.3	164.6	2.29	21.5	11.35	107.4

* Calculation according to Lusk (16); protein equivalent to 4.24 calories; carbohydrate 4.18 calories; and fat 9.46 calories per gram.

† A, before operation, 42.6 per cent of the glucose ingested was burned during 4 hours; protein contributed 8.9 per cent, carbohydrate 85.0 per cent, and fat 6.1 per cent of the total energy metabolism during 4 hours subsequent to glucose administration.

‡ P, after operation, 23.7 per cent of the glucose ingested was burned during 4 hours; protein contributed 13.8 per cent, carbohydrate 52.1 per cent, and fat 34.1 per cent of the total energy metabolism during 4 hours subsequent to glucose administration.

the gastro-intestinal tract drove the blood sugar down to the low level. The curve obtained after operation was markedly different in that the peak of 214 mgm. per cent was reached in half an hour and a level between 133 and 169 mgm. per cent was maintained during the subsequent 3 hours. The high maximum and sustained hyperglycemia indicate an impaired mechanism for the removal of glucose suggestive of the prediabetic state, although the fasting blood sugar was normal and urinary sugar was absent.

The metabolic rate increased after the administration of glucose, the extent of the increase (specific dynamic action) being greater before (12 per cent) than after operation (8 per cent). During the period of hyperinsulinism the respiratory quotient before glucose (0.883) was higher than normal and went up nearly to unity after glucose administration, while after operation the quotient before glucose (0.765) was lower than normal and rose only to 0.914 during the fourth hour after the ingestion of this substance. The marked lowering of the respiratory quotient after operation indicates the profound changes in the composition of the metabolic mixture brought about by the removal of the pancreatic adenoma.

Prior to operation and during the 4 hours following the ingestion of 170 grams of glucose, 71.4 grams carbohydrate, 7.4 grams protein and 2.3 grams fat were burned; while after operation,

40.3 grams carbohydrate, 10.2 grams protein and 11.4 grams fat were metabolized under comparable conditions (Table III, Figure 8). In other words, prior to operation, when there was an excess of insulin the metabolism of carbohydrates played a more dominating rôle and proceeded at a faster rate in contrast to the situation after operation in which carbohydrate was used more slowly and protein and fat were drawn upon to a greater extent.

Linder, Hiller and Van Slyke (15) fed 90 to 100 grams of glucose to normal fasting men, and determined their respiratory quotients and total metabolism. In four hours only 20 to 30 per cent of the glucose had been burned, although apparently all had been absorbed. In our patient glucose combustion prior to operation was 42.6 per cent, exceeding normal limits; while after operation it amounted to 23.7 per cent, which was fairly normal.

The sparing of fat and protein as a result of the predominant utilization of carbohydrate by virtue of the excess insulin, together with overeating, probably accounts for the marked obesity this patient exhibited prior to surgical treatment.

COMMENT

The hypoglycemic syndrome is a symptom complex associated with abnormally low blood sugar. The level of blood sugar at which symptoms occur varies from case to case. Of the large series of cases of hyperinsulinism compiled by Whipple and Frantz (25), the minimal blood sugar ranged from 4 to 58, with the majority falling between 30 and 45 mgm. per cent. The wide range is accounted for partly by the different methods used in the determinations and partly by individual susceptibility to the effects of hypoglycemia. This susceptibility apparently varies not only with age but with other factors as well, so that different responses may be obtained from the same individual on different occasions. Moreover, the ascending threshold for clear consciousness is lower than the descending threshold. There was a difference of over 15 mgm. per cent in our patient.

The symptoms associated with hypoglycemia are protean. If a careful history is taken, the attacks are found almost always to be associated with omission or delay of meals. Overpowering hunger and weakness frequently initiate the trouble, and the patients or their relatives discover sooner or later that food aborts or relieves attacks. Often larger and more frequent meals are taken to prevent symptoms. Overeating together with the protein- and fat-sparing action of insulin results in obesity.

The symptoms of hypoglycemia, though variable, are chiefly vasomotor, such as sweating, flushes, and an increase in the pulse rate and blood pressure; and psychic disturbances, such as drowsiness, excitement, delirium, maniacal seizures, convulsions and coma. Weakness and fatigue are prominent. Rynearson and Moersch (20) tabulated the symptoms. The picture during an attack may vary in individual cases.

From the extensive literature on carbohydrate metabolism reviewed by Cori (4) and Shaffer and Ronzoni (22), it has become generally accepted that the blood sugar is maintained normally at a concentration of approximately 100 mgm. per cent mainly through the interplay between insulin and epinephrine. A rise in blood sugar elicits a secretion of insulin which accelerates conversion of glucose into glycogen and carbohydrate oxidation in the liver, muscles and presumably all tissues, while a fall in blood sugar is followed by a discharge of epinephrine which increases the rate of hydrolysis of liver glycogen to glucose and conversion of muscle glycogen lactate. The latter is reconverted into glycogen by the liver thereby contributing indirectly to the sugar of the blood. Macleod (18) postulates a sugar regulating center in the pons. Its stimulation by hyperglycemia causes the secretion of insulin by way of the vagus; while hypoglycemia results in sympathetic stimulation and the outpouring of epinephrine.

Wauchope (24) has summarized the causes of hypoglycemia under four main headings: First, hyperinsulinism which may be functional, or on the basis of adenoma, carcinoma or hyperplasia of pancreatic islets; or therapeutic, as a result of an overdosage of insulin. Second, lack of opposing hormones, as in Addison's disease, myxedema, and pituitary cachexia. Third, deficient glycogen store due to liver disease (13, 14), severe exercise, excessive drain (renal diabetes or lactation), or starvation. Fourth, disturbances of the regulating center in the pons (vagotonia).

Before a diagnosis of hyperinsulinism is made, all the other conditions enumerated above should be considered and excluded. This was done in our case without much difficulty. The finding of an adenoma of the pancreas composed of cells of the islands of Langerhans, the abatement of symptoms after excision of the tumor and finally the presence of large amounts of insulin in the biological assay of the tumor tissue established beyond doubt that the anatomical basis of the hypoglycemia in our patient was an islet cell adenoma.

As regards treatment, frequent meals rich in carbohydrate usually suffice to avert the symptoms when these are slight and infrequent. Harris (11), however, considers that a diet relatively poor in carbohydrate and rich in fat, with moderate protein, is more effective in reducing the production of insulin by the pancreas. Suprarenal extract by mouth was given in three cases as an adjuvant (19), but it did not appear to offer much advantage over diet alone. Thyroid has been tried without benefit (23).

For emergency treatment during an attack, epinephrine administered hypodermically and glucose by mouth constitute two potent therapeutic measures. Both act promptly. While glucose has a more lasting effect, epinephrine possesses the advantage of being administered easily during coma or convulsions which may render the ingestion of glucose impossible. It is important to remember that glucose per rectum is ineffective. The effect of levulose is doubtful, and presumably that of galactose as well. Pituitrin, pitressin and ephedrine are unreliable.

When the symptoms persist and increase, surgical attack on the pancreas becomes the treatment of choice. In all cases in which an adenoma has been found at operation and removed, relief from symptoms has been complete. Of the 15 cases without demonstrable tumor (25) in which a partial resection of the pancreas was carried out, improvement was noticed in 5. These were instances in which a large portion of the gland was removed. Graham and Hartmann (9) and more recently McCaughan (17) have advocated subtotal pancreatectomy for cases of hyperinsulinism in which a tumor is not demonstrable. It seems reasonable to believe that, as in the case of the thyroid, satisfactory results may not be obtained unless a subtotal excision of the gland is carried out.

It does not seem necessary to go into the details of surgical technic, as these are available elsewhere (8, 17, 25). It should, however, be emphasized that exposure must be adequate and exploration of the pancreas thorough, as multiple adenomata were found in four of the seventeen cases reported previously (8, 25). In our case a long left rectus incision and division of the gastrocolic omentum allowed satisfactory access to the gland. Others have preferred to use a transverse incision (25) or to approach the pancreas by the supragastric route (9). In instances in which mobilization or partial resection of the pancreas is attempted and serious difficulty is encountered due to hemorrhage from branches of the splenic vessels, we would like to suggest simple ligation of the splenic artery near its point of origin as a satisfactory means of controlling the flow of blood. Experience with this procedure as a substitute for splenectomy in certain instances has convinced us that ligation of this vessel is by no means an indication for subsequent removal of the spleen.

SUMMARY

A case of chronic postabsorptive hypoglycemia associated with coma and convulsive seizures is reported. On surgical exploration a small tumor of the pancreas was found, the excision of which led to complete relief of the symptoms. The tumor was composed of cells of the islands of Langerhans, and yielded considerably more insulin than normal pancreatic tissue. Detailed studies of the blood sugar and metabolism before and after operation are presented. Evidence is adduced showing that the hypoglycemia was, in a large measure, related to the fact that the combustion of carbohydrate proceeded at a faster rate and played a more dominating rôle in energy metabolism than is normal, thus sparing fat and protein. This action, combined with overeating, produced obesity. Glucose by mouth and adrenalin hypodermically were promptly efficacious in combating the hypoglycemia. Pituitrin, pitressin, ephedrine, levulose by mouth and glucose per rectum were ineffective.

BIBLIOGRAPHY

1. Banting, F. G., and Best, C. H., The internal secretion of the pancreas. J. Lab. and Clin. Med., 1922, 7, 251.
2. Best, C. H., Jephcott, C. M., and Scott, D. A., Insulin in tissues other than the pancreas. Am. J. Physiol., 1932, 100, 285.
3. Cori, C. F., The fate of sugar in the animal body. III. The rate of glycogen formation in the liver of normal and insulinized rats during the absorption of glucose, fructose and galactose. J. Biol. Chem., 1926, 70, 577.
4. Cori, C. F., Mammalian carbohydrate metabolism. Physiol. Rev., 1931, 11, 143.
5. Derick, C. L., Newton, F. C., Schulz, R. Z., Bowie, M. A., and Pokorny, N. A., Spontaneous hyperinsulinism. Report of a case of hyperinsulinism cured by surgical intervention. New England J. Med., 1933, 208, 293.
6. Fiske, C. H., and Subbarow, Y., The colorimetric determination of phosphorus. J. Biol. Chem., 1925, 66, 375.
7. Folin, O., and Wu, H., A system of blood analysis, Supplement 1. A simplified and improved method for determination of sugar. J. Biol. Chem., 1920, 41, 367.
8. Graham, E. A., and Womack, N. A., The application of surgery to the hypoglycemic state due to islet tumors of pancreas and to other conditions. Surg., Gynec. and Obst., 1933, 56, 728.

9. Graham, E. A., and Hartmann, A. F., Subtotal resection of the pancreas for hypoglycemia. Surg., Gynec. and Obst., 1934, **59**, 474.

10. Harris, S., Hyperinsulinism and dysinsulinism. J. A. M. A., 1924, **83**, 729.

11. Harris, S., Hyperinsulinism, a definite disease entity. J. A. M. A., 1933, **101**, 1958.

12. Howland, G., Campbell, W. R., Maltby, E. J., and Robinson, W. L., Dysinsulinism: convulsions and coma due to islet cell tumor of pancreas with operation and cure. J. A. M. A., 1929, **93**, 674.

13. Judd, E. S., Kepler, E. J., and Rynearson, E. H., Spontaneous hypoglycemia: Report of two cases associated with fatty metamorphosis of the liver. Am. J. Surg., 1934, **24**, 345.

14. Kramer, B., Grayzel, H. G., and Solomon, C. J., Chronic hypoglycemia in childhood. J. Pediat., 1934, **5**, 299.

15. Linder, G. C., Hiller, A., and Van Slyke, D. D., Carbohydrate metabolism in nephritis. J. Clin. Invest., 1925, **1**, 247.

16. Lusk, G., The Science of Nutrition. Saunders, Philadelphia, 1923, 3d ed., p. 60.

17. McCaughan, J. M., Subtotal pancreatectomy for hyperinsulinism. Operative technic. Ann. Surg., 1935, **101**, 1336.

18. Macleod, J. J. R., The control of carbohydrate metabolism. Bull. Johns Hopkins Hosp., 1934, **54**, 79.

19. Nielsen, J., and Eggleston, E. L., Functional dysinsulinism with epileptiform seizures. J. A. M. A., 1930, **94**, 860.

20. Rynearson, E. H., and Moersch, F. P., Neurologic manifestations of hyperinsulinism and other hypoglycemic states. J. A. M. A., 1934, **103**, 1196.

21. Scott, E. L., and Zweighaft, J. F. B., Blood sugar in man following the rectal administration of dextrose. Arch. Int. Med., 1932, **49**, 221.

22. Shaffer, P. A., and Ronzoni, E., Carbohydrate metabolism. Annual Rev. Biochem., 1932, **1**, 247.

23. Tedstrom, M. K., Hypoglycemia and hyperinsulinism. Ann. Int. Med., 1934, **7**, 1013.

24. Wauchope, G. M., Critical review: Hypoglycemia. Quart. J. Med., 1933, **2**, 117.

25. Whipple, A. O., and Frantz, V. K., Adenoma of islet cells with hyperinsulinism. A review. Ann. Surg., 1935, **101**, 1299.

26. Wilder, R. M., Allan, F. N., Power, M. H., and Robertson, H. E., Carcinoma of the islands of the pancreas. Hyperinsulinism and hypoglycemia. J. A. M. A., 1927, **89**, 348.

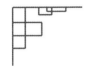
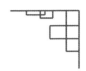

第四编　骨病深耕

　　第四编是本选集收录论文最多的一部分，是北京协和医院内分泌与肾脏病学团队在 20 世纪三四十年代对于骨软化症的钙磷代谢系列研究。这一系列包括了以"骨软化症的钙磷代谢"为题的 13 篇论文，后来被加拿大内分泌医生、钙磷代谢研究权威帕菲特（A.M. Parfitt）誉为"20 世纪人类认识维生素 D 缺乏性疾病的知识宝库"。限于篇幅，本论文选集主要收录了刘士豪教授为第一作者的相关论文，可供读者参考。

Chinese Medical Journal, 48: 623-636, 1934.

CALCIUM AND PHOSPHORUS METABOLISM IN OSTEOMALACIA

I. THE EFFECT OF VITAMIN D & ITS APPARENT DURATION*

R. R. HANNON, S. H. LIU, H. I. CHU, S. H. WANG,
K. C. CHEN, AND S. K. CH

Department of Medicine, Peiping Union Medical College, Peiping.

In the course of our studies on the calcium and phosphorus metabolism in osteomalacia, it seemed important to us to determine not only the effect of vitamin D, but also the duration of its effect. Patients with obviously advanced osteomalacia were encountered, who on study showed marked ability to conserve calcium and phosphorus. These patients had often received cod liver oil or other vitamin D preparations previous to the study. Therefore the question arose as to whether previous vitamin D administration, even though in small doses and for a short period, would exert its corrective influence on calcium and phosphorus metabolism for a long time afterwards, and thereby explain the apparent discrepancy between the clinical condition and the metabolic behavoir. We were unable to find any information in the literature that might help to answer this question. The main purpose of the present communication is to direct attention to the striking and prolonged effect of vitamin D in correcting calcium and phosphorus metabolic abnormality in osteomalacia as exemplified in the following patient who received no vitamin D preparation prior to the studies.

CASE REPORT

C. C., a Chinese girl of 18, was admitted to the Peiping Union Medical College Hospital on December 20, 1932 for pain in both thighs and knees for 22 months and weakness of legs and difficulty in walking for 16 months prior to admission. Patient came from a very poor family. Their dietary staples consisted of corn bread, cabbage, turnip, bean curd and salted vegetables. Rice and flour were occasionally taken. Patient was said to have developed normally

---

* Presented at the Second Biennial Conference of the Chinese Medical Association, Nanking. March 31 to April 7, 1934.

and enjoyed good health until March 1931 when she began to have spontaneous, intermittent pain at the inner aspect of left thigh radiating downwards to the leg. There were usually 6 to 8 attacks a day, each lasting 2 to 5 minutes. Exertion aggravated the pain. About 2 to 3 months later similar pain was also noticed in the right thigh as well as in the medial aspects of both knees. In September 1931, pain extended to the lower back, and she began to notice some weakness of legs with a limp to her gait. A little later the knees began to knock against each other. She frequently noticed numbness of legs after standing for some time, and stooping caused pain in the back. These complaints persisted at a fairly stationary level up to the time of admission. There were no spastic attacks of her hands and feet suggestive of tetany as far as she could remember. Her menstrual function was established at 16 and was very irregular. Pain in the thighs and back was aggravated during the periods.

On examination the patient was well nourished and in no obvious discomfort. Development was considered normal for her age except for the absence of pubic and axillary hair. Weight 36.8 kg. Height 148.5 cm. Teeth normal except for a slight degree of mobility. No obvious deformity of skull or thoracic cage. The spinal column showed slight scoliosis at lower thoracic region with convexity toward right. Slight tenderness over the dorso-lumbar junction. Upper extremities normal except for slight enlargement at the wrists. The lower extremities showed marked genu vulgum, and the legs were spread wide apart with eversion of ankles. The pubic arch appeared to be narrow and rostrated. Pelvic measurements as follows: Interspinous diameter 19.5 cm, intercristal diameter 22.0 cm, external conjugate 17.0 cm, and transverse outlet 7.0 cm. Other incidental findings were mild papillary trachoma, chronic tonsillitis, and deviation of nasal septum.

Examination for neuro-muscular irritability showed positive Chvostek's sign, but negative Trousseau's sign. Galvanic stimulation of facial and ulnar nerves revealed no increased irritability.

Routine laboratory examinations of urine, stool and blood showed nothing remarkable. Serum calcium 8.9 mg and inorganic phosphorus 3.5 mg per 100 cc.

Roentgenologic survey of the entire skeleton showed general osteoporosis and coarse trabeculation. The pelvis was approximately normal in shape except for slight narrowing of pubic arch. The anterior curvature of the lumbo-sacral spine and the posterior curvature of the sacrum were increased with slight shortening of the vertical diameter of all the vertebrae. There was a healed fracture of right fibula and incomplete fracture in each tibia. The epiphyseal line at the lower ends of femora appeared somewhat clouded suggestive of remnants of old rickets. Roentgenologic findings in general, however, were in favor of osteomalacia as the main diagnosis.

METABOLIC PROCEDURE

The patient was studied on the Metabolism Ward from Dec. 24, 1932 to June 9, 1933 during which time her diets (Table 1) were quantitatively prepared and served and excreta completely collected. The general procedure about the preparation of diets and collection of specimens has been described previously (19). Distilled water was used for drinking and cooking. The metabolic periods were 4 days each, and 0.1 gm of carmine was taken at the beginning of each period so as to mark off the stools. Urinary calcium was determined by the method of Shohl and Pedley (28), total phosphorus by the method of Fiske and Subarrow (10). Dried powdered stool was ashed in platinum, and the ash dissolved in

TABLE I. *Composition of diets per day. (Vitamin D content taken from Wu (30), + indicates presence, + + good amount, + + + excellent amount, ± no appreciable amount, and * presence doubtful.)*

Articles of food	Vitamin D content	Diet 1. Periods 1-3	Diet 2 Periods 4-28	Diet 3 Periods 29-34
Millet, *gm.*	±	40	80	80
Flour, *gm.*	±	160	200	200
Rice, *gm.*	±	120	80	80
Pork, *gm.*	*	80	40	40
Egg, *number*	+ +		1	1
Apple, *gm.*	*	40	80	80
Potato, *gm.*	*	80		
Onion, *gm.*	*	40		
Chinese lettuce, *gm.*	*	40		
Pai-ts'ai, *gm.*	±		80	80
Small cabbage, *gm.*	+ + +			80
Kai-ts'ai, *gm.*	+ +		80	
Celery, *gm.*	±		80	80
Sugar, *gm.*	o	60	41	41
Sesame oil, *gm.*	o	32	32	32
Sodium chloride, *gm.*	o	4	4	4
Protein, *gm.*		50	56	56
Carbohydrate, *gm.*		337	331	331
Fat, *gm.*		50	51	49
Calories,		2000	2000	2000
Nitrogen, calculated, *gm.*		7.95	8.88	8.88
Calcium, determined, *mg.*		78	221	218
Phosphorus, determined, *mg.*		583	859	901

5 per cent hydrochloric acid, and aliquot portions taken for the determination of calcium and phosphorus by the same methods. Stool nitrogen was estimated by wet ashing (19). Diet calcium and phosphorus were analysed in the same way as the stool. Nitrogen of diet was calculated from the food values compiled by Wu (30). Venipunctures were done before breakfast, usually on the first day of each period. Serum calcium and phosphorus were determined by the methods of Clark and Collip (7) and Fiske and Subarrow (9) respectively.

RESULTS

Calcium metabolism. As indicated in Table 2 and Figure 1, for the first 3 periods, the patient received a diet (Diet 1) containing a minimal

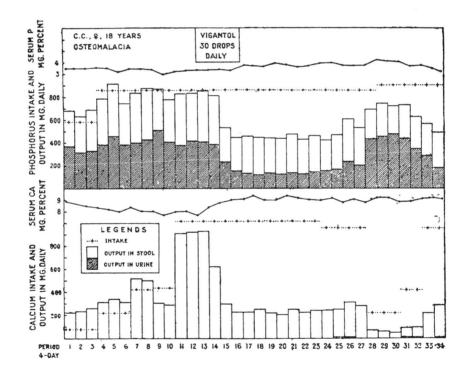

Fig. 1. Calcium and phosphorus metabolism.

第四编 骨病深耕

TABLE 2. *The effect of Vigantol and different levels of calcium intake on calcium, phosphorus and nitrogen metabolism, and serum calcium and phosphorus*

Period (4-day)	Average daily Calcium				Average daily Phosphorus				Serum		Nitrogen balance	Comment
	Intake mgm.	Urine mgm.	Stool mgm.	Balance mgm.	Intake mgm.	Urine mgm.	Stool mgm.	Balance mgm.	Ca mgm. Per 100 cc.	P mgm. Per 100 cc.	gm.	
I	78	1	222	−145	583	368	315	100	8.9	3.5	−0.32	Diet 1
2	78	2	235	−159	583	316	314	−47	8.5	3.5	+0.52	
3	78	0	260	−182	583	325	364	−106	8.4	3.6	+0.57	
4	221	0	312	−91	859	380	406	+73	8.2	3.5	+0.79	Diet 2
5	221	0	340	−119	859	460	455	−56	8.0	3.2	+0.77	
6	221	1	311	−91	859	383	360	+96	8.4	3.4	+0.99	
7	422	1	518	−97	859	398	440	+21	8.0	3.5	+0.30	Diet 2 + calcium chloride by mouth
8	422	1	498	−77	859	428	447	−16	8.0	3.4	+0.24	
9	435	0	304	+131	859	513	358	−12	7.7	3.0	+1.30	Diet 2 + calcium chloride intravenously
10	435	1	289	+145	859	408	368	+83	8.0	3.2	+0.61	
11	1016	0	909	+107	859	377	452	+30	8.0	3.3	+0.79	Diet 2 + calcium lactate by mouth
12	1016	0	920	+96	859	416	414	+29	7.6	3.3	+0.87	
13	1016	0	930	+86	859	409	444	+6	8.3	3.3	+0.76	
14	1016	1	622	+393	859	385	425	+49	8.7	3.4	+0.16	Diet 2 + calcium lactate by mouth + VIGANTOL 30 drops daily
15	1016	0	296	+720	859	232	299	+328	9.0	3.3	+0.61	
16	1016	0	228	+788	859	152	291	+416	9.1	3.7	+0.96	
17	1016	0	224	+792	859	131	324	+404	9.4	3.7	+1.30	
18	1016	0	252	+764	859	116	332	+411	9.0	3.6	+1.16	
19	1016	0	217	+799	859	134	304	+421	9.0	3.9	+1.58	
20	1016	0	201	+815	859	125	309	+425	9.4	3.8	+1.21	
21	1016	0	250	+766	859	138	335	+386	9.2	3.5	+1.12	
22	1016	0	223	+793	859	128	296	+435	9.0	3.6	+1.21	Diet 2 + calcium lactate by mouth
23	1016	1	243	+773	859	144	316	+399	8.9	3.8	+1.09	
24	954	1	244	+710	859	155	264	+440	9.1	3.9	+2.17	
25	954	5	250	+699	859	164	302	+393	8.8	3.7	+1.31	
26	954	4	314	+636	859	233	374	+252	9.0	3.7	+1.33	
27	954	2	280	+672	859	204	322	+333	8.7	3.7	+1.58	
28	221	1	68	+152	859	428	261	+170	9.2	4.0	+0.87	Diet 2
29	218	2	60	+156	901	453	289	+159	9.2	4.0	+0.66	Diet 3
30	218	0	49	+169	901	471	246	+184	8.8	4.0	+0.80	Diet 3 + calcium chloride by mouth
31	419	7	90	+322	901	434	294	+173	8.9	3.6	+1.32	
32	419	6	94	+319	901	347	280	+274	9.1	3.7	+1.93	Diet 3 + calcium lactate by mouth
33	951	1	220	+730	901	285	282	+334	9.2	3.4	+1.78	
34	951	4	288	+659	901	181	309	+411	9.0	3.2	+2.63	

intake of calcium (78 mg) and moderate phosphorus (583 mg). Both the calcium and phosphorus balances were negative. There was on the average a deficit of 160 mg of calcium daily. The extent of negative calcium balance was not excessive as compared with that of normal persons on a similar regime (2), but the point of interest is that practically all the calcium eliminated was in the stool, urinary calcium being almost nil.

During periods 4-28, the patient remained on a constant diet (Diet 2) having 221 mg of calcium and 859 mg of phosphorus per day. The first three periods (4-6) served as a control on her calcium and phosphorus elimination on this diet alone. The extent of negative balance in calcium (average 100 mg daily) though less than previously, remained considerable, while phosphorus balance was even. Again stool calcium constituted the sole outlet for calcium.

In the next two periods (7 and 8) the daily calcium intake was raised to 422 mg by the addition of calcium chloride taken by mouth. The added intake failed to maintain the patient in calcium balance (average calcium balance -86 mg daily), the result being simply increased calcium in the stool. It became of interest to administer the same amount of calcium chloride intravenously. This was done in the succeeding two periods (9 and 10). For the first time the calcium balance became positive to the extent of approximately 140 mg, indicating that most of the injected calcium was retained and the previous failure was mainly due to poor absorption.

From period 11 to 27 the calcium intake was increased to approximately 1 gm by giving a concentrated solution of calcium lactate (7.7 per cent). On this regime the first two periods (11 and 12) gave a slightly positive balance in both calcium and phosphorus. The extent of positive calcium balance (about 100 mg daily or 10 percent of the intake) was very small, especially in view of the fact that the decalcified state of the skeleton of the patient was such as requires urgent reparation.

In periods 13 to 16 the patient received vitamin D in the form of Vigantol 30 drops daily (a preparation containing irradiated ergosterol dissolved in oil, equivalent to 5000 rat units per cc or 60 drops). The effect of Vigantol did not begin in the first period of its administration, but from the second to the fourth there was a striking staircase-like decrease in calcium excretion in stool with a corresponding increase in calcium balance. During the last period of Vigantol medication the positive calcium balance was 788 mg per day representing approximately 78 percent of the intake. The effect on phosphorus retention of Vigantol was slight but noticeable in the second period of its administration, but in the third and fourth periods it was marked and comparable to the calcium retention.

The beneficial effect of Vigantol in promoting both calcium and phosphorus retention persisted in subsequent periods when the medication was stopped. From period 17 to 27 (44 days) while on the same calcium and phosphorus intake without Vigantol, the positive balance of both these elements remained approximately the same as that during the last two periods (15 and 16) of Vigantol administration.

Period 28 when the patient was still on Diet 2 but without added calcium in the form of calcium lactate, and periods 29 and 30 when she was on Diet 3 with approximately the same calcium and phosphorus content as Diet 2, are a contrast to periods 4-6 showing the striking difference in behavior on the part of the patient toward the same calcium and phosphorus intake *before* and *after* vitamin D administration. Now with the effect of vitamin D still operative, it was possible for the organism to retain about 160 mg (or 73 percent) out of 220 mg of calcium given in the diet, whereas previously on the same intake the calcium balance was negative to the extent of 100 mg daily. A normal person is not expected to retain calcium on an intake of 220 mg daily. The fact that this patient retained 73 percent of the calcium on this limited intake after Vigantol suggests that vitamin D is also operative in conserving endogenous calcium elimination.

Periods 31 and 32, when calcium intake was raised to 419 mg by oral administration of calcium chloride, are to be compared with periods 7 and 8 when the same procedure was employed. Again the good absorption and retention of calcium (average calcium balance +320 mg daily) *after* Vigantol contrasts sharply with the calcium deficit (average calcium balance -86 mg daily) *before* Vigantol administration. Thus vitamin D enabled the patient to economize approximately 400 mg of calcium on a moderate level of calcium intake (about 420 mg). This economy is apparently assisted by increased absorption through intestine as well as by decreased endogenous excretion.

The results of periods 33 and 34 indicate that the effect of previous vitamin D administration still continued unabated. This is true of the data obtained for the subsequent 8 periods (not included in this paper). Therefore after the administration of irradiated ergosterol in relatively small dosage for 16 days to this patient, the beneficial effect on calcium and phosphorus metabolism continued for at least 4 months, and perhaps longer, but we had not the opportunity to follow the studies further.

Phosphorus metabolism. It is well known that phosphorus balance depends on calcium and nitrogen balance. The ratio of nitrogen to phosphorus metabolized may be taken as 17.4 : 1 as used by Gargill, Gilligan and Blumgart (11): The mineral composition of bone, according to Roseberry, Hastings and Morse (25), corresponds to dahlite, $CaCO_3 \cdot Ca_3 (PO_4)_2$, with a Ca:P ratio of 2.26: 1. From these ratios a theoretical phosphorus balance can be calculated from the calcium and

TABLE 3. *Comparison of actual phosphorus balance with the theoretical phosphorus balance calculated from calcium and nitrogen balances*

Period	Theoretical, calculated from Ca	Theoretical, calculated from nitrogen	Total theoretical balance	Actual	Deviation actual – theoretical
	mg.	mg.	mg	mg.	mg.
1	− 64	− 19	− 83	− 100	− 20
2	− 70	+ 30	− 40	− 47	− 7
3	− 80	+ 33	− 47	− 106	− 59
4	− 40	+ 45	+ 5	+ 73	+ 68
5	− 53	+ 44	− 9	− 56	− 47
6	− 40	+ 57	+ 17	+ 96	+ 79
7	− 43	+ 17	− 26	+ 21	+ 47
8	− 34	+ 14	− 20	− 16	+ 4
9	+ 58	+ 75	+ 133	− 12	− 145
10	+ 64	+ 35	+ 99	+ 83	− 16
11	+ 47	+ 45	+ 92	+ 30	− 62
12	+ 42	+ 50	+ 92	+ 29	− 63
13	+ 38	+ 44	+ 82	+ 6	− 76
14	+ 174	+ 9	+ 183	+ 49	− 134
15	+ 319	+ 35	+ 354	+ 328	− 26
16	+ 349	+ 55	+ 404	+ 416	+ 12
17	+ 350	+ 75	+ 425	+ 404	− 21
18	+ 338	+ 67	+ 405	+ 411	+ 6
19	+ 354	+ 91	+ 445	+ 421	− 24
20	+ 301	+ 70	+ 431	+ 425	− 6
21	+ 339	+ 64	+ 403	+ 386	− 17
22	+ 350	+ 70	+ 420	+ 435	+ 15
23	+ 342	+ 63	+ 405	+ 399	− 6
24	+ 314	+ 125	+ 439	+ 440	+ 1
25	+ 310	+ 75	+ 385	+ 393	+ 8
26	+ 281	+ 76	+ 357	+ 253	− 104
27	+ 297	+ 91	+ 388	+ 333	− 55
28	+ 67	+ 50	+ 117	+ 170	+ 53
29	+ 69	+ 38	+ 107	+ 159	+ 52
30	+ 75	+ 46	+ 121	+ 184	+ 63
31	+ 142	+ 76	+ 218	+ 173	− 55
32	+ 141	+ 111	+ 252	+ 274	+ 22
33	+ 323	+ 102	+ 425	+ 334	− 91
34	+ 292	+ 151	+ 443	+ 411	− 32

nitrogen balances. Table 3 contains the results of such calculations. A comparison of the calculated with the actual phosphorus balance shows good general agreement, when the limits of experimental error are taken into consideration. The agreement in periods 15-25 is particularly close when the balances were large and a constant regime was kept up for a relatively long time. This indicates that during those periods at least calcium was retained with phosphorus in a ratio approximating that in bone.

In view of the good general agreement, occasional discrepancies may or may not be significant. In period 9, considerably more phosphorus was eliminated than was theoretically expected. This was the first of the two periods in which calcium chloride was administered intravenously. It seems that a sudden flooding of the blood stream and tissues with calcium may not affect immediately the phosphorus elimination that has been going on at a certain rate. During periods 13 and 14 when irradiated ergosterol was first given, change in phosphorus balance did not keep pace with that in calcium balance. It is possible that vitamin D acts primarily on the calcium metabolism and the secondary effect on phosphorus metabolism may conceivably be slower.

Serum calcium and phosphorus observations. Observations on serum calcium and phosphorus showed no striking variations. From period 1 to 12, serum calcium tended to decrease. The lowest serum calcium, namely, 7.6 mg was reached during period 12 just before Vigantol was given. Following the administration of Vigantol serum calcium level was gradually raised so that a maximum value of 9.4 mg was reached during the first period after Vigantol was stopped. Most of the subsequent serum calcium determinations were slightly lower than the maximum level attained. Serum phosphorus level fluctuated between 3 and 4 mg per 100 cc. As a whole higher levels were found after Vigantol administration.

Clinical and roentgenologic observations. The patient made no improvement in her condition until after the institution of vitamin D. In fact shortly before its administration when her serum calcium was at its lowest level, she complained of occasional transient spasm of hands and the Chvostek's sign became more easily demonstrable. However these disappeared promptly after the administration of Vigantol. Somewhat later the pain in her thighs, legs and back was also relieved and walking was accomplished without difficulty. Her weight was 42.7 kg during period 34, representing a gain of 6 kg compared with the beginning of the studies. Roentgenologic survey of the skeleton was repeated on April 17 approximately three months after the institution of treatment. The roentgenograms showed definite increase in the density of the bones as compared with that on admission, although a moderate degree of osteoporosis was still present.

COMMENT

From the results presented it seems evident that the principal metabolic abnormality in this patient with osteomalacia is defective absorption of calcium from the intestine. This was inferred from the earlier metabolic studies by Maxwell and his colleagues (20-23), but the marked retention of calcium injected intravenously as shown in the present study seems to offer direct evidence that it is the defective absorption, and not an increased endogenous calcium excretion that is responsible for the decalcification of bones in osteomalacia. That endogenous calcium elimination is not augmented in this patient is further shown by the entirely normal degree of negative balance on minimal intake. Perhaps the absence of calcium in the urine in this patient may be taken as a measure of conserving calcium on the part of the organism, as it can not be correlated with the level of serum calcium which was within normal limits most of the time. However this endogenous calcium excretion, even though conservative, will eventually lead to decalcification of skeleton, if the loss can not be replaced by entrance through the intestinal tract of ingested calcium. This we believe represents the essential pathologic physiology of osteomalacia.

Vitamin D acts in promoting calcium absorption. This is in accord with the observations of various workers on the effects of cod liver oil (26, 27, 29), sunlight and other sources of ultraviolet radiation (17, 18, 24), and irradiated ergosterol (13, 14, 16) in rickets; as well as those of more recent workers on irradiated ergosterol in osteomalacia (5, 8, 11). The fact that after vitamin D administration the patient was able to retain more than 70 percent of a daily intake as low as 220 mg suggests that vitamin D also acts to diminish endogenous calcium elimination, a phenomenon heretofore not emphasized. Both factors contribute to the marked calcium and phosphorus retention and their deposition in the bones. The remarkable effect of vitamin D in favoring calcium retention is in distinct contrast to its relative ineffectiveness in normal individuals (4, 12). Various workers (1, 15, 31) have reported in individuals with rickets receiving vitamin D a change of reaction of stools from alkaline to acid as an explanation of the increased calcium absorption. Bauer and his co-workers (3) found no increase in the acidity of the gastric and pancreatic juices during ergosterol therapy to account for the increased absorption of calcium or the increased acidity of the stool. Our data do not permit any remarks as to the mechanism of action of vitamin D in increasing calcium absorption and decreasing endogenous calcium excretion in osteomalacia.

The prolonged action of vitamin D supplied in small doses and for a limited period is of considerable interest. If a similar case is observed for the first time after previous vitamin D administration (and cases of calcium deficiency are liable to be given such treatment), difficulty may arise as to the interpretation of the conservative calcium and phosphorus balance in the presence of marked deficiency of lime salts in the bones. If the sustained after-effect of vitamin D exhibition as demonstrated in our patient is taken into consideration, this discrepancy can readily be explained. It takes a long time for the bones to become normal, even if the abnormality in calcium and phosphorus metabolism has been corrected. In this connection it is of interest to mention the recent report of Crawford and Cuthbertson (8) on a patient with osteomalacia who showed "amazing capacity for the absorption and retention of calcium and phosphorus" corresponding to "the capacity of a breast-fed child", and practically no response to irradiated ergosterol. In view of the marked differences in metabolic behavior exhibited by this patient as compared with cases of either late rickets or osteomalacia which showed practically no calcium and phosphorus retention with the same "basal diet", the authors preferred to call their case one of hunger osteopathy, indicating mineral starvation and not vitamin D deficiency as the primary cause of the condition. In the light of our results, this may be an ordinary case of osteomalacia in a reparative state initiated possibly by the vitamin D in the "basal diet", or possibly by previous vitamin D administration, although no mention of previous therapy is made in the history.

We have no explanation to offer for the prolonged action of irradiated ergosterol in our patient. Two possibilities suggest themselves. First, the irradiated ergosterol may be stored. We have been unable to find in the literature any information definitely confirming the storage of vitamin D. Beumer (6) gave an infant 400 mg of irradiated ergosterol for a period of 4 days. Within those 4 days and subsequent 5 days, a total of 147 mg of ergosterol was recovered from the stools, and thereafter practically no ergosterol was found in the stools. The balance of ergosterol was considered either stored or destroyed, but in view of the ease with which ergosterol disintegrated, the author favored destruction rather than storage as the more likely explanation. The second possibility, which in our opinion more probably accounts for the prolonged action of irradiated ergosterol, is related to the vitamin D content of the diets served to the patient. The diets given, though low in vitamin content were by no means devoid of vitamin D (Table 1). The minimal amount of vitamin D in the diet, though insufficient to bring about the reparative process, may suffice to maintain normal calcium and phosphorus metabolism as soon as the initial deficiency is made up by irradiated ergosterol therapy.

SUMMARY

1. Data on calcium, phosphorus, and nitrogen metabolism for 34 periods of 4 days each are presented from a case of relatively early osteomalacia in which no vitamin D therapy had been given prior to the studies.

2. The essential metabolic abnormality in this patient is a lack of absorption of calcium through the intestinal tract, there being no increase in endogenous calcium excretion. The absence of calcium in the urine in the presence of approximately normal serum calcium level is taken as evidence of conservation of endogenous calcium elimination.

3. Vitamin D administered in relatively small dosage and for a limited period increased remarkably calcium absorption and decreased endogenous calcium elimination, thus resulting in striking calcium and phosphorus retention and deposition in the bones. The beneficial action of vitamin D was sustained for at least four months after its administration was discontinued.

LITERATURE

1. *Abrahamson, E. M. and Miller, E. G.* Hydrogen-ion concentration in the gastrointestinal tract of the albino rat. Proc. Soc. Exp. Biol. Med., **22**: 438, 1925.

2. *Bauer, W., Albright, F., and Aub, J. C.* Studies of calcium and phosphorus metabolism. II. The calcium excretion of normal individuals on a low calcium diet, also data on a case of pregnancy. J. Clin Invest., **7**: 75, 1929.

3. *Bauer, W., Marble, A., Maddock, S. J., and Wood, J. C.* The effect of irradiated ergosterol on the composition of gastric and pancreatic juices. Am. J. Med. Sci., **181**: 399, 1931

4. *Bauer, W., Marble, A., and Claflin, D.* Studies on the mode of action of irradiated ergosterol. I. Its effect on the calcium, phosphorus and nitrogen metabolism of normal individuals. J. Clin. Invest., **11**: 1, 1932.

5. *Bauer, W., and Marble, A.* Studies on the mode of action of irradiated ergosterol. II. Its effect on the calcium and phosphorus metabolism of individuals with calcium deficiency diseases, J. Clin. Invest., **11**: 21, 1932.

6. *Beumer, H.* Uber den Versuch einer Ergosterinbilanz, Klin. Wchnschr., **6**: 941, 1927.

7. *Clark, E. P. and Collip, J. B.* A study of Tisdall method for the determination of blood serum calcium with a suggested modification. J. Biol. Chem., **63**: 461, 1925.

8. *Crawford, A. M. and Cuthbertson, D. P.* Clinical and biochemical observations on hunger osteopathy, juvenile and late rickets (osteomalacia). Quart. J. Med., **3**: 87, 1934.

9. *Fiske, C. and Subbarow, Y.* The colorimetric determination of phosphorus. J. Biol. Chem., **66**: 375, 1925.

10. *Folin, O. and Wright, L. E.* A simplified Macro-Kjeldahl method for urine. J. Biol. Chem., **38**: 461, 1919.

11. *Gargill, S. L., Gilligan, D. R. and Blumgart, H. L.* Metabolism and treatment of osteomalacia. Arch. Int. Med., **45**: 879, 1930.

12. *Hart, M. C., Tourtellotte, D. and Heyl, F. W.* The effect of irradiation and cod liver oil on the calcium balance in adult human. J. Biol. Chem., **76**: 143, 1928.

13. *Hess, A. F. and Lewis, J. M.* Clinical experience with irradiated ergosterol. J. A. M. A., **91**: 783, 1928.

14. *Hess, A. F.* Rickets including osteomalacia and tetany. Lea and Febiger, Philadelphia, 1929.

15. *Irving, L. and Ferguson, J.* The influence of acidity in the intestine upon the absorption of calcium salts by the blood. Proc. Soc. Exp. Biol. Med., **22**: 527, 1925.

16. *Karelitz, S.* Activated ergosterol in the treatment of rickets. Am. J. Dis. Child., **36**: 1108, 1928.

17. *Kneschke, W.* Blutkalk und Lichtbehandlung der Rachitis. Klin. Wchnschr., **2**: 1935, 1923.

18. *Kramer, B., Casparis, H., and Howland, J.* Ultraviolet radiation in rickets. Effect on the calcium and inorganic phosphorus concentration of the serum. A. J. Dis. Child., **24**: 20, 1922.

19. *Liu, S. H., Chu, H. I., Wang, S. H., and Chung, H. L.* Nutritional edema. I. The effect of the level and quality of protein intake on nitrogen balance, plasma proteins and edema. Chinese J. Physiol., **6**: 73, 1932.

20. *Maxwell, J. P.* Osteomalacia in China, China Med. J., **37**: 625, 1929.

21. *Maxwell, J. P. and Miles, L. M.* Osteomalacia in China. J. Obs. and Gyn. Brit. Emp., **32**: 433, 1925.

22. *Maxwell, J. P.* Further studies in osteomalacia. Proc. Roy. Soc. Med., **23**: 19, 1930.

23. *Miles, L. M. and Feng, C. T.* Calcium and phosphorus metabolism in osteomalacia. J. Exp. Med., **41**: 137, 1925.

24. *Orr, W. J., Holt, L. E., Wilkins, L., and Boone, F. H.* The calcium and phosphorus metabolism in rickets, with special reference to ultraviolet ray therapy. Am. J. Dis. Child., **26**: 362, 1923.

25. *Roseberry, H. H., Hastings, A. B., and Morse, J. K.* X-ray analysis of bone and teeth. J. Biol. Chem., **90**: 395, 1931.

26. *Schabad, J. A.* Die Behandlung der Rachitis mit Lebertran, Phosphor und Kalk. Ihr Einfluss auf den Kalk u..d Phosphor-stoffwechsel bei Rachitis. Ztschr. klin. Med., **68**: 94, 1909.

27. *Sjollema, B.* Studies in inorganic metabolism. I. The influence of cod liver oil upon calcium and phosphorus metabolism. J. Biol. Chem., **57**: 255, 1923.

28. *Shohl, A. T. and Pedley, F. G.* A rapid and accurate method for calcium in urine. J. Biol. Chem., **50**: 537, 1922.

29. *Telfer, S. V.* Studies on calcium and phosphorus metabolism. Part V. Infantile rickets. The excretion and absorption of the mineral elements and the influence of fats in the diet on mineral absorption. Quart. J. Med., **20**: 7, 1926-27.

30. *Wu, H.* Nutritive value of Chinese foods. Chinese J. Physiol., R. S. **1**: 153, 1928.

31. *Zucker, T. F. and Matzner, M. J.* On the pharmacological action of the antirachitic active principle of cod liver oil. Proc. Soc. Exp. Biol. Med. **21**: 186, 1924.

THE
CHINESE MEDICAL JOURNAL

VOLUME 49   JANUARY 1935   NUMBER 1

CALCIUM AND PHOSPHORUS METABOLISM IN OSTEOMALACIA

II. FURTHER STUDIES ON THE RESPONSE TO VITAMIN D OF PATIENTS WITH OSTEOMALACIA

S.H. LIU, R.R. HANNON, H.I. CHU, K.C. CHEN, S.K. CHOU, AND S.H. WANG

Department of Medicine, Peiping Union Medical College, Peiping.

In a previous communication (1), the data of a patient with relatively early osteomalacia were presented, showing very striking and prolonged response to the corrective influence of vitamin D in calcium and phosphorus metabolism. Since then we have studied four other patients with osteomalacia whose clinical features were more complicated, and whose response to vitamin D therapy showed further points of interest. It seems worthwhile to report these cases for comparison. The methods employed in the metabolism ward and laboratory are the same as those given in our previous paper.

CASE 1. ADVANCED OSTEOMALACIA. TETANY. PREGNANCY.
COMPLICATED CATARACT. CHRONIC NEPHRITIS.

Mrs. C. T. L., a Chinese woman of 24, para 3, about 8 months pregnant, was admitted to the Obstetrical Service December 26, 1932 for spastic attacks of extremities, blurring of vision and swelling of legs. In January 1928 she gave birth to her first child. The confinement and parturition were normal, but a month after delivery she was taken ill with fever, diplopia and blurring of vision, followed by attacks of generalized muscular spasm. Fever subsided after 5 or 6 days, but the spastic attacks recurred daily for a month and occasionally for the following two years. Her second pregnancy was complicated during its later months by blurring of vision and swelling of legs, and was terminated in January 1931 by prolonged labor and stillbirth. In addition to severe spastic attacks, she sustained a fracture of her left femur. This resulted in her confinement to bed for two months before she could get up and walk with a limp. Her present pregnancy was uneventful until two months prior to admission when the same train of symptoms began to recur.

Her diet consisted of rice, noodles, and vegetables in season such as pai-ts'ai, spinach, celery, beans, and bean-curd. Rarely were meat and eggs taken. Appetite poor. She had little chance to get out into the sunshine.

On examination the patient was found to be undernourished and in discomfort. Both lower extremities were flexed at hip and knee-joints and could not be straightened out without causing pain. Adductor muscles in spasm and all the bones tender to touch. Both Chvostek's and Trousseau's signs strongly positive. Irritability to galvanic stimulation increased in facial and ulnar nerves. Both lenses cataractous with spokes and patches in the cortical and central parts. Both fundi indistinct on account of lenticular opacities; disks hyperemic with peripapillary edema; retinal vessels normal. Lungs and heart normal. B.P. 96/72. Abdomen enlarged to about eight months' pregnancy. Fetus in L.S.A. position; heart rate 140. Pelvis and sacrum distorted with rostration of pubis. Pelvic measurements as follows: interspinous 22.5 cm, intercristal 26.5 cm, external conjugate 19 cm, and transverse outlet 7 cm.

Roentgenologic survey of skeleton showed generalized osteoporosis and coarse trabeculation. The pelvic bones were markedly deformed on the right side with ilium, pubis, and ischium crushed inward and upward. Pathological fractures of right pubis, ischium, and femur were present.

Blood hemoglobin 11 gm and R.B.C. 3.5 millions. Serum calcium 3.8 and inorganic phosphorus 3.9 mg per cent. Serum phosphatase 0.42 units. Blood N.P.N. 20 and uric acid 3.7 mg per cent. Serum albumin 2.52 and globulin 2.15 per cent. Urine contained one plus albumin, some W.B.C. and occasional hyaline casts. Phenolsulphonphthalein excretion 65 per cent in two hours. Urea clearance approximately 50 per cent of normal.

Metabolic Study 1. Through the courtesy of Dr. J. P. Maxwell, the patient was transferred to Metabolism Ward, where the first series of studies covering 5 periods of 3 days each was carried out. As shown in Table 1 and Fig. 1, during the first two periods on a minimal calcium intake of 76 mg, and during the third period on a moderate intake of 533 mg daily, the balance was negative, on the average -132 and -50 mg respectively. The fourth and fifth periods on high calcium intake of 1805 mg a day exhibited a positive balance of 172 mg, less than 10 per cent of the intake, the remainder being eliminated entirely through the stool. The very slight calcium retention on high intake in presence of extensive decalcification seems characteristic of active osteomalacia. Phosphorus balance remained slightly positive throughout, and could be accounted for by the positive nitrogen balance. Serum calcium fluctuated between 2.9 and 3.8, and inorganic phosphorus between 4.5 and 3.8 mg per cent. There was slight clinical improvement in that muscular spasms became less frequent and bone pains less severe.

In view of the poor retention of calcium, in spite of large amounts given orally, it was of interest to administer calcium intravenously. On January 13, 20 cc of sterile 20 per cent solution of calcium gluconate of pH 7.1 were given through the cubital vein. An hour later the patient began to have chills followed by fever, palpitation of heart, epigastric distress, nausea and vomiting, abdominal pain, and diarrhea. Skin hot and flushed. B.P. 74/46. Adrenalin and digipuratum hypodermically gave some relief and the acute reaction subsided in 6 hours. The uterus, however, was strongly contracted and fetal heart could not be heard. A Caesarean section was done in the evening by Dr. J. P. Maxwell, using novocaine, gas and oxygen. The uterus was in a state of tonic contraction, and on opening the organ, amniotic fluid spurted out to a height of 2 to 3 feet. A dead male child was extracted by the breech. This on X-ray examination showed fetal rickets. After operation she developed

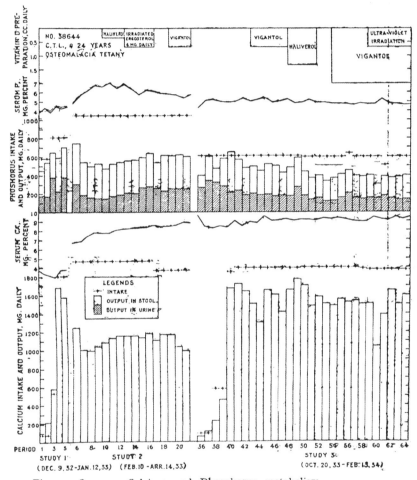

Fig. 1. Case 1. Calcium and Phosphorus metabolism.

bronchopneumonia with fever and cough, lasting for two weeks, after which she slowly convalesced. On February 8, about 4 weeks after operation she was transferred again to Metabolism Ward for further studies.

Metabolic Study 2. While on the Obstetrical Service the patient received in addition to liberal diet and calcium lactate, 15 drops of Haliverol daily from January 14 to 28, and 20 cc of cod liver oil and 2 mg of Irradiated Ergosterol daily from January 29 to February 8. On January 28, serum calcium

4 THE CHINESE MEDICAL JOURNAL

TABLE I.

CASE I. *Data on calcium and phosphorus metabolism and the effect of vitamin D*

Date	Period	Average daily calcium				Average daily phosphorus				Serum*		Treatment†
		Intake mg	Urine mg	Stool mg	Balance mg	Intake mg	Urine mg	Stool mg	Balance mg	Ca mg per cent	P mg per cent	
1932					*Study 1*							
Dec. 29	1- 2	78	2	209	− 133	583	177	319	+ 87	3.8 3.1	3.9 3.8	
1933												
Jan. 4	3	553	0	583	− 50	812	382	269	+ 161	2.9	4.5	
Jan. 7	4- 5	1805	0	1579	+ 171	912	304	340	+ 168	3.7 3.8	4.3 4.5	
					Study 2							
Feb. 10	6- 9	1969	0	1074	+ 895	1048	202	376	+ 470	6.7 7.8	4.8 6.8	
Feb. 26	10-12	1969	0	1126	+ 843	1048	168	346	+ 534	7.7 8.2	7.0 6.9	Haliverol 15 drops daily
Mar. 10	13-16	1969	0	1085	+ 884	1048	240	347	+ 461	8.2 8.6	6.4 6.1	Irradiated Ergosterol 4 mg daily
Mar. 26	17-18	1869	1	1139	+ 729	1048	248	329	+ 471	8.4 8.5	5.9 5.7	Vigantol 30 drops daily
Apr. 3	19-21	1869	0	1068	+ 801	1048	256	358	+ 434	8.8	5.4	
					Study 3							
Oct. 21	36-37	92	0	86	+ 6	608	308	196	+ 104	9.6 8.2	4.3 5.2	

Date										Regimen
Oct. 29	578	0	344	+ 234	608	306	225	+ 77	8.5 / 5.0	
									8.3 / 4.9	
Nov 6	1876	1	1644	+ 231	608	215	355	+ 36	9.0 / 5.0	Vigantol 30 drops daily
									8.9 / 5.1	
Nov 18	1892	2	1494	+ 396	598	191	291	+ 126	8.8 / 5.2	Haliverol 60 drops daily
									9.2 / 5.3	
Dec. 8	1895	0	1650	+ 245	603	174	278	ɿ 151	9.1 / 4.8	
									9.1 / 4.9	
Dec. 24	1898	0	1543	+ 355	598	139	231	+ 228	9.3 / 4.9	
									9.2 / 4.8	
1934 Jan. 1	1898	0	1520	+ 378	606	160	245	+ 201	9.4 / 4.9	Vigantol 90 drops daily
									9.0 / 4.8	
Jan. 21	1862	0	1448	+ 414	583	154	223	+ 206	9.5 / 4.7	Vigantol 90 drops daily + ultraviolet radiation
									9.5 / 4.7	

*Values at beginning and end of each regimen.
†Haliverol, Parke, Davis, contains halibut liver oil with Irradol—250 D. 1 cc=45 drops.
‡Irradiated Ergosterol Burroughs Wellcome & Co., in mg. tablets.
*Vigantol, E. Merck contains irradiated ergosterol in oil. 1 cc (45 drops) equivalent to 5000 rat units.

was 4.2, and inorganic phosphorus 2.9 mg per cent. These values increased to 6.7 and 4.8 respectively on February 10, when the second series of metabolic studies was commenced. This consisted of 16 consecutive periods of 4 days each on a constant diet with added calcium lactate. Calcium intake 1969 mg and phosphorus intake 1048 mg daily. The first four periods (periods 6 to 9) without added vitamin D gave an average daily positive balance of 895 mg calcium and 470 mg phosphorus. This represents retention of 45 per cent of the intake and a marked improvement over the 10 per cent retention during periods 4 and 5. The improvement was undoubtedly related to the vitamin D that the patient received during the interval, although the termination of pregnancy may have played a minor role. Serum calcium rose to 7.7 and inorganic phosphorus to 6.6 mg per cent within the 4 control periods. During the following 12 periods, Haliverol, Irradiated Ergosterol, and Vigantol were administered in succession without making any difference in the calcium and phosphorus balance which had already attained a satisfactory level during the control periods. Serum calcium, however, continued to rise slowly to a maximum of 8.8 mg per cent during the last period, and inorganic phosphorus fluctuated between 7.0 and 5.4 mg per cent.

By this time the clinical condition was very much improved. The patient gained weight and was able to be up and about. Chvostek's and Trousseau's signs had been negative for some time. Radiograms of skeleton in April 1933 showed increased density of all the bones with callus formation in the previous fractures of right femur and pelvic bones, although compared with those of a normal person of her age and sex taken on the same films at the same time, the bones were still deficient in lime salts. Patient was discharged to her home June 12, 1933.

Metabolic Study 3. The patient returned October 18, 1933 after spending the summer in the country. She was doing well. Further improvement was noticeable particularly in two directions. First, radiograms made at this time showed more calcium deposition than those made in April, although slight osteoporosis was still present in comparison with a normal person. Second, vision in both eyes was very much improved. Both lenses were clearer than before, although some lenticular opacities were denser. Her renal condition remained stationary. Although there were no symptoms referable to any renal disease, she continued to excrete a faint trace of albumin and a slightly higher number of casts in sediment counts according to Addis' technic, and urea clearance was consistently approximately 50 per cent of normal.

Her metabolic behaviour on minimal calcium intake of 92 mg (periods 36 and 37), and on moderate calcium intake of 578 mg (periods 38 and 39) showed good conservation in that a positive balance was maintained. However, when placed on a high calcium intake of 1876 mg (periods 40 and 42), she retained only 231 mg approximately 12 per cent of the intake. Subsequent intensive vitamin D therapy did not make much difference in the calcium balance, although Vigantol administration alone or in combination with ultraviolet radiation (periods 43-47, 54-58, 59-64) led to higher calcium retention than during the control periods (periods 40-42) and the Haliverol periods (periods 48-51). Therefore, the relatively poor retention of calcium during Metabolic Study 3 probably was not related to depletion of vitamin D after a lapse of several months, but was a matter of lessened demand on the part of the steadily replenished skeletal store as shown by roentgenologic examinations. Whether latent chronic nephritis had anything to do with her poor calcium retention during the later periods remains an open question. Serum calcium stayed between 9.0 and

9.5 mg per cent; and inorganic phosphorus between 4.3 and 5.4 mg per cent. Roentgenologic examination of skeleton in May 1934 showed further improvement so that all the bone now appeared approximately normal in density and texture.

Comments. This patient is an illustration of advanced osteomalacia with striking hypocalcemia. Tetany and cataract are probably the results of hypocalcemia. Pregnancy and chronic nephritis are aggravating factors. It is remarkable that this patient made an almost complete recovery after a severe and stormy course of events. After the termination of pregnancy and institution of vitamin D and high calcium therapy, clinical improvement and disappearance of hypocalcemia and tetany were fairly prompt. The skeletal system was sufficiently replenished in lime salts to approach normal in a year and half.

The metabolic studies on this patient reveal the following points of interest:

(1) Like low-calcium rickets, osteomalacia may be accompanied by hypocalcemia. The hypocalcemia may be of extreme degree with severe tetany and cataract.

(2) The metabolic defects in osteomalacia consist of lack of conservation of calcium on minimal or moderate intake and poor retention on high intake, so that in presence of low intake, to which these patients are often subjected in view of their limited diets, they will lose calcium. If calcium loss is maintained sufficiently long, osteomalacia inevitably follows. Lack of absorption of ingested calcium has been shown in a previous paper (1) to be the principal cause of the metabolic defects.

(3) Such defects are readily amenable to vitamin D therapy. While vitamin D is operative, balance is maintained even on minimal intake, and large amounts are retained on high intake so that the bony stores are made up.

(4) The low serum calcium is slowly, but steadily, raised to normal as the bony stores are replenished under vitamin D therapy.

(5) The action of vitamin D appears to be maximal in ordinary therapeutic doses, and further addition does not seem to exert any additive effect.

(6) Its action is prolonged and a course of vitamin D in therapeutic doses may be expected to exert its influence at least for several months under the conditions of our studies.

(7) As the demand of the bony stores for replenishment, decreases calcium retention also decreases in spite of large vitamin D intake.

CASE 2. MILD OSTEOMALACIA. TETANY. PREGNANCY. COMPLICATED CATARACT. ACUTE BACILLUS COLI CYSTITIS AND PYELITIS. ACUTE BACILLARY DYSENTERY SHIGA. VITAMIN B DEFICIENCY.

Mrs. W. C. C., a Chinese housewife of 25, was admitted on March 4, 1933 to the Obstetrical Ward for pregnancy and "convulsions." For 5 years previously she had been subject to spastic attacks coming on at intervals of several months and usually after some emotional upset. Such attacks consisted of tonic muscular contractions, starting from the extremities and spreading to the whole body, lasting for several hours, and leaving her weak and numb for several days afterwards. She had her first and second pregnancies in 1930 and 1932 respectively, both of which miscarried at 5 or 6 months. Her third and present pregnancy of approximately 7 months' duration was uneventful until three weeks prior to admission when she again began to suffer from spastic attacks. These were more frequent and lasted longer than before, with numbness all the time.

Routine diet at home consisted of 6 oz of flour, 4 oz of rice and a few vegetables (chiefly *pai-ts'ai* and spinach) cooked in sesame oil. Such a diet gave approximately 32 gm of protein, 23 gm of fat and 230 gm of carbohydrate with 1200 calories; calcium 0.25 gm and phosphorus 1.00 gm practically no vitamin D.

General appearance: undernourished, prostrated and sick-looking. Cough frequent and voice hoarse. Active Chvostek's and Trousseau's signs. Galvanic stimulation of facial, ulnar and peroneal nerves showed marked hyperexcitability. Vision normal, but fundi hyperemic; apparently associated with lenticular opacities demonstrable on slit-lamp examination. Lips fissured at corners. Tongue raw and red with many prominent papillae, and irregular patches of superficial ulceration. Pyorrhea alveolaris marked. Submaxillary and submental lymph-nodes palpably enlarged. Lungs and heart normal. B.P. 82/50. Abdomen enlarged by pregnant uterus which came up 24 cm above symphysis pubis. Fetus in R.O.A. position; heart rate 144. All tendon reflexes absent and vibratory sensation diminished over the right lower leg. No bony deformities or tenderness on pressure. Pelvic measurements: interspinous 21, intercristal 25, external conjugate 17.5, and transverse outlet 9-10 cm.

Urine contained one plus protein with numerous W.B.C. and yielded B. Coli on culture. Blood showed slight anemia with 11 gm hemoglobin, and 3.8 millions R.B.C. Serum calcium 3.0, and inorganic phosphorus 3.4 mg per cent. Phosphatase 0.13 unit. Plasma N.P.N. 17 mg per cent, albumin 2.52, and globulin 3.69 per cent. On X-ray examination the long bones, spine and pelvis showed slight osteoporosis, but no deformities or fractures.

Metabolic Study. After admission the patient felt more comfortable and the glossitis disappeared rapidly, but tetanic attacks kept recurring. She was transferred to Metabolism Ward and studies commenced on March 10. The first four periods were devoted to a study of the effects of parathyroid therapy, hypophosphite being excreted as such through the urine, in conformity with the present communication. It may be mentioned that during periods 2 and 3 small doses of parathormone were given with definite relief of symptoms, but without marked changes in serum calcium or phosphorus.

METABOLISM IN OSTEOMALACIA 9

The data from periods 5 to 11 are presented in Table 2 and Figure 2. During period 5 on a calcium intake of 1162 mg and phosphorus intake of 706 mg per day, the patient retained only 134 mg of calcium, approximately 12 per cent of the intake, and lost small amounts of phosphorus. Period 6 was different from period 5 in that the phosphorus intake was raised to 1254 mg through the addition of a mixture of hypophosphites. This made no significant

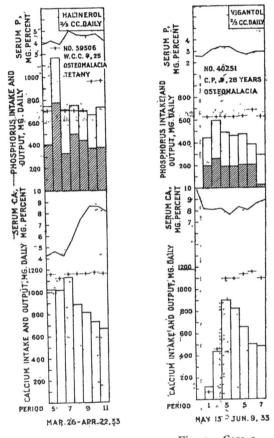

Fig. 2. Case 2. Fig. 3. Case 3.

Calcium and phosphorus metabolism.

difference to either calcium or phosphorus balance, almost the entire amount of hypophosphite being excreted as such through the urine, in conformity with the results of Marriott (2) and Shelling (3). In periods 7 to 11, the patient received daily 30 drops of Haliverol. Serum calcium rose from 4.2 to 8.6 mg per cent within the 12 days of Haliverol administration, but its beneficial effect on calcium retention was not evident until the second period. From then on there was a

TABLE 2.

Case 2. Data on calcium and phosphorus metabolism and the effect of vitamin D

Date 1933	Period	Average daily calcium				Average daily phosphorus				Serum		Treatment
		Intake	Urine	Stool	Balance	Intake	Urine	Stool	Balance	Ca	P	
		mg	mg	mg	mg	mg	mg	mg	mg	mg per cent	mg per cent	
Mar. 26	5	1162	2	1026	+ 134	706	410	338	− 42	4.2	3.8	
30	6	1127	6	1013	+ 108	1254	776	392	+ 86	4.6	4.2	⎫ Hypophosphite
Apr. 3	7	1162	2	1131	+ 29	706	331	381	− 6	4.2	3.9	⎬ P = 548 mg
7	8	1162	0	888	+ 274	706	501	253	± 48	5.7	5.0	⎭
11	9	1162	0	814	+ 348	706	444	256	+ 6	7.5	4.6	⎫ Haliverol 30
15	10	1173	0	730	+ 443	961	371	296	+ 294	8.6	4.6	⎬ drops daily
19	11	1159	11	668	+ 480	965	380	352	+ 232	8.6	4.7	⎭

slight but steady increase in calcium retention so that during period 11, the maximum amount of calcium retained was 480 mg about 41 per cent of the intake. Though not strictly comparable, the rise in serum calcium in this patient was much more rapid than in Case 1, while the increase in calcium balance was not as marked. Serum inorganic phosphorus was raised somewhat, and phosphorus balance remained even during the first three periods of Haliverol therapy and moderately positive during the last two periods.

The last two periods of study were complicated by daily remittent fever with pain and tenderness in right lumbar region. Urine contained less W.B C. than before. It was believed that the patient was suffering from pyelitis with obstruction on the right ureter presumably on account of pressure due to the gravid uterus. After the institution of hexylresorcinol and the knee-chest position, fever began to subside. Before the fever entirely disappeared, dysentery developed, whereupon the metabolic studies had to be discontinued. Stool cultures positive for the dysentery bacillus of Shiga. With dietary and sodium sulphate therapy, the enteric disturbance cleared up in about 10 days. After that the patient remained fairly well and was given 2 mg Irradiated Ergosterol a day.

The pelvis was measured again on May 14, and all measurements remained about the same except the transverse outlet which decreased from 9-10 cm to 6 cm. X-ray examination of pelvis, however, demonstrated no appreciable changes from that of March. On May 25, very near to the expected date, the patient started to have labor pains. Caesarean section was immediately performed by Dr. J. P. Maxwell. A full term normal male child was delivered. The post-operative course was smooth. On July 4 serum calcium was 9.8 and inorganic phosphorus 5.8 per cent. The patient was discharged in good condition on July 10, 1933.

Comment. As was the preceding patient, this is an instance of osteomalacia with pronounced hypocalcemia giving rise to tetany and lenticular opacities. But the absence of marked decalcification and deformities suggests mild or early osteomalacia, although the underlying pathologic physiology of poor calcium conservation is distinctly evident. Besides the complicating factors of pregnancy, urinary tract infection and dysentery, the findings of glossitis, absence of tendon reflexes and diminution of vibratory sense point to vitamin B deficiency, a condition not at all unlikely to be present in view of the frequency of multiple dietary deficiencies. The study of this patient in regard to her response to vitamin D seems to give the following additional information.

(8) In a patient with mild osteomalacia, but with severe hypocalcemia, the rise of serum calcium in response to vitamin D therapy is marked and rapid.

(9) In such a patient the increase in calcium retention, though appreciable, may not be very striking.

CASE 3. ADVANCED OSTEOMALACIA. BACILLARY DYSENTERY, M. F. GROUP.

Mrs. C. P., a Chinese married woman of 28 entered on May 9, 1933 for dull aching pain in the back and lower extremities. Seven years prior to admission while pregnant for the first time, she began to notice pain in the right hip, but it was slight and inconstant, and did not interfere with the delivery which was normal. Since then similar pain had recurred and lasted 3 to 6 months every winter, disappearing with the onset of summer. Two and half years later her second pregnancy began, the later months of which, being in the winter, were accompanied by pain in the back and lower extremities. The pain was considerably disabling, so that she was confined to bed; but again the delivery of her child was attended with no unusual difficulty. Summer came and her symptoms gradually disappeared, but with the onset of winter, all the previous trouble began again with increasing severity. Pain was exaggerated by motion, such as walking, stooping, or changing position in bed. As a result, she sat in bed most of the time working with her hands. Marital relations became difficult. For the last two years there had been general weakness, loss of flesh, and shortening of stature.

The patient's living conditions were unsatisfactory. Apparently she subsisted on approximately 8 oz of cornmeal a day with a little vegetable cooked in sesame oil. Eight ounces of cornmeal contain about 22 gm protein, 2 gm fat, 187 gm carbohydrate, 0.048 gm calcium, and 0.458 gm phosphorus.

On examination the patient appeared undernourished and fairly comfortable, lying on her left side with spine and legs flexed. Standing height 132 cm, sitting height 69 cm, weight 29 kg. Spinal column kyphotic in the thoracic region and markedly lordotic in the lumbo-sacral region. Thoracic cage barrel-shaped with widening at the base. Pelvis extensively rostrated so that the iliac crests were pushed upward and flattened out, and symphysis pubis became prominent. The distance between costal margin and iliac crest was shortened to about 1 cm. Pelvic measurements: interspinous 5, intercristal 24, external conjugate 17.5 and transverse outlet 2 cm. Bones of the extremities not deformed. With the exception of the skull, all the bones were tender on pressure. No evidence of tetany.

Routine urine and blood examinations essentially normal. Serum calcium 9.9, and inorganic phosphorus 2.6 mg per cent. Plasma phosphatase 0.21 unit. Plasma N.P.N. 16 mg per cent, albumin 3.12, and globulin 1.97 per cent.

Roentgenologic survey of skeleton showed varying degrees of osteoporosis in various bones, especially marked decalcification being evident in the spine, pelvis, and long bones. All the vertebral bodies were markedly concave on their superior and inferior surfaces. The pelvis was funnel-shaped and its outlet narrowed. The cortices of the long bones were thin. Fractures were noted in both ulnae, tibiae, fibulae, and left 7th and 8th ribs near the axillary region.

Metabolic Study. The first series of studies lasted 7 periods of 4 days each (Table 3 and Figure 3). The calcium balance on a low intake of 71 mg was slightly negative, and that on a moderate intake of 462 mg was almost even. While on a high intake of 1096 mg she gained only 197 mg, or 18 per cent of the intake. With calcium intake kept at the high level, the patient was given Vigantol 30 drops daily for the remaining four periods. The beneficial effect of Vigantol in promoting calcium gain was noticeable during the first period of its exhibition, and more so with each succeeding period. During the last period calcium retention amounted to 716 mg daily, or 65 per cent of the intake. Phosphorus balance in general corresponded with calcium balance.

TABLE 3

Case 3. Data on calcium and phosphorus metabolism and the effect of vitamin-D

Date of 1933	Period	Average daily calcium				Average daily phosphorus				Serum		Treatment
		Intake	Urine	Stool	Balance	Intake	Urine	Stool	Balance	Ca	P	
		mg	mg	mg	mg	mg	mg	mg	mg	mg per cent	mg per cent	
May 13	1	71	2	112	− 43	627	200	246	+ 181	8.2	2.6	
17	2	462	0	436	+ 26	627	262	335	+ 30	8.1	3.2	
21	3	1096	5	894	+ 197	627	192	301	+ 134	8.2	3.4	
25	4	1096	4	818	+ 274	627	191	270	+ 166	7.6	3.4	
29	5	1135	0	655	+ 480	633	207	269	+ 157	8.3	3.0	
June 2	6	1156	0	399	+ 757	687	207	189	+ 300	8.0	2.7	Vigantol 30 drops daily
6	7	1096	0	380	+ 716	627	27	268	+ 332	8.6	2.9	

Serum calcium came down from 9.9 on admission to 7.6 mg per cent at the end of period 3, while inorganic phosphorus went up from 2.6 to 3.4 mg per cent during the same interval, apparently in association with the low calcium and relatively high phosphorus intake. The period with lowered serum calcium was marked by slightly positive Chvostek's and Trousseau's signs. Signs of latent tetany disappeared after Vigantol medication, coinciding with a tendency of serum calcium to increase and of inorganic phosphorus to decrease.

During period 5 patient had a mild attack of dysentery with 5 to 10 stools a day, but without much systemic disturbance. Rectal swab positive for *B. dysenteriae*, mannite-fermenting group. With a change of diet to softer form and administration of sodium sulphate solution, dysentery cleared up in 4 to 5 days.

At the expiration of the first series of metabolic studies, patient was transferred to a general medical ward where she remained from June 11 to September 18, receiving a full diet, calcium 1 gm (calcium lactate 7.7 gm) and cod liver oil 45 cc daily. On the latter date her standing height had increased to 134 cm and weight to 39.5 kg. Serum calcium 10.0, and inorganic phosphorus 4.4 mg per cent. Radiograms made in September showed healing of all the fractures. The ribs became normal in density, and spine, pelvis and long bones appeared much less porous than before. General improvement was likewise great. Bones were no longer tender and the patient was able to walk about freely.

From September 18, 1933 to May 24, 1934 patient underwent another series of metabolic observations, the results of which will appear in a separate communication. All this time she remained in good condition. Roentgenologic examination on discharge showed a normal skeleton except for the deformities of spine and pelvis and thining of cortices of long bones. Standing height 135 cm, sitting height 68.5 cm, and weight 40.6 kg.

Comments. This is apparently a frank case of osteomalacia with relatively few complications, but the process must be very far-advanced to give rise as it did to extensive skeletal decalcification with marked pelvic and spinal deformities and shortening of stature. The metabolic abnormality was similar to that of the preceding cases, but in this instance serum calcium was within normal limits, while inorganic phosphorus was low. A diet low in calcium and high in phosphorus for a short time seemed capable of raising the serum inorganic phosphorus and depressing the serum calcium sufficiently to produce latent tetany.

The susceptibility of serum calcium and phosphorus to change under the influence of such dietary manipulations suggests that the hypocalcemia of Cases 1 and 2 may be related to the low calcium and high phosphorus content of their previous diets, as in the experimental production of rickets in rats (4). But it is difficult to explain the normal serum calcium and low inorganic phosphorus in the present patient on the same basis, as the nature of the mineral deficiency (low calcium) in the diet is apparently the same in all these instances. It seems possible that the parathyroid glands of different individuals may react differently toward the serum calcium-lowering effect of vitamin D deficiency. In the first two cases the parathyroids may have failed to respond, allowing hypocalcemia to be manifest; while in the present as well as in the following case they may be sufficiently active to maintain serum calcium at a normal level in the face of calcium shortage. While the biochemical criteria for clinical hyper- and hypo-parathyroidism are well defined (5, 6) and absent here, there is at present no available method to gauge subclinical deviation of para-thyroid function; and so the role that the parathyroid glands may play in influencing the level of serum calcium and phosphorus in vitamin D deficiency is as yet problematical.

The response of this patient to vitamin D therapy was particularly prompt and marked in regard to calcium and phosphorus balance, but not in regard to serum inorganic phosphorus. The progress of this patient as followed for a year was gratifying. It seemed that she might regain stature.

In the metabolic study of this patient the following additional points seem worth recording:

(10) As in rickets uncomplicated by tetany, active osteomalacia may be accompanied by normal serum calcium, but low inorganic phosphorus.

(11) In such a patient, serum calcium and phosphorus seem relatively labile in that the former may be depressed and latter raised by a low calcium and high phosphorus diet.

(12) Administration of vitamin D bring about very prompt and marked increase in calcium and phosphorus retention.

(13) Changes in serum calcium and phosphorus, however, may be slight with vitamin D therapy.

CASE 4. ADANCED OSTEOMALACIA

Mrs. Y.W.L., a Chinese woman of 42 was brought to the hospital on October 27, 1933 for pain in the bones and debility of three years' duration. In July 1930 she gave birth spontaneously to her fourth child. Three weeks later an attack of dysentery was followed by dull aching pain in lower limbs and back. It became worse during the winter and made her stay in bed for four months before she could get up and walk about with support. After that pain recurred every winter with great regularity and necessitated her confinement in bed for 4 to 6 months. During the winter of 1932-1933 not only the back and lower extremities, but also the chest, shoulders and arms were affected; and slight movements in bed could not be accomplished without excruciating pain. She preferred to lie on her left side. The condition persisted to a lesser degree throughout the summer up to admission. Marked weakness and impairment of appetite. Deformity of spine and pain on marital intercourse were noticed.

Past illnesses of note were amputation of left leg in 1914 on account of tuberculosis of ankle, excision of tuberculous lymph glands of neck in 1915, and traumatic injury of left eye in 1921, resulting in blindness of that eye.

Her diets were deficient, consisting of 2 ounces of flour, and 6-7 ounces of rice with some cabbage cooked in sesame oil. By approximation, such a diet contains 25 gm protein, 12 gm fat, 208 gm carbohydrate, 0.16 gm calcium, and 0.56 gm phosphorus. Caloric intake 1140.

On examination the patient looked emaciated and miserable, and complained of pain even on gentle touching of her trunk and extremities. Spine deformed with marked kyphosis in thoracic region and lordosis at lumbo-sacral junction. Chest barrel-shaped with protruding sternum, and somewhat asymmetrical with depression of left lower portion. Pelvis rostrated with prominent symphysis pubis and marked narrowing of transverse outlet. Left leg absent below the upper third. Eyes no cataract, but trachoma, phlyctenular keratitis and paralysis of abducens nerve, O. U.; macula of cornea, myopia and presbyopia, O.D.; cyst of upper lid and optic atrophy, O.S. Heart and lungs normal. B.P. 90/60. Examination for neuromuscular irritability showed slightly positive Chvostek's but negative Trousseau's and Erb's signs.

Routine examinations of urine, blood and stool negative. Serum calcium 8.8 mg per cent and inorganic phosphate 2.2 mg per cent.

Radiograms of all the bones showed marked decalcification. Intercostal spaces on the left side narrowed, and the 4th, 5th, and 6th ribs fractured at the posterior portions. Pelvic bones deformed and outlet narrowed. Scoliosis of thoracic and lumbar spine with convexity toward right side and increased concavity of sacrum. Vertebral bodies biconcave with widening of intervertebral spaces. Long bones markedly rarefied with coarse trabeculation and thin cortices. Both ulnae fractured.

Metabolic Studies. Before studies were begun the patient received a total of 110 cc of cod liver oil and 3 mg Irradiated Ergosterol in the 4 days of October 28-31. Balance experiments were started on November 2, 1933 and ended on June 6, 1934. The data on the first 22 periods concerning the response of the patient to various levels of calcium intake and vitamin D are presented in Table 4 and Figure 4; those of the second part will be reported in a later paper. During the first four periods on minimal calcium intake of 58-77 mg per day, the patient lost calcium for the first two periods, but was able to maintain balance for the second two periods, showing good conservation. In periods 5 to 10, calcium intake was successively augmented by calcium lactate; and each addition elicited an increase in calcium balance so that on an intake of 1581 mg (periods 9 and 10), 618 mg, or 39 per cent, were retained. The ability to retain satisfactory amounts of calcium on high intake and to maintain balance on minimal intake represents a reparative stage of osteomalacia undoubtedly initiated by the small amount of vitamin D in the cod liver oil and Irradiated Ergosterol given prior to the studies. Such a small amount of vitamin D, though having a distinctly appreciable effect on calcium metabolism, was not sufficient to produce the best performance of which the patient was capable, as seen from the following observations.

METABOLISM IN OSTEOMALACIA.

During periods 11 to 22 calcium intake remained the same as in periods 9 and 10, but phosphorus intake was raised so that Ca : P ratio in the intake was nearly 2 : 1. Periods 11 and 12 served as a control in which calcium retention amounted to 408 mg per day, or 26 per cent of the intake. Vigantol 1 cc daily was given for the subsequent 10 periods. The effect of Vigantol in increasing calcium retention became plainly visible from the 4th period of its administration so that during periods 16 to 22, the average daily calcium retention amount

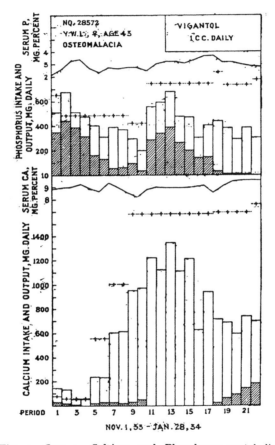

Fig. 4. Case 4. Calcium and Phosphorus metabolism.

ed to 897 mg or about 57 per cent of the intake. This probably represents the maximal effect of therapeutic doses of vitamin D on this patient with the given level of intake.

In contrast to what happened in the preceding cases, calcium appeared in the urine in small amounts during most of the periods, and increased gradually with the administration of Vigantol. During the last period urinary calcium amounted to 184 mg daily, or 26 per cent of the total excretion.

TABLE 4.

Case 4. Data on calcium and phosphorus metabolism and the effect of vitamin D

Date 1933-34	Period	Average daily calcium				Average daily phosphorus				Serum		Treatment
		Intake	Urine	Stool	Balance	Intake	Urine	Stool	Balance	Ca	P	
		mg	mg	mg	mg	mg	mg	mg	mg	mg per cent	mg per cent	
Nov. 2	1	77	28	118	− 69	651	348	164	+ 139	8.8	2.2	
6	2	58	17	116	− 75	488	440	238	− 190	9.0	2.6	
10	3	58	8	48	+ 2	488	387	124	− 23	9.0	3.2	
14	4	58	1	54	+ 3	488	314	163	+ 11	9.2	3.4	
18	5	558	20	220	+ 318	488	163	240	+ 85	8.9	2.7	
22	6	558	27	209	+ 322	488	131	180	+ 177	8.6	2.4	
26	7	1008	28	576	+ 404	488	56	336	+ 96	9.4	2.7	
30	8	1008	19	594	+ 395	488	63	307	+ 118	9.0	2.6	
Dec. 4	9	1581	32	920	+ 629	422	96	201	+ 125	8.5	2.7	
8	10	1581	48	926	+ 607	422	37	164	+ 221	8.2	2.7	
12	11	1581	0	1222	+ 359	747	288	271	+ 188	8.8	2.5	
16	12	1581	1	1122	+ 458	747	341	252	+ 154	9.0	3.0	
20	13	1581	0	1348	+ 233	747	390	292	+ 65	8.9	3.2	
24	14	1581	0	1111	+ 470	747	254	223	+ 270	8.9	3.2	
28	15	1581	0	1214	+ 367	747	201	270	+ 276	8.9	3.1	
Jan. 1	16	1581	0	628	+ 953	742	142	162	+ 438	9.0	3.3	Vigantol 1 cc. daily
5	17	1581	0	944	+ 637	742	144	263	+ 335	9.1	3.6	
9	18	1596	26	693	+ 877	838	30	410	+ 397	8.5	3.7	
13	19	1596	62	628	+ 906	738	8	376	+ 354	9.1	3.2	
17	20	1596	91	505	+ 1000	738	9	284	+ 445	9.4	3.2	
21	21	1596	142	601	+ 853	738	6	380	+ 352	9.5	3.0	
25	22	1660	184	515	+ 961	779	3	300	+ 476	9.6	2.9	

Phosphorus balance was in general parallel to calcium balance. Toward the end of Vigantol administration, phosphorus retention increased to keep pace with the increased calcium retention. This increased phosphorus balance was associated with a slight increase of stool phosphorus, but with the disappearance of urinary phosphorus, while, as has been said, there was an increase of calcium in the urine.

Serum calcium remained fairly stationary throughout the periods of observation, but inorganic phosphorus fluctuated between 2.2 and 3.7 mg per cent. The first peak of phosphorus occurred during periods 2 and 3 when the phosphorus intake was relatively high as compared with the minimal calcium intake. The second peak appeared during periods 16 and 17, in association with increased phosphorus intake and Vigantol administration.

. Subjectively gradual improvement was noticed, and bone pain disappeared entirely before the course of Vigantol was completed. In February 1934, 5 months after admission the patient was up in a wheel-chair, and in May she could walk a few steps. X-ray examination of skeleton on June 7, the day before discharge, revealed a definite increase in density of all the bones, especially the ribs, and healing of all the fractures; but the deformities were not changed and sufficient degree of osteoporosis was still present to justify the diagnosis of low-grade osteomalacia from the roentgenologic standpoint.

Comment. The clinical features of this patient resemble closely those of the preceding patient. Both had advanced osteomalacia with bone tenderness and deformities as their presenting symptoms. Further resemblance lies in the low serum inorganic phosphorus and fairly normal calcium. After having received minute doses of vitamin D prior to the studies, the patient exhibited satisfactory conservation of calcium, but the maximum degree of calcium retention did not occur until considerably more Vigantol was given. When calcium retention reached its maximum, phosphorus retention also increased, mainly at the expense of urinary phosphorus. The disappearance of phosphorus from the urine coincided with the appearance of increasing amounts of urinary calcium. As in the third case, serum inorganic phosphorus was elevated by a diet low in calcium and relatively high in phosphorus, but serum calcium remained unchanged. The stability of serum calcium is again probably the result of the small amount of vitamin D given previous to the studies. With further administration of vitamin D (Vigantol), serum calcium remained unchanged, but serum phosphorus tended to rise, a tendency already evident when phosphorus intake of the diet was raised.

Biochemical studies on this patient bring to light the following additional points:

(14). A minute dose of vitamin D may make its effect felt on the calcium and phosphorus metabolism, but the maximum effect requires considerably more vitamin D.

(15) Under the influence of vitamin D and with a ratio of calcium to phosphorus intake not less than 2:1, large retention of these elements may be accompanied by disappearance of phosphorus from urine and appearance of calcium in large amounts in urine.

SUMMARY

While their basic abnormality of poor calcium conservation because of vitamin D deficiency remains identical, two types of osteomalacia are recognizable by the levels of serum calcium and inorganic phosphorus. In one type serum calcium is low, but inorganic phosphorus normal; and in the other type inorganic phosphorus is decreased, but calcium normal. In low calcium osteomalacia tetany is the predominant feature and lenticular opacities are often present, while in low phosphorus osteomalacia the presenting symptoms are bone tenderness and skeletal deformities. Osseous decalcification in the first type may be mild or early, whereas in the second type it is more likely to be advanced.

In low phosphorus osteomalacia the normal serum calcium may be lowered and the low inorganic phosphorus raised by diets low in calcium and high in phosphorus.

Both types of osteomalacia respond readily to vitamin D therapy. When skeletal decalcification is extensive, the improvement in calcium and phosphorus retention is prompt and marked. When skeletal decalcification is slight, such improvement may not be striking. Likewise calcium and phosphorus retention slackens as the bony stores are replenished under treatment.

After the administration of vitamin D, serum calcium, when low, is raised to normal, and its rise is more rapid in the case of slight skeletal osteoporosis than in the case of pronounced decalcification. Serum inorganic phosphorus, when low, rises rather slowly, being susceptible to the influence of factors other than vitamin D.

Minute doses of vitamin D are effective in promoting calcium gain, but maximal action cannot be obtained until ordinary therapeutic doses are given. Moderate doses usually give a maximal action, and further vitamin D does not seem to exert any additional effect. The therapeutic effect persists long after its exhibition is discontinued, at least under the conditions of our studies.

The underlying basis for the divergent behavior of serum calcium and inorganic phosphorus in the two types of osteomalacia remains problematical. It cannot be determined in the present state of our knowledge whether this difference is related to the kind of mineral deficiency in the previous diet or to the state of the parathyroid glands.

LITERATURE

1. Hannon, R. R., Liu, S. H., Chu, H. I., Wang, S. H., Chen, K. C. and Chou, S. K., Calcium and phosphorus metabolism in osteomalacia. I. The effect of vitamin D and its apparent duration. Chinese Med. J., **48**: 623, 1934.

2. Marriott, W. McK., The therapeutic value of the hypophosphites. J.A.M.A., **66**: 486, 1916.

3. Shelling, D. H., Calcium and phosphorus studies. I. The effect of calcium and phosphorus of the diet on tetany, serum calcium, and food intake of parathyroidectomized rats. J. Biol. Chem., **96**: 195, 1932.

4. Bethke, R. M., Kick, C. H. and Wilder, W., The effect of the calcium-phosphorus relationship in growth, calcification, and blood composition of the rat. J. Biol. Chem., **98**: 389, 1932.

5. Hunter, D. and Turnbull, H. M., Hyperparathyroidism: Generalized osteitis fibrosa with observations upon the bones, the parathyroid tumors, and normal parathyroid glands. Brit. J. Surg., **19**: 203, 1931-1932.

6. Albright, F. and Ellsworth, R., Studies on the physiology of the parathyroid glands. I. Calcium and phosphorus studies in a case of idiopathic hypoparathyroidism. J. Clin. Invest., **7**: 183, 1929.

CALCIUM AND PHOSPHORUS METABOLISM IN OSTEOMALACIA. III. THE EFFECTS OF VARYING LEVELS AND RATIOS OF INTAKE OF CALCIUM TO PHOSPHORUS ON THEIR SERUM LEVELS, PATHS OF EXCRETION AND BALANCES

S. H. LIU, R. R. HANNON, S. K. CHOU, K. C. CHEN, H. I. CHU AND S. H. WANG

(From the Department of Medicine, Peiping Union Medical College, Peiping)

Chinese Journal of Physiology, 1935, Vol. 9. No. 2, pp. 101—118.

Chinese Journal of Physiology, 1935, Vol. **9**. *No. 2, pp. 101—118.*

CALCIUM AND PHOSPHORUS METABOLISM IN OSTEOMALACIA. III. THE EFFECTS OF VARYING LEVELS AND RATIOS OF INTAKE OF CALCIUM TO PHOSPHORUS ON THEIR SERUM LEVELS, PATHS OF EXCRETION AND BALANCES

S. H. LIU, R. R. HANNON, S. K. CHOU, K. C. CHEN,
H. I. CHU AND S. H. WANG

(From the Department of Medicine, Peiping Union Medical College, Peiping)

Received for publication October 15, 1934

It is well-known that three dietary factors, namely, vitamin D, calcium, and phosphorus, are especially concerned in the pathogenesis of rickets and osteomalacia. In the absence of vitamin D, rickets can be produced in animals with great ease by diets deficient or disproportionate in their calcium and phosphorus content [Sherman and Pappenheimer, 1921; Pappenheimer, McCann and Zücker, 1922; McCollum and co-workers, 1921, 1922; Karelitz and Shohl, 1927; Schultzer, 1927; Brown and co-workers, 1932]. The addition of vitamin D renders such diets non-rachitogenic. Although calcium and phosphorus can be conserved to a remarkable degree under the influence of vitamin D, there is considerable evidence to show that adequate amounts of calcium and phosphorus in proper ratio are at the same time necessary to secure optimum retention of these elements and normal ash content of bones [Brown and Shohl, 1930; Templin and Steenbock, 1932; Bethke, Kick and Wilder, 1932].

In a previous communication [Hannon et al, 1934] it has been shown that the primary metabolic abnormality in osteomalacia seems to be a lack of absorption of calcium through the intestinal tract. Such a defect can be readily remedied by the administration of vitamin D. In the studies to be reported presently, attempt is made to evaluate the importance of dietary calcium and phosphorus in the therapy of patients with osteomalacia after healing is initiated by vitamin D administration.

101

Attention is directed to (1) the serum level, (2) the paths of excretion, and (3) the extent of retention of calcium and phosphorus while the levels and ratios of intake of these elements are varied.

EXPERIMENTAL

Procedure.

The two experimental subjects, C.P. and Y.W.L., were respectively Cases 3 and 4 of paper II of this series [Liu et al, 1934] where their clinical histories were fully described. They were cases of advanced osteomalacia with normal serum calcium and low inorganic phosphorus. During the present experiment and for sometime before, they were symptom-free and retaining satisfactory amounts of calcium and phosphorus, a reparative state brought about by the vitamin D therapy given prior to the study. That such reparative state, once initiated by adequate vitamin D administration, would continue for a long time without further dosage has been demonstrated previously [Hannon et al., 1934]. Therefore during the present study although no vitamin D preparation was given, the influence of its previous administration on calcium and phosphorus metabolism should be considered still operative.

While being presumably under the influence of vitamin D, the patients were placed on various diets the composition of which is given in table 1. The diets contained 46-67 grams of protein and 1500-2000 calories with low potential acidity and low vitamin D content. While the diets were uniformly low in calcium, they differed in phosphorus content. On each diet, therefore at each level of dietary phosphorus, calcium lactate was given in desired amounts to vary the calcium intake. Usually two four-day periods were devoted to each level of calcium and phosphorus intake. For patient C.P., there were five levels each of calcium and phosphorus intake, giving 25 combinations; while for patient Y.W.L. there were four levels each, with 16 combinations.

Urine and stools were quantitatively collected for each period and analysed for calcium, phosphorus, and nitrogen. Each diet was analysed once or twice for calcium and phosphorus by taking half aliquot portions of one day's diet. Urinary calcium was determined by the method of Shohl and Pedley [1922], and total phosphorus by the method of Fiske and Subbarrow [1925]. Stools of each period were dried, mixed, ground to fine powder, and ashed in platinum or porcelain crucibles in a muffle furnace; and the ash dissolved in 5 percent hydro-

TABLE 1.

Composition of diets per day

Articles of food (1)	(2) Vitamin D	Diets for subject C. P.					Diets for subject Y.W.L.			
		1	2	3	4	5	1	2	3	4
Flour	±	160	250	160	150		150	130	50	
Millet	±			40	40	40		70	100	50
Rice	±	40		140	60	100	100	100	170	80
Rice, glutinous	±	40	40				60			
Oatmeal	±							30		
Potato, white	±			80						
Aroid	*				100	200				200
Turnip	±	50	100							
Beets	*							50		
Rape	+ +							100		
Lotus roots	*			40						
Bamboo shoots	*							150		
Cauliflower	*						25			
Soybean sprouts	±				100	100				
Peas	±								200	50
P'ai-tsai	±				100	80		100		80
Chinese lettuce	*			40			40			
Spinach	±	50	50				50	55		
Celery	±	50	50		100		50	100		
Pear	*			50		100	50	50		
Egg white	0	200	100				120			
Egg yolk	+ +				20	20				50
Pork	*		10	80	50	100		50	20	100
Fish	*					100			50	50
Sesame oil	0	70	53	41	33	30	70	54	61	19
Butter	+ +							10		
Sugar		94	50	24		10	43	25	11	
Sodium chloride		6	6	4	6	6	6	6	6	6
Protein		50	50	51	47	67	46	48	59	61
Carbohydrate		281	315	315	214	167	289	281	283	157
Fat		73	58	59	52	63	73	76	70	69
Calories		1981	1982	1995	1512	1503	1997	2000	1998	1493
Calcium (mg)		121	220	77	202	200	173	210	137	205
Phosphorus (mg)		293	444	651	776	962	421	779	810	978

(1) Amount in grams except Ca and P, which are in mg and actually determined.

(2) + + = good amount; ± = No appreciable amount; * = doubtful.

chloric acid; and aliquot portions taken for calcium and phosphorus analysis by the same methods. Food was treated, and calcium and phosphorus determined in the same manner as stools. Urine and dried powdered stool were analysed for nitrogen by Folin and Wright's method [1919]. Venepuncture was done on the first day of each period before breakfast. Serum calcium and inorganic phosphorus were determined by the methods of Clark and Collip [1925] and Fiske and Subbarrow [1925] respectively.

Serum calcium and inorganic phosphorus.

The trend of serum calcium and inorganic phosphorus in relation to dietary variations can best be appreciated graphically. In fig. 1,

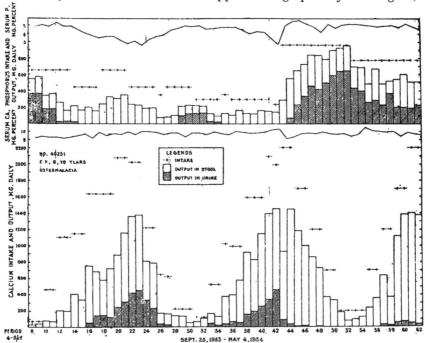

Fig. 1. Subject C. P. Calcium and phosphorus metabolism and their serum levels in relation to varying intake of calcium and phosphorus.

subject C.P. maintained a fairly stationary level of serum calcium. Throughout the whole period of 220 days, all the values remained within the accepted limits of normal with a maximum at 10.5 and a minimum at 9.1 mg percent. There were no remarkable changes in the level of serum calcium except for a slight ascending tendency during periods 8-23 when calcium intake was progressively stepped up, and an abrupt but temporary drop between periods 42 and 44, apparently associated with the change from low to high phosphorus diet and the consequent sudden rise of serum inorganic phosphorus.

... Serum inorganic phosphorus level, on the other hand, showed wide excursions between 2.6 and 5.6 mg percent, a variation of 3 mg percent. During periods 8-42 on low or moderate phosphorus intake, there were two major drops in the level of serum phosphorus, coinciding respectively with the two occasions when calcium intake was brought up to the maximum. The first drop was followed by a gradual rise to the original level as calcium intake was gradually reduced, while the rise after the second drop was more prompt and marked, probably on account of the abrupt increase of phosphorus intake. Subsequently, however, when the phosphorus intake was kept high, a similar elevation of calcium intake failed to depress the serum phosphorus level.

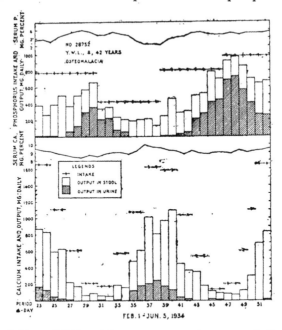

Fig. 2. Subject Y.W.L. Calcium and phosphorus metabolism and their serum levels in relation to varying intake of calcium and phosphorus.

As shown in fig. 2, the serum levels of calcium and inorganic phosphorus of subject Y.W.L. behaved similarly to those of subject C.P. The maximum variation in serum calcium was 1.6 mg percent, namely,

106   S. H. LIU ET AL.

from 8.4 to 10.0 mg percent. There seemed to be a more distinct
tendency for the serum calcium to vary directly with the level of
calcium intake, compared with the preceding case. The values during
periods of maximum calcium intake were all above 9.0 mg percent,
while these during periods of minimum intake were either on or below
that level.

In this patient the general level of serum inorganic phosphorus
(average 3.3, maximum 4.0 and minimum 2.2 mg percent) was somewhat lower, and its variations less marked than in the first patient.
Nevertheless, the same trend was present, namely, the tendency for the
serum phosphorus to rise with a diminishing calcium intake and to
fall with an increasing calcium intake, when diet phosphorus was kept
low or moderate; and to maintain a constant normal level regardless
of variations in calcium intake, when diet phosphorus was high.

Thus these experiments demonstrate clearly the relative mobility
of the level of serum inorganic phosphorus even under the influence of
vitamin D. Whenever the ratio of intake of calcium to phosphorus
is raised to a maximum (tables 2 and 3), serum phosphorus is brought
down to a level below normal; and conversely a reduction of the ratio
produces an opposite change. Serum calcium under the conditions of
our experiment, though more stable, tends very often to reciprocate
the variations in the concentration of inorganic phosphorus.

While our observations serve to emphasize the importance of
adequate calcium and phosphorus intake in proper ratio in maintaining normal serum levels of these elements in osteomalacia under reparation, it is of interest to inquire whether the observed lability of the serum
levels is characteristic of healing osteomalacia, or similar variations are
reproducible in normal individuals under similar regimen. Although
there are no available data to answer the question directly, it is well
established that the fasting values for serum calcium and phosphorus
of healthy individuals remain unvaried over long periods with ordinary
variations in diet and activities [Farquharson and Tibbetts, 1931].
Temporary changes in serum calcium and phosphorus have been noticed
in animals and men after ingestion or injection of large quantities
of calcium or phosphate [Salvesen, Hastings and McIntosh, 1924;
Hjört, 1925; Irving, 1926; Kahn and Roe, 1926; Bauer and Ropes,
1926], but they do not bear on the problem of more permanent changes
as seen in our patients in relation to dietary variations. It is likely that

TABLE 2.

Subject C.P. Calcium and phosphorus metabolism, phosphorus balance corrected for nitrogen balance and serum levels of calcium and inorganic phosphorus, averaged and grouped in order of increasing intake

Period No.	Intake			Output				Balance					Serum	
				Urinary		Fecal								
	Ca	P	Ratio Ca:P	Ca	P	Ca	P	Ca	P	N2	P corrected	Ratio Ca:P corr.	Ca	P
	mg	mg		mg	mg	mg	mg	mg	mg		mg		mg per cent	mg per cent
31-32	121	293	0.41	1	126	90	93	30*	74	1.50	-12	—	9.7	4.8
33-34	521	293	1.78	36	22	114	85	371	186	2.07	68	5.46	9.8	4.8
36-37	991	292	3.38	63	5	452	127	476	160	0.18	149	3.20	10.0	4.6
38-40	1591	292	5.46	178	4	698	116	715	158	1.00	191	6.19	9.8	4.2
41	2091	292	7.16	343	3	1054	148	694	141	1.28	67	10.36	10.2	3.0
28-30	220	444	0.50	3	73	110	197	107	264	1.96	152	0.70	9.6	5.0
27	620	444	1.40	31	5	135	74	454	365	2.56	218	2.07	9.7	4.2
14-15, 24-25	1182	444	2.66	145	10	420	182	617	253	1.23	182	3.37	9.9	3.7
16-17	1632	444	3.67	102	5	620	173	910	267	1.21	196	4.64	9.6	3.6
22-23	2020	444	4.55	438	4	933	229	649	211	1.24	140	4.63	9.8	2.8
8-9	77	651	0.12	0	370	43	197	34	84	0.99	27	1.17	9.3	5.0
10-11	467	651	0.72	1	182	79	171	387	298	1.32	222	1.74	9.3	5.2
12-13	1100	651	1.69	2	26	204	205	894	420	1.54	332	2.69	9.2	4.9
18-19	1635	651	2.51	136	5	519	282	980	364	0.95	310	3.16	9.6	3.7
20-21	2077	651	3.19	280	4	771	327	1026	320	1.62	226	4.54	9.8	3.0
53-54	202	776	0.26	0	422	116	274	86	80	-0.34	100	0.86	10.0	5.2
55-56	702	776	0.90	6	278	296	306	400	192	-0.31	210	1.90	10.0	5.0
57-58	1202	776	1.55	33	305	473	204	696	267	0.34	247	2.80	10.0	5.0
59-60	1702	776	2.20	70	207	1189	371	443	198	-1.24	265	1.67	9.5	5.0
61-62	2202	776	2.84	49	213	1345	303	808	260	-1.42	338	2.38	9.6	4.8
51-52	200	962	0.21	0	649	134	300	66	13	-1.39	-67	—	9.6	5.2
49-50	700	962	0.73	0	548	354	301	346	113	1.46	29	11.90	9.6	5.0
47-48	1200	962	1.25	10	444	789	402	401	116	1.28	43	9.30	9.8	4.6
45-46	1700	962	1.77	16	286	1079	406	605	270	2.60	121	5.00	9.8	5.4
43-44	2200	962	2.29	66	37	1120	387	1014	538	2.61	446	2.25	9.2	5.2

TABLE 3.

Subject. Y.W.L. Calcium and phosphorus metabolism, phosphorus balance corrected for nitrogen balance and serum levels of calcium and inorganic phosphorus, averaged and grouped in order of increasing intake

Period Number	Intake			Output				Balance					Serum	
	Ca	P	Ratio Ca:P	Urinary		Fecal		Ca	P	N_2	P corrected	Ratio Ca:P corrected	Ca	P
				Ca	P	Ca	P							
	mg	mg		mg	mg	mg	mg	mg	mg	mg	mg		mg per cent	mg per cent
31-32	173	421	0.41	4	215	50	132	119	74	1.32	-2	—	8.9	3.6
33-34	573	421	1.36	8	66	165	151	400	204	1.82	100	4.00	8.9	3.4
35-36	1073	421	2.55	149	4	395	195	529	222	2.48	138	3.85	9.6	2.4
37-38	1623	421	3.86	226	2	684	172	713	247	0.92	194	3.68	9.6	2.2
29-30	219	779	0.27	0	325	74	299	136	164	0.60	129	1.11	8.6	3.6
27-28	610	779	0.78	5	94	191	339	414	346	1.40	266	1.56	8.4	3.9
25-26	1110	779	1.42	34	7	578	436	498	336	1.18	270	1.84	8.8	3.4
23-24	1660	779	2.13	148	7	672	316	840	456	1.06	396	2.12	9.2	2.8
45-46	137	810	0.17	13	432	91	317	33	61	1.12	-3	—	9.0	3.4
43-44	537	810	0.66	0	249	264	261	273	300	1.53	212	1.29	8.8	3.6
41-42	1037	810	1.28	28	41	378	253	631	516	2.10	395	1.60	9.0	3.4
39-40	1587	810	1.95	151	8	884	348	552	454	2.66	302	1.83	9.2	3.0
47-48	205	978	0.21	0	709	75	239	139	30	0.36	11	11.80	9.1	3.5
49	605	978	0.61	0	564	124	297	481	117	0.71	76	6.30	9.0	3.6
50	1105	978	1.13	0	406	302	301	803	271	0.35	251	3.20	9.2	3.6
51-52	1655	978	1.67	8	262	756	400	891	316	0.71	275	3.23	9.4	3.7

in normal individuals similar dietary variations are not easily reflected in the fasting serum levels of calcium and phosphorus, in view of their steady rate of endogenous metabolism whereby excesses in supply are excreted, and in view of their large skeletal stores from which deficiencies in intake are made up. On the other hand the situation in healing osteomalacia is quite-different in that the streams of calcium and phosphorus are almost unidirectional towards the bones in a definite ratio and at great speed. Under such circumstances any retardation or acceleration in supply may easily influence the height of the streams, especially when one element is lacking and the other supplied in relative abundance.

Paths of excretion.

Data on calcium and phosphorus metabolism chronologically charted in figs. 1 and 2 were rearranged in order of increasing levels of intake and the averaged results are presented in tables 2 and 3 respectively. As seen in the tables, the urinary calcium and phosphorus output exhibited a marked reciprocal relationship. At a constant level of dietary phosphorus, progressive increment of calcium intake so as to raise the ratio of calcium: phosphorus, increased urinary calcium from nil or negligible amounts to figures as high as 438 mg for subject C. P. and 226 mg daily for subject Y.W.L., amounting to 32 and 25 percent respectively of the total excretion. Furthermore, it can be stated that the tendency for urinary calcium to appear or to increase in quantity varies indirectly with the level of phosphorus intake. Thus with 776 and 962 (table 2) and 978 mg (table 3) phosphorus intake, where additions of calcium did not raise the ratio of calcium to phosphorus intake as much as when phosphorus intake was lower, changes in urinary calcium were either absent or slight.

The behavior of urinary phosphorus under like circumstances was just the opposite of that of urinary calcium. A rising ratio of calcium to phosphorus intake was invariably associated with a falling urinary phosphorus. When the ratio rose to above a certain point (say, 2.5 in subject C.P. and 2.0 in subject Y.W.L.), and when the absolute level of phosphorus intake was low, urinary phosphorus decreased to insignificant amounts. The disappearance of urinary phosphorus usually coincided with the occurrence of relatively large amounts of calcium in urine.

Fecal calcium increased consistently with increased calcium intake. On the other hand, fecal phosphorus, while showing parallelism with phosphorus intake, seemed to vary directly with calcium intake, and consequently with fecal calcium, suggesting that a large amount of calcium in the intestine required a correspondingly large amount of phosphorus for elimination as pointed out by Telfer [1922].

The rise in fecal phosphorus associated with increasing calcium intake, together with the tendency to greater retention of phosphorus when calcium intake is raised, as shown in the next section, would adequately account for the low or negligible urinary phosphorus under such a regimen. Likewise the low or absent urinary calcium accompanying a low ratio of calcium to phosphorus intake may be accounted for by the fact that under such circumstances all the absorbed calcium, being accompanied by more than the corresponding amount of phosphorus needed for bone formation, is retained, and no need arises for elimination of calcium in the urine.

Therefore the absence of urinary calcium very often seen in osteomalacia, whether in active or reparative stage, represents a measure of conservation in the face of limited absorption or supply of calcium in relation to phosphorus. Similarly the low urinary calcium in normal children observed by Sherman and Hawley [1922] and Telfer [1922], and the absence of calcium in urine of a child with healing late rickets reported by Stearns, Oelke and Boyd [1931], should perhaps be regarded in the same light. The theory of a renal threshold for calcium excretion advocated by Albright and Ellsworth [1929], while useful in explaining the low urinary calcium in hypoparathyroidism, would not be adequate here, as the level of serum calcium in our cases was consistently within normal limits and did not vary sufficiently to give rise to the marked changes in the urinary calcium.

Balances.

While calcium retention may be considered as an index of its deposition in the bones, phosphorus metabolism is under the dual influence of calcium and nitrogen metabolism. For every 17.4 g of nitrogen retained or lost, 1 g of phosphorus is also retained or lost. In our patients who were actively repairing their skeletal systems as well as their soft tissues, the portion of phosphorus retained in relation to nitrogen was considerable. Accordingly the phosphorus balance associated with nitrogen metabolism is subtracted from the observed phosphorus balance, and the resulting corrected phosphorus balance is considered to represent the portion actually involved with calcium in the metabolism of bone. However, in case of phosphorus shortage it is not known whether both the bones and soft tissues bear equally the deficiency in phosphorus, or phosphorus enters in the stated ratio with nitrogen into the formation of soft tissues in deference to its deposition with calcium in the bones.

To facilitate comparison, calcium and corrected phosphorus balances are tabulated in relation to intake in tables 4 and 5. In the first portion of table 4 (Subject C.P.), it will be noted that calcium balance increased with rising calcium intake. This was true whether the phosphorus intake was as low as 293 mg or as high as 962 mg. Consequently when calcium balances at the same level of calcium intake were averaged regardless of phosphorus intake, the results showed strikingly the proportionality between calcium intake and retention. That calcium retention did not depend so much on phosphorus intake was seen when calcium balances at the same level of phosphorus intake but different levels of calcium intake were averaged. The averaged calcium balances exhibited a slight tendency to increase with greater phosphorus intake, but it was neither marked nor consistent.

When phosphorus balances were treated in the same way as calcium balances, as seen in the second part of table 4, phosphorus retention seemed also to depend more upon calcium than phosphorus intake. While phosphorus retention increased consistently with greater calcium intake, it rose with increased phosphorus intake up to 776 mg and fell off unaccountably on further raising the intake to 962 mg.

The results set forth in table 5 for subject Y.W.L. were essentially the same as described for subject C.P. Retention of both calcium and phosphorus was limited by calcium intake, while the limitation of either calcium or phosphorus retention by phosphorus intake was not marked nor consistent, except, of course, in instances of extremely low phosphorus intake where phosphorus retained was slight.

Bone may be considered as an organic framework in which $Ca_3(PO_4)_2$ and $CaCO_3$ are deposited in such manner as to form an orderly structure. Analyses of bone by Howland, Marriott and Kramer [1926] yield a ratio of calcium to phosphorus of about 2, and x-ray examination by Roseberry, Hastings and Morse [1931] suggests that the mineral composition of bone corresponds to dahlite, $CaCO_3.2Ca_3(PO_4)_2$

with a ratio of Ca:P of 2.26. A comparison of the ratios of Ca:P intake with those of retention (tables 2 and 3) shows general correspondance, except during the later periods for each patient while on the high level of phosphorus intake, when the ratios of retention were unaccountably high as compared with the ratios of intake. The consistently high ratios of retention noted during periods of low

TABLE 4

Subject C. P. The effect of calcium and phosphorus intake on their balances

Calcium intake		Calcium balance at phosphorus intake of:					Average Ca balance at same Ca intake regardless of P intake
Range	Level	293 mg	444 mg	651 mg	776 mg	962 mg	
mg	mg	mg	mg	mg	mg	mg	mg
77- 220	164	30	107	-34	86	66	64
467- 720	602	371	454	387	400	346	392
991-1202	1135	476	617	894	696	401	617
1591-1702	1652	715	910	980	443	605	731
2020-2202	2118	694	649	1026	808	1014	838
Average Ca balance at same P intake regardless of Ca intake		457	547	664	487	486	

Calcium intake		Phosphorus balance at phosphorus intake of:					Average P balance at same Ca intake regardless of P intake
Range	Level	293 mg	444 mg	651 mg	776 mg	962 mg	
77- 220	164	12	152	27	100	67	40
467- 720	602	68	218	222	210	29	150
991-1202	1135	149	82	332	247	43	191
1591-1702	1652	101	196	310	265	121	198
2020-2202	2118	67	140	226	338	446	244
Average P balance at same P intake regardless of Ca intake		74	178	223	232	114	

TABLE 5.

Subject Y.W.L. The effect of calcium and phosphorus intake on their balances

Calcium intake		Calcium balance at phosphorus intake of:				Average Ca balance at same Ca intake regardless of P intake
Range	Level	421 mg	779 mg	810 mg	978 mg	
mg	mg	mg	mg	mg	mg	mg
58- 210	181	119	136	33	130	104
537- 610	581	400	414	273	481	192
1008-1073	1081	529	498	631	803	615
1581-1660	1631	713	840	552	891	749
Average Ca balance at same P intake. regardless of Ca intake		440	472	372	376	
Calcium intake		Phosphorus balance at phosphorus intake of:				Average P balance at same Ca intake regardless of P intake
Range	Level	421 mg	779 mg	810 mg	978 mg	
58- 210	181	- 2	129	- 3	11	34
537- 610	581	100	266	212	76	164
1008-1073	1081	138	270	395	251	264
1581-1660	1631	194	396	302	275	292
Average P balance at same P intake regardless of Ca intake		108	265	226	153	

phosphorus intake, suggest that considerably more calcium may be deposited as carbonate than is found in dahlite. It was only when both calcium and phosphorus were supplied at fairly high levels that the ratios of retention began to approach 2.26, the ratio of calcium to phosphorus that apparently normally exists in bone. There were two ratios of retention noted in subject C.P., namely, 2.38 during periods 61-62 and 2.25 during periods 43-44, which may perhaps be considered as optimal ratios of retention. One such ratio occurred in subject Y.W.L., namely, 2.12 during periods 23-24. All these optimal ratios of retention were obtained when both calcium and phosphorus were fed at fairly high levels in ratios of 2.84, 2.29 and 2.13 respectively.

Thus, while limitation of phosphorus intake does not necessarily result in limited calcium retention, it is important to supply sufficient phosphorus in the diet to make the ratio of intake of calcium to phosphorus approximately 2:1 in order to secure the normal relationship of these elements for deposition in the bones.

DISCUSSION

Under normal conditions the skeletal system is constantly undergoing destruction and repair, but the rates of the two processes are equal so that the net condition in the bones remain stationary. In osteomalacia while the destructive activity may not be increased, as is suggested by the relatively low endogenous calcium excretion on minimal intake [Hannon et al., 1934], the reparative process is handicapped by defective absorption of calcium through the gastrointestinal tract. The result is osseous decalcification. When healing is brought about by vitamin D therapy, anabolic activities predominate and large amounts of calcium and phosphorus are capable of being deposited in the bones. The actual amounts of calcium and phosphorus deposited depend on the level and ratio of intake of these elements, which, therefore, bear close study in order to promote optimal retention and rapid reparation.

Calcium retention varies directly with its intake. But there is a limit to the intake. As ordinary Chinese dietaries are low in calcium, the greater part of the high calcium intake desired in the therapy of osteomalacia has to be supplied by medication; a practical upper limit of calcium intake seems to be about 2 g which is the maximal level used in our experiments. At this level of calcium intake 0.7-1.0 g can be retained. While calcium retention does not depend very much on phosphorus intake, it is important to supply adequate amounts of phosphorus to insure that sufficient phosphorus is retained to approach the ratio of Ca:P that normally exists in bone. Therefore if 2 g be considered as an optimal calcium intake, this should be accompanied by 1 g of phosphorus which can be easily supplied in ordinary Chinese dietary staples.

Besides these practical considerations, the present study brings out the remarkable manner in which calcium and phosphorus are conserved in the reparative stage of osteomalacia under the influence of vitamin D. When calcium intake is limited in relation to phosphorus (low Ca:P ratio), practically all the calcium absorbed is deposited, none appearing in the urine. When phosphorus supply is short as compared with calcium (high Ca:P ratio), likewise 'all the available phosphorus is retained, and urinary phosphorus vanishes. It is only when either calcium or phosphorus is absorbed in excess, one over the other, of the necessary ratio for bone formation that the element in excess begins to be excreted through the kidneys.

Conservation of excretion through the urinary tract and efficient absorption through the gastro-intestinal canal account admirably for the ability of patients with healing osteomalacia to maintain positive balance even when calcium and phosphorus supplies are at a minimum. Likewise they explain the protective influence of vitamin D on experimental animals when fed rickets-producing diets.

SUMMARY

1. In two patients with healing osteomalacia the serum levels of calcium and phosphorus, the paths of excretion and the retention of calcium and phosphorus were studied in relation to the level and ratio of their intake.

2. Serum calcium showed a slight tendency to vary directly with calcium intake, while serum inorganic phosphorus fluctuated widely under dietary influence. A high ratio of intake of calcium to phosphorus was invariably associated with low serum phosphorus, and vice versa.

3. Fecal calcium varied directly with calcium intake; and fecal phosphorus, while parallel with phosphorus intake, tended to increase with increasing calcium intake. On lowering the ratio of intake of Ca:P, urinary calcium tended to disappear, while urinary phosphorus appeared in relatively large amounts. On the other hand when the ratio of Ca:P intake was raised, calcium appeared in urine in large quantities, while urinary phosphorus became negligible.

4. Whereas phosphorus retention was limited by both phosphorus and calcium intake, considerable calcium might be retained without an equivalent amount of phosphorus for bone formation. However to insure normal relationship between calcium and phosphorus in the bones, both elements should be supplied in optimal ratio.

LITERATURE

ALBRIGHT, F. AND ELLSWORTH, R.   (1929)   J. clin. Invest., **7**, 183.

BAUER, W. AND ROPES, M. W.   (1926)   J. Amer. med. Ass., **87**, 1902.

BETHKE, R. M., KICK, C. H. AND WILDER, W.   (1932)   J. biol. Chem., **98**, 389.

BROWN, H. B. AND SHOHL, A. I.   (1930)   Ibid, **86**, 245.

BROWN, H. B., SHOHL, A. T., CHAIMAN, E. E., ROSE, C. S. AND SAURWEIN, E. M.   (1932)   Ibid, **98**, 207.

CLARK, E. P. AND COLLIP, J. B.   (1925)   Ibid, **63**, 461.

FARQUHARSON, R. F. AND TIBBETTS, D. M.   (1931)   J. clin. Invest., **10**, 271.

FISKE, C. AND SUBBAROW, Y.   (1925)   J. biol. chem., **66**, 375.

FOLIN, O. AND WRIGHT, L. E.   (1919)   Ibid, **38**, 461.

HANNON, R. R., LIU, S. H., CHU, H. I., WANG, S. H., CHEN, K. C. AND CHOU, S. K.   (1934)   Chinese med. J., **48**, 623.

HJÖRT, A. M.   (1925)   J. biol. Chem., **65**, 783.

HOWLAND, J., MARRIOTT, W. McK. AND KRAMER, B.   (1926)   Ibid, **68**, 721.

IRVING, L.   (1926)   Ibid, **68**, 513.

KAHN, B. S. AND ROE, J. H.   (1926)   J. Amer. med. Ass., **86**, 1761.

KARELITZ, S. AND SHOHL, A. T.   (1927)   J. biol. Chem., **73**, 655, 664.

LIU, S. H., HANNON, R. R., CHU, H. I., CHEN, K. C., CHOU, S. K., AND WANG, S. H.   (1935)   Chinese med. J., **49**, 1.

McCOLLUM, E. V. AND SIMMONDS, N.   (1921)   J. biol. Chem., **47**, 1921.

McCOLLUM, E. V., SIMMONDS, N., KINNEY, M., SHIPLEY, P. G. AND PARK, E. A.   (1922)   Amer. J. Hyg. **2**, 97.

PAPPENHEIMER, A. M., McCANN, G. F. AND ZÜCKER, T. F.   (1922)   J. exp. Med., **35**, 421.

ROSEBERRY, H. H., HASTINGS, A. B. AND MORSE, J. K.   (1931)   J. biol. Chem., **90**, 395.

SALVESEN, H. A., HASTINGS, A. B. AND McINTOSH, J. F.   (1924)   Ibid, **60**, 311, 327.

SCHULTZER, P.   (1927)   Biochem. Z., **188**, 435.

SHERMAN, H. C. AND PAPPENHEIMER, A. M.   (1921)   J. exp. Med., **34**, 189.

SHOHL, A. T. AND PEDLEY, F. G.   (1922)   J biol. Chem. **50**, 537.

STEARNS, G., OELKE, M. J. AND BOYD, J. D.   (1931)   Amer. J. Dis. Child., **42**, 88.

TELFER, S. W.   (1922)   Quart. J. Med., **16** 45

TEMPLIN, V. M. AND STEENBOCK, H.   (1933)   J. biol. Chem., **100**, 209, 217

WU, H.   (1928)   Chinese J. Physiol., Rep. Ser. 1, 153

骨質輕化症中鈣與燐之新陳代謝

其三・飲食中鈣與燐之成分及其比率，對於血清中鈣與燐之濃度，尿
糞內鈣與燐之排泄，以及其存留於骨骼內數量之影響

劉士豪　韓　恩　周壽愷　陳國楨　朱憲彝　王叔咸

北平協和醫學院內科學系，北平

按著者已往研究之結果，骨質輕化症，其主要原因為飲食內缺少維生素丁，因之腸壁失去吸收鈣質之能力，體內鈣質之消耗不能彌補，而骨骼逐呈變態・但除丁種維生素以外，飲食中所含鈣與燐之數量，以及鈣與燐之比率，對骨質之代謝亦甚有關係・本篇所述即為此種研究・其法為選擇患骨質輕化症者二人，先用維生素丁治療之，使其腸壁完全恢復吸收與應用鈣燐二質之功能・然後改變（增或減）其飲食中之鈣與燐，而同時檢定（定量分析）其血清以及尿糞中之鈣與燐質・今將其重要結果略述於下・

（一）血清：飲食中鈣質加增或減少時，血清中鈣質隨之略為增減・但飲食中之燐質增減時，則血清中無機燐質變化甚著・此外飲食中鈣與燐之比率，亦能影響血清之燐質・如鈣比燐多，血清中之燐質降低・反之則增高・

（二）尿糞中之排泄：糞中排出之鈣與燐，均隨其飲食中成分之多寡而變・鈣與燐二者並同時增減，如鈣質排出量增加，燐質排出量亦多・但由尿中泄出之鈣與燐，則不然・每於食物中鈣與燐之比率增高時，尿中泄出之鈣質漸增，而燐質減少・如鈣與燐之比率減低時，則尿中鈣質漸減，而燐質漸增・故由尿中泄出之鈣與燐，其數量適成反比率・

（三）存留於骨骼之分量：存貯於骨骼內鈣質之量，全由飲食內鈣質之量而定・但燐質之存留量，非特與進食之燐質有關，且與鈣質亦有密切之關係・正常骨質含 $CaCO_3 \cdot 2Ca_3(PO_4)_2$，其鈣與燐之比率為2.3：1，故如飲食中之燐過多時，其過量之燐質均由尿糞中排出，但飲食中如含過多鈣質時，此過量之鈣質大半仍存留體中・足見燐質缺乏時，骨質所含之 $CaCO_3$ 可比上列方式為多・雖然，在治療骨質輕化症時，飲食中之鈣與燐・除須充足外・其比率亦不能與2.3：1相差甚遠，俾使新愈後骨質含有正常鈣與燐之成分・

Reprinted from THE JOURNAL OF CLINICAL INVESTIGATION, Vol. XVI, No. 4, pp. 603–611, July, 1937.
Printed in U. S. A.

CALCIUM AND PHOSPHORUS METABOLISM IN OSTEOMALACIA. V. THE EFFECT OF VARYING LEVELS AND RATIOS OF CALCIUM TO PHOSPHORUS INTAKE ON THEIR SERUM LEVELS, PATHS OF EXCRETION AND BALANCES, IN THE PRESENCE OF CONTINUOUS VITAMIN D THERAPY

BY S. H. LIU, C. C. SU, S. K. CHOU, H. I. CHU, C. W. WANG AND K. P. CHANG

(Department of Medicine, Peiping Union Medical College, Peiping, China)

(Received for publication January 8, 1937)

Osteomalacia is a bone disease more commonly seen and with greater clinical implications in North China than elsewhere (1, 2, 3). The principal cause of the skeletal demineralization resides in vitamin D deficiency, a combination of its lack in the diet and exclusion of sunlight. By reason of such deficiency, calcium given by mouth fails to be absorbed. Poor intestinal absorption rather than excessive elimination is incriminated because it has been demonstrated by the studies of Hannon et al. (4) that the endogenous calcium metabolism in patients with osteomalacia on low intake is within normal limits and that calcium administered parenterally is largely retained. Under such circumstances while the endogenous destructive activity in the bones may not be excessive, the reparative process is very much interfered with through defective intestinal absorption so that skeletal decalcification inevitably ensues. The limited intake of calcium in common Chinese dietaries (5), and periods of mineral stress incident to pregnancy and lactation are some of the contributing factors that enter into the pathogenesis of osteomalacia.

Studies of the effect of vitamin D in the treatment of osteomalacia (4, 6) demonstrate the remarkable conserving action of vitamin D on calcium and phosphorus metabolism. As a result of its administration, intestinal absorption is promoted and endogenous elimination is decreased so that large quantities of calcium and phosphorus are available for deposition in the bones. The actual amount of calcium and phosphorus retained depends upon the level and ratio of intake of these elements. It has been shown in two patients with osteomalacia undergoing reparation initiated by vitamin D (7) that calcium retention varied directly with calcium intake while phosphorus retention was limited by both calcium and phos-

phorus intake. Fecal calcium likewise varied directly with calcium intake while fecal phosphorus was parallel with both calcium and phosphorus intake. When calcium supply is limited in relation to phosphorus (low Ca : P ratio) practically all the calcium absorbed is deposited, none appearing in the urine. On the other hand, when phosphorus supply is short compared with calcium (high Ca : P ratio), all the available phosphorus is retained and urinary phosphorus vanishes. Conservation of excretion through the urinary tract and efficient absorption through the intestinal canal account for the markedly positive balances in osteomalacia when reparation is brought about under the influence of vitamin D.

Similar observations on the effects of variations of the levels and ratios of calcium to phosphorus intake on their serum levels, paths of excretion and balances have been made on another patient with healing osteomalacia. But in contrast to the previous patients who received vitamin D only prior to the observations, the present subject was given vitamin D throughout the entire study so as to obviate any uncertainty in ascribing the metabolic results obtained to vitamin D action. Moreover, attempt was made in the present study to secure more nearly metabolic equilibrium by using three 4-day periods for each level or ratio of dietary intake. The data obtained from this patient, together with those from another subject having syphilitic osteitis of right radius and tibia without general metabolic disturbance, taken as a control, constitute the basis of discussion in the present communication.

PROCEDURE

The clinical histories of the two subjects are briefly described in the appendix. Subject 1, H. F. M., was a woman of 32 with advanced osteo-

603

malacia of seven years' duration. While skeletal rarefaction and deformities were marked, her serum calcium and phosphorus were within normal limits. She was placed on various diets, the compositions of which are given in Table I. All the diets were low in calcium but contained varying amounts of phosphorus. The desired high levels of calcium intake were attained by giving appropriate quantities of a saturated solution of calcium lactate (7.7 per cent). At a given level of calcium intake, the phosphorus level was progressively increased by giving Diets 5, 2, 3 and 4 in that order. There were altogether 3 levels of calcium and 4 levels of phosphorus intake, making a total of 12 different ratios. Three four-day pe-

riods were devoted to each ratio of calcium to phosphorus intake. The first five periods concerned preliminary observations without vitamin D, but after that 1 cc. of Vigantol, an oily solution of irradiated ergosterol containing 15,000 international units of vitamin D per cc., was given daily.

Subject 2, L. Y. H., was a man of 24 with syphilitic osteitis of right radius and tibia, the rest of the skeleton showing normal density and texture on x-ray examination. As localized bone involvement by infection usually does not give rise to general metabolic disturbances, the patient may be regarded as a control for the present purpose. He was given Diets 1, 2 and 3 in that sequence. With each diet, namely, with each level of phos-

TABLE I

Composition of diets in grams per day †

Articles of food	Vitamin D	Subject 1 (H. F. M.)						Subject 2 (L. Y. H.)		
		Diet 1	Diet 2	Diet 3	Diet 4	Diet 5a	Diet 5b	Diet 1	Diet 2	Diet 3
Millet	±	50		50	50					100
Rice	±		50			20	16		200	100
Glutinous rice									50	
Oatmeal	±				100					
White wheat flour	+	50	150	200	75	150	120	300	200	150
Mung bean flour	*				25	100	80			
Peanut				30	30					
Egg	+					300	240	300	100	
Egg white	±									
Pork	*	150	75	50	25				25	100
Chicken	*	100	50	50	75					100
Beef	±			50	75	75				
Aroid	*	50	50	50						100
Potato	*	50							50	50
Sweet potato	±				50					
Carrot	±				50					
Turnip	±		50	100		100	80			
Cabbage	±	100	100	150	100					100
Onion	*								50	
Chinese lettuce									100	
Spinach	±							100		
Apple	*	50	50	50						50
Banana	*					50	40			
Orange	*					50	40			
Lard								50	31	
Butter	++							30	20	
Sesame oil		32	45	50	50	70	56	40	20	50
Table salt		4	4	4	4	4	3.2	4	6	6
Sugar		21	20	20	24	50	40	60	24	
Soy bean sauce		5	5	5	5	5	4			
Protein		65	59	69	77	58	46	71	62	80
Carbohydrate		102	192	232	211	284	227	286	392	307
Fat		63	70	79	94	73	58	120	76	76
Calories		1235	1642	1923	2000	2022	1614	2508	2500	2232
Calcium		0.138	0.140	0.191	0.181	0.176	0.140	0.178	0.118	0.173
Phosphorus		0.914	0.627	0.925	1.163	0.324	0.259	0.402	0.582	1.094
Nitrogen		10.40	9.12	10.68	12.39	8.28	6.64	10.82	8.69	11.51

† Calcium, phosphorus and nitrogen values are actually determined, and vitamin D values taken from Wu (8); ++ good amount; + fair amount; ± no appreciable amount; * doubtful or undetermined. Approximate computation of the acid base balance of the diets according to Sherman (9) gives potential acidities ranging from 19 to 35 cc. of normal acid for Subject 1, and 30 to 44 cc. for Subject 2.

phorus intake, calcium was raised by the addition of desired amounts of calcium lactate. With this patient, 3 levels each of calcium and phosphorus were studied, giving 9 combinations. No vitamin D was administered.

Calculation of the acid base balance of the diets according to Sherman (9) showed that all the diets were potentially acid with relatively small variations, but the computation should be considered only approximate, because of the uncertainty of the applicability of Sherman's figures to local foodstuffs.

Stool and urine respectively of each period were pooled for analysis. Venepuncture was done before breakfast at the beginning of each period. Metabolic ward routine and analytical methods for calcium, phosphorus and nitrogen of food, urine, stool and blood were described previously (7).

RESULTS

Serum calcium and phosphorus. As seen from Figure 1, Subject 1 maintained a fairly stationary level of serum calcium throughout the period of 212 days of continuous observation, the range be-

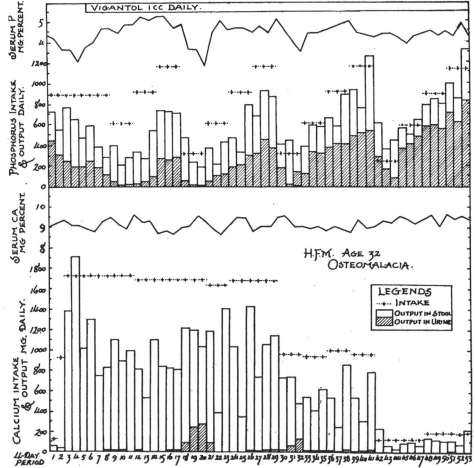

FIG. 1. CALCIUM AND PHOSPHORUS METABOLISM AND THEIR SERUM LEVELS IN RELATION TO VARYING INTAKE OF CALCIUM AND PHOSPHORUS IN SUBJECT 1

ing from 8.7 to 9.6 mgm. per 100 cc. and the trend bearing no apparent relation to the dietary changes. The serum inorganic phosphorus level, however, varied from 2.9 to 5.3, a difference of 2.4 mgm. per 100 cc. The phosphorus level, beginning at 4.3 mgm. per 100 cc., gradually went down to 3.0 as calcium intake in the diet was stepped up to 1.7 grams (Period 4). While the calcium intake was maintained at this high level, the phosphorus curve began to climb as vitamin D was given, and rose to a maximum of 5.3 as the phosphorus intake was progressively raised (Period 15). The phosphorus curve showed a second drop in Periods 18 to 20 when the phosphorus intake was suddenly decreased to a minimum, and a subsequent recovery to the high level in Periods 27 to 29 when high phosphorus intake was restored. When calcium intake was maintained at a lower level, namely, 1.0 gram as in Periods 30 to 41, similar changes in the phosphorus intake brought about a repetition of the cycle of events in the serum phosphorus curve, but to a lesser extent. But when the calcium intake was kept minimal (Periods 42 to 53), lowering of the phosphorus intake failed to elicit any significant change in serum phosphorus. In other words, serum phosphorus varied more with the ratio of calcium to phosphorus than with their actual levels in the intake. Whenever the ratio is high serum phosphorus drops.

In Subject 2 (Figure 2) the serum calcium level was also relatively constant, varying from a minimum of 9.0 to a maximum of 10.2 mgm. per 100 cc., irrespective of the calcium and phosphorus intake. The serum phosphorus, compared with that of Subject 1, showed much less fluctuation, ranging as it did between 3.9 and 5.1 mgm. per 100 cc. Moreover, the trend of variation with dietary intake seemed to be opposite in direction to that seen in Case 1. When the calcium supply was short in relation to phosphorus (low Ca:P ratio), the serum phosphorus tended to fall with a subsequent rise when calcium intake was stepwise increased. However, the changes observed were not sufficiently pronounced to render their significance indubitable.

From the above observations it may be concluded that dietary variations of calcium and phosphorus are not significantly reflected in the serum calcium level. This is true in osteomalacia, as·

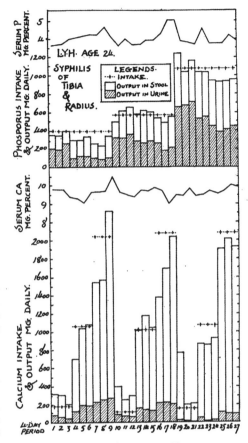

FIG. 2. CALCIUM AND PHOSPHORUS METABOLISM AND THEIR SERUM LEVELS IN RELATION TO VARYING INTAKE OF CALCIUM AND PHOSPHORUS IN SUBJECT 2

well as in the control case, probably on account of the protective influence of vitamin D, as in its absence the serum calcium and inorganic phosphorus reflect remarkably the ratio of these elements in the diet as shown by Shohl (10) in experimental rickets in rats. Dietary changes may cause fluctuations in serum phosphorus, however, even when vitamin D is added to the diet. In healing osteomalacia, for example, where there is marked deposition of calcium and phosphorus in the bones, a deficiency in intake of phosphorus relative to calcium intake results in a fall in serum phosphorus; and excess phosphorus intake relative to calcium intake may result in a rise in serum phosphorus. On the other hand, in the case of localized bone disease and presumably in normal individuals where excesses in supply are excreted and deficiencies in intake are made up from the large skeletal store, serum phosphorus level is less subject to fluctuation.

Paths of excretion. The data from Subject 1 as presented in Figure 1 and as averaged in Table II demonstrate a general reciprocal relationship between urinary calcium and phosphorus. At a constant level of calcium intake, progressive increment of phosphorus supply tended to decrease the urinary calcium sometimes to the point of disappearance, and at the same time to augment the urinary phosphorus.

If the results at the same level of dietary phosphorus are taken for comparison successive addition of calcium intake increased the urinary calcium coincident with a gradual and steady diminution of urinary phosphorus. In general, the magnitude of urinary excretion of calcium was small or negligible but it became considerable when calcium was supplied far in excess of the dietary phosphorus (Periods 18 to 20). Likewise, urinary excretion of phosphorus was very much limited on low phosphorus diet, but became dominant

when phosphorus supply was far in excess of dietary calcium (Periods 51 to 53).

Fecal calcium increased consistently with the calcium intake, having little relation with the phosphorus supply, while fecal phosphorus was directly related not only with dietary phosphorus, but also with dietary calcium. Intestinal elimination of phosphorus, then, depends not only on its supply in the diet, but also on the amount of calcium presented in the intestine for excretion.

In Subject 2 (Figure 2 and Table III) similar results were obtained. The magnitude of urinary calcium excretion was greater, and it never disappeared, even when the supply was minimal in the presence of large phosphorus intake (Periods 19 to 21). Likewise, when phosphorus intake was minimal in the presence of excessive dietary calcium, urinary phosphorus, though decreased, was still considerable, compared with that in healing osteomalacia. The fecal elimination of calcium and, to a lesser degree, of phosphorus in Subject 2 was greater also, but the correlation between the intake of calcium and phosphorus and their output in the stool was just as close. In addition to the tendency for fecal phosphorus to vary directly with calcium intake, there was a

TABLE II

Subject 1. Average daily calcium and phosphorus metabolism

Period number	Diet number	Intake			Output					Balances				
		Ca	P	Ratio Ca : P	Urinary		Fecal			Ca	P	N₂	P corrected	Ratio Ca : P corrected
					Ca	P	Ca	P	Dry weight					
		mgm.	*mgm.*		*mgm.*	*mgm.*	*mgm.*	*mgm.*	*grams*	*mgm.*	*mgm.*	*grams*	*mgm.*	
3– 5	1	1738	914	1.90	0	222	1444	420	19.4	294	272	1.05	212	1.39
*6– 8	1	1738	914	1.90	5	190	956	238	12.7	777	486	1.43	404	1.93
9–11	2	1740	627	2.14	19	25	962	283	17.0	759	319	1.22	249	3.05
12–14	3	1691	925	1.83	7	62	822	328	17.9	862	535	2.24	406	2.12
15–17	4	1681	1163	1.45	6	297	829	438	22.8	846	428	2.40	287	2.94
18–20	5	1676	324	5.18	209	23	945	287	20.1	522	14	0.98	— 44	
21–23	2	1640	627	2.60	31	85	970	261	18.9	639	281	0.71	239	2.67
24–26	3	1691	925	1.83	4	238	935	296	18.3	752	391	1.56	301	2.50
27–29	4	1681	1163	1.45	19	393	960	444	22.2	702	326	2.17	201	3.49
30–32	5	976	324	3.01	77	37	582	318	19.7	313	— 31	1.59	—124	
33–35	2	940	627	1.50	6	252	545	249	15.9	389	126	0.22	113	3.44
36–38	3	994	924	1.08	8	413	535	301	16.5	451	210	2.17	82	5.50
39–41	4	981	1163	0.84	6	528	540	408	19.0	435	227	1.50	139	3.13
42–44	5a	141	259	0.54	3	184	111	299	18.4	27	—224	—0.01	—223	
45–47	2	140	627	0.22	4	436	78	157	11.6	58	34	0.70	— 6	
48–50	3	194	924	0.21	1	593	129	242	18.3	64	89	1.40	7	
51–53	4	181	1163	0.16	4	744	137	335	20.2	40	84	1.11	20	2.00

* Vigantol 1 cc. daily started from this period and continued throughout.

第四编　骨病深耕

TABLE III

Subject 2. Average daily calcium and phosphorus metabolism

Period number	Diet number	Intake			Output					Balances			
		Ca	P	Ratio Ca : P	Urinary		Fecal			Ca	P	N₂	P corrected
					Ca	P	Ca	P	Dry weight				
		mgm.	*mgm.*		*mgm.*	*mgm.*	*mgm.*	*mgm.*	*grams*	*mgm.*	*mgm.*	*mgm.*	*mgm.*
1– 3	1	178	402	0.44	73	232	207	153	20.3	−102	28	1.65	−69
4– 6	1	1058	402	2.63	189	158	736	155	20.5	133	89	2.27	−45
7– 9	1	2043	402	5.08	252	104	1561	183	18.2	230	115	2.33	−22
10–12	2	118	582	0.20	79	341	241	255	16.5	−202	−14	1.16	−82
13–15	2	1023	582	1.76	153	282	928	323	21.4	58	−23	1.09	−87
16–18	2	2080	582	3.58	211	221	1495	319	21.2	374	42	1.16	−26
19–21	3	173	1094	0.16	19	695	373	471	21.0	−219	−72	0.60	−107
22–24	3	1078	1094	0.99	36	519	859	492	20.7	183	83	0.50	54
25–27	3	2084	1094	1.91	116	414	1812	525	25.4	156	155	0.48	127

discernible but slight tendency for the fecal calcium to vary directly with phosphorus intake.

As the average daily dry fecal weights in both cases varied only slightly on the various diets, it is unlikely that variations in roughage were sufficiently large to play an important rôle in the intestinal elimination of calcium and phosphorus.

Balances. While calcium balance may be taken to represent the state of bone metabolism, phosphorus balance is under the dual influence of bone and soft tissue metabolism. For every 17 grams of nitrogen retained or lost, 1 gram of phosphorus is retained or lost. To calculate the amount of phosphorus actually involved with calcium in bone metabolism, the total phosphorus balance is corrected by an amount equivalent to nitrogen balance. The corrected phosphorus balances are set forth in Tables II and III. In Table II it may be of interest to note the remarkable effect of vitamin D on calcium balance in osteomalacia. Prior to vitamin D administration the patient retained 294 mgm. of calcium on an intake of 1738 mgm. per day (Periods 3 to 5), but after its administration the retention increased to 777 mgm. on the same intake (Periods 6 to 8), the improvement being mainly due to lessened elimination in the stool.

To facilitate comparison, Tables IV and V are constructed in which calcium and corrected phosphorus balances are grouped according to intake. Subject 1 (as seen in the upper part of Table IV) exhibited a striking dependence of calcium balance on calcium intake. Calcium retention on the aver-

age increased steadily from 47 to 654 mgm. per day as calcium intake was progressively raised from 164 to 1672 mgm. per day, regardless of phosphorus intake. On the other hand, at a given

TABLE IV

Subject 1. The effect of calcium and phosphorus intake on their balances

Calcium intake		Calcium balance at the phosphorus intake of				Average Ca balance at same Ca intake regardless of P intake
Range	Level	324 mgm.	627 mgm.	922 mgm.	1163 mgm.	
mgm.	*mgm.*	*mgm.*	*mgm.*	*mgm.*	*mgm.*	*mgm.*
140–194	164	*0.52** 27	*0.22* 58	*0.21* 64	*0.16* 40	47
940–994	973	*3.01* 313	*1.50* 389	*1.08* 451	*0.84* 435	397
1640–1691	1672	*5.18* 522	*2.60* 639	*1.83* 752	*1.45* 702	654
Average of Ca balance at same P intake regardless of Ca intake		287	362	422	392	

Calcium intake		Phosphorus balance at the phosphorus intake of				Average P balance at same Ca intake regardless of P intake
Range	Level	324 mgm.	627 mgm.	922 mgm.	1163 mgm.	
140–194	164	*0.52* −223	*0.22* −6	*0.21* 7	*0.16* 20	−50
940–994	973	*3.01* −124	*1.50* 113	*1.08* 82	*0.84* 139	52
1640–1691	1672	*5.18* −44	*2.60* 239	*1.83* 301	*1.45* 201	174
Average P balance at same P intake regardless of Ca intake		−130	115	130	120	

* Figures in italics are ratios of calcium to phosphorus intake.

level of calcium intake, progressive increment of dietary phosphorus up to 922 mgm. per day resulted in a slight ascending tendency in the calcium balance, but further increase to 1163 mgm. failed to improve the calcium balance which, in fact, fell somewhat at the latter level of phosphorus intake. Corrected phosphorus balance likewise depended more on calcium than on phosphorus intake. When calcium intake was raised from 164 to 1672 mgm., the average phosphorus balance increased from — 50 to + 174 mgm.; whereas various levels of phosphorus intake made no striking difference to the phosphorus balance except in the case of minimal phosphorus intake where negative balance prevailed.

Balance data on Subject 2, summarized in Table V, show essentially the same findings, namely, the greater importance of calcium as the limiting factor in both calcium and phosphorus balances. However, on a minimal calcium intake of 145 mgm. he lost on the average 174 mgm. per day in

contrast to Subject 1 who gained 47 mgm. on an intake of 164 mgm. The degree of calcium loss on a minimal intake in Subject 2 was within normal limits (11), while the behavior of Subject 1 was usually conservative. Thus the latter stored approximately 95 grams of calcium and 43 grams of phosphorus in the period of 200 days, equivalent to 15 per cent of the stores which should be in the body, in contrast to the control patient who retained only 5.9 grams of calcium and 4.8 grams of phosphorus in 108 days.

Examination of the ratios of calcium to corrected phosphorus balance (Table II) shows that they are above 2 in the majority of instances, and above 3 in several instances, bearing no close relationship with the ratios of intake. If we accept the mineral composition of normal bone as $CaCO_3.2Ca_3(PO_4)_2$ according to the x-ray analysis of Roseberry, Hastings and Morse (12), then the ratio of Ca : P should be 2.26. The fact that the ratios of retention in Subject 1 were usually higher than that prescribed for normal bone would suggest that more calcium was deposited as $CaCO_3$ than $Ca_3(PO_4)_2$ in the new bone formation or that calcium suffered to a greater extent than phosphorus during the prior demineralization. As to the actual amount of calcium retained, the maximum was 752 mgm. (or 45 per cent of intake) on an intake of 1672 mgm. calcium and 922 mgm. phosphorus giving a ratio of 1.83 (Table IV). This happens to be also the level and ratio of intake associated with the largest retention of phosphorus, namely, 301 mgm. (or 32 per cent of intake). Thus both calcium and phosphorus have to be given at fairly high levels with a ratio approaching 2 in order to secure maximal retention of both elements. Otherwise, the ratio made very little difference to the calcium balance which depended mainly on the level of intake, in conformity with the work of Shohl (10).

TABLE V

Subject 2. The effect of calcium and phosphorus intake on their balances

Calcium intake		Calcium balance at the phosphorus intake of			Average Ca balance at same Ca intake regardless of P intake
Range	Level	402 mgm.	582 mgm.	1094 mgm.	
mgm.	*mgm.*	*mgm.*	*mgm.*	*mgm.*	*mgm.*
112–178	145	*0.44* -102	*0.20* -202	*0.16* -219	-174
1012–1078	1040	*2.63* 113	*1.76* -58	*0.99* 183	86
2012–2084	2055	*5.08* 230	*3.58* 374	*1.91* 156	253
Average Ca balance at same P intake regardless of Ca intake		87	38	40	

Calcium intake		Phosphorus balance at the phosphorus intake of			Average P balance at same Ca intake regardless of P intake
Range	Level	402 mgm.	582 mgm.	1094 mgm.	
112–178	145	*0.44* -69	*0.20* -82	*0.16* -107	-86
1012–1078	1040	*2.63* -45	*1.76* -87	*0.99* 54	-26
2012–2084	2055	*5.08* -22	*3.58* -26	*1.91* 126	26
Average P balance at same P intake regardless of Ca intake		-45	-65	24	

* Figures in italics are ratios of calcium to phosphorus intake.

DISCUSSION

The present results obtained with the patient with osteomalacia receiving continuous administration of vitamin D are in entire agreement with those of previous studies on patients whose treatment with vitamin D was discontinued after relatively short periods of 4 to 6 weeks when its maximum effect had been attained. The behavior of serum calcium and phosphorus, the manner of conservation of these elements through the urinary and intestinal tracts, the ability of the patients to maintain positive calcium balance on minimal intake and to retain large amounts of it on higher levels of intake, and finally the relatively greater importance of calcium intake rather than phosphorus intake as the limiting factor in both calcium and phosphorus retention are essentially the same in both instances. Thus vitamin D, once given to the extent of its maximum effect, will maintain its action unabated for at least several months after its discontinuation, and its continuous administration in the treatment of osteomalacia does not seem to offer any substantial advantage.

In the therapy of osteomalacia, while vitamin D administration corrects the basic metabolic defect, it is essential that both calcium and phosphorus be given at fairly high levels, preferably with a ratio of approximately 2 in order to promote large retention of both elements and therefore rapid restoration of the mineral contents of the depleted osseous system. With ordinary Chinese dietaries which are low in calcium and fairly high in phosphorus, the desired high level of calcium intake has to be supplied as calcium salts, while that of phosphorus intake can easily be taken care of by the diet.

The behavior of the patient without skeletal decalcification resembles that of patients having healing osteomalacia in respect to the reciprocal relationship between urinary calcium and phosphorus, the approximately parallel relationship between stool calcium and phosphorus, the dependence of both calcium and phosphorus balances on calcium intake, and the slight effect of phosphorus intake as a limiting factor in both calcium and phosphorus retention. On the other hand, he differs in that the serum phosphorus is relatively more stable toward dietary changes, and in that the magnitudes of urinary and stool excretion of calcium and phosphorus are greater, resulting in negative balance on low intake and only slight retention on higher levels of intake. These differences are but an expression of the fact that in a relatively normal individual measures of mineral conservation are less urgently in need of application.

SUMMARY

1. In two patients, one with osteomalacia under reparation and the other with syphilitic osteitis of radius and tibia, the serum levels of calcium and phosphorus, paths of excretion and retention of these elements were studied in relation to their levels and ratios of intake.

2. Serum calcium was fairly constant in both cases, while serum inorganic phosphorus tended to lower with a higher ratio of Ca : P intake in the first patient. No such variations were demonstrable in the second patient.

3. A reciprocal relationship between calcium and phosphorus in urine was shown in both instances. Whenever the Ca : P ratio in the diet was high, urinary calcium increased, while urinary phosphorus diminished. An opposite change in the ratio resulted in a diminution of urinary calcium coinciding with a rise of urinary phosphorus.

4. Fecal calcium and phosphorus varied with their respective level of intake, while fecal phosphorus was also partly dependent on calcium intake.

5. Retention of either calcium or phosphorus depended more on the calcium than phosphorus intake, although both had to be supplied in fairly large quantities with a Ca : P ratio of approximately 2 in order to realize maximal retention of both elements to promote efficient repair of skeletal demineralization in osteomalacia.

6. The present study with prolonged administration of vitamin D revealed no essential difference from the previous work with limited vitamin D therapy, showing that the effect of vitamin D lasts long after its discontinuation.

CASE HISTORIES

Case 1. H. F. M., a Chinese housewife of 32, was admitted on August 28, 1935 for pain in back and legs and difficulty in walking. These began 7 years prior to admission when she had her first pregnancy. Labor was spontaneous but lasted for more than 24 hours. After that she had periodical exacerbations of the above symptoms in winter and spring when she kept herself indoors. The second pregnancy occurred 4 years after the first and resulted in a seven months' premature labor lasting more than 48 hours. Henceforth symptoms became worse. She could neither stand on her feet nor walk without support. Her diet had always been extremely poor. In the cold months she lived on cereals and salted vegetables. In the warmer months some fresh vegetables were available. Meat was seldom taken and eggs only occasionally.

Examination on admission confirmed her statement about her inability to stand or walk without support. Body weight was 40 kgm. and height 136 cm. On lying down, the right thigh was slightly flexed and abducted, with the knee joint held in 30° flexion. Movement at the hip joint caused pain. There was no tenderness along the lower extremities. The pelvis was of the funnel type. Symphysis pubis protruded and sacrum was prominent. Tenderness was marked over the sacro-iliac joints, pelvic bones, lower ribs and lumbar vertebrae. The right upper molar teeth and lower incisors were loose. Other physical findings were normal. X-ray showed a deformed pelvis and general osteoporosis and some pleural thickening with adhesions in the right lower chest. Blood calcium was 8.92, phosphorus 3.29 mgm. per cent, and plasma phosphatase 4.9 units (Bodansky). Blood counts and urinalysis were essentially normal. Stool was positive for ova of ascaris. Metabolic studies were carried out in four-day periods for 212 days from October 4, 1935 to May 2, 1936. Besides the dietary treatment and vitamin D administration she also received physiotherapy in the form of exercises for extension of the hip and spine and infra-red irradiation. At the time of discharge she could walk fairly well without support, and x-ray of bones revealed definitely increased density.

Case 2. L. Y. S., a Chinese man of 24, entered on July 13, 1934 for swelling and lengthening of the right leg of 8 years' duration and of the right forearm of two years' duration. Onset was insidious without history of injury. He had occasional low grade fever and pain after prolonged walking. He had had venereal exposures.

The patient was found to be slightly undernourished. Body weight was 42.2 kgm. and height 159 cm. His right leg was 5.5 cm. longer than the left and also bigger especially in the lower part. There was slight tenderness over the right tibia, and the overlying skin was slightly warmer than that of the left side. The knee and ankle were not involved. Right forearm was 1.5 cm. longer than the left. The elbow and wrist were free. Other physical findings were essentially normal. X-ray of the bones showed irregular areas of condensation and rarefaction in the cortex involving the entire length of right tibia and radius. The rest of the skeleton appeared normal. Blood and urine examinations revealed no significant findings. Stools contained ova of ascaris. Blood calcium was 9.7 and phosphorus 4.2 mgm. per cent. Basal metabolic rate was + 8.4 per cent. Blood Wassermann

and Kahn tests were strongly positive. Metabolic studies were carried on for 108 days (27 four-day periods from September 18, 1934 to January 3, 1935). Subsequent intensive antisyphilitic treatment to date has given rise to marked improvement in the bone lesions.

BIBLIOGRAPHY

1. Maxwell, J. P., Osteomalacia in China. China M. J., 1923, **37**, 625.
2. Maxwell, J. P., Further studies in osteomalacia. Proc. Roy. Soc. Med. (Section Obst. and Gynec.), 1930, **23**, 19.
3. Maxwell, J. P., and Miles, L. M., Osteomalacia in China. J. Obst. and Gynec. Brit. Emp., 1925, **32**, 433.
4. Hannon, R. R., Liu, S. H., Chu, H. I., Wang, S. H., Chen, K. C., and Chou, S. K., Calcium and phosphorus metabolism in osteomalacia. I. The effect of vitamin D and its apparent duration. Chinese Med. J., 1934, **48**, 623.
5. Wu, H., and Wu, D. Y., Dietaries of Peking. Chinese J. Physiol. (Report Series), 1928, **1**, 135.
6. Liu, S. H., Hannon, R. R., Chu, H. I., Chen, K. C., Chou, S. K., and Wang, S. H., Calcium and phosphorus metabolism in osteomalacia. II. Further studies on the response to vitamin D of patients with osteomalacia. Chinese Med. J., 1935, **49**, 1.
7. Liu, S. H., Hannon, R. R., Chou, S. K., Chen, K. C., Chu, H. I., and Wang, S. H., Calcium and phosphorus metabolism in osteomalacia. III. The effects of varying levels and ratios of intake of calcium to phosphorus on their serum levels, paths of excretion and balances. Chinese J. Physiol., 1935, **9**, 101.
8. Wu, H., Nutritive value of Chinese foods. Chinese J. Physiol. (Report Series), 1928, **1**, 153.
9. Sherman, H. C., Chemistry of Food and Nutrition. Macmillan Co., New York, 1928, 3d ed.
10. Shohl, A. T., Rickets in rats. XV. The effect of low calcium-high phosphorus diets at various levels and ratios upon the production of rickets and tetany. J. Nutrition, 1936, **11**, 275.
11. Bauer, W., Albright, F., and Aub, J. C., Studies of calcium and phosphorus metabolism. II. The calcium excretion of normal individuals on a low calcium diet, also data on a case of pregnancy. J. Clin. Invest., 1929, **7**, 75.
12. Roseberry, H. H., Hastings, A. B., and Morse, J. K., X-ray analysis of bone and teeth. J. Biol. Chem., 1931, **90**, 395.

Chinese Journal of Physiology, 1937, Vol. 11, No. 3, pp. 271—294.

CALCIUM AND PHOSPHORUS METABOLISM IN OSTEOMALACIA. VI. THE ADDED DRAIN OF LACTATION AND BENEFICIAL ACTION OF VITAMIN D

S. H. LIU, C. C. SU, C. W. WANG AND K. P. CHANG

(From the Department of Medicine, Peiping Union Medical College, Peiping)

Received for publication September 13, 1936

In a previous report [Hannon et al., 1934] it has been demonstrated that the primary metabolic defect in osteomalacia is lack of intestinal absorption of calcium on account of vitamin D deficiency. The low level of calcium intake that prevails in common Chinese dietaries accentuates the difficulty. Pregnancy and lactation both exert a drain on the maternal mineral supplies and must be also important factors in the pathogenesis of osteomalacia especially when the dietary constituents concerned are restricted. The fact that symptoms of osteomalacia often begin with pregnancy and become worse with each succeeding reproductive cycle corroborates that supposition [Liu et al., 1935].

Quantitative measurement of calcium and phosphorus metabolism during pregnancy and lactation in osteomalacia is not available in the literature. However, certain reported studies of apparently normal women may bear on the present problem. Coons and Blunt [1930] observed that in nine pregnant women on a calcium intake of 0.6 - 1.7 g per day the mineral retention often fell short of the requirement of the fetus. Macy, Hunscher, Nims and McCosh [1930] frequently obtained negative calcium balances on three normal women during pregnancy with intake varying from 1.5 to 2.7 g per day. Toverud and Toverud [1931] made 44 periods of metabolic observations on 17 expectant mothers receiving the usual diet of the home. Negative calcium and

271

phosphorus balances were found in the majority of the cases. No woman showed a positive calcium balance in the last two months of pregnancy unless the intake reached the value of 1.6 g per day.

During lactation the mineral requirement seems to be even greater. Hunscher [1930], and Hummel, Sternberger, Hunscher and Macy [1936] failed to maintain actively nursing women in calcium balance on very high intake (3-4 g per day) during the first part of lactation. Only during late lactation when milk flow diminished was calcium stored [Donelson, Nims, Hunscher and Macy, 1931]. Supplementing the usual home diets with cod liver oil, although improving the calcium balance, did not always change a negative to a positive balance [Macy, Hunscher, McCosh and Nims, 1930]. Garry and Stiven [1936] who have reviewed the recent literature on dietary requirements in reproduction recommend 1 to 2 g of calcium per day for milk yields of from 500 cc to 1 liter and calcium contents from 20 to 30 mg per 100 cc milk.

Thus the adult maintenance requirement of 0.68 g of calcium per day [Sherman, 1932] is evidently insufficient for periods of mineral stress. In the case of Chinese women whose diet does not contain more than 0.3 g calcium per day [Wu and Yen, 1928], the mineral shortage would be especially acute during periods of reproduction, and its bearing on the pathogenesis of osteomalacia would be equally obvious. The present communication presents the results of studies of calcium, phosphorus and nitrogen metabolism of Chinese lactating women, with or without osteomalacia, in an attempt to evaluate the added drain of lactation on low calcium intake and the beneficial effect of vitamin D.

EXPERIMENTAL

Procedure.

Of the five experimental subjects available for this investigation, the first three suffered from varying degrees of osteomalacia. Case 1 had very low serum calcium and inorganic phosphorus with manifest tetany, and Case 2 moderately low serum calcium and inorganic phosphorus with latent tetany; while Case 3 showed normal serum calcium and phosphorus as a result of previous vitamin D administration during her pregnancy. Cases 4 and 5 were lactating women without evident osteomalacia on x-ray examination, intended as controls. All the subjects came from families whose income was below basic necessities. Their diet consisted of cereals such as corn meal, millet, and rarely flour and rice. Vegetables were mainly salted turnip and cabbage with small amounts of other vegetables in season. Eggs and meat were seldom, if ever, eaten. Such a diet is known to be deficient in several respects. It is poor in fat-soluble vitamins particularly vitamin D. These people must rely largely on exposure to sunshine for the protective effect of vitamin D. The mineral content of such a diet is notably low in calcium, but relatively high in phosphorus.

The plan was to place each subject on a constant diet simulating her diet at home (table 1). The resemblance must be considered only approximate, as more pork was used and better cooking and serving employed in the hospital diets to render them sufficiently attractive to insure their quantitative consumption for long periods of time. Distilled water was used for drinking and preparation of diet. Vitamin D preparation given was Vigantol, an oily solution of irradiated ergosterol containing 15,000 international units of vitamin D per cc.

Metabolic periods were four days each, carmine being used to mark off the stools of each period. Stools and urine respectively of each period were pooled for analysis. Breasts were emptied with an electric pump five or six times a day and an aliquot was taken of each milking. The 24-hour composite milk was analysed. Venepuncture was done before breakfast at the beginning of each period.

Analytical methods for calcium, phosphorus and nitrogen of food, urine, stool and blood were described previously [Liu, et al., 1935]. For milk, 3 cc were ashed in platinum and the ash dissolved in 15 cc of 0.1 N HCl. Calcium was determined by the method of Clark and Collip [1925] on 10 cc of the ash solution with the addition of 1 cc of 20 per cent sodium acetate solution. The pH of such a mixture was found to be approximately 5.0, optimal for the precipitation of calcium oxalate. It was also found necessary to add a drop of decalcified serum to the precipitate before washing with 2 per cent ammonia water in order to prevent the precipitate from floating on top of the fluid. Fiske and Subbarow's method [1925] was used for the determination of total phosphorus of milk, 2 cc of the ash solution being employed.

Results.

Data on lactation and composition of milk are presented in table 2. By far the most actively lactating subject was Case 3. Not only did she produce more than a liter of milk per day, but also her milk excelled in calcium, phosphorus and nitrogen contents, when compared with other subjects. She spent the last seven months of her pregnancy in the Hospital where she received diets adequate in all respects, including vitamin D, and 2 g of calcium and 1 g of phosphorus per day for the treatment of osteomalacia. Such excellent preparation probably accounts for her superior performance during lactation.

All the rest of the subjects are relatively poor nursing mothers from the viewpoint of milk flow as well as its mineral contents. While the late stage of lactation may account for the low figures in some instances, particularly in case 5, the real explanation probably lies in the inadequacies of their previous dietaries, the nature of which may be gleaned from table 1.

Metabolic data during lactation may best be presented individually.

Case 1. This patient had relatively mild osteomalacia, but marked hypocalcemia and severe tetany. Studies were commenced during the 7th month of lactation. She was on a constant diet throughout the 19 periods of metabolic study (fig. 1 and table 3). During the first five

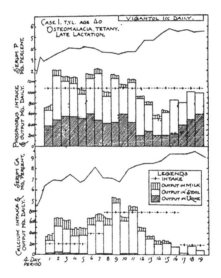

Fig. 1. Case 1. Calcium and phorphorus metabolism in lactation and effect of vitamain D administration.

periods on a calcium intake of 193 mg per day the balance was markedly negative, averaging 339 mg per day. Of the total output, stool calcium amounted to 69 per cent, milk 26 per cent and urine 5 per cent. It appeared that the most important source of calcium loss was through the intestine, and that the amount of calcium secreted in the milk, though constituting an added drain, was not nearly as important as the excessive loss through the stool.

The intake of calcium during periods 6 and 7 was increased to 393 mg by the addition of calcium lactate. Almost all the added calcium was eliminated in the stool. Further augmentation of the calcium supply to 793 mg during periods 8 and 9 did not seem to rectify the situation materially. Then from the 10th period onward while calcium intake remained the same, vitamin D as Vigantol was given in 1 cc daily doses. The stool elimination of calcium decreased promptly and progressively so that an increasingly positive balance was obtained. The maximum effect of vitamin D was reached during period 14, the 5th period of its administration. During that period the patient was able to retain 533 mg of calcium per day, namely, 67 per cent of the intake.

Weaning was begun in period 15 and completed in period 16 when calcium retention was even greater. During the last three periods, calcium lactate was withdrawn so that the patient was receiving the same minimal calcium intake as during the beginning of the investigation. She was able to maintain a distinctly positive balance. Had lactation been allowed to continue, it would be possible for her to maintain balance during some of the periods of low intake. This study demonstrates the remarkable value of vitamin D in conserving calcium. Under the influence of vitamin D, lactation may be accomplished with relatively little calcium loss to the mother even on minimal calcium intake.

Phosphorus balances in general were parallel with calcium balances. On a liberal phosphorus intake (1082 mg per day) the balance was negative as long as calcium balance remained so. Shortly after the exhibition of vitamin D, phosphorus began to be retained and the retention increased progressively corresponding to the degree of calcium retention. The maximum retention was attained during period 14 amounting to 514 mg per day, nearly 50 per cent of the intake. The striking dependence of phosphorus upon calcium metabolism renders the large phosphorus intake of no avail to the organism as long as the calcium supply is the limiting factor.

Serum calcium showed an initial prompt rise from 4.55 to 7 mg per cent level and remained there until after vitamin D administration when it gradually rose above 9 mg per cent. Serum inorganic phosphorus behaved similarly. There was an initial rise from 1.68 to 4, and then, as a result of vitamin D therapy, a further rise to 5.95 mg per cent.

Case 2. Moderately marked osteomalacia was represented by this patient, who was admitted for study during her 8th month of lactation. The quantitative diet on which she was placed contained 377 mg calcium and 1197 mg phosphorus per day. As seen in the first two periods (fig. 2 and table 4) the calcium balance was slightly negative,

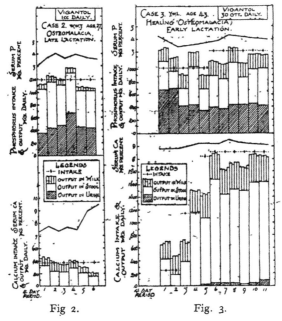

Fig 2.   Fig. 3.

Figs. 2 and 3. Cases 2 and 3. Calcium and phosphorus metabolism in lactation and effect of vitamin D administration.

while phosphorus balance was even. In contrast to Case 1, this patient exhibited greater power of conserving calcium, although her intake was higher. But in agreement with the behavior of Case 1, the calcium loss in the stool in the present subject accounted for 70 per cent, and milk secretion only 30 per cent of the total output.

Again calcium in stool is quantitatively more important than that in milk. While the diet was kept the same, vitamin D was added (Vigantol 1 cc daily) during periods 3-6. This was followed in periods

5. and 6 by substantial calcium and phosphorus retention. Under the influence of vitamin D the limited supply of calcium in the diet was sufficient not only for the metabolic needs during lactation but also for deposit in the tissues for the repair of skeletal decalcification. Such behavior is characteristic of patients with osteomalacia undergoing reparation brought about by vitamin D administration.

This patient had latent tetany with serum calcium level at 7.5 mg per cent; but after vitamin D administration, the signs of neuromuscular hyper-irritability disappeared coinciding with the elevation of serum calcium to 9.5 mg per cent.

Case 3. This patient with osteomalacia was under continuous observation during the last two-thirds of her pregnancy and received a well balanced diet with high calcium and phosphorus intake supplemented by Vigantol. She was retaining approximately 800 mg calcium and 400 mg phosphorus per day during gestation. Observation on the effects of lactation began 18 days post partum (fig. 3 and table 5). On a low calcium intake of 247 mg per day, her balance was markedly negative. In view of the large volume of milk secretion containing more calcium than what the diet supplied, balance, as expected, could not be maintained even though vitamin D effect were operative. Milk calcium accounted for 47 per cent of the total output. When the calcium intake was raised to 1147 mg per day, her balance was first positive, and then negative. On averaging the results of the two periods (periods 3 and 4), a slightly positive balance was obtained. When the calcium intake was further raised to a little over 2000 mg per day, calcium retention became somewhat greater, but it was much less than that during gestation. It was thought that the poor retention might be explained by the wearing out of the effect of vitamin D given during pregnancy. Therefore Vigantol was given again from period 7 on. No distinct improvement in calcium balance could be discerned during the five periods in which vitamin D was administered indicating that the patient was not deficient in vitamin D.

This patient, then, differs from the two previous patients in that relatively large amounts of calcium are required for maintaining balance even in the presence of vitamin D. Although no clear explanation for the difference in behavior is available, it seems likely that during early lactation with relatively abundant milk flow calcium metabolism is

greatly stimulated so that conservation through other channels of elimination becomes very difficult even though there is no vitamin D
deficiency. Moreover, the marked calcium retention during gestation,
as shown by this patient, has sufficiently replenished the skeletal store
of calcium to render conservation during lactation less urgent than in
cases where preparation during pregnancy is less adequate.

Case 4. This lactating woman, without any clinical or roentgenologic evidence of osteomalacia, was observed during her third month
of lactation. While on a diet containing 275 mg calcium and 1425 mg
phosphorus, she showed a negative calcium balance to the extent of
159 mg daily (fig. 4 and table 6). As her milk yield was not abundant

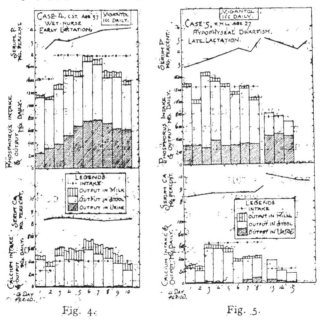

Fig. 4.   Fig. 5.

Fig. 4. Case 4. Calcium and phosphorus metabolism in lactation and
effect of vitamin D administration.

Fig. 5. Case 5. Calcium and phosphorus metabolism in lactation and
effect of vitamin D administration.

during the first two periods the amount of calcium loss through lactation
averaged only 68 mg per day, approximately 16 per cent of her total
output (periods 1 and 2), and fecal calcium was quantitatively much
more important.

On raising the calcium intake to 408 mg. per day during subsequent periods, the amount of calcium loss was not decreased, as calcium elimination was augmented both in the milk and in the feces. Vigantol was given during periods 8-10, when fecal calcium gradually diminished so that a slightly positive balance was obtained during the third period of vitamin D administration.

The above described metabolic behavior is very much like that of Cases 1 and 2. The calcium metabolism of strictly normal individuals is relatively indifferent to the effects of irradiation, cod liver oil [Hart, Tourtellotte and Blumgart, 1928] and irradiated ergosterol [Bauer, Marble and Claflin, 1932]. Therefore, the susceptibility of calcium metabolism to the conserving effect of Vigantol suggests that the present subject, although without clinical and roentgenologic evidence of osteomalacia, is nevertheless deficient in vitamin D as well as in skeletal store of calcium. This observation demonstrates the existence of what may be termed subclinical vitamin D and calcium deficiencies which are probably more widespread than commonly realized.

This patient maintained a positive phosphorus balance throughout all the metabolic periods. This is largely due to the marked retention of nitrogen which amounted to 3 to 5 g per day. She gained considerable bodily tissue as evidenced by her weight increase of 7.5 kg. within the 10 periods of study.

Her serum calcium was maintained at 8.5, while inorganic phosphorus increased from 2.45 to 4.05 mg. per cent.

Case 5. Aside from hypophyseal dwarfism this subject showed no evidence of calcium deficiency in the skeleton. Observations on her were made during late lactation when milk output was rather small (fig. 5 and table 7). While on a diet with 271 mg calcium and 1257 mg. phosphorus, her calcium balance was slightly negative (periods 1 and 2). Again the intestine was much more important as path of elimination (70 percent) than the breasts (23 percent). Calcium intake was then increased to 671 mg. per day, whereupon the balance became slightly positive (periods 3 and 4). During periods 5-8 Vigantol was given, to which the patient responded by diminishing stool calcium and consequent substantial calcium retention.

After a lapse of 17 days, during which lactation was allowed to stop, the patient was again studied for 3 periods (periods 13-15). The diet was changed, and the calcium content (251 mg per day) was slightly less than the initial calcium intake. While the balance was negative during the first of the periods, some calcium gain was shown during later periods indicating conservation of calcium metabolism, probably the result of prior administration of vitamin D.

What has been said about Case 4 holds true in the present case. While there is no gross calcium deficiency in the bones, the patient shows evidence of vitamin D deficiency and calcium shortage. The administration of Vigantol resulted in considerable improvement in her state of calcium metabolism. Both serum calcium and inorganic phosphorus showed distinct rise after Vigantol exhibition.

Discussion.

From the foregoing observations several points bear discussion. The common Chinese diet is admittedly low in calcium. The dietary survey of Wu and Yen [1928] shows that the average calcium content of diets in Peiping is 0.337 g and phosphorus content 1.178 g; and our experience with the diets of individual patients corroborate their findings. These figures are lower than those proposed by Sherman for adult maintenance, let alone the increased requirements for pregnancy and lactation suggested by various investigators. The low calcium intake would account for the somewhat greater prevalence of calcium-deficiency diseases in North China and would also explain the calcium loss by the nursing women in the present study. But that does not seem to represent the complete picture as seen from the following considerations.

With calcium intake ranging between 193 and 377 mg per day in our cases, the extent of negative balance varied from 31 to 339 mg per day. As compared with the studies by Hunscher [1930] on three American women who showed during the 26 to 27th week of lactation negative calcium balances from 0.749 to 2.154 g on an intake of 3.399

to 4.424 g per day, the calcium loss sustained by the Chinese subjects during lactation was relatively slight. The comparison suggests that the human organism is able to conserve calcium, when the supply is limited. Conservation was brought about by diminished elimination through all the channels, but more particularly through urine and milk Urinary output of calcium was negligible in all the cases. Milk yield did not exceed 500 cc with calcium content from 68 to 138 mg in 4 out of the 5 subjects. Calcium secreted in the milk amounted to 16 to 30 per cent of the total output. Therefore lactation though constituting an added drain to the maternal mineral supply, accounts for only a small part of the calcium loss. The safety mechanism of reduction in milk yield has been demonstrated in animal experiments and does not seem to come into action until 20 per cent of the total body calcium is lost [Schmidt and Greenberg 1935].

The beneficial effect of vitamin D as demonstrated in our studies is remarkable. As a result of its administration all but one of the subjects maintained a positive calcium balance even when the supply was restricted. While vitamin D was operative, the limited intake was sufficient not only for the metabolic needs of lactation, but also for storage to replenish the skeletal deprivation. Therefore the calcium loss in lactation in all but Case 3 is to be attributed more to vitamin D deficiency than to the low calcium intake. Moderate augmentation of calcium intake as in Cases 1 and 4 prior to vitamin D therapy failed to rectify the calcium loss.

From the above considerations it seems fair to conclude that with low calcium intake, a safety mechanism comes into play by which milk production is reduced so that the extent of calcium loss becomes much less than it would be otherwise; and that vitamin D deficiency is a more important factor than low calcium intake in accounting for the mineral stress in lactation.

While a woman may do well on low calcium diet supplemented by vitamin D when milk yield is low, it is essential to supply larger quantities of calcium to maintain balance in case of abundant milk secretion, or to promote large milk yield. As shown in Case 3 where the milk output was high, even though prior vitamin D had been given, calcium intake had to be increased to a little over 1 g before a slightly positive balance was obtained. It seems as if the physiological adjustment at the height of lactation is such that relatively large quantities of calcium must be allowed to run to waste in order that requisite amounts of the mineral may be constantly at the disposal of the mammary gland.

A word may be said about the so-called calcium requirement. Current conception about calcium requirement implies that it is a fixed quantity below which there is danger of running into negative balance; whereas it must be a very variable affair. Aside from the increased demand in growth and reproduction, many other modifying factors may be operative. The requirement may seem to be greater when dietary habits accustom the subject to larger intake, and when there is a larger prior store in the body. On the other hand vitamin D when present in adequate amounts will conserve calcium metabolism to such an extent as to render the usually quoted requirement superfluous. Therefore in defining calcium requirement for a given period of life, such factors as the previous dietary custom, the state of skeletal store and the amount of vitamin D must be taken into consideration. Therefore Chinese diet is inadequate not so much from its low calcium content as from its vitamin D deficiency. However, the low calcium intake is pathogenetically important in that it renders the effect of vitamin D deficiency more easily or acutely felt than when the calcium supply is more liberal.

SUMMARY AND CONCLUSIONS

Data on calcium, phosphorus and nitrogen metabolism of five Chinese lactating women were presented. Three had osteomalacia and two showed no clinical evidence of bony decalcification.

Four of the subjects on low calcium intake had relatively small milk yield. The negative balance in calcium was not excessive and calcium loss through lactation accounted for a small fraction of the total output.

Moderate addition of calcium failed to rectify materially the calcium loss, but vitamin D administration was efficacious in reducing the stool elimination of the element so that a markedly positive balance was obtained.

CA AND P IN OSTEOMALACIA

In one subject whose milk yield was high, calcium intake had to be considerably increased to maintain balance even in presence of vitamin D.

The two subjects without clinical skeletal decalcification behaved similarly to, and showed as marked response to vitamin D exhibition as those with osteomalacia, suggesting the existence of subclinical states of vitamin D deficiency and calcium shortage in the bones.

LITERATURE

BAUER, W., MABBLE, A. AND CLAFLIN, D.   (1932) J. Clin. Invest., **11**, 1.

CLARK, E. P. AND COLLIP, J. B.   (1925) J. biol. Chem., **63**, 461.

COONS, C. M. AND BLUNT, K.   (1930) Ibid, **86**, 1.

DONELSON, E., NIMS, B., HUNSCHER, H. A. AND MACY, I. G.   (1931) J. biol. Chem., **91**, 675.

FISKE, C. AND SUBBAROW, Y.   (1925) Ibid, **66**, 375.

GARRY, R. C. AND STIVEN, D.   (1936) Nutrition Abstr. Rev., **5**, 855.

HANNON, R. R., LIU, S. H., CHU, H. I., WANG, S. H., CHEN, K. C. AND CHOU, S. K.   (1934) Chinese med. J., **48**, 623.

HART, M. C., TOURTELLOTE, D. R. AND BLUMGART, H. L.   (1928) J. biol. Chem., **76**, 143

HUMMEL, F. C., STERNBERGER, H. R., HUNSCHER, H. A. AND MACY, I. G.   (1936) J. Nutrition, **11**, 235.

HUNSCHER, H. A.   (1930) J. biol. Chem., **86**, 37.

LIU, S. H., HANNON, R. R., CHU, H. I., CHEN, K. C., CHOU, S. K. AND WANG, S. H.   (1935) Chinese med. J., **49**, 1.

LIU, S. H., HANNON, R. R., CHOU, S. K., CHEN, K. C., CHU, H. I. AND WANG, S. H.   (1935) Chinese J. Physiol., **9**, 101.

MACY, I. G., HUNSCHER, H. A., NIMS, B. AND MCCOSH, S. S.   (1930) J. biol. Chem., **86**, 17.

MACY, I. G., HUNSCHER, H. A., MCCOSH, S. S. AND NIMS, B.   (1930) Ibid, **86**, 59.

MCLEAN, F. C. AND HASTINGS, A. B.   (1935) Amer. J. med. Sci., **189**, 601.

SCHMIDT, C. L. A. AND GREENBERG, D. M.   (1935) Physiol. Rev., **15**, 297.

SHERMAN, H. C.   (1932) Chemistry of food and nutrition, 4th ed., New York.

TOVERUD, K. U. AND TOVERUD, G.   (1931) Acta Pediat. (Supp. 2), **12**, 1.

WU, H.   (1928) Chinese J. Physiol., Rep. Ser., **1**, 153.

WU, H. AND WU, D. Y.   (1928) Ibid, **1**, 135.

ABSTRACTS OF CASE HISTORIES

Case 1. T.Y.L., a Chinese woman of 40, was admitted to the Hospital on February 10, 1936 for spastic attacks of hands and feet. She came from a poor family with income below basic necessities. Her diet consisted almost exclusively of corn meal and millet with cabbage and salted turnip. She was married at 20 and subsequently gave birth to six children. The fifth child was born 2 years and the sixth child 6 months prior to admission. All pregnancies were without complications and deliveries easy and spontaneous. The older children were breast fed up to 8 months, but after the birth of the last child she was not only nursing the new born, but also the 2-year old child.

About one month prior to admission the patient began to have general weakness, numbness of lower limbs and soreness of teeth. The numbness usually came in the evening after a day's work, disappearing in the morning. Four days before admission, following several days of fever, cough and sputum, she was suddenly seized with spasm and rigidity of all the extremities, accompanied by dyspnea and palpitation of heart, but no loss of consciousness. The attack wore off in 3 hours after massage. Similar attack recurred on the day of entry to the Hospital.

On examination, the patient appeared in severe pain with carpo-pedal spasm. Chvostek's sign was strongly positive. Temp. 37.6°C. Weight 41.4 kg. Eye lids were puffy, face flushed and pharynx injected. Several teeth were carious. Lungs were clear except for scattered rhonchi. Heart was normal. B.P. 120/74. Abdomen was soft and non-tender. Spleen and liver were not palpable. Tendon reflexes were normal. Bones were not tender on pressure.

Blood withdrawn prior to treatment showed serum calcium 4.55, inorganic phosphorus 1.68 mg per cent, albumin 3.43 and globulin 2.34 mg per cent. Calculation according to McLean and Hastings' nomogram [1935] gave calcium ions 2.1 mg per cent, well within the "tetany level". Serum phosphatase was 9.8 units (Bodansky). Blood counts gave R.B.C. 4.13 millions, W.B.C. 6.400, and hemoglobin 11 g per 100 cc. Urine on several occasions contained sugar which proved to be lactose. Stool contained ova of ascaris. Roentgenograms of chest suggested minimal pulmonary tuberculosis in both upper areas. Roentgenologic survey of the skeleton showed mild degree of osteoporosis. The pubic bones tended to rostration. Transverse outlet measured 7.5 cm. Eye ground examination showed mild hypertensive type of vascular disturbance of retinal vessels, and slit-lamp examination revealed dust-like opacities in the cortical layer of both lenses, although her vision was not disturbed.

On admission, the patient was given intravenously 20 cc of 2 per cent calcium chloride solution which brought immediate relief of acute symptoms. She took a quantitative diet which resembled her diet at home, and cooperated exceedingly well throughout the period of 76 days of metabolic observations (from February 14 to April 29 inclusive). Shortly after admission, her serum calcium rose to 7 and inorganic phosphorus to 4 mg per cent. She was symptom free, although Trousseau's and Chvostek's signs remained positive,

After the administration of vitamin D there was a prompt further increase of serum calcium to 9.3 and inorganic phosphorus to 5.5 mg per cent. She was then discharged well on May 2, 1936. Prior to discharge she was allowed to stop lactation. Follow-up x-ray examination before discharge showed healing of pulmonary tuberculosis, and no change in the density of the skeleton compared with the findings on entry.

Case 2. W.W.J. This patient, a lactating women of 27, para IV, came in on May 16, 1936 for pain in lumbo-sacral region and thighs for 6 years. She has lived all her life in a country district and subsisted on corn meal, millet and occasionally wheat with cabbage, salted turnip, and rarely meat or eggs. However, she had frequent access to sunshine. Marriage occurred at 19, and her first child was born at 20, second child at 21, third child at 24 and fourth child at 27, namely, seven months prior to admission. All pregnancies were said to be smooth and confinements easy and spontaneous. All the children were breast-fed; and after the birth of her second child the patient was suckling two babies at one time. It was at that time when pain in the lower back and extremities began. It was a continuous dull ache aggravated by movement and locomotion. Occasionally attacks of numbness and spasm of hands and feet were noticed. The lower ribs became tender to touch and spine stiff. Stature was said to have shortened somewhat shortly after the onset of illness. The symptoms were worse during spring and summer and better during autumn and winter, and showed no apparent downward progression during subsequent pregnancies and lactations.

When examined, the patient appeared comfortable. She walked with small steps with head somewhat bent forward. Weight 43.5 kg. Height 151 cm. Thoracic cage was slightly narrowed at its lower portion and the lower ribs were tender on pressure. Symphysis pubis was slightly rostrated, and the arch narrowed. Transverse outlet measured 6.5 cm. Trousseau phenomenon was positive, but Chvostek not elicited. The remaining physical findings were normal except for trachoma in both eyes and loosening of one of the lower incisors.

Serum calcium was 7.34, inorganic phosphorus 3.03 mg per cent, and phosphatase 13.5 units (Bodansky). Erythrocyte count was 5.48 millions with hemoglobin 14.9 g, and leukocyte count 8200 with normal differential pattern. Fasting blood sugar was 95 mg per cent. Urine contained sugar which was probably lactose. On x-ray examination, the bones showed slight general osteoporosis with retraction of the ribs of the lower thoracic cage and increased biconcavity of the body of lower thoracic and lumbar vertebrae.

While on a constant diet the composition of which simulated that of her diet at home, metabolic studies were carried out for six 4-day periods (May 19 to June 12 inclusive). After the administration of vitamin D her pains gradually disappeared coinciding with a rise of serum calcium to 9.53 and inorganic phosphorus to 3.58 mg per cent, whereupon she was discharged home.

Case 3. Y.W.L. This patient, aged 43, was Case 4 of Paper II [Liu, Hannon, Chu, Chen, Chou and Wang, 1935] and Case Y.W.L of Paper. III [Liu, Hannon, Chou, Chen, Chu and Wang, 1935] of this series where her clinical history and calcium and phosphorus metabolism were described in detail. During that admission (October 1933), she had advanced osteomalacia with symptoms dating back three years when her fourth child was born. With treatment with vitamin D and adequate amounts of calcium and phosphorus intake in proper ratio, her metabolic defect was corrected with subjective improvement. On discharge in June 1934, x-ray examination of skeleton revealed definite increase in the density of all the bones, although the deformities were not changed and sufficient degree of osteoporosis was still present to justify the diagnosis of low-grade osteomalacia from the roentgenologic standpoint. In August, pain in the back began to return and she was readmitted on September 17. She was found to be pregnant for two months, her expected date of confinement being on April 18, 1935. Her calcium and phosphorus metabolism was studied throughout the remaining seven months of pregnancy and will be reported in a separate communication. The patient had gastrointestinal upset with pain and gaseous distension several times in the course of pregnancy. She also developed a moderate macrocytic anemia beginning with the fourth month of pregnancy. The lowest hemoglobin reached was 8.6 g per 100 cc, and the lowest erythrocyte count 2.8 millions. Treatment with large doses of ferric ammonium citrate, intramuscular liver extract and hydrochloric acid, alone or in combination, did not seem to improve the anemia. However the pregnancy was successfully brought to term and a Caesarian section was performed on April 13, 1935 and a living male child was delivered. The puerparium was uneventful. Lactation commenced shortly after delivery. Balance study consisted of 11 four-day periods from April 30 to June 13 inclusive: She was discharged on June 15 in good condition.

Case 4. C.S.T. A chinese wet-nurse of 37, Para VI, was admitted on January 16, 1936 for study. There were no complaints. She was married at 19 and gave birth to six full term children without any complication during any of the reproductive cycles. The last child was born two months prior to admission. Although she gave the child away, she kept nursing another child as its wet nurse. Her diet consists of corn meal, millet and rice with cabbage and salted turnip and rarely pork.

Examination showed no distinct abnormality except for trachoma and slight undernutrition. Weight 45.8 kg B.P. 114/66. Urine normal, Stool contained ova of ascris. Blood hemoglobin 11.4 g per 100 cc, R.B.C. 4.4 millions, and W.B.C. 4,800. Roentgenograms of skull, hands and pelvic bones were normal with no evidence of osteoporosis or osteomalacia.

She was placed on a diet which simulated closely her diet at home (table 1), and observed for 10 four-day periods (January 17 to February 26 inclusive) during which calcium, phosphorus and nitrogen metabolism was studied. On discharge her weight was 53.0 kg, a gain of 7.2 kg.

Case 5. K.M.L. A Chinese lactating women of 28 was admitted for study on March 11, 1936. She presented no complaints, but the striking abnormality was her dwarfism. She was born and brought up in the country. Not much was known about her early developmental history, but she ceased gaining stature at the age of 14 when she was already much shorter and smaller than other girls of the same age. Her diet consisted of cornmeal, flour, millet, salted vegetables, cabbage, spinach, beans, bean sprouts and sometimes soybean milk. Her parents, sister and two brothers were tall or of medium stature. Menstrual periods commenced at 17 and were always irregular. Pubic and axillary hairs' did not appear until 24. She was married at 21 and gave birth to a child at 26, namely, two years prior to admission. Labor was prolonged and delivery was accomplished by means of forceps. The puerperium was complicated by dysentery and abscess of right breast which cleared up promptly. However the left breat lactated satisfactorily and the child was breast fed up to admission.

On examination, the patient appeared much younger than her age. Weight 26.3 kg. Height 131.5 cm. Span 126.8 cm. Upper measurement 68.2 cm. Lowever measurement 63.3 cm. Her stature is that of an average 10-year old girl with retention of infantile proportions. Skin was of fine texture; pubic and axillary hair scanty. Eye grounds and visual fields revealed no abnormality. Heart and lungs were normal. B.P. 90/50. The right breast was scarred and not lactating, while the left breast was engorged. Pelvic examination showed short vagina and undersized uterus. Transverse outlet measured 8 cm. Blood showed no anemia. Lactosuria was present. Stool contained ascaris ova. Basal metabolic rate was plus 15 per cent. On x-ray examination, the sella turcica was small and of the closed type. The rest of the skeleton showed no abnormality except for undersize. Serum calcium was 8.42 and inorganic phosphorus was 2.82 mg per cent.

While on a constant diet the patient was subjected to metabolic studies for 8 four-day periods from March 12 to April 12 inclusive. Toward the end milk secretion was diminishing and after the completion of the metabolic observation it was allowed to stop. Shortly after the commencement of the quantitative studies, the patient began to run daily remittent fever with occasional peaks up to 39.8°C. No subjective discomfort was complained of. No cause for the fever was discovered, save for the suggestive enlargement of tracheo-branchial lymph glands as seen on chest roentgenograms. The temperature curve, however, became normal after April 22 Further metabolic observations were made for 3 four-day periods (April 29 to May 10) after lactation had already ceased. Patient was discharged in good condition on May 19.

288   S. H. LIU, C. C. SU, C. W. WANG AND K. P. CHANG

APPENDIX

TABLE 1.

Composition of diets per day

Articles*	Vitamin D **	Case 1	Case 2	Case 3		Case 4			Case 5	
		Diet 1	Diet 1	Diet 1	Diet 2	Diet 1	Diet 2	Diet 3	Diet 1	Diet 2
Rice	±	100	90	50	62	160	160	160	60	50
Millet	±	120	60	50	62	120	120	120	120	25
Flour	±	200	150	150	188	200	200	200	100	150
Oatmeal	±			30	38					
Cornmeal	±	100	200			200	200	200	200	
Soybean	±		20							
Peanut	***									30
Egg	+		30	30	38					60
Beef	±			50	62					50
Pork	***	50	40	100	125		200	200	50	
Chicken	***			50	62					
Pai Ts'ai	±	120				120	120	120	120	
Small cabbage	+ + +			50	62					
Spinach	±		100							60
Turnip	±		100							
Bean sprout	±			100	125					60
Salted turnip	±	30	10			60	60	60	60	20
Pear	***			100	125					100
Orange juice	o					1000				
Sugar	o	30	40	19	12	54	54	54	40	
Sesame oil	o	30	30	42	52	40	40	40	20	40
Butter	+ +			10	12					
Table salt		4	4	6	7.5	4	4	4	5	3
Protein		64	65	89	100	70	97	87	59	58
Carbohydrate		442	429	234	293	591	699	591	412	169
Fat		37	48	82	103	48	67	67	37	47
Calories		2357	2408	1994	2499	3076	3787	3315	2257	1415
Calcium(mg)		193	377	247	309	275	498	283	271	251
Phosphorus(mg)		1082	1197	1025	1281	1425	1792	1606	1257	750
Nitrogen		9.65	10.78	11.58	14.50	10.85	15.05	13.53	9.21	9.23

*   Amount in grams except Ca and P which are in mg and actually determined; nitrogen also actually analysed.

**   + + + excellent amount, + + good amount, + presence, ± no appreciable amount,

***   evidence lacking.

TABLE 2.

Data on lactation and composition of milk

Case	Age	No. of preg- nancy	No. of lactation	Milk flow cc. per day			Calcium content mg percent			Phos. content mg per cent			Nitrogen content mg per cent			Remarks
				Max.	Min.	Av.	Max.	Min.	Av.	Max.	Min.	Av	Max	Min.	Av.	
1	40	6	7-9	642	221	452	27.15	20.40	23.15	16.56	13.12	14.71	381.8	130.8	147.1	Mild osteo- malacia, ac- tive tetany
2	27	4	8	696	212	458	24.11	21.28	22.52	10.51	12.28	15.19	200.0	(64.3)	181.5	Mild osteo- malacia, la- tent tetany
3	43	5	1-2	1426	744	1165	34.26	27.58	30.95	24.40	15.62	18.67	295.0	201.7	235.7	Healing osteomalacia
4	37	6	3	587	244	446	32.01	21.60	27.33	17.48	11.85	15.57	214.6	171.2	196.5	Wet ourse
5	28	1	24	384	155	228	23.52	16.02	18.14	23.28	13.34	17.97	251.8	156.0	199.6	Hypophyseal dwarfism

TABLE 3.

Case 1. Calcium, phosphorus and nitrogen metabolism

Period	Calcium, mg daily					Phosphorus, mg daily					Nitrogen, g daily					Serum, mg per cent	
	Intake	milk	urine	stool	bal.	Intake	milk	urine	stool	bal	intake	milk	urine	stool	bal.	Ca	P
1	193	117	26	220	−170	1082	74	392	295	+321	9.66	0.81	5.80	0.40	2.65	6.40	2.85
2	193	144	48	488	−487	1082	95	505	809	−327	9.66	0.81	4.98	1.63	2.24	6.92	3.32
3	193	147	35	451	−440	1082	92	574	627	−211	9.66	0.83	7.01	1.29	0.53	6.86	3.72
4	193	143	18	325	−293	1082	86	571	608	−183	9.66	0.87	6.86	1.22	0.71	7.42	4.05
5	193	138	9	349	−303	1082	84	511	468	+19	9.66	0.82	6.30	0.89	1.65	6.70	4.07
6	393	129	4	552	−292	1082	70	618	647	−259	9.66	0.78	6.88	1.43	0.57	6.86	4.15
7	393	116	8	618	−349	1082	68	497	856	−339	9.66	0.69	5.71	1.72	1.55	8.10	4.07
8	393	117	7	554	−115	1082	70	446	502	+74	9.66	0.70	6.23	0.87	1.86	7.16	3.68
9	793	89	4	969	−260	1082	53	600	812	−249	9.66	0.54	4.97	1.54	2.61	7.06	3.62
*10	793	79	5	611	+98	1082	51	436	501	−70	9.66	0.50	8.52	1.23	−0.59	6.78	3.45
*11	793	73	2	823	−105	1082	46	204	759	−152	9.66	0.48	6.78	1.52	0.96	7.96	3.70
12	793	64	4	436	+280	1082	43	280	683	+150	9.66	0.47	7.04	1.26	0.95	8.26	3.68
13	293	60	1	296	+436	1082	43	108	499	+260	9.66	0.49	7.59	1.19	0.39	8.45	4.74
14	793	67	2	191	+533	1082	51	215	319	+514	9.66	0.57	4.71	0.81	3.57	8.43	4.76
15	793	44	2	209	+538	1082	30	230	426	+411	9.66	0.34	6.66	1.27	1.39	8.68	5.44
16	793	—	0	151	+642	1082	—	230	632	+220	9.66	—	5.87	1.84	1.95	9.31	5.95
17	193	—	0	33	+160	1082	—	394	415	+273	9.66	—	5.98	1.29	2.39	9.31	5.71
18	193	—	0	161	+32	1082	—	503	516	+63	9.66	—	6.39	1.89	1.38	9.34	5.85
19	193	—	0	84	+109	1082	—	603	391	+88	9.66	—	7.67	1.30	0.69	9.52	5.58

* From this period on Vigantol 1 cc daily was given.

TABLE 4.

Case 2. Calcium, phosphorus and nitrogen metabolism

Period	Calcium, mg daily					Phosphorus, mg daily					Nitrogen, g daily					Serum mg per cent	
	Intake	milk	urine	stool	bal.	Intake	milk	urine	stool	bal.	Intake	milk	urine	stool	bal	Ca	P
1	377	120	3	337	−83	1197	72	358	695	+72	10.78	0.87	5.46	2.02	2.43	7.34	3.03
2	377	133	1	254	−11	1197	87	439	720	−49	10.78	1.03	6.92	1.87	0.96	7.77	3.69
*3	377	114	1	246	+16	1197	79	486	628	+4	10.78	0.93	6.70	1.82	1.33	7.40	4.00
4	377	107	0	298	−28	1197	76	672	632	−183	10.78	0.86	6.12	2.11	1.69	7.66	3.65
5	377	88	0	216	+73	1197	61	448	570	+118	10.78	0.78	6.57	2.01	1.42	7.46	3.93
6	377	57	0	161	+159	1197	40	436	582	+136	10.78	0.48	6.65	2.02	2.63	8.95	3.70

* Vigantol 1 cc daily started from this period.

TABLE 5.

Case 3. Calcium, phosphorus and nitrogen metabolism.

Period	Calcium, mg daily					Phosphorus, mg daily					Nitrogen, g daily					Serum mg per cent	
	Intake	milk	urine	stool	bal.	Intake	milk	urine	stool	bal.	Intake	milk	urine	stool	bal.	Ca	P
1.	247	253	3	427	-434	1025	188	681	440	-284	11.58	2.28	7.01	1.26	1.03	8.76	4.23
2.	247	287	1	178	-219	1025	213	702	265	-155	11.58	2.57	7.06	0.93	1.02		
3.	1147	308	11	370	+458	1025	214	422	274	+115	11.58	2.70	7.33	0.64	0.91	8.80	3.40
4.	1147	339	8	1162	-354	1025	217	430	602	-233	11.58	2.78	7.65	1.14	0.01		
5.	2047	351	25	1062	+609	1025	214	348	341	+122	11.58	2.59	6.64	1.08	1.27	9.23	3.60
6.	2109	385	46	1635	-43	1281	215	398	505	+163	14.50	2.78	7.89	1.69	1.73		
7.	2109	396	40	1398	+275	1281	218	382	473	+207	14.50	2.78	8.82	1.43	1.47	9.20	3.88
8.	2109	399	51	1483	+176	1281	212	450	663	-59	14.50	2.84	9.72	1.72	0.22	9.32	
9.	2109	416	39	1422	+241	1281	222	444	435	+199	14.50	2.80	9.43	1.45	0.82		
10.	2109	426	44	1591	+48	1281	219	461	548	+50	14.50	2.87	9.26	1.71	0.66		
11.	2109	414	85	1544	+66	1281	219	434	576	+52	14.50	2.99	9.40	1.78	0.42	9.07	3.99

* Vigantol 30 drops (0.6 cc) daily was started from this period.

TABLE 6.

Case 4. Calcium, phosphorus and nitrogen metabolism

Period	Calcium, mg daily					Phosphorus, mg daily					Nitrogen, g daily					Serum mg per cent	
	Intake	milk	urine	stool	bal.	Intake	milk	urine	stool	bal.	Intake	milk	urine	stool	bal.	Ca	P
1	275	66	2	441	−234	1425	38	237	890	+260	10.84	0.48	4.81	2.27	3.28	8.40	2.45
2	275	71	2	327	−125	1425	42	319	757	+307	10.84	0.53	5.85	1.83	2.63	8.50	3.11
3	408	108	9	497	−206	1792	69	383	880	+460	15.05	0.82	6.13	2.65	5.45		
4	408	151	4	437	−184	1792	86	521	946	+239	15.05	1.07	6.30	2.30	5.38	8.58	3.10
5	408	145	8	428	−173	1792	80	667	793	+252	15.05	1.03	6.77	2.01	5.24		
6	408	156	17	585	−350	1779	85	747	945	+2	13.80	1.08	6.96	2.22	3.54		
7	408	154	10	522	−278	1779	82	760	885	+52	13.80	1.08	7.38	1.99	3.35	8.28	3.96
*8	408	156	9	450	−207	1779	82	705	732	+260	13.80	1.08	6.63	1.83	4.26		
9	408	134	20	364	−110	1779	77	618	822	+262	13.80	0.98	6.30	2.16	4.36	8.44	4.05
10	408	106	13	258	+31	1779	63	610	715	+391	13.80	0.78	5.99	2.12	4.91		

* Vigantol 1 cc. q.d. was given during periods 8-10 inclusive

TABLE 7.

Case 5. Calcium, phosphorus and nitrogen metabolism

Period	Calcium, mg daily					Phosphorus, mg daily					Nitrogen, g daily					Serum mg per cent	
	Intake	milk	urine	stool	bal.	Intake	milk	urine	stool	bal.	Intake	milk	urine	stool	bal.	Ca	P
1	271	68	16	224	−37	1257	51	310	932	−36	9.21	0.54	4.18	3.12	1.37	8.42	2.82
2	271	71	27	197	−24	1257	60	312	667	+218	9.21	0.64	4.30	2.29	1.98		
3	671	60	34	549	+28	1257	59	258	1158	−218	9.21	0.63	4.65	3.64	0.29	8.70	3.45
*4	671	62	25	548	+36	1257	56	382	951	−132	9.21	0.60	4.63	3.08	0.90		
*5	671	56	19	502	+94	1257	47	308	941	−39	9.21	0.54	5.02	3.61	0.04	8.75	4.31
6	671	45	3	362	+261	1257	41	313	815	+83	9.21	0.46	5.09	3.06	0.60	8.74	4.05
7	671	39	64	339	+229	1257	37	338	885	−3	9.21	0.38	5.14	2.74	0.95	9.25	5.02
8	671	42	105	306	+218	1257	39	326	701	+191	9.21	0.45	4.94	3.01	0.81	10.23	5.14
13	251	—	61	317	−127	750	—	451	364	−65	9.23	—	6.39	1.44	1.40		
14	251	—	43	168	+40	750	—	483	287	−20	9.23	—	6.48	1.43	1.32		
15	251	—	22	149	+80	750	—	439	238	+73	9.23	—	6.57	1.24	1.42	9.70	4.78

* Vigantol 1 cc q.d. was given during periods 5-8 inclusive

鈣與燐之新陳代謝

其六・乳哺期間之特殊消耗及維生素丁之效用

劉士豪　蘇啓楨　王季午　張光璧

私立北平協和醫學院內科學系，北平

　　婦女哺乳期中，消耗異常，吾國通常膳食，能否維持鈣與燐之平衡，頗屬疑問・爲研究起見，著者選擇乳婦五人（其中三人患骨質軟化症，其餘二人依愛克斯光檢察骨質正常），進以定量飲食，質量與彼等日常家居所食者相等・各人規定之每日飲食，據分析結果，含鈣由193至377公絲，燐質由1025至1425公絲，氮質由9.66至11.58公分・同時檢定其乳，尿及糞中之鈣，燐及氮，以求各質之平衡・

　　進以上述低度鈣質膳食後，其中四人產乳量較小者（骨質軟化二例，骨質正常二例），鈣平衡雖均呈負性，而由乳中失去之鈣只佔總排泄量之百分之十六至三十・增加鈣質之供給，亦不能矯正其消耗・但服以維生素丁之製劑，糞中鈣質逐漸低減，反負平衡爲正・有此維生素之保護作用，雖膳食含鈣甚少，而自身之鈣亦能保持・吾國普通飲食含鈣較低，授乳期間，加維生素丁，有特殊之必要・

　　以上四例中，二例依愛克斯光檢驗骨質正常，而其鈣質之代謝，及其對于維生素丁之感應，與患骨質軟化症者無異，顯見該二例雖未罹臨證的骨病，而其鈣質及丁種維生素，均屬缺如・想此種隱症，未經發覺者，必甚普遍・

　　所餘一乳婦，原係骨質軟化症患者，在未作乳哺研究之先，常食以優良之膳食，富于鈣燐等質，以及丁種維生素，迨授乳期至，產量特大（每日約1200公撮），且鈣質成分濃厚，故其由乳中分泌之鈣量超出低量鈣質膳食之供給・是以欲此種乳婦之鈣質平衡呈正性，除丁種維生素充足外，亦須給以多量之鈣質・

　　普通膳食含燐甚多，而平衡結果各異，其中一人呈負平衡，一人呈正平衡，其餘三人出入相等，服丁種維生素後，每人均能存留多量燐質・氮質平衡，在所有試驗期間，各人均能保持正平衡或出入相等・

Reprinted from The Journal of Clinical Investigation, Vol. XIX, No. 2, pp. 327–347, March, 1940
Printed in U. S. A.

CALCIUM AND PHOSPHORUS METABOLISM IN OSTEOMALACIA
IX. METABOLIC BEHAVIOR OF INFANTS FED ON BREAST MILK FROM MOTHERS SHOWING VARIOUS STATES OF VITAMIN D NUTRITION

By S. H. LIU, H. I. CHU, C. C. SU, T. F. YU and T. Y. CHENG

(*From the Department of Medicine, Peiping Union Medical College, Peiping*)

(Received for publication October 24, 1939)

It is generally recognized that the nutritional state of the mother has an important influence upon that of the infant. This influence is exerted during the antenatal period as well as during infancy when breast feeding constitutes the only or main source of nutrients. Among the numerous nutritive factors, those concerned in bone metabolism, namely, calcium, phosphorus and vitamin D, have recently received considerable attention. It has long been suspected that mothers with osteomalacia may give birth to children showing evidence of disturbed calcium and phosphorus metabolism *in utero* or in early infancy. In 1930 Maxwell and Turnbull (16) reported 2 cases of fetal rickets. The mothers of both children were suffering from advanced osteomalacia with marked pelvic deformities necessitating cesarean section. The infants showed evidence of rickets by x-ray, and one of them, on histological examination of the bones, exhibited deficiency in provisional calcification, irregularity of endochondral ossification from the diaphysis and slight fibrosis in the metaphysis characteristic of rickets. This is the first demonstration of the existence of fetal rickets in infants born of osteomalacic mothers. Subsequent collections of Maxwell and co-workers (17, 18, 19) have added 15 more such cases, establishing beyond doubt the causal relationship between osteomalacia in the mother and rickets in the newborn. In fact, Maxwell (18) says that fetal rickets is certainly to be looked for where the product of serum calcium and phosphorus in the mother is below 20, especially if the calcium factor is distinctly low.

Tetany, another manifestation of vitamin D deficiency, tends to occur early in infancy among the cases observed here. In Chu and Sung's analysis (3) of 45 cases of infantile tetany, 30 cases or 66.7 per cent appeared within the first three months of life. In view of the fact that in Europe and America spasmophilia, the identity of which with infantile tetany has been controversial, is more frequently seen after the age of six months, the much earlier age incidence of this condition in North China is probably significant. In looking for an explanation of this unusual observation, they investigated the diet, mode of living and health condition of the mothers, and found that the majority of these women subsisted on diets deficient, among other things, in calcium and vitamin D, or had frank osteomalacia or tetany. This finding suggests to Chu and Sung that the high incidence of tetany in the early months of infancy may be accounted for by a congenital deficiency of vitamin D and calcium. While the importance of antenatal deficiency in the manifestation of the disease cannot be denied, neonatal nutrition as influenced by the condition of the milk of the mother probably also has a significant bearing on the problem.

In order to determine how the state of vitamin D nutrition of the mother during lactation affects that of the infant, opportunity has been taken to study the calcium, phosphorus and nitrogen metabolism of both the mother and the infant simultaneously in four instances. The results from the four sets of cases, though similar in demonstrating the intimate relationship between infantile and maternal metabolism during the nursing period, are sufficiently varied to be useful in illustrating the different aspects of the problem:

1. The behavior of calcium and phosphorus metabolism of an infant receiving milk from its mother who, having had osteomalacia, had been adequately treated with large doses of vitamin D and calcium during gestation.

2. The state of mineral metabolism of an infant

327

S. H. LIU, H. I. CHU, C. C. SU, T. F. YU AND T. Y. CHENG

TABLE 1

Composition of diets in grams per day

(Values for calcium, phosphorus, and nitrogen are actually analyzed)

	Case 1a		Case 2a	Case 3a′			Case 4a		
Periods (four-day)	1–5	6–11	1–12	1–2 10–14 16–17	3–9	19–20	1–10	11–16	17–26
Diet number	1	2	1*	1	2	3	3	4	5
Rice	50	62	180	150	100	460	190	190	190
Wheat flour	150	188	300	500†	400		150	300	400
Corn meal			100						
Millet	50	62					80	80	80
Oat meal	30	38							
Egg	30	38				90			
Beef	50	62	30						
Pork	100	125	30	30	30	50	100	100	100
Chicken	50	62		30	30	60			
Soy bean curd					100	200			
Gram bean					50				
Mung bean						20			
Potato, sweet							100		100
Lotus root starch				10	10				
Turnip					100		100	100	100
Turnip, salted			40			10			
Cucumber, salted							10	10	10
Wosun				100					
Cabbage, large			100	50			300	400	
Cabbage, small	50	62				100			400
Celery					100				
Spinach						100			
Bean sprouts	100	125		100					
Hai tai					20				
Apple						50			
Banana					100				
Crabapple					50				
Pear	100	125		100					
Tangerine							100	100	100
Molasses					40				
Sugar	10	12	20	20	20	20			
Butter	10	12							
Sesame oil	42	52	30	50	50	60	50	50	50
Sauce, soybean				10	10	10			
Sodium chloride	6	7.5	5	6	9	8	10	10	12
Baking powder				20‡	20‡				
Protein	80	100	74	86	88	102	70	88	100
Carbohydrate	234	293	479	557	509	411	374	489	561
Fat	82	103	35	62	65	88	73	75	76
Calories	1994	2499	2528	3125	2972	2844	2435	2980	3329
Calcium, *mgm.*	247	309	227	186	505	421	207	292	456
Phosphorus, *mgm.*	1025	1281	932	930	1157	1174	812	1065	1006
Nitrogen	11.58	14.50	11.34	12.35	13.76	16.25	10.61	12.96	14.84

* Half portion of this diet was used for periods 2–4, and two-thirds portion for periods 5–6 and 10–12 inclusive.

† Only 400 grams of flour were used for periods 10–14; and 300 grams for periods 16–17, inclusive. Flour on analysis gave 21 mgm. calcium, 133 mgm. phosphorus, and 1.63 grams nitrogen per 100 grams.

‡ Baking powder on analysis contained 986 mgm. calcium, and 1,587 mgm. phosphorus in 20 grams. This was used during periods 7–9 (diet 2) and 10–11 (diet 1) only, accounting for the exceedingly high intake of calcium and phosphorus during those periods.

with tetany and rickets, breast-fed by its mother who also had tetany as well as osteomalacia; and the changes brought about both in the infant and in the mother after the latter alone received vitamin D.

3. The response of an infant, born of an osteomalacic mother and itself having tetany and rickets, to breast feeding from a presumably normal wet nurse before and after vitamin D administration to the wet nurse.

4. The effect on an infant of variations in the state of vitamin D nutrition in the mother who had osteomalacia: a limited dose of vitamin D during the latter part of pregnancy, depletion for a period after parturition, and finally replenishment.

PROCEDURE

All the patients were studied in the metabolism ward where the routines for the preparation and serving of constant diets and collection of excreta for quantitative purposes have been standardized (7, 13, 14). The composition of the diets is shown in Table I. While the fuel values are calculated from the compilation of Wu (25) and from *Outline of Diets* of the Peiping Union Medical College Hospital, 3rd edition, Peiping, 1937, the calcium, phosphorus and nitrogen contents were analyzed, 50 per cent of the day's food being used for the purpose. Where the same diet was used for a relatively long period of time, the analyses were repeated at intervals.

Stools and urine were collected in four-day periods, 0.1 gram of carmine being used to mark off the stools every four days. For the quantitative collection of excreta from infants, the special metabolism cots, described by Tso (23), were used. As all the infants studied were male, the urine collection was satisfactory and complete. It is usually a good plan, if time permits, to interpose periods of rest between periods of study so as to avoid maceration of the skin of the perineum and possible ill effects of continuous restriction of activities of the infant.

Stools were passed directly into tared enamel pans, dried in an oven at 90 to 100° C., and weighed. All the stools of the period were ground in a mill into a fine homogeneous powder, and accurately weighed portions ashed in a muffle furnace at approximately 500° C. The ash was extracted with hot 5 per cent hydrochloric acid and portions taken for analysis of calcium and phosphorus. The four-day pooled collection of urine was preserved by the addition of 5 cc. of concentrated hydrochloric acid per liter and analyzed for the same elements.

Breasts were emptied five or six times every twenty-four hours by means of a hand or electric breast pump. A measured amount of each milking was fed to the infant from a feeding bottle, and a small aliquot was saved. The pooled specimens of one or four days were used for analysis. Venipunctures were done before breakfast at the beginning of each period, but less frequently in the case of infants.

The analytical procedures for calcium and phosphorus in stool, urine, blood, milk and food have been given previously (7, 13, 14). The macro-Kjeldahl method was used for nitrogen determinations.

RESULTS

Composition of milk. All the lactating women included in this study were good milk-providers.

TABLE II

Composition of breast milk

Four-day period	Case 1a				Case 2a				Case 3a'				Case 4a			
	Volume	Calcium	Phosphorus	Nitrogen	Volume	Calcium	Phosphorus	Nitrogen	Volume	Calcium	Phosphorus	Nitrogen	Volume	Calcium	Phosphorus	Nitrogen
	cc.	mgm. per cent	mgm. per cent	mgm. per cent	cc.	mgm. per cent	mgm. per cent	mgm. per cent	cc.	mgm. per cent	mgm. per cent	mgm. per cent	cc.	mgm. per cent	mgm. per cent	mgm. per cent
1	819	30.95	22.92	277.9	922	35.30	16.21	180.5	558	32.28	13.69	217.4	498	25.74	16.51	241.0
2	936	30.67	22.83	274.8	952	31.48	15.00	154.7	623	34.20	14.32	215.0	581	27.90	16.85	232.6
3	1041	29.68	20.62	259.9	904	33.20	14.88	167.0	654	34.18	14.25	221.7	680	27.80	17.85	235.7
4	1116	30.56	19.52	249.5	877	34.20	15.36	203.0	739	30.76	15.62	221.4	780	26.80	17.02	226.7
5	1146	30.62	18.64	225.4	907	32.34	15.68	167.0	798	30.96	13.95	206.6	867	30.16	16.44	215.2
6	1230	31.30	17.45	226.0	908	31.80	16.83	177.5	837	33.39	13.28	213.8	928	30.40	17.12	212.3
7	1236	32.06	17.76	222.8	906	29.00	15.84	165.2	870	30.78	12.38	203.0	981	29.30	16.00	205.3
8	1274	31.35	17.16	222.7	902	31.98	14.98	188.6	794	28.04	12.48	199.7	1009	27.80	16.00	198.0
9	1309	31.70	16.25	214.0	906	32.07	16.20	197.5	800	28.63	11.68	199.0	1070	29.50	14.36	192.0
10	1353	31.46	16.38	210.3	976	32.52	15.70	189.8	927	33.68	15.18	194.0	1079	29.25	14.52	185.2
11	1367	30.32	16.00	210.2	1030	31.94	14.90	190.0	1016	30.83	13.06	194.0	1145	27.89	14.02	170.8
12					1118	32.20	15.51	165.3	1007	33.59	12.08	196.9	1184	27.30	13.96	172.2
13									980	29.85	11.88	181.5	1175	29.60	14.68	176.4
14									946	31.15	11.50	176.0	1183	29.40	13.45	168.5
15									966	30.34	11.63	183.3	1200	28.96	14.70	165.6
16									992	28.60	11.50	1.843	1229	27.63	13.08	161.4
17									996	29.81	12.60	1.760	1256	27.19	13.15	156.8
18													1248	25.02	12.84	148.0
19									1087	27.90	13.42		1248	26.09	12.14	157.8
20									1132	27.09	12.28		1248	25.63	12.28	160.0
21									1066	27.00	11.44	152.0	1268	24.41	12.34	164.8
22									1008	27.69	11.48	159.0	1156	26.06	12.31	161.6
23													1236	26.59	12.91	169.9
24													1138	25.29	12.56	159.1
25													1251	25.09	11.92	157.3
26													1310	22.53	12.46	145.2

Note: Studies of milk started eighteen days postpartum in Case 1a, two months in Case 2a, one month in Case 3a', and seventeen days in Case 4a. Values are expressed as daily averages for each four-day period.

They were all in early stages of lactation. The milk yield, starting from 500 to 900 cc. per day, gradually increased so that eventually it exceeded 1 liter in Cases 2a and 3a′ and 1.3 liters in Cases 1a and 4a (Table II). The average calcium content varied from 27 to 32 mgm. per 100 cc. in the 4 cases. Slight fluctuations in calcium content from period to period were noticeable, but these could not be definitely correlated with progression of time, with the institution of vitamin D, or with the different levels of calcium intake. However, a descending tendency with the lapse of time was discernible in both the phosphorus and nitrogen content, particularly in Cases 3a′ and 4a, in which the studies extended over eighty-eight and one hundred and four days respectively. The average phosphorus content was from 13 to 18 mgm. per 100 cc. and the average protein was from 1.7 to 2.2 per cent. The figures for calcium and phosphorus were within the limits of normal variation in the composition of human milk as compiled by Leitch (11).

Case 1a. Mother Y. W. L. While anatomical evidence of osteomalacia was still present during this study, the disease was considered to be at the healing stage due to the large intake of calcium, phosphorus and vitamin D given during the last seven months of pregnancy. Studies began eighteen days postpartum. As seen from Figure 1 and Table III, calcium intake had to be raised to over 2 grams before a slight positive balance could be obtained. As discussed in a previous communication (12), this rather "extravagant" behavior was not the result of vitamin D deficiency, as Vigantol given during periods 7 to 11 made no difference to the calcium balance. It was considered very likely that the physiological requirements during active lactation rendered conservation very difficult and that the large amounts of calcium gained during pregnancy made further storage less urgent than in cases with less adequate preparation during pregnancy. Phosphorus metabolism was parallel to calcium metabolism. Serum calcium and inorganic phosphorus remained within low normal levels throughout the period of observations.

Case 1b. Infant Y. W. L. This infant was normal in every way. He was fed solely on the mother's milk. Metabolic observations were made for 7 four-day periods (periods 3 to 9). The intake of calcium increased progressively from 280 to 363 mgm. per day as milk consumption increased (Figure 1 and Table IV). The urinary and fecal excretion of calcium was equal in extent, and both were minimal so that marked positive calcium balances were obtained, the average daily retention amounting to 74 per cent of the intake with very little variation from period to period. The same may

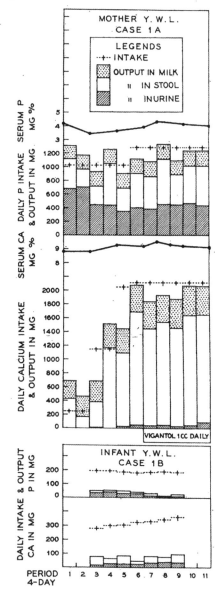

Fig. 1. Calcium and Phosphorus Metabolism of Cases 1A and 1B

The lactating mother had healing osteomalacia with adequate prior store and subsequent administration of vitamin D. The infant exhibited remarkably good retention of calcium and phosphorus throughout the periods of observation.

TABLE III

Mother Y. W. L. Case Ia. Calcium, phosphorus and nitrogen metabolism in a case of healing osteomalacia during lactation with adequate vitamin D supply

Date 1935	Period four-day	Calcium, average per day					Phosphorus, average per day					Nitrogen, average per day					Serum	
		Intake	Urine	Stool	Milk	Balance	Intake	Urine	Stool	Milk	Balance	Intake	Urine	Stool	Milk	Balance	Calcium	Phosphorus
		mgm.	mgm.	mgm.	mgm.	mgm.	mgm.	mgm.	mgm.	mgm.	mgm.	mgm.	mgm.	mgm.	mgm.	mgm.	mgm. per cent	mgm. per cent
IV30–V3	1	247	1	427	253	−434	1025	681	440	188	−284	11.58	7.01	1.26	2.28	+1.03	8,76	4.23
V 4–7	2	247	1	178	287	−219	1025	702	265	213	−155	11.58	7.06	0.93	2.57	+1.02		
V 8–11	3	1147	11	370	308	+458	1025	422	274	214	+115	11.58	7.33	0.64	2.70	+0.91	8.80	3.40
V12–15	4	1147	0	1162	339	−354	1025	439	602	217	−233	11.58	7.65	1.14	2.78	+0.01		
V16–19	5	2047	25	1062	351	+609	1025	348	341	214	+122	11.58	6.64	1.08	2.59	+1.27	9.23	3.60
V20–23	6	2109	46	1635	385	+ 43	1281	398	505	215	+163	14.50	7.89	1.60	2.78	+2.23		
V24–27	7*	2109	40	1398	396	+275	1281	382	473	219	+207	14.50	8.82	1.43	2.78	+1.47	9.20	3.88
V28–31	8	2109	51	1483	399	+176	1281	450	663	218	− 50	14.50	9.72	1.72	2.84	+0.22		
VI 1–4	9	2109	30	1422	416	+241	1281	444	435	212	+190	14.50	9.43	1.45	2.80	+0.82	9.32	
VI 5–8	10	2109	44	1591	426	+ 48	1281	461	548	222	+ 50	14.50	9.26	1.71	2.87	+0.66		
VI 9–12	11	2109	85	1544	417	+ 66	1281	434	576	219	+ 52	14.50	9.40	1.78	2.90	+0.42	9.07	3.99

This table is reproduced from Chinese J. Physiol., 1937, 11, 292 (12), for convenience.
* Vigantol 0.6 cç. daily was started from this period.

also be said of the phosphorus metabolism, the average daily retention being 80 per cent. Nitrogen balance was likewise positive, approximately 50 per cent of the intake being retained. Both the calcium and phosphorus balances were much more than normal, as discussed later.

The results on this infant show the remarkable manner in which the mineral elements of human milk were utilized with very little wastage. It is very likely that the vitamin D present in the milk, together with the store of the vitamin acquired during the antenatal period, was responsible for the extreme degree of conservation in calcium and phosphorus exchange exhibited by the infant. Extra ingestion of Vigantol by the mother did not further improve the degree of mineral conservation.

Case 2a. Mother C. S. Y. This patient had tentany and mild osteoporosis of the visualized long bones at the time of metabolic observation. As shown in Figure 2 and Table V, while on a minimal calcium intake of 227

mgm. per day, the patient exhibited a moderately negative balance (period 1). With the intake raised to over 900 mgm., the loss of calcium was rectified (periods 2 and 3), but no substantial retention of the element took place until vitamin D was given (periods 4 to 12). The first 2 periods of Vigantol administration (1 cc. per day, equivalent to 12,000 international units) were without effect, but from the third period on, retention amounted to from 30 to 40 per cent of the intake. This retention was brought about entirely by a reduction in the fecal calcium output, the secretion of calcium in the milk being maintained. At the height of vitamin D action (periods 10 to 12) small amounts of calcium appeared in the urine, indicating that intestinal absorption had improved to such an extent as to be more than sufficient for the needs of the body.

Phosphorus balance was markedly negative in the beginning but with vitamin D administration considerable

TABLE IV

Infant Y. W. L. Case Ib. Calcium, phosphorus and nitrogen metabolism of a presumably normal infant fed exclusively on mother's milk

Date 1935	Period four-day	Breast milk intake	Calcium, average per day					Phosphorus, average per day					Nitrogen, average per day					Body weight
			Intake	Urine	Stool	Balance	Retention	Intake	Urine	Stool	Balance	Retention	Intake	Urine	Stool	Balance	Retention	
		cc.	mgm.	mgm.	mgm.	mgm.	per cent	mgm.	mgm.	mgm.	mgm.	per cent	mgm.	mgm.	mgm.	mgm.	per cent	kgm.
V 8–11	3	944	280	18	60	+202	72	195	35	15	+145	74	2.45	1.03	0.24	+1.25	51	3.82
V12–15	4	985	301	28	36	+237	79	192	42	11	+139	72	2.46	1.18	0.12	+1.16	47	3.97
V16–19	5	995	305	26	60	+219	72	185	30	18	+137	74	2.24	0.93	0.27	+1.04	46	4.13
V20–23	6	1034	324	26	20	+278	86	180	23	7	+150	83	2.34	1.25	0.10	+0.99	42	4.30
V24–27	7*	1027	329	36	47	+246	75	182	15	17	+150	82	2.28	1.02	0.19	+1.07	47	4.45
V28–31	8	1102	346	41	36	+269	78	189	6	9	+174	92	2.44	1.09	0.11	+1.24	51	4.73
VI1–4	9	1142	363	36	62	+265	73	185	10	17	+158	85	2.45	1.12	0.11	+1.22	50	4.97

* Mother started to receive renewed vitamin D supply.

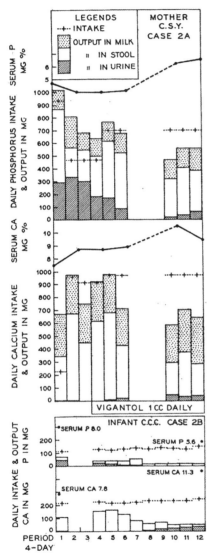

FIG. 2. CALCIUM AND PHOSPHORUS METABOLISM OF CASES 2A AND 2B

The lactating osteomalacia mother showed poor calcium and phosphorus balances which were subsequently improved by Vigantol therapy. A similar state of affairs was reflected in the infant (with rickets and tetany) via breast milk.

amounts of phosphorus were stored. The conservation of phosphorus, in contrast to that of calcium, was brought about mainly by a diminution in the urinary phosphorus output. Serum calcium, rather low to start with, was raised to normal after vitamin D therapy; and inorganic phosphorus was increased from a normal level on admission to a level higher than normal toward the end of the experiment.

This patient, then, differs from the first patient in that vitamin D therapy was capable of conserving the calcium and phosphorus metabolism so that not only were the extensive requirements of active lactation covered, but also considerable amounts of these minerals were retained in her own tissues and skeleton, which were probably in urgent need of reparation.

Case 2b. Infant C. C. C. The metabolism of the infant (Figure 2 and Table VI) reflects that of the mother. He was likewise admitted for tetany with evidence of rickets. The calcium retention of 48 per cent (period 1), as compared with that of the first infant, was poor, and it remained so during periods 4 to 6 when the mother began to receive vitamin D. But from period 7 on, the fecal output of calcium showed progressive reduction so that retention attained 80 per cent, comparable to the best performance of the first infant. The reduction of fecal calcium was accompanied by the appearance and increase of calcium in the urine.

Phosphorus balance was small in the beginning but it was very much increased after vitamin D therapy. The average retention of phosphorus during the last 5 periods was 88 per cent of the intake. Nitrogen retention, however, remained around 50 per cent. Serum calcium increased from 7.8 mgm. at the beginning to 11.32 mgm. at the end of the experiment, while inorganic phosphorus decreased from 8.0 mgm. to 5.61 mgm. The rachitic bone changes present on admission, however, were not altered on discharge, the period during which the infant was fed the breast milk of the mother receiving vitamin D being only thirty-six days.

Although on roentgenologic examination there was no obvious evidence of healing in the rickets of the infant within thirty-six days, the metabolic defects characteristic of rickets and tetany were corrected. This shows that the amount of vitamin D given to the mother was sufficient to enrich her milk and to render it effective in correcting the faulty mineral metabolism of the infant. Were the period of observation extended, healing of the rachitic bone changes would have followed eventually.

Case 3a'. Wet nurse W. C. S. This was presumably a normal lactating woman. Her metabolic behavior (Figure 3 and Table VII) may be taken to represent a normal state of affairs during lactation and it is closely comparable to that of Case 1a with healed osteomalacia. Marked negative balances in calcium were obtained on intakes of from 186 to 505 mgm. per day (periods 1 to 6). It was only after the calcium intake was raised to about 1,500 to 2,000 mgm. that slightly positive balances began to appear (periods 7 to 11). Vitamin D in the form of Vigantol 1 cc. or 12,000 international units per

TABLE V

Mother C. S. Y.   Case 2a.   Calcium, phosphorus and nitrogen metabolism in a case of tetany and osteomalacia during lactation before and after vitamin D therapy

Date 1937	Period four-day	Calcium, average per day					Phosphorus, average per day					Nitrogen, average per day					Serum	
		In-take	Urine	Stool	Milk	Bal-ance	In-take	Urine	Stool	Milk	Bal-ance	In-take	Urine	Stool	Milk	Bal-ance	Cal-cium	Phos-phorus
		mgm.	mgm.	mgm.	mgm.	mgm.	mgm.	mgm.	mgm.	mgm.	mgm.	mgm.	mgm.	mgm.	mgm.	mgm.	mgm. per cent	mgm. per cent
IV 6–9	1	227	6	340	326	−445	932	296	571	150	− 85	11.34	5.92	2.31	1.67	+1.44	7.46	4.70
IV10–13	2	958	5	671	300	− 18	466	336	331	143	−344	5.67	5.99	1.42	1.47	−3.21		
IV14–17	3	914	4	446	300	+164	466	302	245	134	−215	5.67	4.24	0.57	1.51	−0.65	8.72	4.05
IV18–21	4*	914	4	613	300	− 3	466	183	317	135	−169	5.67	4.66	0.57	1.89	−1.45		
IV22–25	5	970	9	674	293	− 6	699	172	442	142	− 57	8.52	5.44	0.96	1.51	+0.61	8.70	4.03
IV26–29	6	970	21	407	288	+254	699	89	436	153	+ 21	8.52	5.27	1.85	1.61	−0.21		
IV30																	8.95	4.11
V12–15	10	970	46	223	318	+383	699	20	299	153	+227	8.52	5.09	0.97	1.85	+0.61		
V16–19	11	970	34	342	329	+265	699	37	370	154	+138	8.52	5.22	1.44	1.96	−0.10	10.45	6.24
V20–23	12	970	38	244	360	+328	699	62	324	174	+139	8.52	4.70	1.50	1.85	+0.47	9.42	6.52

* Vigantol 1 cc. started from this period.

TABLE VI

Infant C. C. C.   Case 2b.   Calcium, phosphorus and nitrogen metabolism of a breast-fed rachitic infant and its response to vitamin D administration to the mother

Date 1937	Pe-riod four-day	Breast milk intake	Calcium, average per day					Phosphorus, average per day					Nitrogen, average per day					Serum		Body weight
			In-take	Urine	Stool	Bal-ance	Re-ten-tion	In-take	Urine	Stool	Bal-ance	Re-ten-tion	In-take	Urine	Stool	Bal-ance	Re-ten-tion	Cal-cium	Phos-phorus	
		cc.	mgm.	mgm.	mgm.	mgm.	per cent	mgm.	mgm.	mgm.	mgm.	per cent	mgm.	mgm.	mgm.	mgm.	per cent	mgm. per cent	mgm. per cent	kgm.
IV 6–9	1	656	232	5	105	+122	48	106	46	26	+ 34	31	1.18	0.61	0.24	+0.33	28	7.8	8.0	4.97
IV18–21	4*	648	247	0	156	+ 91	37	118	22	19	+ 77	65	1.34	0.33	0.26	+0.75	56			4.92
IV22–25	5	720	233	0	165	+ 68	29	113	16	25	+ 72	61	1.20	0.37	0.29	+0.54	45			4.97
IV26–29	6	720	229	0	131	+ 98	43	121	5	33	+ 83	68	1.28	0.43	0.29	+0.56	44			5.18
IV30–V3	7	810	235	3	79	+153	65	128	5	51	+ 72	56	1.34	0.38	0.28	+0.68	51			5.15
V 4–7	8	810	259	7	51	+201	78	122	2	13	+107	88	1.53	0.35	0.26	+0.92	60			5.34
V 8–11	9	810	260	18	51	+191	74	131	2	14	+115	88	1.60	0.44	0.32	+0.84	52			5.53
V12–15	10	810	264	25	28	+211	80	127	2	13	+112	88	1.54	0.50	0.28	+0.76	49			5.55
V16–19	11	810	259	31	27	+201	78	121	1	14	+106	88	1.54	0.45	0.27	+0.82	53			5.70
V20–23	12	900	289	32	24	+233	81	144	1	15	+128	89	1.48	0.42	0.30	+0.76	51	11.32	5.61	5.94

* Mother starting to receive Vigantol 1 cc. per day from this period on.

day was given from periods 5 to 15, and from periods 16 to 20 the dosage was raised to 1.5 cc. or 18,000 international units per day. All this vitamin D supply did not seem to produce obvious changes in the calcium metabolism, balances being approximately even on levels of intake varying from 1,000 to 2,000 mgm. No significant amounts of calcium appeared in the urine, the paths of excretion being mainly through the bowel and breasts during most of the periods. The absence of calcium in the urine was possibly related to the very high phosphorus intake (periods 7 to 11). While no substantial gain in calcium or phosphorus was evident after vitamin D administration, such therapy was probably important in enabling the subject to maintain mineral balance in spite of heightened requirements during lactation.

The phosphorus metabolism followed closely the calcium metabolism, although the urinary tract constituted by far the largest channel of phosphorus elimination. Nitrogen gain prevailed during most of the experimental periods. Serum calcium and inorganic phosphorus showed no remarkable changes, although a slight ascending tendency was discernible in both, as time went on.

From the observations on this experimental subject, it may be stated that a normal woman with intact skeletal calcification is able to maintain herself in calcium and phosphorus balance in the face of mineral stress incident to lactation, provided that the level of intake is sufficiently high and vitamin D supply is adequate. However, significantly positive balance is not expected, as there is presumably no need for it.

Case 3b. Infant T. N. T. This infant, born of a mother having osteomalacia and tetany, was admitted at the age of three months. He presented evidence of moderate rickets with very low serum calcium and high inorganic phosphorus. During periods A, B and C

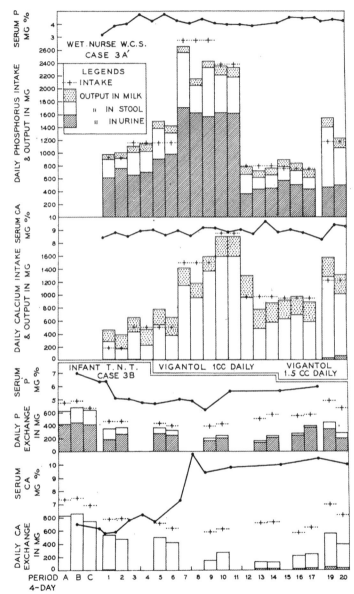

FIG. 3. CALCIUM AND PHOSPHORUS METABOLISM OF CASES 3A′ AND 3B

　　The wet nurse was presumably normal, although the Vigantol given probably helped her in maintaining mineral balance. The infant with rickets and tetany did poorly on Klim and on breast milk of the wet nurse until vitamin D was given to the latter. Then remarkably good mineral retention occurred in the infant.

TABLE VII

Wet nurse W. C. S. Case 3a . Calcium, phosphorus and nitrogen metabolism of a presumably normal lactating woman before and after vitamin D therapy

Date 1938	Period four-day	Calcium, average per day					Phosphorus, average per day					Nitrogen, average per day					Serum	
		Intake	Urine	Stool	Milk	Balance	Intake	Urine	Stool	Milk	Balance	Intake	Urine	Stool	Milk	Balance	Calcium	Phosphorus
		mgm.	mgm.	mgm.	mgm.	mgm.	mgm.	mgm.	mgm.	mgm.	mgm.	grams	grams	grams	grams	grams	mgm. per cent	mgm. per cent
I19–22	1	186	8	278	180	−280	930	616	288	76	−50	12.35	7.69	1.62	1.21	+1.83	8.42	3.15
I23–26	2	186	5	170	213	−202	930	760	156	89	−75	12.35	7.15	1.32	1.34	+3.54	8.80	3.87
I27–30	3	505	12	422	223	−152	1157	666	350	93	+48	13.76	8.39	1.59	1.44	+2.34	8.49	4.08
I31–II3	4	505	5	238	227	+35	1157	708	331	116	+2	13.76	7.92	1.60	1.64	+2.60	8.94	4.82
II 4–7	5*	505	5	533	247	−280	1157	910	472	111	−336	13.76	7.44	2.01	1.65	+2.66	8.99	4.25
II 8–11	6	505	5	371	280	−151	1157	986	327	111	−267	13.76	8.25	1.66	1.79	+2.06	8.63	4.82
II12–15	7	1491	4	1144	268	+75	2744	1708	853	108	+75	13.76	8.10	2.28	1.77	+1.61	8.93	4.33
II16–19	8	1491	5	951	223	+312	2744	1624	428	99	+593	13.76	6.90	2.09	1.58	+3.19	8.54	4.14
II20–23	9	1491	2	1361	229	−101	2744	1568	762	93	+321	13.76	7.40	2.52	1.59	+2.25	9.18	4.43
II24–27	10	1951	5	1587	312	+47	2384	1630	585	141	+28	10.72	6.49	1.65	1.80	+0.78	9.15	4.08
II28–III3	11	1951	4	1591	303	+52	2384	1620	556	133	+75	13.76	5.84	1.41	1.97	+1.50	8.67	3.99
III 4–7	12	965	1	960	338	−334	797	366	301	122	+8	10.72	7.27	1.38	1.98	+0.09	8.97	3.99
III 8–11	13	965	4	479	293	+189	797	436	181	116	+64	10.72	7.29	0.84	1.78	+0.81	8.69	3.91
III12–15	14	965	2	574	295	+94	797	453	200	109	+35	10.72	6.68	0.84	1.64	+1.56	9.69	4.28
III16–19	15	948	2	623	293	+30	725	577	210	112	−174	8.92	7.74	0.98	1.77	−1.57	8.82	4.62
III20–23	16	948	0	690	284	−26	725	508	214	114	−111	8.92	6.87	1.26	1.83	−1.04	9.01	4.49
III24–27	17	948	1	592	297	+58	725	436	177	126	−14	8.92	6.12	1.01	1.75	+0.04	8.80	4.16
III28–31	18																8.30	4.30
IV 1–4	19	1221	28	1249	303	−359	1174	469	937	146	−378	16.25	9.11	2.26	2.51	+2.37	9.41	4.46
IV 5–8	20	1221	60	948	307	−94	1174	501	575	139	−41	16.25	10.45	1.58	2.56	+1.66	9.30	4.36

* Vigantol 1 cc. daily starting from this period on.

TABLE VIII

Infant T. N. T. Case 3b. Calcium, phosphorus and nitrogen metabolism of a rachitic infant on cow's milk, breast milk from the wet nurse and combinations thereof

Date 1937–1939	Period four-day	Milk intake		Calcium, average per day					Phosphorus, average per day					Nitrogen, average per day					Serum			Medication (3)		Body weight
		Breast (1)	Klim (2)	Intake	Urine	Stool	Balance	Retention	Intake	Urine	Stool	Balance	Retention	Intake	Urine	Stool	Balance	Retention	Calcium	Phosphorus	Phosphatase	Calcium	Phosphorus	
		cc.	cc.	mgm.	mgm.	mgm.	mgm.	per cent	mgm.	mgm.	mgm.	mgm.	per cent	grams	grams	grams	grams	per cent	mgm. per cent	mgm. per cent	units	mgm.	mgm.	kgm.
XII22–25	A	68	798	1072	0	826	+246	23	755	418	204	+133	18	4.06	2.66	0.42	+0.98	24			13.74			5.72
XII26–29	B	46	820	1095	2	860	+233	21	774	439	242	+93	12	4.44	2.66	0.45	+1.33	30	5.50	7.07				5.79
XII30–12	C	29	703	938	1	744	+193	21	662	411	226	+25	4	3.52	2.16	0.42	+0.94	27						5.97
I 7																			5.19	6.34	7.56			5.96
I19–22	1	420	420	772	9	524	+239	31	460	180	168	+112	24	2.98	1.23	0.54	+1.21	41	4.77	6.40		90		5.81
I23–26	2	420	420	780	2	465	+313	40	462	263	106	+93	20	2.97	1.82	0.40	+0.75	25	4.88	5.07		90		6.12
I27																			5.88	5.02				6.10
I31																			6.16	4.73				6.33
II 4–7	5*	420	391	711	0	494	+217	30	432	289	93	+70	16	3.04	1.55	0.35	+1.14	38	5.60	4.64		73		6.25
II 8–11	6	420	353	633	1	420	+212	32	491	248	74	+69	14	2.62	1.04	0.38	+0.60	23	7.24	5.02		70		6.59
II19																			10.82	4.85				6.33
II20–23	9	359	366	579	1	147	+431	73	393	165	36	+192	49	2.52	1.31	0.25	+0.96	38	9.40	4.16				6.35
II24–27	10	402	375	624	2	275	+347	56	421	204	43	+174	41	2.64	1.50	0.38	+0.76	29	9.80	5.53	4.47			6.34
III 8–11	13	780	0	716	18	112	+586	82	499	137	28	+334	67	1.79	0.79	0.23	+0.77	43	10.01	5.56		480	422	6.28
III12–15	14	780	0	727	17	105	+605	83	586	214	25	+327	58	1.68	0.62	0.27	+0.79	47				480	422	6.45
III20–23	16	622	0	565	16	98	+451	80	544	254	27	+263	48	1.39	0.58	0.28	+0.53	38	10.49	5.97		383	422	6.68
III24–27	17	701	0	644	23	122	+499	78	560	371	28	+161	29	1.47	0.56	0.24	+0.67	46				432	422	6.52
IV 1–4	19	0	768	994	52	509	+433	44	779	346	108	+325	42	3.98	2.32	0.37	+1.29	32						6.52
IV 5–8	20	0	644	836	37	361	+438	52	663	205	81	+377	57	3.38	2.06	0.23	+1.09	32	10.00					6.73

(1) The small amounts of breast milk given during periods A, B and C were from the mother (Case 3a), and the breast milk for the rest of the periods was supplied by the wet nurse (Case 3a′, Table II).

(2) "Klim" used for periods A, B and C was analyzed to contain 132.5 mgm. calcium, 93.9 mgm. phosphorus and 0.492 grams nitrogen per 100 cc.; while that used for the remaining periods, 129.2 mgm. calcium, 94.4 mgm. phosphorus and 0.484 grams nitrogen per 100 cc. The formula was made up by dissolving one part of Klim whole milk powder in eight parts of water.

(3) Calcium given in periods 1–2 was in the form of 10 per cent gluconate intramuscularly; that in periods 5 and 6, 3 per cent gluconate by mouth; and that in periods 13–17, 7.7 per cent lactate by mouth. Phosphorus was given as disodium phosphate solution per os.

* Wet nurse starting to receive vitamin D from this period.

(Figure 3 and Table. VIII) while on a Klim formula (with small amounts of breast milk from the mother) providing about 1,000 mgm. of calcium, large amounts of calcium came out in the stools, leaving a net retention of only 21 to 23 per cent of the intake. Phosphorus retention was even poorer, being 4 to 18 per cent. Serum calcium went down to as low as 4.77 mgm. per cent, whereupon convulsive seizures occurred. Evidently the infant, like the mother, was markedly deficient in vitamin D.

After the manifest tetany was brought under control by means of parenteral calcium therapy, metabolic observations were resumed, and breast feeding from the wet nurse was begun. Periods 1 and 2 served as control for a regimen of "half breast milk and half Klim formula" furnishing from 600 to 800 mgm. of calcium and from 400 to 500 mgm. of phosphorus. On this regimen the retention of both elements was distinctly poor, though slightly better than during periods A to C when Klim constituted almost the sole source of nutrients. This indicates that the wet nurse prior to vitamin D supplements, while capable of maintaining her skeleton intact for a time, was probably unable to secrete milk of sufficiently high antirachitic potency to correct the metabolic defect of the infant.

From period 5 on the wet nurse received vitamin D. The effect of this supplement to the milk provider on the infant's metabolism was not evident during the first 2 periods (periods 5 and 6), but subsequently considerable improvement was noticed. During periods 9 and 10, calcium retention rose to 56 to 73 per cent and phosphorus retention to 41 to 49 per cent. The best performance came during periods 13, 14, 16 and 17, when breast milk from the wet nurse alone was. fed with additions of calcium lactate and disodium phosphate to maintain the calcium and phosphorus intake. Here the average calcium retention of the 4 periods amounted to 81 per cent, and the average phosphorus retention to 50 per cent of the intake. The high degree of retention of calcium was brought about entirely by a reduction in the stool elimination, while that of phosphorus was caused by a reduction in both the urine and stool excretion.

The last 2 periods were devoted to a study of the effects of feeding Klim alone comparable to the regimen in periods A to C. While vitamin D was still operative, as it was presumably so during periods 19 and 20, both calcium and phosphorus retention were decidedly better than during periods A to C when marked vitamin D deficiency had existed. However, the degree of retention was not as good as during the exclusive breast-feeding periods, possibly suggesting certain peculiarities in the cow's milk that rendered its mineral contents less readily absorbable.

The behavior of serum calcium is worth noting. After it reached its lowest ebb with the onset of convulsions, parenteral calcium was capable of raising it only just enough to stop the convulsions; but with the feeding of "vitaminized" breast milk it rose precipitously to normal in the course of twelve days, and remained so throughout the balance of the experiment. Serum inorganic phosphorus, high to start with, went down to below normal when serum calcium reached the normal level, and subsequently it also rose to normal.

Coinciding with the correction of the biochemical abnormalities, there was clinical improvement. as well as roentgenologic evidence of healing of the rachitic bone changes in the course of a little over two months.

Case 4a. Mother W. H. S. This patient had active osteomalacia with slightly low serum calcium and markedly low serum inorganic phosphorus. She was admitted at the eighth month of pregnancy, and metabolic observation during the latter part of gestation showed that even balances were obtained on high levels of calcium intake and that the administration of Vigantol, 5 cc. daily for four days, was followed by progressive and marked retention of calcium and phosphorus, and a return of serum calcium and inorganic phosphorus to normal. The Vigantol given for the above-stated period, together with cod liver oil in 30 cc. daily doses for six days immediately postpartum, constituted the only supply of vitamin D prior to the studies on lactation.

As shown in Figure 4 and Table IX, metabolic observations, begun seventeen days postpartum, were continued for 26 four-day periods on intakes of calcium ranging from 1,407 to 1,656 mgm. per day. No vitamin D was supplied until the 19th period when Vigantol was started in daily doses of 2 cc. or 24,000 international units and continued for the remainder of the experiment. During the first 18 periods without vitamin D, the calcium balances showed considerable fluctuation. However, the trend is one of progressive loss of calcium from the body. If the 18 periods are divided into 3 series of 6 periods each, and the balances in each series averaged, one obtains a daily calcium balance of $+9$ mgm., -19 mgm. and -70 mgm. for periods 1 to 6, 7 to 12 and 13 to 18, respectively. This progressive weakening of calcium balance indicates most probably that the limited amount of vitamin D received prior to the studies was gradually being depleted in the course of three or four months. Another sign of vitamin D depletion, or rather deficient intestinal absorption, is the diminution and disappearance of urinary calcium with a correspondingly increased stool calcium.

After vitamin D therapy (beginning with period 19), the situation was entirely reversed. Stool calcium gradually decreased while urinary calcium returned. But the conservation through the bowel was much greater in extent than the loss through the urinary tract and, as a result, the balance became increasingly positive. The average daily calcium retention for the 8 periods amounted to 133 mgm. Thus vitamin D administration during lactation in a woman with skeletal decalcification, similar to Case 2a, was capable of conserving the metabolism of calcium to such an extent as to enable her not only to meet the. strenuous requirements of lactation, but

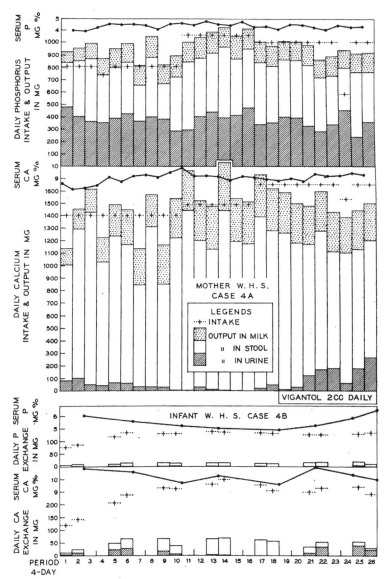

FIG. 4. CALCIUM AND PHOSPHORUS METABOLISM OF CASES 4A AND 4B

The mother with osteomalacia had a limited amount of vitamin D prior to study, but showed increasing mineral loss as observation proceeded until Vigantol was given. The infant exhibited good retention of calcium and phosphorus throughout, but a decrease, and later, disappearance of urinary calcium with corresponding increase of fecal calcium occurred while the mother was being depleted of vitamin D. Reinstitution of vitamin D therapy in the mother brought about a reversal in the partition of calcium between urinary and fecal elimination.

S. H. LIU, H. I. CHU, C. C. SU, T. F. YU AND T. Y. CHENG

TABLE IX

Mother W. H. S.   Case 4a.   Calcium, phosphorus and nitrogen metabolism in a case of osteomalacia during lactation at various states of vitamin D nutrition

Date 1938	Four-day period	Calcium, average per day					Phosphorus, average per day					Nitrogen, average per day					Serum		
		Intake	Urine	Stool	Milk	Balance	Intake	Urine	Stool	Milk	Balance	Intake	Urine	Stool	Milk	Balance	Calcium	Phosphorus	Phosphatase
		mgm.	mgm.	mgm.	mgm.	mgm.	mgm.	mgm.	mgm.	mgm.	mgm.	grams	grams	grams	grams	grams	mgm. per cent	mgm. per cent	units
II24–27	1	1407	83	924	128	+272	812	480	360	82	−110	10.61	6.70	1.34	1.19	+1.38	8.64	5.97	
II28–III3	2	1407	103	1191	162	−49	812	405	452	98	−143	10.61	6.10	1.60	1.45	+1.46	8.16	4.00	
III 4–7	3	1407	51	1378	189	−211	812	364	507	121	−180	10.61	6.15	1.81	1.60	+1.05	8.23	3.97	3.61
III 8–11	4	1409	45	982	209	+174	743	352	389	133	−131	9.95	5.69	1.20	1.77	+1.29	8.44	4.22	
III12–15	5	1407	67	1167	261	−88	812	390	418	142	−138	10.61	5.72	1.41	1.86	+1.62	9.10	4.56	
III16–19	6	1407	60	1108	282	−43	812	426	417	159	−190	10.61	5.72	1.10	1.97	+1.82	8.74	4.48	
III20–23	7	1407	34	812	287	+274	812	364	290	159	−1	10.61	5.79	0.89	2.01	+1.92	9.20	4.50	2.76
III24–27	8	1407	33*	1280	281	−187	812	401	481	167	−237	10.61	5.77	1.27	2.00	+1.57	9.31	4.40	
III28–31	9	1407	31	819	316	+241	812	381	287	154	−10	10.61	7.63	0.64	2.05	+0.29	9.08	4.04	
IV 1–4	10	1407	6	1218	318	−135	812	287	433	157	−65	10.61	6.72	1.24	2.00	+0.65	9.48	4.53	
IV 5–8	11	1492	4	1443	319	−274	1065	294	553	161	+57	12.96	7.19	1.75	1.96	+2.06	9.80	4.64	3.28
IV 9–12	12	1492	31	1168	323	−30	1065	402	474	165	+24	12.96	6.86	1.53	2.04	+2.53	9.24	4.48	
IV13–16	13	1492	11	1120	348	+13	1065	441	474	173	−23	12.96	8.76	1.36	2.07	+0.77	9.24	4.78	
IV17–20	14	1492	6	1478	348	−340	1065	396	570	159	−60	12.96	7.40	1.55	2.00	+2.01	9.20	4.53	
IV21–24	15	1492	3	1192	348	−51	1065	413	459	176	+17	12.96	8.10	1.42	1.99	+1.45	8.93	4.22	2.24
IV25–28	16	1492	0	1176	340	−24	1065	475	474	161	+35	12.96	9.90	1.45	1.98	−0.37	9.19	4.72	
IV29–V2	17	1656	21	1374	341	−80	1006	340	502	165	−1	14.84	8.40	1.78	1.97	+2.69	9.10	4.27	
V 3–6	18	1656	48	1233	321	+63	1006	354	458	160	+34	14.84	8.14	1.86	1.85	+2.99		4.39	
V 7–10	19*	1656	13	1250	326	+67	1006	401	466	152	−13	14.84	8.81	1.99	1.97	+2.07	8.84	4.07	
V11–14	20	1656	31	1151	320	+154	1006	396	463	153	−6	14.84	8.94	1.75	1.99	+2.16	9.02	4.54	
V15–18	21	1656	124	1048	310	+174	1006	328	494	156	+28	14.84	8.92	2.28	2.09	+1.55	8.80	4.44	
V19–22	22	1656	173	1105	323	+55	1006	284	428	153	+241	14.84	8.24	1.86	2.01	+2.73	9.38	4.24	2.86
V23–26	23	1656	182	933	329	+112	1006	339	398	160	+109	14.84	8.62	1.72	2.10	+2.40	9.19	4.00	
V27–30	24	1537	62	1042	287	+146	587	457	342	143	−355	8.42	6.43	1.08	1.81	−0.90	9.24	4.43	1.85
V31–VI3	25	1656	180	954	314	+208	1006	241	425	149	+191	14.84	7.89	1.57	1.97	+3.41	9.44	4.20	
VI4–7	26	1656	268	943	295	+150	1006	363	401	163	+79	14.84	8.38	1.61	1.90	+2.95	9.31	4.35	2.18

* Vigantol 2 cc. daily starting from this period.

also to retain considerable amounts of the mineral for the replenishment of the skeletal store.

Phosphorus balances were mainly negative, especially during periods 1 to 10 when the intake was relatively low. But after vitamin D therapy substantial amounts of phosphorus were retained. Serum calcium and inorganic phosphorus were maintained at fairly steady levels.

Case 4b. Infant W. H. S. This was a normal baby. Although his mother (Case 4a) had active osteomalacia during pregnancy, the vitamin D given during the latter part of gestation, albeit limited in amount, might have contributed to the relative wellbeing of the infant from the standpoint of mineral metabolism. While exclusively fed on the mother's milk, the calcium, phosphorus and nitrogen balances of the infant were studied *pari passu* with those of the mother, although with him 2 periods of actual study were alternated with 2 "rest" periods. Comparable to the normal infant (Case 1b) and the 2 rachitic infants (Cases 2b and 3b) following feeding with breast milk "vitaminized" via the mother, this infant showed such avidity in retaining calcium and phosphorus that he left only small amounts of these elements to be eliminated in the urine and stool. As shown in Figure 4 and Table X approximately 80 per cent of the calcium and 90 per cent of the phosphorus in the milk were retained.

As the mother was being depleted of vitamin D, the infant began to show a slight decrease in calcium retention (periods 13 to 18). What is more striking is

the behavior of the urinary and stool calcium. As impoverishment of vitamin D proceeded in the mother, there was in the infant a progressive decrease in the urinary calcium to the point of disappearance, coinciding with a steady increase in the stool calcium.

This phenomenon was interpreted as an early sign of vitamin D deficiency, because when the mother began to be replenished with vitamin D, the infant showed a return of urinary calcium with a corresponding decrease of stool calcium. The net gain of calcium was somewhat better during the last 4 periods (periods 21 to 22 and 25 to 26) of observation when the mother was receiving Vigantol.

It is of interest to note that throughout the entire 26 periods, the phosphorus retention was maintained at the uniform high level of 90 per cent with very little variation in the partition of phosphorus between the urine and the stool, suggesting that phosphorus metabolism was possibly a less sensitive index of vitamin D nutrition than calcium metabolism.

Both the serum calcium and inorganic phosphorus were maintained within normal limits throughout the periods of observation. However, there seemed to be a decline in both elements toward the end of the depletion period in the mother, with a return to the initial levels subsequently when the mother was being replenished with vitamin D.

Roentgenograms of the wrists taken periodically revealed that the epiphyseal lines, normal to start with, began to be fuzzy with "lipping" at the end of the period of depletion in the mother. After the infant had received for a month breast milk from the mother being given vitamin D, x-ray showed improvement in what were considered to be the early changes of rickets.

DISCUSSION

Observations made simultaneously on the calcium, phosphorus and nitrogen metabolism of the lactating mother and of the breast-milk-fed infant of the type recorded in the present communication have not been reported in the literature as far as we are aware. Yet such experiments are of importance in throwing light on the nature and extent of the relationship between the maternal and infantile nutrition by way of the breast milk. From the results presented, several points of interest may be mentioned.

Maternal metabolism during lactation. It is generally accepted that considerable difficulty exists in maintaining women in mineral balance during lactation. Hunscher (10) and Hummel and associates (9) failed to maintain actively nursing women in calcium balance on very high intake (3 to 4 grams per day) during the early part of lactation. Only during late lactation, when milk flow diminished, was calcium stored (5). Supplementing the usual home diets with cod liver oil, although improving the calcium balance, did not always change a negative to a positive balance (15). Garry and Stiven (6), who have reviewed the recent literature on dietary requirements in pregnancy and lactation, recommend 1 to 2 grams of calcium for milk yields of from 500 to 1,000 cc. and calcium contents from 20 to 30 mgm. per 100 cc. milk.

To insure the proper utilization of the above-recommended amount of calcium intake, vitamin D must be added. Thus all the 4 lactating women studied maintained themselves in calcium balance on intakes between 1 to 2 grams when vitamin D was operative. These data are especially significant when it is remembered that they were obtained from women in early lactation with milk yields exceeding one liter a day and calcium content more than 25 mgm. per 100 cc. On the other hand, when vitamin D was deficient (Case 2a), or being depleted (Case 4a), negative balance prevailed. Therefore, some of the reported difficulties in maintaining calcium balance in lactation on relatively high intake can be as justly attributed to vitamin D undernutrition as to the heightened requirements of this phase of the reproductive cycle.

To the woman with prior vitamin D and calcium deficiency, as in osteomalacia, the administration of vitamin D has the added importance of making it possible for her to store calcium for her skeletal replenishment in the face of extra drain of lactation. This is amply illustrated by the data obtained from Cases 2a and 4a.

The situation in late lactation, when the milk flow diminishes, may be less stringent. Of the

TABLE X

Infant W. H. S. Case 4b. Calcium, phosphorus and nitrogen metabolism of a presumably normal breast-fed infant showing changes due to the varying state of vitamin D nutrition in the mother

Date 1939	Period four-day	Breast milk intake	Calcium, average per day					Phosphorus, average per day					Nitrogen, average per day					Serum			Body weight
			In-take	Urine	Stool	Bal-ance	Re-ten-tion	In-take	Urine	Stool	Bal-ance	Re-ten-tion	In-take	Urine	Stool	Bal-ance	Re-ten-tion	Cal-cium	Phos-phorus	Phospha-tase	
		cc.	mgm.	mgm.	mgm.	mgm.	per cent	mgm.	mgm.	mgm.	mgm.	per cent	grams	grams	grams	grams	per cent	mgm. per cent	mgm. per cent	units	kgm.
II24–27	1	466	120	4	8	+108	90	77	0	6	+71	92	1.07	0.35	0.17	+0.55	51				3.01
II28–III3	2	510	142	12	12	+118	83	86	1	9	+76	88	1.19	0.82	0.20	+0.17	14	10.88	6.03	8.21	3.08
III12–15	5	720	217	23	25	+169	79	118	2	8	+108	92	1.55	0.55	0.21	+0.79	51				3.57
III16–19	6	780	237	28	39	+170	72	134	2	13	+119	89	1.66	0.73	0.25	+0.68	41	10.55	5.56	17.00	3.70
III28–31	9	900	256	17	50	+199	75	129	1	15	+113	88	1.73	0.62	0.24	+0.87	50				4.15
IV 1–4	10	900	263	6	32	+225	86	131	2	11	+118	90	1.67	0.61	0.19	+0.87	52	9.70	5.18	15.42	4.40
IV13–16	13	945	280	3	64	+213	76	139	1	14	+124	89	1.67	0.62	0.24	+0.81	48				4.85
IV17–20	14	1020	300	1	67	+232	77	137	1	14	+122	89	1.72	0.62	0.22	+0.88	51	10.25	5.00		4.97
IV29–V2	17	1020	277	1	62	+214	77	134	1	13	+121	90	1.56	0.57	0.24	+0.75	48	9.58	4.86		5.67
V 3–6	18*	1020	255	0	57	+198	78	131	1	11	+119	91	1.51	0.57	0.17	+0.77	51				5.76
V15–18	21	1020	249	9	25	+215	86	126	1	16	+109	94	1.68	0.47	0.25	+0.86	51	11.17	5.24	5.08	6.24
V19–22	22	1020	266	34	19	+213	80	126	3	15	+108	93	1.65	0.55	0.27	+0.83	50	10.34	5.87	13.93	6.39
V31–VI3	25	1080	271	39	15	+217	80	129	5	14	+110	92	1.70	0.67	0.24	+0.79	48				6.80
VI 4–7	26	1080	243	30	7	+206	85	135	2	10	+123	91	1.57	0.55	0.14	+0.88	56	10.01	6.49	10.60	6.77

* Mother starting to receive Vigantol 2 cc. per day right after the completion of this period.

TABLE XI

Data selected and averaged from Tables IV, VI, VIII and X to show the calcium retention of the infants in the present study for comparison with the maximum recorded retention of breast-fed infants compiled from the literature by Leitch (11)

Age	Leitch				Case 1b				Case 2b				Case 3b				Case 4b			
	Intake	Balance	Retention	Ideal retention	Period	Intake	Balance	Retention	Period	Intake	Balance	Retention	Period	Intake	Balance	Retention	Period	Intake	Balance	Retention
months	mgm.	mgm.	per cent	mgm.		mgm.	mgm.	per cent		mgm.	mgm.	per cent		mgm.	mgm.	per cent		mgm.	mgm.	per cent
0–1	208	82	39	130	3–4	290	220	76									1–2	131	113	86
1–2	127	85	67	310	5–9	336	255	76									5–10	246	191	78
2–3	149	102	68	250													13–18*	278	228	82
3–4	235	109	46	240					8–12	266	207	78					21–26	257	213	83
4–5	236	142	60	220																
5–6	221	65	29	170									13–17	663†	535	81				

* Beginning vitamin D deficiency may be present during these periods.
† Intake raised by the addition of calcium lactate.

5 lactating women reported on in a previous paper (16), 4 were in relatively late lactation with milk yields ranging from 280 to 460 cc. per day, and it was possible for them to store calcium on intakes varying from 400 to 700 mgm. However, this was possible only after the exhibition of vitamin D.

Metabolism of breast-fed infants. In 1937 Leitch (11) assembled all available recent data on calcium metabolism of normal infants fed exclusively on breast milk. The maximum recorded retention for the entire series was shown for each monthly period from the first to the sixth month. This ranged from 65 to 142 mgm. per day or from 29 to 68 per cent of the intake. In each instance the amount of calcium retained fell very much short of the requirement of 170 to 310 mgm. calculated for skeletal growth to maintain the calcium content of the body at 10 grams per kgm. Should such a state prevail, a skeleton of more inferior grade of calcification than that at birth would be built up, leading to rickets and osteoporosis. Leitch finds it difficult to reconcile his calculation with the anomalous situation where feeding of breast milk, the natural food for the infant, would lead to deterioration of the skeleton.

A review of the data on the 4 infants included in the present work (rearranged in Table XI) suggests that such an anomalous position need not arise if milk intake is adequate and if vitamin D is operative. When such was the case, each of the 4 infants showed an average daily retention approaching the ideal calculated by Leitch and exceeding the maximum retention recorded in the literature. The explanation for such excellent retention in our infants is probably two-fold. First, the quantities of breast milk consumed were sufficient to provide a total intake of calcium to meet the requirement. Second, by virtue of the conserving and absorption-promoting action of vitamin D, the retention of calcium became exceedingly efficient, from 76 to 86 per cent of the intake being retained. It is true that 2 of the infants (Cases 2b and 3b) had rickets in which vitamin D treatment should give rise to extraordinary retention to restore the depleted skeletal store. However, the other 2 infants, who had no rickets to start with, exhibited the same high degree of calcium retention, suggesting that breast feeding in adequate amounts, fortified by vitamin D, would lead to normal skeletal growth of the infant.

Vitamin D in human milk. The position of the vitamin D content of human milk is rather vague. Hess (8) has demonstrated that, whereas 25 cc. of ordinary human milk daily failed to cure rickets in rats, the same could be made effective by treating the mother with ultraviolet irradiation. Outhouse, Macy and Brekke (22) reported that pooled milk from wet nurses on an average American dietary in amounts of 25, 30, or 40 cc. daily contained no antirachitic factor as tested on rachitic rats, although 30 cc. of cow's milk fed daily induced marked healing. Bunker, Harris and Eustis (2) found that milk of human mothers fed previously on "vitamin D" milk of the cow was potent in the antirachitic factor for the rat.

When the antirachitic potency of breast milk

from mothers receiving vitamin D supplements is tested on the infant, it is generally believed that some, though uncertain, degree of protection is transferable to the suckling children. Weech (24), in a survey of 47 infants breast fed by mothers given cod liver oil, found that the degree of intensity of the rachitic process, as judged by roentgenograms of wrists and the product of serum calcium and phosphorus, was inversely proportional to the amount of cod liver oil administered. Even in the group of 4 women receiving the largest amount of cod liver oil (50 to 60 ounces in six months), 2 of the infants had x-ray evidence of rickets. Barnes, Cope, Hunscher and Brekke (1) studied a woman whose diet was superior in quality and, in addition, was fortified with 2 quarts of cow's milk daily in which 300 units of a vitamin D concentrate was incorporated. It was found that the milk secreted was not sufficiently enriched by vitamin D to heal rickets in 3 colored infants, or in experimental rachitic rats. Her own breast-fed baby, however, showed no signs of rickets throughout the investigation.

From the observations presented in this paper, there is no doubt that the administration of vitamin D to the mother in ordinary therapeutic doses (12,000 to 24,000 international units) is capable of sufficiently enriching her milk by vitamin D to prevent (Cases 1b and 4b) or cure (Cases 2b and 3b) rickets in the infant. When vitamin D is withheld from the mother for a period of three months or so, as in Case 4a, her milk will be sufficiently impoverished to produce early evidence of vitamin D deficiency in the infant. This demonstrates, in a somewhat novel way, the dependence of the infant on the mother from the standpoint of vitamin D nutrition via breast milk.

Importance of vitamin D supplement to the mother during lactation. It is usually recommended that infants be started with vitamin D supplements in the early months of life, while nursing mothers receive relatively scant attention in this respect. This work should give credence to the view that it is just as important to supplement the mother as the child, if not more so. Vitamin D administration to the lactating mother is necessary to maintain her in balance in case her skeletal store is normal, and to enable her to store calcium if she has prior skeletal depletion as in osteomalacia. In adequate doses, the administra-

tion of vitamin D to the mother would supply her milk with antirachitic properties sufficient for the care of the child.

The minimal dosage for the mother that would be efficacious both for the mother and for the infant is not determined. The daily dosage of 12,000 to 24,000 international units is probably more than the minimal effective dose. Nor is there evidence to indicate that such dosage need be kept up uninterruptedly throughout the nursing period. However, to render a relatively small dosage of vitamin D effective, it is important that the level of calcium intake be raised over the ordinary requirement. The recommended amount of 1 to 2 grams of calcium per day will likely be sufficient for the purpose.

SUMMARY

1. Data on calcium, phosphorus and nitrogen metabolism were obtained on 4 women while they were supplying breast milk to 4 infants from whom similar data were secured at the same time, showing intimate relationship in the state of vitamin D nutrition between the mother and the infant during the nursing period.

2. In the first set of cases, the mother had healing osteomalacia with good retention of calcium and abundant store of vitamin D during gestation, and the infant was born normal. During lactation the mother maintained herself in mineral balance on relatively high intake, while the infant retained the major portion of the calcium and phosphorus intake in the milk.

3. The second pair of cases consisted of a mother with osteomalacia and tetany and her infant with rickets and tetany. Both showed poor retention of calcium and phosphorus, but after vitamin D administration to the mother, the metabolic defects of the mother as well as the infant were corrected. The mother, as a result of vitamin D therapy, was able to absorb sufficient minerals not only for the heightened requirements of lactation but also for the reparation of her depleted skeletal store. The infant, after receiving the "vitaminized" milk, showed markedly improved mineral retention.

4. The third experiment was on a presumably normal wet nurse supplying breast milk to a rachitic infant born of an osteomalacic mother. The wet nurse had to have her calcium intake

raised to 1.5 to 2.0 grams before she was able to maintain balance. The vitamin D given subsequently probably contributed to this favorable state of affairs. The infant showed poor calcium and phosphorus retention while on a Klim formula and on breast milk prior to vitamin D administration to the wet nurse; but after such supplement, the infant was very much improved in mineral retention as well as in the rachitic bone changes.

5. The last series of observations was made on an osteomalacic mother and her infant. The mother had a limited period of vitamin D therapy during gestation with sufficient improvement in her metabolic disorder to give birth to a normal baby. During lactation while vitamin D was being withheld, she began to show negative mineral balance on relatively high intake; and subsequently, when vitamin D therapy was reinstituted, good retention of calcium and phosphorus. The infant exhibited excellent mineral retention throughout the period of study, but as the mother was being depleted of vitamin D, the urinary calcium excretion diminished and disappeared, corresponding with an increase in the stool. This phenomenon was interpreted as an early sign of vitamin D deficiency, for subsequent supply of vitamin D to the mother induced a reversal in the partition of calcium elimination between the urine and stool in favor of the former.

CASE ABSTRACTS

Case 1a. Mother, Mrs. Y. W. L. (Hospital Number 28572), a Chinese woman of 42 was first seen in October 1933 for pain in the bones and debility of three years' duration. Her detailed history was reported in paper II (12) of this series. Briefly stated, she presented a case of advanced osteomalacia with marked skeletal decalcification, deformities and fractures dating back to July 1930 when she gave birth to her fourth child. Her serum calcium was 8.8 and inorganic phosphorus 2.2 mgm. per 100 cc., findings that justify the classification of her case as one of low-phosphorus osteomalacia.

She went through detailed metabolic studies from November 1933 to June 1934. Her dramatic response to vitamin D therapy from the symptomatic, roentgenologic and metabolic standpoints was given in paper II (12) and her behavior toward varying levels and ratios of calcium to phosphorus intake was presented in paper III. (13).

In September 1934 the patient was readmitted with a slight recurrence of the pain in the bones and difficulty in walking. Her appetite was poor, with occasional nausea and vomiting. She was found to be pregnant

with the expected date of confinement on April 15, 1935. Although slight tenderness was present over the lumbar spine and ribs, roentgenologic examination of the skeleton showed no evidence of exacerbation in osteomalacia. Serum calcium was 8.92 and inorganic phosphorus 2.82. There was minimal pulmonary tuberculosis at right upper lung. A slight degree of anemia developed shortly after admission. Hemoglobin remained at 10 grams, and erythrocyte count at 3.2 millions, in spite of the administration for prolonged periods of ferric ammonium citrate and hydrochloric acid by mouth, and liver extract intramuscularly. Her calcium, phosphorus and nitrogen metabolism was studied throughout pregnancy. From December 1934 to April 1935 her calcium intake was approximately 2 grams per day, and vitamin D in the form of Vigantol was given in doses of from 1 to 3 cc. a day (1 cc. is equivalent to 12,000 international units of vitamin D). During this period of four months, 40 to 50 per cent of the intake of calcium was retained. This would enable her not only to meet the fetal requirements, but also to replenish her own skeletal store of calcium.

The course of gestation was fairly smooth except for an attack of abdominal pain in the latter part of the pregnancy. In view of the pelvic deformities, a cesarean section was performed by Dr. J. P. Maxwell on April 13, 1935, and a normal male baby (weighing 2,885 grams) was delivered. The postoperative course was satisfactory. The patient was studied again from the viewpoint of lactation. The studies began eighteen days *postpartum*, and were continued for 11 four-day periods. This part of the studies, together with observations on other patients during lactation, was reported in Paper VI (14).

The patient was discharged on June 15, 1935 in good condition. She remained well and nursed her baby until September 1936 when she began to have diarrhea, abdominal distension and swelling of legs. On reentry into the hospital in November, although her diarrhea subsided, her general condition deteriorated considerably. There was anasarca with ascites and enlarged liver. Plasma proteins were 1.31 per cent albumin and 2.72 per cent globulin. The pulmonary tuberculosis at right upper lung showed extension. In the right breast there was a firm mass measuring $10 \times 8 \times 5$ cm. associated with enlarged axillary lymph nodes. There had been a firm nodule in her breast for eight years, showing no tendency to grow until four months prior to admission when rapid enlargement commenced. Biopsy of the tumor and axillary lymph gland revealed carcinoma in both, and the section of the sediment of the ascitic fluid withdrawn also exhibited malignant tumor cells. As radical operation was not considered advisable in view of the advanced stage of the disease and of the patient's poor general condition, a course of intensive deep radiotherapy was given to the breast and axilla. Although the tumor masses diminished in size, the general condition of the patient went downhill. Death took place at home in February 1937.

Case 1b. Infant, Y. W. L. (Hospital Number 49062),

was the fifth child of the mother described above. Although the mother had osteomalacia, this was largely healed, and she received large amounts of calcium and vitamin D during gestation. The child delivered at term on April 13, 1935 by cesarean section weighed 2,885 grams and measured 53 cm. in length. He was normal in every respect. There was no clinical evidence of rickets. Cord blood serum calcium was 11.1 mgm. per cent. Roentgenologic examination of the bones of the upper and lower extremities showed normal size, contour and density. He was fed exclusively on mother's milk. Metabolic studies commenced on the twenty-sixth day after birth and proceeded smoothly for 7 four-day periods. General condition remained excellent and weight gain was uninterrupted. On discharge on June 12, he weighed 5,600 grams, almost doubling birth weight.

Case 2a. · *Mother, Mrs. C. S. Y. (Hospital Number 58397)*, age 31, was admitted on April 4, 1937 for general bodily ache, tingling and spasm of extremities for a year and a half. In December 1934 she gave birth to her first·baby, which was breast fed until June 1936, when it died. In November 1935, while lactating, she began to have bony aches, followed by numbness and spasticity of the limbs. Active tetanic attacks occurred usually after exposure to cold or prolonged pressure on the limbs. The condition cleared up in April 1936 when she became pregnant for the second time. The bony aches and numbness began to recur in October and became progressively more debilitating. The second child was delivered spontaneously in February 1937. Spastic attacks returned after parturition.

After the birth of the second child, bowels were constipated and bleeding from rectum was frequently noticed on defecation. There was an attack of dysentery in September 1936. Diet consisted of corn, millet, wheat flour, rice and vegetables in season. Meat and eggs were very rarely eaten.

On admission the patient appeared well developed, fairly well nourished and not in acute distress. Temperature 37.4° C., pulse 88, blood pressure 110/70, weight 48 kgm. Breasts were lactating with marked venous engorgement. Spleen was just palpable. Hemorrhoids, both external and internal, were present and bled on digital examination. There were no skeletal deformities, although pain was complained of in the shoulders, lumbar spine and thighs on motion. The patella tendon reflexes were hyperactive; and both Chvostek's and Trousseau's signs were positive. Urine was normal except for the presence of sugar which proved to be lactose. Blood picture was not remarkable. Serum calcium was 7.46 and inorganic phosphorus 4.70 mgm. per 100 cc.; phosphatase was 12.9 Bodansky units. On x-ray examination slight osteoporosis was present in all the visualized bones, but no deformities.

Metabolic studies were started on April 6. The patient developed dysentery with 7 to 10 blood and mucus-containing stools a day. Low-grade fever was present. Tetany at times became manifest, requiring calcium gluconate intramuscularly for relief. *B. dysenteriae*, mannite-fermenting group, was isolated from the stools.

Fortunately, the attack subsided in six days and was not sufficiently serious to interrupt the metabolic regime.. After 3 control periods Vigantol 1 cc. daily was given, and marked symptomatic improvement in the bony aches, numbness and spasticity was noticed.

After 6 periods of metabolic studies, there was a recurrence of dysentery necessitating suspension of the rigid quantitative regime. While the administration of Vigantol and high calcium intake were maintained, a semi-liquid diet and doses of sodium sulphate were given. In twelve days the bowel condition returned to normal. Metabolic studies were then resumed for 3 periods before the patient was discharged in good condition on May 25, 1937.

Case 2b. *Infant, C. C. C. (Hospital Number 58396)*, a male baby, aged 57 days, was admitted on April 4, 1937 for convulsive attacks for four days prior to entry. Although the mother had tetany and osteomalacia as stated above, the birth of the baby was spontaneous and easy. Feeding was exclusively on breasts. The onset of convulsive seizures was sudden without any previous illness. They were generalized with retraction of head, deviation of mouth, upward rolling· of eyeballs and spastic and clonic contractions of all extremities. Each attack lasted from five to ten minutes.

Examination showed good development and nutrition. Although no convulsions were noticed, both hands and feet were held in spasm, and Trousseau's and Chvostek's signs were present. The anterior fontanelle was wide open, but craniotabes, rosary· and enlargement of the wrists were absent. Liver and spleen were palpable and hydrocele of tunica vaginalis was noted on both sides.

Urine and blood count were normal and stools contained some mucus. Blood serum calcium was 7.8 and phosphorus 8.0 mgm. per cent; phosphatase was 19.6 units (Bodansky). Plasma proteins were 3.11 per cent albumin and 1.62 per cent globulin. X-ray films showed a slight condensation, haziness and lipping at the distal ends of radii, ulnae, tibiae and fibulae. The bones were slightly osteoporotic. These changes were suggestive of mild rickets, but over the lateral aspects of both femurs there was considerable periosteal thickening.

After admission the spastic phenomenon was promptly controlled by doses of calcium gluconate intramuscularly and calcium chloride orally. Metabolic experiments were started at the same time as those on the mother whose milk constituted the sole form of feeding. The studies went on well for 1 period, but during the second and third periods they had to be discontinued on account of a severe local vaccinia reaction to smallpox vaccination, accompanied by fever and return of convulsive attacks. The latter were again controlled by parenteral calcium gluconate and oral calcium chloride, and the whole episode subsided in three or four days. The baby was put on the metabolic regimen again from the fourth period on, and satisfactory studies were carried on for 9 more periods.

The infant was discharged in good condition on May 25, 1937. Serum calcium and phosphorus were 11.32 and 5.61 mgm. per cent, respectively. X-ray examination, repeated on the day of discharge, showed no obvious changes in the bones from that on admission. The weight gain was from 4,900 to 6,100 grams in the course of seven weeks.

Case 3a. Mother, Mrs. T. W. T. (Hospital Number 61219), a Chinese woman of 38, was admitted on November 29, 1937 with the chief complaint of pain in the lumbar region for thirteen months and in both thighs for five months. She began to have pain in the lower back soon after the onset of her eighth pregnancy thirteen months prior to admission. The pain gradually increased in severity, resulting in difficulty in walking throughout the first and second trimesters of pregnancy. In the latter part of pregnancy the pain also involved the thighs. She was completely bedridden shortly before parturition and has remained so since. Her parturition which took place in August 1937 was slow but spontaneous. The baby (Case 3b) was found to have rickets at the same time that the mother was seen. He was breast fed by the mother but the milk secretion was extremely poor. The patient had attacks of numbness and spasm of hands throughout the course of present illness. She was married at 17, and gave birth to eight children, the eldest one being 20 years of age. She had tingling sensation, spasm of hands and pain in the lower back during her sixth and seventh pregnancies six and four years prior to admission, respectively. Her husband, being a peddler, could scarcely earn enough to feed a family of seven. The diet was extremely inadequate and the patient led a secluded life.

Examination revealed that she was completely disabled in bed, complaining of pain in the muscles and bones whenever she was moved. She had marked muscle spasm and tenderness in the thighs and over the lower ribs. Slight scoliosis and kyphosis of lumbar spine, slight rostration of the symphysis pubis and very narrow pubic arch were present. Signs of Chvostek and Trousseau were positive. Head organs were normal. Thyroid was slightly enlarged. There were no important abnormal findings in the chest and abdomen. Routine laboratory studies, including blood Wassermann test, blood counts, urinalysis and stool examinations were all negative except for a slight transient lactosuria. Fasting blood sugar and non-protein nitrogen were within normal range. Serum calcium was 6.87 and inorganic phosphorus 2.75 mgm. per cent. Plasma proteins were 2.51 per cent albumin and 5.66 per cent globulin. Basal metabolic rate was + 21.2 per cent. X-ray examination revealed marked osteoporosis of all the bones, exceedingly marked biconcave deformity of the vertebral bodies, eversion and old fractures of the pubic bones. The right upper lung field appeared slightly clouded.

Metabolic observation extended from December 6, 1937 to April 15, 1938. Her response, clinically and metabolically, to ultraviolet irradiation was reported in paper VII (4) of this series. She gained 9 kgm. of weight in four and one-half months, and was discharged on April 16, 1938 much improved symptomatically and roentgenologically.

Case 3a'. Wet nurse, Mrs. W. C. S. (Hospital number

61624), age 23, was admitted on January 14, 1938 as a wet nurse for baby T. N. T. (Case 3b described below). Her past history was irrelevant. She was married a year prior to admission and became pregnant soon afterwards. The course of pregnancy was smooth, and a male child weighing 5 lbs. was delivered spontaneously at term on December 17, 1937. The child was fed on her breast soon after birth. The diet for the past year consisted of rice, wheat flour, millet, corn meal and salted and fresh vegetables, but practically no meat or eggs.

Physical examination showed good development and nutrition. Weight 52.2 kgm., height 161 cm. There were no skeletal deformities, bone tenderness, nor signs of tetany. Both breasts were lactating. Except for moderate gingivitis, pharyngitis and endocervicitis, the rest of the physical findings were normal.

Routine urine, blood and stool examinations were normal. Blood Wassermann reaction was negative. Serum calcium and phosphorus were 9.07 and 4.78 mgm. per cent, respectively (January 15). Calcium, phosphorus and nitrogen balance studies were started on January 19 and carried out for a total of 22 four-day periods. These included observations on the effects of various levels of calcium and phosphorus intake and of vitamin D therapy. The patient was discharged on April 14 in good condition.

Case 3b. Infant, T. N. T. (Hospital Number 61227), male, age three months, was admitted on November 30, 1937 for investigation for possible rickets or tetany on account of advanced osteomalacia in the mother. As mentioned before (Case 3a), this was the eighth child, and his birth was at term and spontaneous but prolonged. As the mother's milk secretion was scanty, breast feeding had to be supplemented by *hsin erh cha* (almond tea), *oufen* (lotus root starch) and *kao kan* (rice flour cake). When two months old the infant had an attack of high fever followed by convulsions lasting for half a day.

Physical development and general nutrition were fair; weight was 5,260 grams. The anterior fontanelle was wide open and the posterior fontanelle partially so. Parietal bosses, Harrison's groove, enlargement of the costochondral junctions and widening of the wrists were noticeable. The head organs were normal except for some nasal discharge and the lungs and heart showed no abnormality. The abdomen was prominent with both spleen and liver palpable at 1 cm. below costal margin.

Urinalysis and stool examinations were normal. Blood showed 10.5 grams hemoglobin, 3.4 million red blood cells, and 11,250 white blood cells with 35 per cent polymorphonuclear leukocytes and 62 per cent lymphocytes. Serum calcium was 5.18 and inorganic phosphorus 5.94 mgm. per 100 cc. and phosphatase was 13.7 Bodansky units. Roentgenograms exhibited moderate osteoporosis of all the bones with slight haziness and cupping of the distal epiphysial ends of all the long bones of the forearms and legs. Slight beading was observed at the anterior aspects of all the ribs. The diagnosis was moderate rickets (Figure 5). This was likely to be of fetal origin.

For 3 four-day periods (designated as A, B, C; December 22, 1937 to January 2, 1938, inclusive) while on a formula of "Klim" with a small amount of breast milk from the mother, the calcium, phosphorus and nitrogen balances were observed.

On January 18 and 19, attacks of generalized convulsions occurred. Serum calcium and phosphorus were respectively 4.77 and 6.40 mgm. per cent. Calcium ion was 2 mgm. per cent, as determined by the frog heart method (20) and 2.4 mgm. per cent by calculation from total calcium and serum proteins (5.56 grams per cent) according to McLean and Hastings (21). It was considered that the convulsive attacks were a manifestation of tetany. Calcium gluconate (Sandoz) 10 per cent 10 cc. (90 mgm. calcium) was given intramuscularly daily from January 19 to 26 (periods 1 and 2), while the feeding consisted of breast milk from the wet nurse and "Klim," 420 cc. each daily, with additions of orange juice.

From January 27 on, calcium gluconate 3 per cent solution was given by mouth in daily doses of 27 cc. (73 mgm. calcium) instead of the 10 per cent solution intramuscularly and the wet nurse received Vigantol 1 cc. (12,000 international units vitamin D) daily. The amount and proportion of "Klim" and breast milk remained approximately the same. While on this regime, balance studies were made on the child for 2 periods from February 4 to 11 (periods 5 and 6).

On February 11 rhinitis developed with purulent discharge from which virulent B. diphtheriae were isolated. There was a low-grade fever. Leukocyte count was 10,-450 with 52 per cent polymorphonuclears. A total dose of 20,000 units of a concentrated form of diphtheria antitoxin was given intramuscularly in divided doses on February 12 and 13. There was some febrile reaction following the serum treatment. Though the nasal discharge cleared up promptly, positive K. L. B. cultures were obtained on several subsequent occasions.

While on essentially the same regime, except for the omission of calcium gluconate by mouth, 2 more periods (periods 9 and 10) of metabolic observations were secured from February 20 to 27. From March 8 to 15 (periods 13 and 14) and from March 20 to 27 (periods 16 and 17), feeding was entirely on the breast milk from the wet nurse and the calcium and phosphorus intake was maintained by the addition of a 7.7 per cent solution of calcium lactate 48 cc. daily (480 mgm. calcium), and a solution of disodium phosphate (422 mgm. phosphorus).

The last 2 periods (periods 19 and 20) of metabolic studies were from April 1 to 8 when the feeding was entirely on "Klim," the calcium lactate being omitted.

Just prior to discharge on April 18, 1938, x-ray examination showed evidence of healing of rickets with increased bony density in the course of four months (Figure 6). Body weight on discharge was 6,700 grams.

Case 4a. Mother, Mrs. W. H. S. (Hospital Number 65376), age 29, was admitted on December 9, 1938 for bony aching, particularly of the pelvis and lumbar region, with occasional carpopedal spasm for eleven years prior to entry. She was married in 1926, led an indoor life in a cave dwelling in Pingyao, Shansi, and subsisted mainly on cereals and vegetables. Her symptoms, which began

shortly before her first pregnancy in 1927, were considerably aggravated during gestation so that she was confined to bed on account of bone pains and spastic attacks. However, the delivery was spontaneous without difficulty, and lactation was abundant. In the course of two years the symptoms were gradually improved. On getting up she noticed that her stature dwindled by several inches with knock-knee and pelvic deformities. In 1933, she became pregnant for the second time, and the gestation was terminated by medication at the third month. Her symptoms were aggravated especially during the winter. She was examined in this hospital for the first time in April 1936, when a course of calcium lactate, cod liver oil and ultra violet radiation gave rise to considerable improvement. She returned to Shansi and was pregnant for the third time in March 1937. The backache and leg pains recurred and the pregnancy was artificially aborted at the fourth month. Her fourth pregnancy started in May 1938 and she was admitted during the eighth month of gestation.

Examination showed undernutrition and stunted stature. Weight 44.2 kgm. and height 154 cm. The lower extremities were particularly short in comparison with the trunk and upper extremities. The gait was unsteady with the pelvis tilted from one side to the other in walking, while only very short steps could be made. The thighs were strongly adducted and internally rotated, and the knees knocked against each other. The right lower extremity was shorter than the left by 4 cm. Definite tenderness was present over the ribs, spine, pelvis and femurs. Chvostek's sign was negative, but Trousseau's sign was positive. The heart and lungs were normal. The blood pressure was 80/50. The abdomen was enlarged by the gravid uterus, the fundus of which came up to 28 cm. above the symphysis pubis. Fetal movements and heart sounds were heard. The pelvis was contracted and the transverse outlet measured 7 cm.

Routine urine and stool examinations were normal. Blood count showed 11.2 grams hemoglobin, 3.3 million red blood cells, and 6,500 white blood cells, with 77 per cent polymorphonuclears. Serum calcium was 8.24 and phosphorus 2.77 mgm. per cent, and phosphatase 2.3 Bodansky units. Plasma non-protein nitrogen was 21 mgm. per cent, and proteins were 2.97 per cent albumin and 3.24 per cent globulin. Basal metabolic rate was plus 6.7 per cent. Blood Wassermann reaction was negative. Roentgenologic survey of the skeleton showed moderate degree of osteoporosis in all the long bones, with slight biconcave absorption of the vertebral bodies with irregular curvature of the sacrum, asymmetry of the pelvis, distortion and compression of the head of the femur into the acetabulum and pathological fracture of the right upper femur.

Metabolic studies commenced on December 26 and proceeded for 10 four-day periods prior to the termination of pregnancy. The first 4 periods served as control on high calcium intake alone, and the fifth period was used for the administration of Vigantol in daily doses of 5 cc. (60,000 international units of vitamin D). During the next 5 periods, definite progressive increase in calcium and phosphorus retention was noticed, with subjective improvement. Serum calcium and phosphorus were 9.46 and 3.86 mgm. per cent, respectively.

Cesarean section was performed by Drs. H. L. Hsu and S. Lin on February 7, 1939, and a normal male child weighing 2,920 grams was delivered. The puerperium was satisfactory and lactation active. She received 30 cc. cod liver oil daily for six days immediately after parturition.

Metabolic observation on lactation and its effect on the infant was started on February 24, and continued for 26 four-day periods (one hundred and four days). The results are presented in the text. The patient was discharged in excellent condition on June 11, 1939.

Case 4b. Infant, W. H. S. (Hospital Number 66085), was a male baby born on February 7, 1939 by cesarean section of an osteomalacic mother who received a limited dose of Vigantol and liberal amounts of calcium during the latter part of pregnancy, as described above. The child weighed 2,920 grams and measured 49.5 cm. in length at birth. He was in every way normal. There were no bony deformities and x-ray of the bones showed normal texture with sharp outline and smooth diaphyseal ends (Figure 7). Urine was normal. Blood count showed 9.8 grams hemoglobin, 4.14 million red blood cells, 7,600 white blood cells, with 53 per cent polymorphonuclears. Serum calcium was 10.8 and phosphorus 6.03 mgm. per 100 cc. and phosphatase 8.2 Bodansky units.

Mother's milk constituted the only form of feeding. Metabolic observations were started on February 24, and continued for 2 four-day periods followed by 2 four-day periods without metabolic studies. Thereafter, 2 "observation" periods alternated with 2 "rest" periods. From May 7, that is, after the elapse of 18 periods, the mother received Vigantol 2 cc. (24,000 international units of vitamin D) per day for 8 periods, during which metabolic observations were continued on the infant to ascertain the effect of "vitaminized" milk. Throughout the course of study, the infant took the prescribed feedings quantitatively, remained in excellent condition and gained weight steadily. On discharge on June 11, he weighed 7,000 grams, almost two and one half times the birth weight in the course of four months, although slight anemia persisted.

BIBLIOGRAPHY

1. Barnes, D. J., Cope, F., Hunscher, H. A., and Brekke, V., Human milk studies. XVI. Vitamin D potency as influenced by supplementing the diet of the mother during pregnancy and lactation with cow's milk fortified with a concentrate of cod liver oil (test on rachitic infants and rats). J. Nutrition, 1934, **8**, 647.

2. Bunker, J. W. M., Harris, R. S., and Eustis, R. S., The antirachitic potency of the milk of human mothers fed previously on vitamin D milk of the cow. New England J. Med., 1933, **208**, 313.

3. Chu, F. T., and Sung, C., Tetany in infancy and childhood: a clinical study of 45 cases seen in North China with especial reference to etiology. J. Pediat. (To be published).

4. Chu, H. I., Yu, T. F., Chang, K. P., and Liu, W. T., Calcium and phosphorus metabolism in osteomalacia. VII. The effect of ultra violet irradiation from mercury vapor quartz lamp and sunlight. Chinese Med. J., 1939, **55**, 93.

5. Donelson, E., Nims, B., Hunscher, H. A., and Macy, I. G., Metabolism of woman during the reproductive period. IV. Calcium and phosphorus utilization in late lactation and during subsequent reproductive rest. J. Biol. Chem., 1931, **91**, 675.

6. Garry, R. C., and Stiven, D, A brief review of recent work on dietary requirements in pregnancy and lactation, with an attempt to assess human requirements. Nutrition Abstr. and Rev., 1936, **5**, 855.

7. Hannon, R. R., Liu, S. H., Chu, H. I., Wang, S. H., Chen, K. C., and Chou, S. K., Calcium and phosphorus metabolism in osteomalacia. I. The effect of vitamin D and its apparent duration. Chinese Med. J., 1934, **48**, 623.

8. Hess, A. F., Weinstock, M., and Sherman, E., The production of antirachitic properties in human milk resulting from irradiation of the mother. Proc. Soc. Exp. Biol. and Med., 1925–26, **23**, 636.

9. Hummel, F. C., Sternburger, H. R., Hunscher, H. A., and Macy, I. G., Metabolism of women during the reproductive cycle. VII. Utilization of inorganic elements; continuous case study of multipara. J. Nutrition, 1936, **11**, 235.

10. Hunscher, H. A., Metabolism of women during the reproductive cycle. II. Calcium and phosphorus utilization in two successive lactation periods. J. Biol. Chem., 1930, **86**, 37.

11. Leitch, I., The determination of the calcium requirements of man. Nutrition Abstr. and Rev., 1937, **6**, 553.

12. Liu, S. H., Hannon, R. R., Chu, H. I., Chen, K. C., Chou, S. K., and Wang, S. H., Calcium and phosphorus metabolism in osteomalacia. II. Further studies in the response to vitamin D of patients with osteomalacia. Chinese Med. J., 1935, **49**, 1.

13. Liu, S. H., Hannon, R. R., Chou, S. K., Chen, K. C., Chu, H. I., and Wang, S. H., Calcium and phosphorus metabolism in osteomalacia. III. The effects of varying levels and ratios of intake of calcium to phosphorus on their serum levels, paths of excretion and balances. Chinese J. Physiol., 1935, **9**, 101.

14. Liu, S. H., Su, C. C., Wang, C. W., and Chang, K. P., Calcium and phosphorus metabolism in osteomalacia. VI. The added drain of lactation and beneficial action of vitamin D. Chinese J. Physiol., 1937, **11**, 271.

15. Macy, I. G., Hunscher, H. A., McCosh, S. S., and Nims, B., Metabolism of women during the reproductive cycle. III. Calcium, phosphorus, and nitrogen utilization in lactation before and after supple-

menting the usual home diets with cod liver oil and yeast. J. Biol. Chem., 1930, **86**, 59.

16. Maxwell, J. P., and Turnbull, H. M., Two cases of fetal rickets with report on histology of bones. J. Path. and Bact., 1930, **33**, 327.

17. Maxwell, J. P., Hu, C. H., and Turnbull, H. M., Fetal rickets. J. Path. and Bact., 1932, **35**, 419.

18. Maxwell, J. P., Further studies in adult rickets (osteomalacia) and fetal rickets. Proc. Roy. Soc. Med., 1935, **28**, 265.

19. Maxwell, J. P., Pi, H. T., Lin, H. A. C., and Kuo, C. C., Further studies in adult rickets (osteomalacia) and fetal rickets. Proc. Roy. Soc. Med., 1939, **32**, 287.

20. McLean, F. C., and Hasting, A. B., Biological method for estimation of calcium iron concentration. J. Biol. Chem., 1934, **107**, 337.

21. McLean, F. C., and Hastings, A. B., Clinical estimation and significance of calcium ion concentration in blood. Am. J. Med. Sc., 1935, **189**, 601.

22. Outhouse, J., Macy, I. G., and Brekke, V., Human milk studies. V. A quantitative comparison of the antirachitic factor in human milk and cow's milk. J. Biol. Chem., 1928, **78**, 129.

23. Tso, E., and Chu, F. T., Nitrogen metabolism in infants on graded intake of soybean milk proteins. Chinese J. Physiol., 1931, **5**, 287.

24. Weech, A. A., The influence of the administration of cod liver oil to the mother on the development of rickets in the infant. Bull. Johns Hopkins Hosp., 1927, **40**, 244.

25. Wu, H., and Yen, D. Y., The nutritive value of Chinese foods. Chinese J. Physiol., 1928, Rep. Ser. **1**, 135.

Reprinted from THE JOURNAL OF CLINICAL INVESTIGATION, Vol. XX, No. 3, pp. 255–271, May, 1941
Printed in U. S. A.

CALCIUM AND PHOSPHORUS METABOLISM IN OSTEOMALACIA. XI. THE PATHOGENETIC RÔLE OF PREGNANCY AND RELATIVE IMPORTANCE OF CALCIUM AND VITAMIN D SUPPLY

BY S. H. LIU, H. I. CHU, H. C. HSU, H. C. CHAO, AND S. H. CHEU

(*From the Department of Medicine, Peiping Union Medical College, Peiping, China*)

(Received for publication November 6, 1940)

Though osteomalacia is fundamentally a disease due to vitamin D deficiency and dietary calcium shortage, it is made manifest or aggravated by a host of predisposing factors among which the processes of reproduction deserve special attention. Pregnancy and lactation, albeit normal physiological phenomena, make additional demands upon the calcium and phosphorus supplies of the mother, so that diets adequate under ordinary circumstances become deficient during reproductive activity. Our previous reports (1, 2) on the metabolic data of eight Chinese lactating women, with or without osteomalacia, have demonstrated that the drain of lactation varies with the stage of lactation and the quantity of milk secretion. During late lactation when milk yield is small, positive balances in calcium and phosphorus can usually be secured with the addition of vitamin D, even when the intake of minerals is moderate or limited. However, in early lactation, especially if abundant, the loss of calcium in milk is so great that a high intake of calcium is essential in addition to adequate vitamin D supply to prevent depletion of skeletal store. Therefore, if nursing is maintained on dietaries deficient in vitamin D and calcium, as is often the case in China, skeletal demineralization will inevitably result.

A similar chain of events probably occurs in pregnancy. In this part of the reproductive cycle nutritional requirements are increased to provide building material for the fetus and its adnexa and for the development of maternal tissues such as the uterus, mammary glands and other organs, in order to meet the demands of labor and parturition and to prepare for milk secretion. The quantitative aspects of the question are not accurately known, but may be approached from the chemical analysis of fetuses at term and at various ages. Givens and Macy (3) and Macy and Hunscher (4) have shown the average calcium content of

the human fetus at birth to be about 21 to 23 grams; Coons *et al.* (5) give similar estimates, while McIlroy (6) puts the figure considerably higher, namely, at 30 grams. The average phosphorus content of the fetus at term is approximately 14 grams. The whole subject has been reviewed by Macy and Hunscher (4) and by Garry and Stiven (7). It is generally accepted that the mineral needs of the fetus are insignificant during the first four months, but from then on they increase rapidly so that about two-thirds of the total are deposited during the last three months. Therefore, a minimum of 200 mgm. of calcium and 100 mgm. of phosphorus per day should be retained by the mother during the last three months of pregnancy in order to satisfy the fetal requirement without drawing upon the maternal mineral store. These estimates, though they are from Western sources, may serve to indicate the magnitude of drain upon the maternal tissues during pregnancy, if living conditions and dietaries are incapable of supporting such a degree of mineral retention, as they appear to be frequently in China.

The primary purposes of the work to be reported in the present communication are to observe the calcium, phosphorus and nitrogen metabolism of patients with osteomalacia during pregnancy, to compare it with that of individuals without skeletal decalcification and to assess the relative importance of vitamin D, calcium and phosphorus intake in securing adequate mineral balances for the added requirements of gestation.

PROCEDURE

All the patients were studied in the metabolism ward where diets were quantitatively prepared and served, and excreta completely collected. The diets were practically free from vitamin D except those containing small amounts of eggs. They were low in calcium but, when desired, the calcium intake was raised by administering

255

TABLE I

Composition of diets in grams per day

(Values for calcium, phosphorus and nitrogen are actually analyzed.)

Case	Periods (4-day)	Diet number	Protein	Carbohydrate	Fat	Calories	Calcium, mgm.	Phosphorus, mgm.	Nitrogen
1	1-2, 5-6, 9-10	1	54	242	42	1562	141	325	7.68
1	3-4, 7-8, 11-13	2	67	263	65	1866	150	674	8.92
2	1-2, 7-8, 13-14	1	60	287	62	1952	189	565	8.50
2	3-4, 9-10, 15-16	2	51	285	70	1899	192	565	7.84
2	5-6, 11-12, 17	3	72	323	42	1953	268	826	9.98
3	1-3, 13-15, 19-21	1	89	457	78	2882	277	1296	14.67
3	4-6, 10-12, 16-18, 22-24	2	81	516	52	2858	314	837	12.34
4	1-3, 7-9, 14-16	1	71	380	55	2300	215	926	9.69
4	4-6, 10-13, 17-18	2	68	403	52	2353	275	692	8.69
5	1-3, 11-13	1	76	404	50	2371	260	1199	12.59
5	4-5, 6-7, 14-16	2	74	402	52	2374	196	782	12.10
6	1-3, 7-9, 13-15	1	91	406	70	2611	212	1078	14.19
6	4-6, 10-12, 16-18	2	76	494	76	2956	257	703	9.42
7	1-2, 7-8, 13-14, 19-20	1	63	360	47	2116	160	1026	10.49
7	3-4, 9-10, 15-16, 21-22	2	63	330	41	1951	205	651	9.30
7	5-6, 11-12, 17-18	3	60	287	62	1952	142	308	8.64
8	1-9	1	68	369	63	2315	273	724	10.39
8	11-14	2	48	272	46	1688	273	514	6.87
8	15-19	3	64	305	45	2042	271	694	9.10
9	1-10	1	71	368	63	2325	283	832	10.52
10	1-4	1	65	165	58	1442	304	974	10.40
10	5-7	2	43	232	45	1505	462	924	6.88
10	8-12	3	51	315	45	2004	118	634	8.16
10	13-16, 20-32	4	75	214	59	1750	126	1041	12.00
10	17-18	5	64	239	58	1743	148	366	10.24
10	36-31	6	76	199	68	1712	145	1108	12.16

a 7.7 per cent solution of calcium lactate. Distilled water was used for cooking and drinking. The diets were quantitatively consumed with the exception of a few instances. The refused food or vomitus, as the case may be, was then separately analyzed and subtracted from the day's intake. The ward routines and chemical methods for the analysis of food, excreta and serum were described previously (1, 2, 8). The metabolic periods were four days each.

RESULTS

This study includes ten Chinese women admitted during various stages of pregnancy. For convenience in presentation, these subjects may be divided into 3 groups according to the condition of their skeletal system. Group I consists of three cases which may be considered, for our purpose, as normal controls, there being no tetany, nor roentgenologic evidence of osteomalacia. Group II contains four subjects, all of whom showed mild osteoporosis, and three of whom had active tetany prior to the metabolic studies. Group III is composed of three patients with advanced osteomalacia, with marked skeletal rarefaction, deformity and fractures. This classification is only approximate because slight depletion of the mineral contents of bones may be passed as normal and small differences in the density of bones from case to case are not detectable by x-ray examination. Moreover, the current state of vitamin D nutrition, as shown by the metabolic behavior at the moment, may not always correspond with the condition of the skeleton. However, there is a general parallelism between the skeletal condition and the state of vitamin D store as revealed by metabolic observation in those patients receiving no prior vitamin D medication.

Group I. Normal

Case 1, K. C. H. This was a 19-year-old primipara with normal serum calcium and inorganic phosphorus and without clinical or roentgenologic evidence of skeletal decalcification. She was observed for 13 four-day periods from the end of the eighth month of gestation to term. Two diets, one low in both calcium and phosphorus and the other low in calcium but moderate in phosphorus, alternated with each other every 2 periods. As seen from Figure 1 and Table II, an intake of 141 to 150 mgm. calcium (Periods 1 to 4) gave

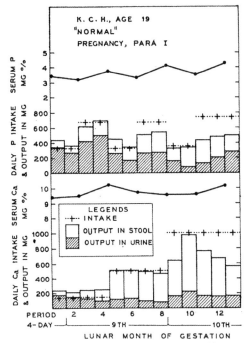

FIG. 1. CASE 1. CALCIUM AND PHOSPHORUS METABOLISM IN A PRESUMABLY NORMAL INDIVIDUAL DURING THE LATTER PART OF PREGNANCY

rise to considerable negative balance, averaging 92 mgm. per day. Raising the intake to 500 mgm. (Periods 5 to 8) elicited barely even balances. On further augmenting the intake to 1000 mgm. (Periods 9 to 13), one notices a considerable calcium gain, namely, 284 mgm. per day. The calcium balance at a given level of calcium intake was not influenced by the different amounts of phosphorus in the two diets.

However, phosphorus balances were naturally dependent on the phosphorus intake. With an intake of 325 to 358 mgm. per day (Periods 1 to 2, 5 to 6 and 9 to 10), the balances were in the main negative, averaging 44 mgm. per day; while an intake of 674 to 741 mgm. (Periods 3 to 4, 7 to 8 and 11 to 13) gave rise to considerable gain, namely, about 160 mgm. per day. The extent of phosphorus retention at a given level of intake also depended upon the calcium intake. As the latter was gradually raised from 150 to 1000 mgm., there was a progressive diminution of the

negative phosphorus balance on the low phosphorus intake and a similar increase of the positive phosphorus balance on the moderate phosphorus intake. This dependence of both calcium and phosphorus balances upon the calcium intake indicates that calcium is a more important limiting factor in the metabolism of the two elements, an observation which has already been described in our previous studies (9, 10).

Nitrogen balances remained fairly satisfactory. Serum calcium did not vary significantly throughout the periods of observation, but there was a tendency for serum inorganic phosphorus to fluctuate with the phosphorus intake.

In a previous communication (11), it has been shown that the earliest sign of vitamin D deficiency is a diminution or disappearance of urinary calcium. Increase of stool calcium, decrease of calcium balance and changes in serum calcium and phosphorus follow in that order as the deficiency is allowed to go on. This patient was able to maintain good amounts of calcium in the urine throughout the 13 periods of study. This, together with the consistently normal serum calcium and phosphorus, indicates that the patient had an adequate store of vitamin D during the studies. Most of that store probably had been acquired prior to admission, as only one of the diets served on the ward contained any vitamin D-containing food, namely egg, and that in small amounts only.

With vitamin D operative, one may perhaps expect this patient to keep definitely postive balances on an intake of 500 mgm. calcium a day. However, only even balances were obtained, and this suggests that her usual intake had been at that level because, as previously pointed out (1), the calcium requirement depends upon, among other factors, the customary dietary level. If 500 mgm. be the usual level of intake, considerably more should be supplied during pregnancy to meet the fetal needs. In this patient an intake of 1000 mgm. of calcium enabled her to retain a sufficient amount for the added requirement.

Case 2, W. T. Though this 17-year-old primipara had a normal skeleton, her serum calcium and phosphorus were somewhat lower than normal. Metabolic studies extended for 17 periods from the sixth to the eighth lunar month of gestation (Table II). This subject was given 3 diets, all low in calcium, but progressively increased in

S. H. LIU, H. I. CHU, H. C. HSU, H. C. CHAO, AND S. H. CHEU

TABLE II

Group 1. Normal calcium, phosphorus and nitrogen metabolism

Case	Date		Period 4-day	Stage of gestation	Calcium, average daily				Phosphorus, average daily				Nitrogen, average daily			
					Intake	Urine	Stool	Balance	Intake	Urine	Stool	Balance	Intake	Urine	Stool	Balance
				lunar months	mgm.	mgm.	mgm.	mgm.	mgm.	mgm.	mgm.	mgm.	grams	grams	grams	grams
1. K.C.H.	March	1937 29–April 5	1–2	8–9	141	164	60	−83	325	306	96	−77	7.68	6.74	0.62	+0.32
	April	6–13	3–4	9	150	116	134	−100	674	459	196	+19	8.92	7.88	0.65	+0.39
		14–21	5–6	9	500	128	376	−4	325	216	182	−73	7.68	5.92	0.70	+1.06
		22–29	7–8	9	500	97	385	+18	674	268	259	+147	8.92	6.52	0.64	+1.76
		30–May 7	9–10	10	1000	200	612	+188	358	122	218	+18	8.45	6.68	0.64	+1.13
	May	8–19	11–13	.10	1015	165	502	+348	741	208	266	+267	9.81	7.68	0.65	+1.48
2. W.T.	December	1936–37 27–January 3	1–2	6	189	39	256	−106	341	327	240	−226	8.50	8.40	1.01	−0.91
	January	4–11	3–4	6–7	192	29	162	+1	565	445	171	−51	7.84	7.29	0.74	−0.19
		12–19	5–6	7	268	20	220	+28	826	491	258	+77	9.98	8.57	0.87	+0.54
		20–27	7–8	7	500	57	380	+63	426	206	295	−75	10.63	7.80	1.13	−1.70
		28–February 4	9–10	7	500	9	414	+77	706	363	247	+96	9.80	7.20	0.86	+1.74
	February	5–12	11–12	8	500	4	444	+52	1032	458	388	+186	12.48	8.21	1.16	+3.11
		13–20	13–14	8	1000	20	682	+298	426	378	350	−302	10.63	7.94	1.26	+1.43
		21–28	15–16	8	1000	4	809	+187	706	288	324	+94	9.80	8.04	0.94	+0.82
	March	1–4	17	8	1000	12	698	+290	1032	329	333	+370	12.48	9.31	1.07	+2.10
3. L.C.P.	March	1940 11–22	1–3	7	277	3	138	+136	1296	544	463	+289	14.67	9.22	1.99	+3.46
		23–April 3	4–6	8	1314	6	939	+369	837	426	294	+117	12.34	9.66	1.15	+1.53
	April	4–15	7–9	8	277	5	507	−235	1296	581	566	+149	14.67	9.15	2.29	+3.23
		16–27	10–12	8–9	1314	7	820	+487	837	457	223	+177	12.34	8.54	0.99	→3.45
		28–May 9	13–15*	9	277	2	326	−51	1296	614	500	+182	14.67	8.89	1.74	+4.04
	May	10–21	16–18	9	1314	297	475	+542	837	281	242	+314	12.34	8.54	1.28	+2.52
		22–June 2	19–21	10	218	21	128	+69	1277	552	504	+221	14.48	8.44	2.05	+3.99
	June	3–14	22–24	10	1257	118	446	+693	708	189	261	+258	12.65	7.91	1.06	+3.68

* Vigantol during Periods 13–16.

phosphorus content. She showed similar metabolic behavior to Case 1 in that negative calcium balances (— 26 mgm. daily) prevailed on an intake of 189 to 268 mgm., slightly positive balances (64 mgm. daily) were obtained on an intake of 500 mgm. and substantial gain (253 mgm. daily) was secured on an intake of 1000 mgm. This is also true with phosphorus balances which varied directly not only with the level of phosphorus intake but also with that of calcium intake.

In comparison with the first case, although this individual exhibited the same degree of conservatism in handling calcium and phosphorus, her store of vitamin D was probably not as adequate, in that the levels of serum calcium and phosphorus were not strictly normal and urinary calcium tended to decrease and disappear even on high intake. Although small amounts of eggs were present in the diet, they were evidently not sufficient to prevent a gradual depletion of the scanty vitamin D store of the body. However, an intake of 1000 mgm. of calcium seemed adequate to fulfill the requirements of pregnancy even if the vitamin D store was somewhat inadequate.

Case 3, Mrs. L. C. P. This pregnant woman, para IV, was considered normal from the standpoint of her skeleton, and her serum calcium and phosphorus on admission were essentially normal. The plan of observation in this case consisted of 3 periods of low calcium-high phosphorus intake followed by 3 periods of high calcium-moderate phosphorus intake; and this cycle was repeated 3 more times. Therefore, the study covered 24 periods from the seventh month to term. The data are set forth in Figure 2 and Table II. During the first 3 periods on low calcium diet (277 mgm.), the patient exhibited extraordinary ability in maintaining positive balance, averaging 136 mgm. per day. During the next 3 periods on high calcium intake (1296 mgm.), the average positive balance of 369 mgm. per day was likewise satisfactory. When the cycle of dietary regime was repeated, though the calcium balance was excellent on high intake (Periods 10 to 12), it was markedly negative on low intake (Periods 7 to 9), indicating poor conservation. This, together with a tendency for the serum calcium to fall during the low calcium periods, suggests the wearing out of whatever vitamin D store the patient might have had at the beginning of the studies.

The supply of vitamin D as Vigantol 1 cc. per day (12,000 international units) for Periods 13 to 16 brought about striking changes. From Period 13 to 15, the first 3 periods of Vigantol administration, when the effect of the therapy could hardly be maximal, the calcium balance on low intake began to show favorable influence. In the next 3 periods (Periods 16 to 18), while on high calcium intake, the stool calcium was much reduced, and the urinary calcium much increased. As the reduction of calcium in the stool was greater than the increase of urinary calcium, the

net balances exceeded those of previous periods on similar high intake. The last 6 periods showed even better calcium retention. During Periods 22 to 24, the average daily retention was 693 mgm., namely, 55 per cent of the intake.

Phosphorus balances remained positive throughout, more so after Vigantol administration. Periods of high phosphorus intake were not necessarily associated with greater phosphorus retention

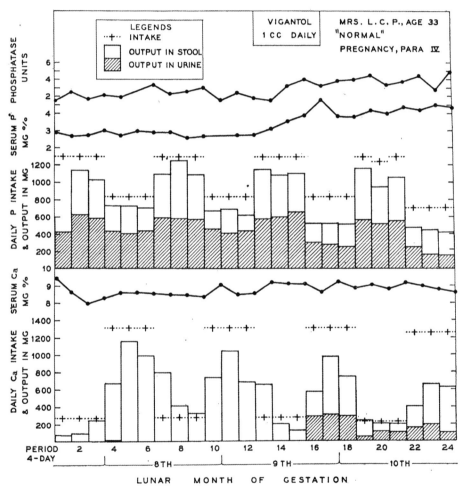

FIG. 2. CASE 3. CALCIUM AND PHOSPHORUS METABOLISM IN A WOMAN DURING THE LATTER PART OF PREGNANCY

Although there was no skeletal decalcification, metabolic behavior showed vitamin D deficiency and responded well to Vigantol therapy.

than periods of moderate phosphorus intake. In fact, the average daily retention during all the moderate phosphorus periods was slightly more than that during all the high phosphorus periods, undoubtedly because of the limiting effect of low calcium intake during the latter.

Serum calcium and phosphorus both showed a tendency to rise after vitamin D therapy. The rise of serum phosphorus was particularly striking. The nitrogen balance remained excellent throughout.

In comparison with the preceding case, this patient probably had even scantier vitamin D store, because the urinary calcium was absent from the beginning of the experiment. The unusual ability to maintain a positive calcium balance on a low intake during the first 3 periods is to be explained by her previous low calcium intake, which was quite likely the case. In agreement with this supposition is her inability to maintain a balance when the low calcium intake periods were repeated immediately after 3 periods of high intake. However, further depletion of the scanty vitamin D store probably played a contributory rôle in the difference in behavior between the first and second series of low calcium intake periods.

In spite of inadequate vitamin D store, an intake of approximately 1300 mgm. of calcium resulted in adequate retention for the heightened requirements of pregnancy. However, the supply of vitamin D constitutes a more fundamental solution to the problem. Thus, after Vigantol administration in this case, not only did the urinary calcium appear, the calcium balances on high intake improve and the serum calcium and phosphorus rise to normal, but also positive balances were maintained on low intake. With adequate vitamin D supply the calcium intake necessary for the requirements of pregnancy could be considerably reduced from 1.3 grams.

Comment. These three patients are alike in possessing normal skeletal mineral store, but they differ in the state of vitamin D nutrition. The first subject apparently had an adequate store of vitamin D so that 13 four-day periods of a diet low in vitamin D failed to elicit any evidence of depletion. The average daily calcium retention on high intake was 284 mgm., namely 28 per cent of the intake. The vitamin D store of the second subject was not so adequate, in that signs of de-

pletion began to occur after a similar period of study. However, the extent of calcium retention was approximately the same, namely 263 mgm. on high intake, or 26 per cent. The third patient showed evidence of depletion even earlier in the course of observation than in Case 2. Still, the extent of calcium retention on high intake remained satisfactory (28 per cent during Periods 4 to 6 and 37 per cent during Periods 10 to 12). These observations indicate the frequency of the existence of early or subclinical vitamin D deficiency as in the second and third patients. Such deficiencies cannot be recognized unless detailed metabolic observations are made. In such cases, however, high calcium intake (1 to 1.3 grams) exerts an ameliorative influence and even promotes sufficient calcium retention for the augmented requirements of gestation. On the other hand, vitamin D is such an economizer of calcium that in the presence of a lower level of calcium, as is the rule here, an adequate supply of vitamin D is imperative, especially during periods of reproductive activity.

Group II. Early or mild osteomalacia

Case 4, Mrs. L. C. F. Though this 19-year-old primipara had no history or clinical evidence of osteomalacia or tetany, a roentgenologic survey of the skeleton showed slight but definite osteoporosis. Similar to Case 3, a low calcium-high phosphorus regimen alternated with a· high `calcium-moderate phosphorus regimen, covering a total of 18 four-day periods from the eighth month of gestation to term. The first series of 6 periods (Table III) witnessed a slightly positive calcium balance on an intake of 215 mgm. per day and a substantial gain (averaging 401 mgm. daily or 31 per cent) on an intake of 1275 mgm. per day. But, as the studies proceeded, a negative balance prevailed on a low intake, and retention on a high intake steadily diminished so that during the last 2 periods hardly any calcium was retained. This extraordinary behavior indicates the markedly defective intestinal absorption of calcium usually seen in advanced vitamin D deficiency.

Phosphorus balances were slightly positive throughout, but they tended to be less so with progress of time, corresponding to the behavior of calcium balances. Serum calcium remained constantly between 8 and 9 mgm., while inorganic phosphorus, slightly above 3 mgm. at the beginning, went down to 2 mgm. per cent towards the latter part of the studies. Phosphatase was slightly above normal, mostly between 4 and 6, but on occasions above 7 Bodansky units.

The point worthy of note in this patient is that, in severe vitamin D depletion, even an intake as high as 1275 mgm. calcium may not enable the patient to maintain a positive balance. This fact may serve to support the contention that adequate vitamin D plays a more important rôle than high calcium intake in promoting calcium gain.

Case 5, Mrs. S. P. S. This subject, aged 29 years, para IV, may be characterized as a case of mild osteomalacia and latent tetany. Her studies during 7 four-day periods between the fifth and sixth months of gestation showed slightly negative calcium balances on an intake of 260 mgm. and an average daily retention of 363 mgm. on an intake of 1197 to 1266 mgm. (Table III). The same dietary regimen was repeated eleven days after spontaneous abortion of twin fetuses. Both the negative balances in calcium on low intake and the positive balances on high intake (averaging 302 mgm. daily) were essentially the same as those during pregnancy. Nor were there pronounced differences in phosphorus retention between the observations during pregnancy and those after delivery. However, there was an unquestionable tendency for both serum calcium and phosphorus to rise after parturition. Whereas before delivery serum calcium varied between 7.14 and 8.47 mgm., its range after delivery was between 7.24 and 8.96 mgm. per cent. Likewise, serum phosphorus, varying between 1.73 and 2.24 during pregnancy, was from 2.11 to 3.47 mgm. per cent after delivery.

In this patient moderate vitamin D deficiency was present, as evidenced by the low serum calcium and phosphorus, the absence of calcium in urine and the failure to retain larger amounts of calcium than she did in the face of mineral shortage in the skeleton.

This patient gave us the opportunity to compare the metabolic behavior of the same individual during pregnancy with her behavior postpartum and uncomplicated by lactation. The results revealed no essential difference between pregnancy at the fifth and sixth months and reproductive rest, as far as the mineral balances were concerned.

Of course, one is aware of the fact that during pregnancy a goodly portion of the retained mineral goes to supply the fetus and its adnexa, while during reproductive rest all remains in the maternal tissues. This is probably the explanation for the tendency of the serum calcium and phosphorus to rise after the termination of the pregnancy without any change in the dietary regimen and without any addition of vitamin D, as shown by this patient.

However, there was no extra demand over and above what was required by the products of conception for growth and development. This is in distinct contrast to the state of affairs in active and early lactation where, it has been demonstrated (1, 2), the metabolic processes are so greatly stimulated that calcium has to be supplied not only to cover what is secreted in the milk, but also to cope with this less well-defined factor of stimulation. This is true even in the presence of adequate vitamin D supply. From this we may infer that the drain of pregnancy, as a rule, is not as great as that of lactation.

Case 6, Mrs. C. W. C. This woman of 31 years of age, with mild osteomalacia, cataract and tetany for many years, was studied during the eighth to tenth months of her fourth pregnancy. Prior to the commencement of metabolic observations, calcium gluconate and small amounts of vitamin D were given so that tetany was controlled. Metabolic behavior for the first 3 periods on a daily intake of 212 mgm. of calcium (Table III) was conservative in that positive balances were observed. With the intake raised to 1257 mgm. per day, the daily calcium retention averaged 416 mgm. (Periods 4 to 6). When the low calcium diet was repeated during Periods 7 to 9 and 13 to 15, negative balances prevailed, partly because of the preceding high calcium regimen and partly because of beginning depletion of the scanty store of vitamin D acquired prior to the studies. However, with high calcium intake during Periods 10 to 12 and 16 to 18, the patient had no difficulty in securing adequate positive balances which were, respectively, 324 and 474 mgm. per day.

Phosphorus balances were, on the whole, positive, the extent of retention varying with the level of phosphorus intake as well as with that of calcium intake. Serum calcium fluctuated irregu-

TABLE III

Group 2. Early or mild osteomalacia. Calcium, phosphorus and nitrogen metabolism

Case	Date	Period 4-day	Stage of gesta-tion	Calcium, average daily				Phosphorus, average daily				Nitrogen, average daily			
				Intake	Urine	Stool	Balance	Intake	Urine	Stool	Balance	Intake	Urine	Stool	Balance
			lunar months	mgm.	mgm.	mgm.	mgm.	mgm.	mgm.	mgm.	mgm.	grams	grams	grams	grams
4 L.C.F.	1939-40 October 30-November 10	1-3	8	215	6	172	+ 37	926	369	426	+131	9.69	5.64	2.21	+1.84
	November 11-22	4-6	8-9	1275	5	868	+402	692	282	249	+161	8.69	5.63	1.58	+1.48
	23-December 4	7-9	9	215	5	319	-109	926	505	419	+ 2	9.69	6.54	1.89	+1.26
	December 5-20	10-13	9-10	1275	4	1066	+205	692	288	308	+ 96	8.69	4.65	1.82	+2.22
	21-January 1	14-16	10	215	4	301	- 90	926	435	377	+114	9.69	5.14	1.59	+2.96
	January 2- 9	17-18	10	1275	4	1252	+ 19	692	267	364	+ 61	8.69	4.57	1.67	+2.45
5 S.P.S.	1940 February 7-18	1-3	5	260	0	314	- 54	1199	500	576	+123	12.59	7.88	2.06	+2.65
	19-26	4-5	5-6	1197	2	786	+409	782	324	436	+ 22	12.10	8.10	1.76	+2.24
	27-March 5*	6-7	6	1266	2	948	+316	753	238	374	-141	11.77	7.92	1.87	+1.98
	March 18-29	11-13		260	2	322	- 64	1199	660	494	+ 45	12.59	9.23	1.52	+1.84
	30-April 10	14-16		1266	4	960	+302	753	256	278	+219	11.77	7.58	1.27	+2.92
6 C.W.C.	1939-40 November 19-30	1-3	8	212	9	145	+ 58	1075	588	349	+138	14.19	7.8	1.93	+2.48
	December 1-12	4-6	8	1257	21	821	+415	703	399	234	+ 70	9.42	7.29	1.37	+0.76
	13-24	7-9	8-9	212	2	342	-132	1075	458	413	+204	14.19	8.23	1.56	+4.40
	25-January 5	10-12	9	1257	2	931	+324	703	281	244	+178	9.42	5.90	1.25	+2.27
	January 6-17	13-15	9-10	222	5	398	-181	1123	509	452	+162	15.06	9.17	1.76	+4.13
	18-29	16-18	10	1257	3	780	+474	703	316	283	+104	9.42	7.12	1.19	+1.11
7 W.E.T.	1937 March 13-20	1-2	5	160	48	163	- 51	1026	402	470	+154	10.49	7.95	1.53	+1.01
	21-28	3-4	5	205	41	82	+ 82	651	388	328	- 65	9.30	6.93	1.27	+1.10
	29-April 5	5-6	5-6	142	48	62	+ 32	308	141	176	- 9	8.64	6.68	1.28	+0.68
	April 6-13	7-8	6	1000	70	640	+290	1026	128	630	+268	10.49	7.52	1.56	+1.41
	14-21	9-10	6	1000	44	872	+ 84	651	274	447	- 70	9.30	7.84	1.20	+0.26
	22-29	11-12	6	1000	74	710	+216	308	84	242	- 18	8.64	6.85	0.95	+0.94
	30-May 7	13-14†	7	160	18	256	-114	1026	280	564	+182	10.49	7.05	1.46	+1.98
	May 8-15	15-16	7	205	33	60	+112	651	326	219	+106	9.30	6.34	1.34	+1.62
	16-23	17-18	7	142	58	46	+ 38	308	136	140	+ 32	8.64	5.87	1.31	+1.46
	24-31	19-20	7-8	1000	188	438	+374	1026	136	579	+311	10.49	6.68	1.74	+2.07
	June 1-8	21-22	8	1000	228	361	+411	651	176	310	+165	9.30	6.02	1.40	+1.88
	9-12	23	8	1000	272	370	+358	308	105	208	- 5	8.64	5.71	1.30	+1.63

* Abortion March 7.   † Vigantol during Periods 13–23.

larly between 8.12 and 9.73 mgm. per cent, while inorganic phosphorus ranged between 3.45 and 4.09 mgm. per cent. Thus, all the serum inorganic phosphorus values were normal, and most of the serum calcium values were within normal limits. Phosphatase was normal throughout.

Though this patient showed more marked anatomical evidence of previous vitamin D deficiency (osteomalacia, tetany and cataract) than the two preceding subjects, her metabolic behavior exemplified a greater degree of conservatism in that her serum calcium and phosphorus were maintained within normal limits, and her calcium balance on high intake was on the average somewhat higher. This more conservative behavior was most likely the result of the limited supply of vitamin D received prior to the studies. However, this supply was inadequate to enable her to maintain a balance on low calcium intake and to eliminate significant amounts of calcium in the urine. In other words, there was room for improvement in her metabolic behavior, as in Case 3,

if a more adequate supply of vitamin D had been available to her.

Case 7, Mrs. W. E. T. Similar to the foregoing case, this was one of mild osteomalacia, cataract and tetany of many years' duration. Likewise, this patient received calcium and cod liver oil prior to the metabolic observation for the treatment of her tetany, so that her serum calcium and phosphorus were within normal limits and her metabolic behavior was conservative by the time the studies were begun (Table III). She was given for the first 2 periods a low calcium-high phosphorus diet, and successively for 2 periods each, two diets similarly low in calcium but progressively lower in phosphorus. On the low calcium intake (142 to 205 mgm. per day) the average balance was slightly positive and a considerable proportion of the calcium output was in the urine, showing that vitamin D action was operative. When this series of diets was repeated, but with the calcium intake raised to 1000 mgm. a day (Periods 7 to 12), the average daily balance was 195 mgm., and the urinary calcium, though smaller in relation to the total output, was still considerable, showing that her response to high intake was fairly satisfactory by reason of the prior vitamin D store. However, that this was not the best performance of which the patient was capable was demonstrated by the observations during the subsequent 11 periods in which vitamin D in daily doses of 1 cc. of Vigantol, or 12,000 international units, was given. The first 6 periods on vitamin D therapy were on low calcium regimen (Periods 13 to 18), and no obvious difference was noted in the calcium balance, but, subsequently, during Periods 19 to 23, while on high calcium diet, definite changes took place. Not only did the average daily retention improve to 386 mgm., but also the urinary calcium increased greatly. The urinary calcium averaged 221 mgm. per day, amounting to 36 per cent of the total output, signifying that intestinal absorption of calcium had improved so that much more calcium was absorbed than could be retained.

Phosphorus balances varied not only with the levels of phosphorus and calcium intake, but also with the state of vitamin D nutrition. All the high phosphorus periods (1 to 2, 7 to 8, 13 to 14 and 19 to 20) were associated with considerable positive balance, especially in periods of high calcium intake and after Vigantol therapy. In periods of moderate phosphorus intake (Periods 3 to 4, 9 to 10, 15 to 16 and 21 to 22), the balances, which were negative prior to vitamin D therapy, became positive afterwards. Low phosphorus periods showed slightly negative balances, the degree of phosphorus loss remaining uninfluenced by the high level of calcium intake or by the vitamin D therapy.

Serum calcium, fairly normal to start with, tended to fall as studies progressed until vitamin D was given. After this it slowly returned to the initial value. A more definite rise occurred in the level of serum inorganic phosphorus after Vigantol administration.

This patient, though clinically similar to the preceding patient, was somewhat different in metabolic behavior, in that urinary calcium persisted in significant amounts, indicating the presence of a greater store of vitamin D. However, that this store was not the optimum was shown by the improvement in calcium balance, the increase in

urinary calcium and the rise in serum phosphorus subsequent to Vigantol administration.

Comment. The four patients in this group are united by the presence of a mild degree of skeletal osteoporosis, but they vary in their metabolic behavior by reason of the varying store of vitamin D. Cases 4 and 5, though presenting less anatomical evidence of vitamin D deficiency than Cases 6 and 7, were nevertheless more deficient in vitamin D, as shown by the metabolic behavior at the time of observation. Obviously, anatomical evidence and metabolic behavior may not necessarily correspond with each other at a given moment. The former is the result of the extent and duration of previous vitamin D deficiency, and once the skeleton is decalcified to an extent to be appreciable by roentgenologic examination, a long period of replenishment is required to eradicate the physical evidence of disease. Some of the evidence, such as cataract, may remain permanently, even if the skeletal lesion is all repaired. On the other hand, metabolic behavior is dynamic, readily influenced by such small amounts of vitamin D as may be introduced by involuntary exposure to sunlight, inclusion in the diet of such items as eggs (11), or the use of limited amounts of cod liver oil for medication, as in Cases 6 and 7. Such factors, often neglected or unrecognized, may make no difference to an individual with an abundant store, but they exert a corrective influence on the metabolic behavior of a patient with vitamin D deficiency, and therefore must be taken into account in interpreting the metabolic data obtained. Furthermore, such vitamin D supply is usually small and, if not continued, can easily be depleted so that metabolic evidence of vitamin D deficiency appears after a varying number of periods of conservative behavior. This was true of Cases 4 and 6 and would have been true of Case 7, had vitamin D been withheld from her. Case 5 was probably deficient in vitamin D from the beginning of the metabolic observations.

Therefore, as a group, these patients all showed mild but definite osseous evidence of previous vitamin D deficiency, but at the time of observation the metabolic behavior indicated a greater current deficiency of the vitamin in Cases 4 and 5 than in Cases 6 and 7, in which some cod liver oil had been given prior to the observations. In severe deficiency (Case 4), high calcium may be of no

S. H. LIU, H. I. CHU, H. C. HSU, H. C. CHAO, AND S. H. CHEU

avail in promoting sufficient calcium gain for the fetal needs, although in moderate deficiency (Case 6), it is capable of doing so. With adequate vitamin D supply, high calcium intake will enable the patient not only to take care of the demands of pregnancy, but also to store enough calcium for the reparation of her depleted skeleton. Thus, in the treatment of this group of patients, adequate vitamin D therapy, as well as high calcium intake, is necessary.

Comparison of this group of patients with mild skeletal decalcification with the previous group without bone lesions shows no essential differences in metabolic behavior except insofar as they are related to the state of vitamin D nutrition. In the first group, absence of bone lesions is associated with an early or a mild grade of vitamin D deficiency, if it is present at all. On the other hand, in the second group where bony decalcification is already recognizable, usually severer grades of vitamin D deficiency are present if not previously treated. Whatever metabolic differences may exist between the two groups are to be accounted for by the differences in vitamin D store

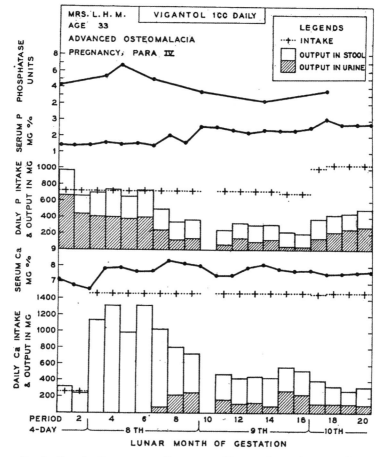

FIG. 3. CASE 8. CALCIUM AND PHOSPHORUS METABOLISM IN ADVANCED OSTEO-MALACIA SHOWING REMARKABLE MINERAL RETENTION AFTER VITAMIN D ADMINISTERED DURING THE LATTER PART OF PREGNANCY

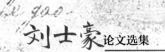

TABLE IV

Group 3. *Advanced osteomalacia. Calcium, phosphorus and nitrogen metabolism*

Case	Date	Period 4-day	Stage of gesta-tion	Calcium, average daily				Phosphorus, average daily				Nitrogen, average daily			
				Intake	Urine	Stool	Balance	Intake	Urine	Stool	Balance	Intake	Urine	Stool	Balance
			lunar months	*mgm.*	*mgm.*	*mgm.*	*mgm.*	*mgm.*	*mgm.*	*mgm.*	*mgm.*	*grams*	*grams*	*grams*	*grams*
	1938–39														
8	November 20–27	1–2	7	273	5	274	– 6	724	556	265	– 97	10.39	8.86	2.00	–0.47
L.H.M.	28–December 9	3–5	8	1473	3	1147	+ 323	724	406	296	+ 22	10.39	7.05	1.55	+1.79
	December 10–25	6–9*	8	1473	140	835	+ 498	724	231	257	+236	10.39	6.42	1.63	+2.34
	30–January 14	11–14	9	1473	125	327	+1021	725	114	188	+423	6.87	4.57	1.24	+1.06
	January 15–22	15–16	9	1471	256	294	+ 921	694	42	178	+474	9.10	5.11	1.34	+2.65
	23–February 7	17–20	10	1468	110	225	+1133	1030	231	214	+585	9.10	5.87	1.54	+1.69
	1938–39														
9	December 26–January 10	1–4	9	1483	60	1268	+ 155	832	405	379	+ 48	10.52	7.47	1.58	+1.47
W.H.S.	January 11–14	5†	10	1438	123	1360	– 45	914	371	381	+162	10.80	7.45	1.77	+1.58
	15–February 3	6–10	10	1398	181	893	+ 324	878	337	282	+259	10.33	6.68	1.70	+1.95
	1934–35														
	September 18–October 3	1–4	3–4	304	6	124	+ 174	974	436	285	+253	10.40	8.12	0.94	+1.34
	October 4–15	5–7	4	458	0	179	+ 279	919	364	324	+231	6.88	5.91	0.93	+0.04
	16–23	8–9	4	118	4	211	– 97	634	281	404	– 51	8.16	5.13	1.35	+1.68
	24–November 4	10–12	5	88	1	65	+ 22	476	240	264	– 28	6.08	3.65	1.19	+1.24
	November 5–20	13–16	5	126	0	97	+ 29	1041	466	414	+161	12.00	8.31	1.28	+2.41
	21–28	17–18	6	1948	233	808	+ 907	323	22	194	+107	9.54	5.98	1.05	+2.51
10	December 3–10	20–21	6	1937	13	1384	+ 540	1041	126	494	+421	12.00	8.40	1.13	+2.42
Y.W.L.	11–18	22–23‡	6	1937	23	1034	+ 880	1041	140	403	+498	12.00	8.38	0.93	+2.69
	19–30	24–26	7	1937	91	888	+ 958	1041	42	468	+531	12.00	8.41	1.19	+2.40
	31–January 15	27–30	7	1937	119	797	+1021	1041	12	422	+607	12.00	8.77	1.22	+2.01
	January 16–23	31–32	8	1937	92	990	+ 855	1041	52	470	+519	12.00	8.82	1.23	+1.95
	February 5–12	36–37	8	1945	202	1030	+ 713	1108	12	658	+438	12.16	8.55	1.32	+2.29
	13–28	38–41	9	1945	202	1086	+ 657	1108	12	736	+360	12.16	9.33	1.42	+1.41
	March 1–12	42–44	9	1943	81	1158	+ 704	1091	165	515	+411	12.00	8.89	1.21	+1.90
	13–24	45–47	10	1945	51	1047	+ 847	1108	214	429	+465	12.16	9.22	0.87	+2.07
	25–April 9	48–51	10	1945	95	1472	+ 378	1108	275	605	+228	12.16	9.24	1.22	+1.70

* Vigantol during Periods 6–13.　　　† Vigantol in this period.　　　‡ Vigantol during Periods 22–51.

rather than by the presence or absence of slight bony rarefaction.

Group III. *Advanced osteomalacia*

Case 8, Mrs. L. H. M. This subject, aged 33 years, was admitted for study at the seventh month of her fourth pregnancy. She had severe osteomalacia with symptoms dating back eleven years, which was shortly after the birth of her first child. The metabolic data of 20 periods are presented in Figure 3 and Table IV. In the first 2 periods on an intake of 273 mgm. of calcium per day, the output, all in the stools, almost balanced the intake. Beginning with Period 3, the intake was raised to 1473 mgm. daily. During the first 3 periods on the augmented intake, there was, on the average, a daily retention of 323 mgm., or 22 per cent of the intake. This degree of retention may not be abnormally low for a person with a normal skeleton, but for a patient like this with such extensive bony decalcification, together with absence of urinary calcium and low serum calcium and phosphorus, it indicates poor intestinal absorption or severe vitamin D deficiency. The correctness of this interpretation is shown by

her response to Vigantol therapy which was given from Period 6 to 13. From Period 7 onward there was a progressive decrease of stool calcium and, at the same time, the appearance of a considerable amount of calcium in the urine. The average daily retention from Period 11 to 20 was over 1 gram or 70 per cent of the intake. If the last 4 periods, in which the phosphorus intake was raised, were considered alone, the retention averaged 1133 mgm. a day or 77 per cent of the intake. The amount retained would enable the patient not only to meet the requirements of pregnancy, but also to repair her depleted skeleton. Her symptoms were considerably improved.

Phosphorus balances were generally parallel with calcium balances. Serum calcium, 6.58 to 7.18 mgm. per cent during the low calcium periods, was raised to a maximum of 7.90 mgm. per cent during high calcium periods. After Vigantol administration, a slight further rise occurred, but the highest figure reached was only 8.36 mgm. per cent. Serum inorganic phosphorus, 1.45 mgm. per cent to start with, remained at this level until vitamin D administration, after which it showed steady elevation, the maximum being

3.06 mgm. per cent. Serum phosphatase, 4.2 to 6.70 Bodansky units per 100 cc., was lowered to 2.35 to 3.54 units after Vigantol therapy.

This patient, who had a severe osteomalacia, showed evidence of vitamin D deficiency in the early part of the metabolic observations. With vitamin D therapy there resulted remarkable calcium and phosphorus retention. Over and above what was required by the fetus, a substantial part of the retained minerals must have been deposited in the depleted skeleton. In this case, serum calcium and phosphorus failed to rise to perfectly normal levels in spite of adequate vitamin D therapy. Thus it seemed as if the urgent requirement of the skeleton, as well as of the fetus, had to be fulfilled at the expense of the serum concentration of these elements.

Case 9, Mrs. W. H. S. This patient, aged 29 years, was observed for 10 four-day periods during the last part of her fourth pregnancy. While the history of osteomalacia and tetany had been of eleven years' duration, and bony deformities were marked, the degree of skeletal rarefaction was not as extensive as in the preceding case, partly on account of previous treatment. As shown in Table IV, the average calcium balance on an intake of 1483 mgm. per day during the first 4 periods was 155 mgm., or approximately 10 per cent of the intake. The poor calcium retention, together with low serum inorganic phosphorus and relatively low calcium, indicates definite vitamin D deficiency. Vitamin D in the form of Vigantol 5 cc. daily was given for four days during Period 5. The response during the subsequent 5 periods consisted of an increase of the average calcium retention to 324 mgm. per day, or 23 per cent of the intake, and a considerable increase of urinary calcium. The response, however, was probably not the best of which the patient was capable in view of the unusual manner in which vitamin D was given. Large doses of Vigantol given for a few days might not be as efficient as smaller doses spread over a longer period of time, although single massive doses of vitamin D have been claimed to be effective in the treatment of rickets (12). It is possible that this patient with a lesser degree of skeletal mineral depletion might not require a higher degree of calcium retention than she showed. However,

this explanation is not likely, because patients with slight skeletal decalcification (Case 7), or without obvious bone lesions (Case 3), exhibited better retention of calcium under adequate vitamin D therapy.

Retention of phosphorus corresponded with that of calcium. Serum calcium was slightly but definitely raised and inorganic phosphorus was markedly elevated after Vigantol therapy.

Case 10, Mrs. Y. W. L. This woman of 43 years of age with severe osteomalacia of four years' duration was observed continuously from the third to the tenth month of her fifth pregnancy. For a year previously she went through detailed metabolic studies during which Vigantol 1 cc. daily (12,000 international units of vitamin D per cc.) was given for forty days (ending January 28, 1934) with considerable improvement in metabolic behavior, as well as clinical symptomatology. Observations during the present pregnancy were begun on September 19, 1935, on a diet containing 304 mgm. calcium per day (Figure 4 and Table IV.) On this diet (Periods 1 to 4) more than half of the intake of calcium was retained. This was true of the next diet containing 461 mgm. calcium per day (Periods 5 to 7), indicating satisfactory circumstances. Even when the diet calcium was reduced to 88 to 126 mgm. per day (Periods 8 to 16), balances, on the whole, were even, showing the remarkable power of conservation of calcium in a patient with osteomalacia when a prior store of vitamin D had been present.

From Period 17 on, the calcium intake was raised to 1959 mgm. per day. During the first 2 periods of high calcium intake, associated with very low phosphorus intake, the calcium retention averaged 907 mgm. per day, or 47 per cent of the intake, and the urinary calcium 233 mgm. per day, or 22 per cent of the total output. In distinct contrast were the results of Periods 20 and 21, during which both calcium and phosphorus intakes were high. Here the calcium retention was not as good and the urinary calcium was negligible. It was thought that at this point the patient might be showing an early vitamin D depletion. Therefore, Vigantol 2 cc. daily was started from Period 22. Subsequently, the calcium balances showed slight improvement and the urinary calcium gradually returned (Periods 22 to 32). Likewise, the phosphorus balances in-

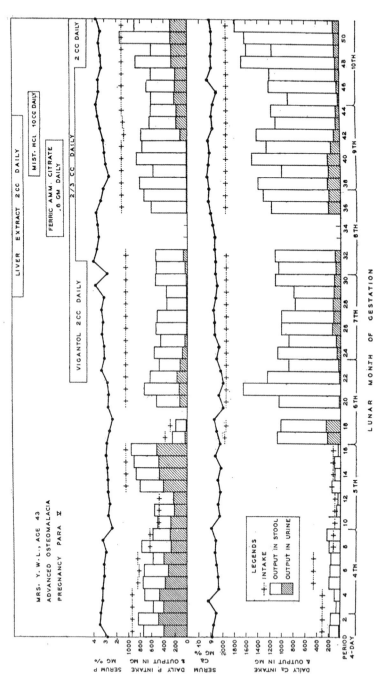

FIG. 4. CASE 4. CALCIUM AND PHOSPHORUS METABOLISM IN A CASE OF ADVANCED OSTEOMALACIA OBSERVED FROM THE THIRD TO THE TENTH LUNAR MONTH OF GESTATION, SHOWING THE EFFECTS OF VITAMIN D ADMINISTRATION, AND THOSE OF FERRIC AMMONIUM CITRATE AND HYDROCHLORIC ACID GIVEN AT THE SAME TIME FOR THE ANEMIA

creased correspondingly, mainly at the expense of urinary phosphorus.

In view of the presence of anemia, ferric ammonium citrate, 6 grams daily, was given during Periods 34 to 41. The anemia did not respond to the iron therapy; both calcium and phosphorus balances were adversely affected by it. The absorption of phosphorus seemed to be particularly impeded by the presence of large amounts of iron in the intestinal tract, probably on account of the formation of insoluble ferric phosphate. Since the absorption of phosphorus was impaired, the calcium balance would decrease mainly on account of a shortage of phosphorus for simultaneous deposition in the bone; hence the undeposited calcium was eliminated in the urine. The discontinuation of iron administration in Period 42 was followed by improved balances both in calcium and in phosphorus, and by decreasing amounts of calcium and increasing amounts of phosphorus in the urine.

The last 4 periods prior to delivery, however, were associated with poorer retention of both calcium and phosphorus. The explanation was not clear, although the discontinuation of hydrochloric acid administration, which had been given during Periods 39 to 45, might conceivably have removed a factor that promoted absorption. An alternative would be that with prolonged high calcium intake the skeletal store was gradually being replenished, rendering mineral retention less urgent. In support of this supposition, there seemed to be a slight general trend toward decreasing retention throughout the periods of high calcium intake.

Both serum calcium and inorganic phosphorus were within lower limits of normal at the commencement of the observations. Serum calcium varied but slightly except for a tendency to decrease during periods of low calcium intake, and a tendency to increase after vitamin D addition and after iron therapy. Serum inorganic phosphorus fluctuated more widely. In general, it varied directly with the phosphorus intake. While the latter was maintained on a constantly high intake, vitamin D administration was associated with a definite rise and iron therapy with a distinct lowering of .serum phosphorus.

There are several points of interest in this patient with advanced osteomalacia. First, while

vitamin D was operative a minimal intake of calcium was associated with an even balance, and a high intake with a retention of 40 to 50 per cent. Second, as observations proceeded, there was a tendency to a decreasing retention. This was considered to be related to a gradual replenishment of the skeletal store rather than to any interference attributable to later stages of pregnancy. Finally, the adverse effects of iron on calcium and phosphorus balances deserve attention. While both calcium and phosphorus retention may be reduced under iron therapy, serum phosphorus may fall with a rise in serum calcium. This phenomenon has been utilized in the treatment of hypocalcemia and hyperphosphatemia associated with chronic advanced renal insufficiency (13).

Comment. The three patients in this group, though they were alike in showing marked skeletal decalcification, deformity and fractures, again varied in their metabolic behavior on admission on account of the varying store of vitamin D acquired prior to the studies. Thus Cases 8 and 9 were deficient in vitamin D, while Case 10 exhibited evidence of a considerable store when the studies were begun. Cases 8 and 10, under adequate Vigantol therapy and high calcium and phosphorus intake, consistently showed a retention of calcium and phosphorus considerably over and above the requirements of pregnancy, proving that in osteomalacia it is possible for the patients under such a regimen to gain sufficient minerals for the skeletal reparation as well. The mineral retention in Case 9 was not as much as expected, probably due to the inefficient manner of administering vitamin D. When large amounts of calcium and phosphorus are required for the growth of the fetus as well as for the replenishment of the depleted skeleton of the mother, as in Case 8, serum calcium and phosphorus may fail to rise to perfectly normal levels in spite of adequate vitamin D and high mineral intake.

The behavior that may be said to characterize this group of patients with extensive bone involvement consists of more marked metabolic evidence of vitamin D deficiency when untreated, unusually high retention of calcium and phosphorus under high mineral and vitamin D intake, and ocasional failure of the serum calcium and phosphorus to rise to normal in spite of such therapy.

刘士豪论文选集

DISCUSSION

Quantitative measurements of calcium and phosphorus metabolism in osteomalacia during pregnancy of the type here presented are not available in the literature except for the two cases which have been briefly reported by us (14). Such data are important in evaluating the rôle of pregnancy in the pathogenesis of osteomalacia in view of the frequent association of the two. A comparison of the metabolic behavior during pregnancy of patients with severe or mild osteomalacia with that of subjects showing no skeletal lesions reveals no essential differences. With adequate vitamin D supply and moderately high intake of calcium and phosphorus, subjects of various skeletal condition have no difficulty in retaining sufficient amounts of the minerals for the needs of gestation. In fact, under similar regimen, osteomalacic patients tend to retain more calcium and phosphorus in an attempt to replenish the depleted maternal store, as well as to provide for fetal growth. In other words, there is no inherent inability on the part of osteomalacic patients during pregnancy to utilize calcium and phosphorus in the midst of plenty of these minerals and vitamin D. Whatever metabolic defect they may show during gestation results from limited vitamin D and mineral supply just as it does during reproductive rest.

Furthermore, in contrast to lactation, where the physiological activity is such that mineral requirement has to be increased much above what is secreted in the milk, even in the presence of adequate vitamin D, there is no such factor in pregnancy. Cases 9 and 10 were subsequently observed during lactation and reported on as Cases 1a and 4a in paper IX of this series (2). In both instances, the mineral balances were much less favorable during lactation than during pregnancy under similar conditions of adequate vitamin D and high calcium intake. Moreover, in Case 5, where the termination of pregnancy was not followed by lactation, mineral retention did not improve after delivery, again showing that pregnancy itself has no excessively deleterious influence on mineral retention.

However, the minimal requirement for fetal growth of 200 mgm. calcium and 100 mgm. phosphorus per day during the last three months of gestation has to be met through the maternal mineral resources. The usual level of calcium intake in Chinese dietary is approximately 0.337 gram and that of phosphorus 1.2 grams (15), although somewhat higher levels of intake have been recorded by others. Such a level of calcium intake, in the presence of vitamin D, may maintain an individual in balance under ordinary circumstances, but in pregnancy it cannot be expected to yield adequate mineral balance for the fetal requirement. The extent of drain on the skeletal store of the mother will depend upon her state of vitamin D nutrition. If there is adequate vitamin D supply—sometimes from the diet, but usually from sunlight (16)—a variable proportion of the total fetal requirement (21 to 23 grams of calcium) may have to be drawn from the maternal store. This alone may not constitute a serious loss to the mother. On the other hand, in the absence of vitamin D, the mineral loss will be much greater than that imparted to the fetus. Under such circumstances, pregnancy plays an important rôle in the causation of osteomalacia. Moreover, pregnancy is usually followed by prolonged lactation, which constitutes a much greater drain upon the maternal skeletal store. Such a reproductive cycle frequently repeated under an inadequate supply of calcium and vitamin D will inevitably lead to the development of osteomalacia.

As to the actual level of calcium that may be considered adequate to meet the needs of gestation, our data do not give a clear-cut answer. In the first subject who was presumably normal from the standpoint of vitamin D nutrition, an intake of 1 gram of calcium was necessary to bring about sufficient retention for the fetal needs. In individuals (Cases 2, 3 and 6) in whom the vitamin D supply was limited, or beginning to be depleted, an intake of 1.0 to 1.3 grams of calcium seemed also adequate for the gestatory requirement. There was evidence that, in the presence of greater supply of vitamin D, they could acquire the same degree of retention on an intake level considerably lower than 1.3 grams (Case 3). However, in severe grades of vitamin D depletion, an intake of 1.3 grams, or higher, of calcium would not maintain the individual in balance (Case 4). These data all go to show that vitamin D is a more important factor than the actual level of

S. H. LIU, H. I. CHU, H. C. HSU, H. C. CHAO, AND S. H. CHEU

calcium intake in determining the extent of renten-tion, provided a reasonable amount of calcium is present in the diet. As to phosphorus, its utili-zation depends a great deal on that of calcium. As Chinese dietaries contain good amounts of phosphorus, adequate calcium retention usually means adequate phosphorus retention. Likewise, there is apparently no difficulty in nitrogen metab-olism with usual Chinese dietaries.

A comparison of the data of these subjects showing varying skeletal condition and vitamin D store with those of presumably normal women in pregnancy available in the literature shows greater degree of mineral conservation in our patients. Toverud and Toverud (17) made short periods of observation on thirty Norwegian women living in a home for expectant mothers during the last two to three months of pregnancy. Negative cal-cium and phosphorus balances were the rule on the usual home diets, but positive balances were sometimes observed after the intake of calcium and phosphorus had been increased to 1.6 to 2.0 grams. Coons et al. (5) reported the results on 2 groups of women, one in Chicago, the other in Oklahoma. With an average intake of 1.4 grams calcium and 1.6 grams phosphorus, adequate re-tention for gestatory needs occurred in the South-ern women, but not in the Chicago women, the difference being attributed to the influence of sun-shine. Macy and Hunscher (4), from a com-pilation of data in the literature on mineral utili-zation during pregnancy, concluded that during the last three months an intake of 1.4 to 1.5 grams of calcium and 2 grams of phosphorus was neces-sary to secure adequate retention for the demands of pregnancy. On the other hand, in our subjects 1.0 to 1.3 grams of calcium seemed adequate for the requirements of pregnancy, even when the supply of vitamin D was limited. With optimum vitamin D nutrition calcium requirement may be lowered.

This relative conservatism shown by our pa-tients cannot be entirely due to the depleted skele-tal store which would cause calcium to be re-tained with great avidity because the patients in the first group without obvious osseous decalci-fication exhibited the same phenomenon. Another important factor seems to lie in the previous level of intake. When the dietary habits accustom the subject to a lower intake, the added requirement

for reproductive activity will be correspondingly lower. Furthermore, vitamin D plays such an im-portant rôle in conserving calcium that its judicious use will make it possible to decrease the usually quoted requirement for a given state of physio-logical activity. The combination of previous low level of intake and existing vitamin D action probably explains the unusual ability on the part of five of the ten subjects in this series to retain calcium on intakes varying from 88 to 277 mgm. per day (Cases 3, 4, 6, 7 and 10). It is plain, then, that the so-called calcium requirement, con-trary to current conception, must be regarded as a variable quantity conditioned by such factors as the prior skeletal store, the previous dietary cus-tom, and the state of vitamin D nutrition.

SUMMARY

Data on calcium, phosphorus and nitrogen me-tabolism during the latter part of pregnancy were obtained on ten subjects showing various states of skeletal store and vitamin D nutrition. Given an adequate supply of vitamin D and calcium, pa-tients with osteomalacia showed no inherent in-ability to retain minerals during pregnancy, com-pared with those with no skeletal depletion. The added requirement during gestation, unlike that in lactation, did not seem to go beyond fetal needs. However, such needs had to be filled at the ex-pense of the maternal tissue, if the supply of vita-min D and minerals was inadequate. Under such circumstances, pregnancy plays an important pathogenetic rôle in osteomalacia inasmuch as it hastens the skeletal demineralization. While high calcium intake tends to ameliorate the effects of vitamin D deficiency, the latter conserves calcium. Of the two, vitamin D is probably more impor-tant, provided a reasonable level of calcium intake is available. The calcium requirement during pregnancy is conditioned by the prior skeletal store, the previous dietary intake, and the state of vitamin D nutrition.

BIBLIOGRAPHY

1. Liu, S. H., and others, Calcium and phosphorus me-tabolism in osteomalacia. VI. The added drain of lactation and beneficial action of vitamin D. Chi-nese J. Physiol., 1937, 11, 271.
2. Liu, S. H., and others, Calcium and phosphorus me-tabolism in osteomalacia. IX. Metabolic behavior of infants fed on breast milk from mothers show-

ing various states of vitamin D nutrition. J. Clin. Invest., 1940, **19**, 327.

3. Givens, M. H., and Macy, I. C., The chemical composition of the human fetus. J. Biol. Chem., 1933, **102**, 7.

4. Macy, I. C., and Hunscher, H. A., An evaluation of maternal nitrogen and mineral needs during embryonic and infant development. Am. J. Obst. and Gynec., 1934, **27**, 878.

5. Coons, C. M., and others, Oklahoma Agric., Mech. Coll., Agric. Exp. Stat., Bull. No. 233, 1935.

6. McIlroy, L., Discussion on diet in pregnancy. Proc. Roy. Soc. Med., 1935, **28**, 1385.

7. Garry, R. C., and Stiven, D., A review of recent work on dietary requirements in pregnancy and lactation, with an attempt to assess human requirements. Nutrition Abstr. and Rev., 1935–36, **5**, 855.

8. Hannon, R. R., and others, Calcium and phosphorus metabolism in osteomalacia. I. The effect of vitamin D and its apparent duration. Chinese M. J., 1934, **48**, 623.

9. Liu, S. H., and others, Calcium and phosphorus metabolism in osteomalacia. III. The effects of varying levels and ratios of intake of calcium to phosphorus on their serum levels, paths of excretion and balances. Chinese J. Physiol., 1935, **9**, 101.

10. Liu, S. H., and others, Calcium and phosphorus metabolism in osteomalacia. V. The effect of varying levels and ratios of calcium to phosphorus intake on their serum levels, paths of excretion and balances, in the presence of continuous vitamin D therapy. J. Clin. Invest., 1937, **16**, 603.

11. Chu, H. I., and others, Calcium and phosphorus metabolism in osteomalacia. X. Further studies on vitamin D action: early signs of depletion and effect of minimal doses. J. Clin. Invest., 1940, **19**, 349.

12. Gunnarson, S., Treatment of rickets with a single massive dose of vitamin D_2. Acta. Paediat., 1939, **25**, 69.

13. Liu, S. H., and others, Unpublished data.

14. Liu, S. H., and others, Calcium and phosphorus metabolism in osteomalacia. II. Further studies on the response to vitamin D of patients with osteomalacia. Chinese M. J., 1935, **49**, 1.

15. Wu, H., and Wu, D. Y., Study of dietaries in Peking. Chinese J. Physiol. (rep. ser.), 1928, no. 1, 135.

16. Chu, H. I., and others, Calcium and phosphorus metabolism in osteomalacia. VII. The effect of ultraviolet irradiation from mercury vapor quartz lamp and sunlight. Chinese M. J., 1939, **55**, 93.

17. Toverud, K. U., and Toverud, G., Studies on the mineral metabolism during pregnancy and lactation and its bearing on the disposition to rickets and dental caries. Acta. Paediat., 1931, **12**, supp. II.

18. Liu, S. H., The rôle of vitamin D in the calcium metabolism in osteomalacia. Chinese M. J., 1940, **57**, 101.

THE
CHINESE MEDICAL JOURNAL

VOLUME 57   FEBRUARY 1940   NUMBER 2

THE RÔLE OF VITAMIN D IN THE CALCIUM
METABOLISM IN OSTEOMALACIA*

S. H. LIU

Department of Medicine, Peiping Union Medical College, Peiping, China

Early in the course of our observations on the calcium and phosphorus metabolism in osteomalacia, we came to recognize that a fundamental defect in this condition is an altered state in the intestinal tract by which calcium is not absorbed or absorbed with great difficulty. With the dietary calcium unabsorbed the mineral balance becomes negative. This calcium loss is due to the calcium that accompanies the secretion of the gastro-intestinal canal. The urinary tract, another channel of calcium loss under ordinary circumstances, is not significant in osteomalacia, because here the amount of calcium in the urine is usually small or nil. Therefore in osteomalacia calcium loss by way of the gastro-intestinal secretion is practically the only way by which skeletal depletion may be brought about. Yet the intestinal secretion of calcium is not excessive in osteomalacia, because the extent of negative balance even on low calcium intake is within normal limits. Although such loss is not great on a daily basis, it will lead, in time, to marked skeletal decalcification. Periods of increased demand for mineral such as occurring during pregnancy and lactation enhance the rate of calcium loss and therefore hasten the development of osteomalacia.

---

*Presented at the Faculty Medical Society, P. U. M. C. November 29, 1939, and at the Biochemistry-nutrition Seminar, Yenching University, December 19, 1939.

This fundamental metabolic defect cannot be materially rectified by increasing the intake of calcium, because that procedure may force the individual to absorb a little calcium to give rise to a slightly positive balance, but it will not circumvent the difficulties of absorption. The more efficient and specific remedy is the supply of vitamin D either as such or in the form of ultraviolet irradiation or sunlight. The beneficial effects of these therapeutic agents in osteomalacia are well known, but the detailed manner of action bears comment.

VITAMIN D ACTS BY PROMOTING CALCIUM ABSORPTION AND THE ACTION IS PROLONGED

This is one of the striking observations made early in the course of our studies.

CASE 1. In 1934, we (1) reported on a girl (C.C.) of 18 with pain in the thighs and knees and difficulty in walking. There were generalized osteoporosis, genu valgum, narrowing of transverse outlet of the pelvis, and tenderness of the dorso-lumbar spine, findings typical of osteomalacia of moderate degree. Serum calcium of 8.9 mg and inorganic phosphorus of 3.5 mg were within normal limits,

On a diet with 78 mg calcium and 583 mg phosphorus, both calcium and phosphorus balances were negative. There was on the average a deficit of 160 mg of calcium daily. The extent of negative calcium balance was not excessive compared with that of normal persons on a similar regime (2), indicating that there was no increased endogenous excretion of calcium.

The dietary intake was then raised to 221 mg per day, and the calcium balance remained negative to the extent of 100 mg. Increasing the calcium intake further to 422 mg by the addition of calcium chloride by mouth also failed to maintain the patient in balance (average calcium balance—86 mg), the result being simply increased calcium in the stool. Instead of oral administration, the added amount of calcium chloride was given intravenously. The result was that the calcium balance, for the first time, became positive to the extent of 160 mg, indicating that most of the calcium injected was retained and that the previous failure was mainly due to poor absorption.

While the patient was on an intake of 1 gm a day, the balance was only slightly positive, namely, about 100 mg. Vitamin D in the form of Vigantol 0.5 cc a day (probably 7,500 international units) was given for 4 periods of 4 days each. The effect of the medication was not evident in the first period but from the second to the fourth period there occurred a striking staircase-like descent in the calcium loss in the stool with a corresponding increase in the calcium balance. During the last period of Vigantol administration the retention amounted to almost 800 mg or 80 per cent of the intake. It seems that once the difficulties of absorption are surmounted, retention can be accomplished with ease. The retained calcium is deposited in the bones, probably also on account of the action of vitamin D.

After the vitamin D therapy was discontinued, the metabolic observations were continued over a period of 3 months during which the beneficial effect of the medication persisted unabated, indicating its remarkably prolonged action.

Toward the latter part of the studies, while vitamin D action was still operative, the intake of calcium was lowered to the original level of 221 mg. The result was in distinct contrast to that obtained before the administration of vitamin D. Instead of a stool elimination of 320 mg, giving a negative balance of about 100 mg, the patient excreted only 60 mg of calcium in the stool with a positive balance of 160 mg. This observation demonstrates the remarkable efficiency of absorption. If the calcium secreted in the gastro-intestinal secretion is not decreased under this circumstance, it will mean a resorption of the secreted calcium. As a result a large proportion of the intake is retained and deposited in the bones for repair.

STORAGE *VERSUS* SUPPLEMENTARY EFFECT OF DIET AS EXPLANA‚
TION FOR THE SUSTAINED EFFECT OF PREVIOUS
VITAMIN D ADMINISTRATION

The explanation for the prolonged action of vitamin D was not clear to us at the time. Two possibilities presented themselves. First, the vitamin D was stored. Second, the vitamin D content of the diet (1 egg daily) used for the experimental studies, although small in amount and incapable of rectifying the metabolic defect, was sufficient to maintain good absorption of calcium and phosphorus, once the initial deficiency was corrected by the relatively large doses of vitamin D medication. At the time we were not certain as to which explanation was the correct one. But in the light of recent work done by others and by us, both factors are important. Heymann (3) demonstrated in rabbits the presence of vitamin D in the liver and blood plasma 12 weeks after a single dose of viosterol equivalent to 200,000 international units. This great capacity for storage of vitamin D by the animal organism was confirmed by Guerrant and associates (4) in growing calves and by Vollmer (5) in human beings. It is evident that part of the vitamin D given must be stored to account for the sustained after-effect.

As to the diet content of vitamin D, observations have shown that the major part of the population in this locality subsists on an essentially cereal-soybean-vegetable diet. This diet is devoid of vitamin D. Patients subsisting on this diet and having no access to the sun will develop in the course of time evidence of vitamin D deficiency. The addition of rather small quantities of vitamin D containing food will result in sufficient improvement in the mineral metabolism to be comparable to that from small doses of vitamin D given as such. This is illustrated by one of the patients recently studied by us (6).

CASE 2: A woman, S. C. C., of 18 was admitted to the Obstetrical Service in October 1938 for prolonged labor due to contracted pelvis. There was a history of pain in the thighs and difficulty in walking for about 3 years and a half. Adductor spasm, bone tenderness, and deformities of the chest, spine and pelvis were present. X-ray showed moderate generalized osteoporosis with multiple pathological fractures; serum calcium was 8.0 mg, inorganic phosphorus 1.9 mg and phosphatase 10.50 Bodansky units. This was evidently a severe case of osteomalacia of the low serum phosphorus type. After admission the child had to be delivered by craniotomy. After considerable puerperal morbidity the patient pulled through. We had the opportunity of studying her after she was well advanced in convalescence.

The patient was placed on vitamin D deficient diets with a calcium intake of 1,400 mg per day. During the first few periods (4 days per period), the calcium retention amounted to an average of 54 per cent of the intake. This excellent mineral retention indicates that the pathological process was in a state of reparation, undoubtedly due to the influence of vitamin D derived from the diet and medication given prior to the metabolic study. She had been on a general hospital diet containing daily one or two eggs and some milk, and, in addition, she had received 40 cc of cod liver oil in 4 doses on two different dates. Although the amount of vitamin D given in the diet and in the medication was small, it apparently was sufficient to bring about a favorable effect on the calcium metabolism of this patient. However, as the metabolic observations progressed, the extent of retention gradually diminished so that by the end of 22 periods (88 days) the balance became almost even. The gradual diminution of positive balance was most likely the result of depletion of the vitamin D store secured during the pre-experimental regimen. The experimental diets (cereals, vegetables, fruits, meats and sesame oil) on which the patient was placed were sufficiently devoid of vitamin D to allow the depletion to take place.

Effect of minimal doses of vitamin D. Vigantol was diluted with olive oil 1 to 24, and 1 cc of this preparation containing 500 international units was given to this patient daily for 4 periods. Immediately the stool calcium began to decrease and urinary calcium began to appear with improvement in the calcium balance. The calcium retention, which averaged not more than 15 per cent of the intake just prior to Vigantol administration, increased progressively reaching a maximum of 64 per cent in the third period (12 days) after the Vigantol was discontinued. Therefore, this part of the study shows that a dose of vitamin D as small as 500 international units a day was effective in bringing about a striking effect on the calcium metabolism.

Effect of one and three hen's eggs. It became of interest to see whether the addition of ordinary vitamin D containing food would exert similar favorable effects. At first one egg was given daily for four periods; no obvious effect was noted, except that immediately after the single egg was withdrawn the calcium retention became poorer. When 3 eggs were included in the diet unequivocal changes in calcium metabolism were observed. The fecal calcium decreased with an increase of calcium retention from 15 per cent in the control periods to about 50 per cent during the 3-egg regimen. These observa→

tions indicate that the small amount of vitamin D contained in the eggs (estimated to be about 60 international units per egg) was effective in promoting calcium gain in osteomalacia.

Although the major portion of the population does not depend on dietary source for vitamin D, the addition of such food as eggs will make up the deficiency.   It confirms our impression that the favorable state of calcium metabolism observed at the start of the study in this patient was due to the vitamin D containing food in the hospital diet such as eggs and milk.   The prolonged action of vitamin D strikingly demonstrated in Case 1, although mainly due to storage, might be partly due to the supplementary effect of the diet.   However, if eggs or other vitamin D containing foods were withdrawn, the diets then became sufficiently devoid of vitamin D to allow depletion to take place.

THE ADDED REQUIREMENTS OF PREGNANCY

During gestation nutritional requirements are increased to provide building materials for the fetus and its adnexa, and to allow for the development of the maternal tissues such as the uterus, mammary glands and other organs in order to take care of the demands of labor, parturition and the preparation for milk secretion.   The quantitative aspects of the question are not accurately known.   According to Macy and Hunscher (7), the calcium content of the fetus at birth is approximately 23 gm, and most of that is acquired during the last trimester of gestation.   The daily accumulation in the fetus and its adnexa is about 50 mg from the third to the seventh months and thereafter it increases to about 120 mg until the tenth month when there is a sharp rise to 450 mg.   With an adequate intake of calcium (1.5 gm daily) and vitamin D, sufficient calcium may be retained to cover the requirements of gestation.   On the other hand, if the dietary calcium is low and in the absence of vitamin D, the fetal requirement has to be met at the expense of the maternal skeletal store.   In this locality where the diet is usually low in calcium and devoid of vitamin D, and the value of sunlight is not appreciated, it is easy to understand that osteomalacia frequently develops or gets worse with gestation.   Our metabolic studies on patients with osteomalacia during pregnancy serve to emphasize the importance of adequate intake of calcium and vitamin D during this part of the reproductive cycle.

CASE 3. L. H. M., a Chinese woman of 33 was admitted in November 1938 at the 7th month of her 4th pregnancy. She had had osteomalacia for 11 years with symptoms coming on after the first child birth. Metabolic studies were made for 19 four-day periods (76 days) from the 7th lunar month to term.

In the first two periods on an intake of 273 mg per day, the output, all in the stool, almost balanced the intake, and whatever the fetus required must have been derived from her own tissue store. From the third period on the intake was raised to 1,473 mg per day. During the first 3 periods on the augmented intake, there was, on the average, a daily retention of 323 mg which, if maintained, would be adequate to meet the fetal demands. However, not much would be left for the replenishment of her own decalcified skeleton. Therefore, vitamin D in the form of Vigantol 1 cc per day was started from period 6 and continued for 8 periods. The response was a progressive and marked decrease of stool calcium and increase of urinary calcium with great improvement in retention. During the last 9 periods of observation the average daily retention was a little over 1 gm. This degree of calcium retention would enable the patient not only to meet the heightened requirements of pregnancy but also to repair her bony depletion. Her symptoms were considerably improved and the child delivered by Cesarean section was normal.

THE ADDED REQUIREMENTS OF LACTATION

The added drain of lactation is more obvious than that of pregnancy, and in cases of active and prolonged lactation, it is more extensive. Among the 8 lactating women observed, 3 were in late lactation yielding 300—500 cc of milk a day containing 60-120 mg of calcium. Such loss does not appear to be great, but when prolonged as it is often the case in Chinese lactating mothers (and instances of lactation for a period of over 2 years are not infrequent), serious drain on the skeletal store will be the result. However, in late lactation with relatively low milk yields, the loss can easily be rectified by the addition of vitamin D even when the intake of calcium is only on a moderate level as exemplified by the following case (8).

CASE 4. W. W. J., a Chinese woman of 27 years of age, was admitted in May 1936 for moderately severe osteomalacia with occasional attacks of tetany for 6 years. Diet was poor, although she had frequent access to sunshine. She gave birth to 4 children, the last about 7 months prior to admission. All children were breast-fed for prolonged periods. Serum calcium was 7.34, inorganic phosphorus 3.03 mg per cent and phosphatase 13.5 Bodansky units.

The quantitative diet on which the patient was placed contained 377 mg calcium and 1,197 mg phosphorus per day. During the first two periods the calcium balance was slightly negative, while the phosphorus balance was even. The calcium loss in the stool accounted for 70 per cent and milk secretion only 30 per cent of the total output; there being no calcium in the urine. Vitamin D (Vigantol 1 cc daily) was added during the next 4 periods. This was followed during the last two periods by substantial calcium and phosphorus retention. Under the influence of vitamin D the limited supply of calcium in the diet was sufficient not only for the metabolic needs during lactation, but also for deposit in the tissues for the repair of skeletal decalcification. After vitamin D administration serum calcium rose to normal with disappearance of tetany.

However, in early lactation, especially when the milk yield is large, a high intake of calcium is essential in addition to adequate vitamin D supply. Of the 5 women studied in early lactation, 4 secreted milk exceeding a liter a day, losing about 250-350 mg of calcium. In these cases a high intake of calcium is imperative not only to cover the large loss of calcium in the milk, but also to cope with a less well understood factor peculiar to active lactation whereby calcium metabolism is so stimulated that conservation through other channels of elimination becomes very difficult even though there is no vitamin D deficiency.

CASE 5. A case in point is Y.W.L., a Chinese woman of 43 with osteomalacia. She was under continuous metabolic observation during the last two-thirds of her 5th pregnancy, and received a well-balanced diet with high calcium and phosphorus intake supplemented by Vigantol. She was retaining approximately 800 mg of calcium a day during gestation. Observation on lactation began 18 days postpartum for 11 four-day periods.

On a low intake of 247 mg of calcium per day, her balances were markedly negative. In view of the large volume of milk produced containing more calcium than what the diet supplied, balance, as expected, could not be maintained even though vitamin D were operative. When the calcium intake was raised to 1,147 mg a day, balances were just even. On further raising the calcium intake to a little over 2,000 mg a day, one began to notice some retention, but it was much less than during gestation. Subsequent administration of Vigantol did not improve the extent of calcium retention, indicating that the patient was then not deficient in vitamin D and that the poor retention was not related to any possible vitamin D deficiency.

This study indicates that in early and active lactation the calcium drain upon the mother is enormous and probably more so than during gestation. It is probable that more patients with osteomalacia date the onset of symptoms from after child-birth than during pregnancy. This is in accord with the view that while both pregnancy and lactation are important predisposing factors in the etiology of osteomalacia, the latter is relatively more important.

THE DEPENDENCE OF INFANT METABOLISM ON THE STATE OF VITAMIN D NUTRITION OF THE NURSING MOTHER

In order to find out how the mineral metabolism of infants may be influenced by the state of vitamin D nutrition of the mother during lactation, we have undertaken a simultaneous study of the mother and infant in four instances (9). One series of observations was made on an osteomalacic mother of 29 years old and her child.

CASE 6. The mother, W.H.S., had osteomalacia and tetany for 11 years. On admission in December 1938 she was in the 8th month of her 4th pregnancy. Marked shortening of stature, waddling gait, and bone tenderness were present. X-ray examination showed general osteoporosis, biconcave absorption of the vertebral bodies, asymmetry of the pelvis, distortion and compression of the heads of the femurs into the acetabulae and pathological fracture of the right femur. Serum calcium was 8.2 and inorganic phosphorus 2.8 mg per cent.

Metabolic studies made during the latter part of pregnancy showed that only even balances were obtained on high calcium intake. After Vigantol in daily doses of 5 cc (60,000 international units) was given for 4 days, mineral retention occurred and became progressively more marked and the serum calcium and phosphorus returned to normal.

The Vigantol given for the above stated period together with some cod liver oil and general hospital diet given postpartum constituted the only supply of vitamin D prior to the studies on lactation.

On resuming metabolic studies 17 days post-partum, observations were continued for 26 four-day periods on calcium intakes ranging from 1,400—1,650 mg per day. The first 18 periods were without vitamin D supplements, and the calcium balances showed considerable fluctuation. At first the balances were barely even, but later on they were distinctly negative. This, together with the diminution and disappearance of urinary calcium indicates that the limited amount of vitamin D given prior to the studies was being gradually depleted in the course of 2 or 3 months. Vigantol 2 cc daily was started from the 19th period on. This was followed by a progressive diminution of stool calcium and an increase of urinary calcium. As the conservation through the bowel was much greater than the loss through the urinary tract, the net result was that the balances became increasingly positive. Thus vitamin D administration during lactation in a woman with skeletal decalcification was capable of conserving the metabolism of calcium to such an extent as to enable her not only to meet the heightened requirements of early and active lactation, but also to retain a small amount of the mineral for the reparation of the bones.

CASE 7. The infant, whose mother was described above, was delivered by Cesarean section. He was normal and the bones showed no rarefaction nor rachitic changes. The protection was probably derived from the vitamin D the mother received during the latter part of pregnancy.

The metabolic observations made while the infant was fed exclusively on the mother's milk showed exceedingly good retention. Approximately 80 per cent of the calcium and 90 per cent of the phosphorus in the milk were retained. The small amounts of calcium eliminated were about equally divided between the urine and the stool. However, as the mother was being depleted of vitamin D the infant began to show a slight decrease in calcium retention. What is more striking is the behavior of the urinary and stool calcium. There was a progressive decrease in the urinary calcium to the point of disappearance coinciding with a steady increase in the stool calcium, most likely related to a decrease of the vitamin D content of the milk as the result of vitamin D depletion in the mother. At this point early changes in the epiphyses of the radii and ulnae appeared. After vitamin D was supplied to the mother, a reversal of the metabolic behavior of the infant was brought about: a return of urinary calcium with a corresponding decrease of stool calcium and a slightly better net retention. At the end of the observation the slight rachitic changes in the wrists also disappeared.

These observations indicate that the metabolism of the infant intimately reflects that of the mother. On account of the variations in the vitamin D content of the breast milk, the infant exhibited period of vitamin D depletion and replenishment corresponding to those of the mother. This intimate relationship between the maternal and infantile metabolism explains the occurrence of fetal rickets in children born of osteomalacia mothers as described by Maxwell (10), and the high frequency of tetany in early months of life in infants breast-fed by mothers whose diet was deficient, as observed by Chu and Sung (11). When the mother has a sufficient store of vitamin D, her milk possesses antirachitic properties. But as the store becomes depleted the child begins to show early signs of rickets. Prior to the development of appreciable changes in the epiphyses, alterations in the calcium metabolism are detectable. These alterations consist of a diminution and disappearance of urinary calcium corresponding to an increase in stool calcium, pointing to defective absorption of the mineral. If this metabolic defect is allowed to proceed further, clinical rickets will inevitably result.

SUMMARY

From the foregoing observations it is clear that the role played by vitamin D in the pathogenesis of osteomalacia is of primary importance. In the absence of vitamin D or when it is being depleted from the bodily store, difficulty arises in the intestinal absorption of calcium. This leads to mineral loss from the body especially when the intake is low, as it is in this part of the world. One of the first signs of vitamin D depletion is a diminution or disappearance of the urinary calcium, to be followed by an increase in the stool calcium. The former may be considered as a measure of mineral conservation. In spite of conservation through the urinary tract, the stool elimination, made up, as it is, of the unabsorbed dietary calcium and of the calcium that accompanies the gastro-intestinal secretion, usually exceeds the intake, giving rise to negative balance. Such loss may not seem to be great on a daily basis, but, if permitted to proceed uninterruptedly for long periods of time, will eventually lead to osteomalacia. While interruption of this pathological process may occur through involuntary exposure to sunshine or accidental introduction of minimal amounts of vitamin D-containing food in the diet, the downward trend may be accelerated during pregnancy and lactation, periods of mineral stress.

With the administration of vitamin D the pathological process can be at once rectified. Intestinal absorption improves with a decrease of calcium output in the stool and appearance of calcium in the urine. At times even the calcium that accompanies the gastro-intestinal secretion may be reabsorbed. As a result, a large proportion of the calcium intake is retained for deposition in the bones, and maintenance of serum concentration. While positive balance may be obtained on a minimal intake, it is necessary to supply a large amount of calcium in the diet to promote rapid reparation of the depleted skeletal store. Therefore in the therapy as well as in the pathogenesis of osteomalacia the importance of calcium is only second to that of vitamin D. High intake of calcium is especially important during the reproductive cycle when the physiological requirements are such as cannot be met without an extra supply even if the conservative action of vitamin D is operative.

Finally an adequate supply of vitamin D and calcium is essential during pregnancy and lactation in order to provide protection to the fetus and child from rickets.

ABSTRACT OF DISCUSSION

Dr. Hsien Wu. Dr. Liu has given a good account of vitamin D in osteomalacia, but the significance of his work goes far beyond this disease. What vitamin D does for the osteomalacia patient, it does also for the normal person. As you all know, the Chinese diet is low in calcium. The average daily Ca intake per person is about 0.34 gram, while the minimum requirement according to Prof. Sherman is 0.45 gram and the amount he recommended is 0.68 gram. According to this standard, there is a widespread calcium deficiency in China, but rickets and osteomalacia are not as prevalent as one would expect. Surely there must be some other factor at work, and that factor is vitamin D which, by increasing the efficiency of calcium absorption from the intestine, decreases the amount of calcium which has to be taken. The actual vitamin D content of the Chinese diet is very low, but sunshine is fortunately abundant in North China. Here lies the possibility of a solution of our calcium problem, but the detailed knowledge needed has yet to be worked out by calcium metabolism experiments on normal persons with known amounts of exposure to sunshine.

While the action of vitamin D on the gastro-intestinal tract has been demonstrated, it is not yet certain whether it has any other action in the body. Now since calcium chloride given intravenously is well utilized, whereas the same substance given orally is little absorbed in vitamin D deficiency as Dr. Liu has shown, it would seem that the bone is able to absorb calcium from blood without the assistance of vitamin D, and we need not assume that vitamin D, at least in physiological doses, has any action other than that on the gastro-intestinal tract.

Dr. I. Snapper. The results of the painstaking investigation of Dr. S. H. Liu and his collaborators are not only highly interesting,— they form at the same time the most exact data available about the calcium metabolism in man, specially in osteomalacia and allied disorders. Every one, who is interested in calcium metabolism and bone diseases, will be indebted to this group of scientists of the P.U.M.C. for the valuable information their publications contain.

As far as the quantitative side of the problem, which Dr. Liu discussed today, is concerned, it has to be pointed out that the adult human skeleton contains about 700 gm of calcium (even for a woman of 50 Kg. the usual average body weight here, it should be about 500 gm) whereas in the human newborn only 23 gm of calcium are found. Thus it becomes evident that osteomalacia during pregnancy will occur, only when the skeleton of the expectant mother has been depleted for a long time before the pregnancy started. Only then the loss of 23 grams of calcium would be a significant last item which changes the latent osteomalacia into a manifest syndrome.

Dr. Liu's figures, however, show that the loss of calcium during one year of lactation is considerably greater than the 23 gm lost during pregnancy. This might imply that during the many months of lactation which are customary in North China, osteomalacia might become even more often manifest than during pregnancy. It would be interesting to know Dr. Liu's experience about this question.

Dr. H. I. Chu. Dr. Liu has well emphasized the difficulty of calcium absorption in the gastro-intestinal tract in osteomalacia. I would like to point out that there is no difficulty of phosphorus absorption in cases of vitamin D deficiency. When phosphorus intake is adequate, there is always a good amount of phosphorus excreted in the urine, indicating good absorption. With a very low calcium intake the proportion of urinary phosphorus is further increased. It is only when calcium intake is very much raised that phosphorus begins to be excreted in the stool in large amounts in proportion to the unabsorbed calcium.

In spite of the fact that dietary phosphorus is well absorbed in cases of osteomalacia many of these patients have low serum inorganic phosphorus like infants with rickets. The cause of this phenomenon is not understood. The state of parathyroid function may play a rôle, but at present there is no data to prove or disprove that hypothesis.

The study on the effect of minimal dose of vitamin D in osteomalacia represents the beginning of an investigation into the quantitative relationship between calcium and phosphorus intake on one hand and vitamin D requirement on the other. This is of theoretical as well as practical significance. The dietaries of the mass of the population in this part of the country are deficient in calcium and vitamin D containing food is scarce and expensive. One way of solving the problem may be to raise the dietary calcium and to encourage exposure to the sun rather than to increase the dietary vitamin D. It is our impression that the mass of the population here cannot afford to have eggs and other vitamin D containing foods in their diet and that they do not get osteomalacia probably because they acquire enough antirachitic ultra-violet rays from sun exposure during the late spring, summer and early fall. This may be enough to prevent any difficulty of calcium and phosphorus metabolism and, by virtue of the prolonged action of vitamin D, to protect the individual through the winter when the natural ultra-violet radiation is negligible.

Although the primary action of vitamin D in osteomalacia is that of promotion of calcium absorption through the intestinal tract, the same is not observed in a perfectly normal individual who is in calcium and phosphorus equilibrium with adequate vitamin D nutrition. It can be demonstrated that a normal individual would not absorb an excessively large amount of calcium when the same therapeutic dose of vitamin D is given as in the case of osteomalacia. Thus we may say that vitamin D, in addition to its action in promoting the absorption of calcium, also exerts a regulatory function in the intestinal absorption of calcium. It augments calcium absorption only when the body is in need of the mineral.

Dr. F. T. Chu. Dr. Liu's observation on the transmission of vitamin D from the lactating mother to the nursing infant is of particular interest to me. That such a transmission is possible in experimental animals has been surmised by previous workers, notably Sontag and his colleagues, but the indubitable evidence of the passage of vitamin D by way of human milk is for the first time demonstrated by Dr. Liu and his associates. This finding has some important bearing on the incidence of rickets and tetany in Chinese children. In a study of 176 cases of rickets seen in the pediatric ward of this hospital, it was found that about 60 per cent had been breast fed, and in a series of 37 cases of tetany seen in first year of life, 57 per cent had been breast fed before the development of active symptoms of spasmophilia. In Western literature the history of artificial feeding is obtainable in a vast majority of cases of either rickets or tetany; but this is not true here. Evidently, the milk of many Chinese mothers, being of inferior quality on account of lack of vitamin D and possibly of calcium, is not able to prevent the development of these deficiency diseases. In view of the prolonged effect of vitamin D therapy as shown by Dr. Liu, and also in view of the fact that many Chinese mothers of the poor class have no means to provide themselves with cod liver oil or eggs, it may be interesting to find out whether it is feasible to rely entirely upon the exposure to sunlight during the warmer season for the protection of such mothers against the vitamin D deficiency throughout the period of pregnancy and lactation.

Dr. H. C. Chang. The work of Dr. Liu and his associates in emphasizing the defective Ca absorption due to the lack of vitamin D in the high cereal diet and indoor living (i.e. lack of sun-shine) as an etiological factor of osteomalacia, and demonstrating the curative rôle of vitamin D in such condition is a distinct contribution.

It was supposed by Mellanby that the cereals contain "toxamin" which is responsible for producing the pathological bone changes in canine rickets, and that this toxic factor can be abolished by boiling the cereal with 1 per cent HCl. According to Bruce and Callow, the cereal diet may produce deficient calcification by virtue of its phosphorus being in a poorly available form, i.e. inositolhexaphosphoric acid. On boiling with HCl, this form of phosphorus is hydrolyzed and rendered biologically available, removing thereby the anticalcifying effect. This is in contrast to the statement made by Dr. H. I. Chu that phosphorus absorption is not hampered in osteomalacia, although a good part of the diet phosphorus is cereal in origin. The availability of cereal phosphorus in human metabolism, I believe, bears study.

That defective absorption of calcium can produce a disturbance in ossification of the bones has been experimentally demonstrated by Ivy and his associates in puppies after gastrectomy. In the absence of the gastric HCl, the less soluble Ca salts cannot be rendered more soluble. Furthermore, the quickened transit of the food in the absence of the stomach may seriously prevent an adequate absorption of the dietary

Ca salts. The experimental condition was described as "osteoporosis", but inasmuch as the softening, pliability and deformities of the bones are concerned, the picture is rather similar to those seen in clinical osteomalacia.

Dr. W. N. Bien. I would like to raise the question why the infant (Case 7) should show evidence of early rickets while his mineral retention remained as excellent as before.

Reply by Dr. S. H. Liu. I am grateful to the speakers for their kind remarks. Dr. Snapper's surmise that lactation constitutes quantitatively a greater mineral drain on the mother than pregnancy is correct. Yet the impression that pregnancy is a more important predisposing factor in osteomalacia prevails. This is probably because the dramatic circumstances of obstructed labor arrest the attention of the clinicians more forcibly than the unobstrusive state of prolonged lactation. Actually when one starts to look into the histories of these patients and analyse them, one finds the majority of them dating their onset of osteomalacia from after child-birth than during pregnancy. This is in accord with the chemical data.

It is certainly true that the major portion of the population in this locality derives antirachitic protection entirely from sunlight. Attempt to put this question on a quantitative basis has been made by Dr. H. I. Chu *et al* (Chu, H. I., Yu, T. F., Chang, K. P. and Liu, W. T. Calcium and phosphorus metabolism in osteomalacia. VII. The effect of ultra-violet irradiation from mercury vapor quartz lamp and sun light. Chinese Med. J. 55: 93, 1939). A total of 25-26 graded daily exposures to direct sun light during April and May, including 9 general exposures of one hour each during the last part of the course of treatment, gave rise to improvement in calcium and phosphorus retention and in symptomatology of osteomalacia and tetany, comparable to the effects of therapeutic doses of vitamin D. Therefore it seems feasible that sunlight utilized to such a degree would provide adequate protection to pregnant and lactating mothers against vitamin D deficiency.

Dr. Bien's query about the occurrence of epiphyseal changes without concomitant diminution of mineral retention may be tentatively answered by saying that as the infant grows, the demand for calcium increases. It is possible that merely maintaining the previous level of calcium retention is not adequate for the need of growth and thereby impaired calcification results. However one can not exclude the additional specific effect of Vitamin D in the regulation of calcium deposition in the bones.

REFERENCES

1. *Hannon, R. R., Liu., S. H., Chu, H. I., Wang, S. H., Chen, K. C., and Chow, S. K.* Calcium and phosphorus metabolism in osteomalacia. I. The effect of vitamin D and its apparent duration. Chinese Med. J., **48**: 623, 1934.

2. *Bauer, W., Albright, F., and Aub, J. C.* Studies of calcium and phosphorus metabolism. II. The calcium excretion of normal individuals on a low calcium intake, also data on a case of pregnancy. J. Clin. Invest., **7**: 75., 1929.

3. *Heymann, W.* Metabolism and mode of action of vitamin D. II. Storage of vitamin D in different tissues in vivo. J. Biol. Chem., **118**: 371, 1937.

4. *Guerrant, N. B., Morck, R. A., Bechdel, S. I., and Hilston, N. W.* Storage of vitamin D in the tissues of growing calves. Proc. Soc. Exp. Biol. and Med., **38**: 827, 1938.

5. *Vollmer, H.* Distribution of vitamin D in body after administration of massive doses. Am. J. Dis. Child., **57**: 343, 1939.

6. *Chu, H. I., Liu, S. H., Yu, T. F., Hsu, H. C., Cheng, T. Y., and Chao, H. C.* Calcium and phosphorus metabolism in osteomalacia. X. Further studies on vitamin D action: early signs of depletion and effect of minimal doses. J. Clin. Invest. **19**: 1940.

7. *Macy, I. G. and Hunscher, H. A.* An evaluation of maternal nitrogen and mineral needs during embryonic and infant development. Am. J. Obs. and Gyn. **27**: 878, 1934.

8. *Liu, S. H., Su, C. C., Wang, C. W., and Chang, K. P.* Calcium and phosphorus metabolism in osteomalacia. VI. The added drain of lactation and beneficial action of vitamin D. Chinese J. Physiol. **11**: 271, 1937.

9. *Liu, S. H., Chu, H. I., Su, C. C., Yu, T. F., and Cheng, T. Y.* Calcium and phosphorus metabolism in osteomalacia. IX. Metabolic behavior of infants fed on breast milk from mothers showing various states of vitamin D nutrition. J. Clin. Invest. **19**: 1940.

10. *Maxwell, J. P., Hu, C. H., and Turnbull, H. M.* Fetal rickets. J. Path. and Bact., **35**: 419, 1932.

11. *Chu, F. T. and Sung, C.* Tetany in infancy and childhood: a clinical study of 45 cases seen in North China with especial reference to etiology. J. Ped., **16**: 1940.

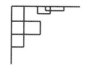
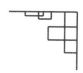

第五编　名世之作

　　第五编仅包括两篇论文，但这两篇论文几乎代表了老协和临床学科所取得的最大成就。北京协和医院的代谢病房在长期用代谢平衡法对骨软化症患者进行代谢研究之后，临床上发现了一类新的骨软化症患者，即慢性肾衰后出现的骨软化症。刘士豪教授和朱宪彝教授对这类患者的代谢数据进行了极为细致的分析，最终得出结论：维生素 D 对这类患者治疗无效而双氢速变固醇（A.T.10）治疗有效。他们首先在《科学》（Science）发表短文提出：这类疾病应该采用一个新的疾病命名，即"肾性骨营养不良"，应使用双氢速变固醇治疗。接着他们在《医学》（Medicine）发表了长达 59 页的论文，详细阐述了所有的数据以及他们对这一现象提出的假说。

SCIENCE

Vol. 95   Friday, April 10, 1942   No. 2467

SCIENCE: A Weekly Journal devoted to the Advancement of Science, edited by J. McKEEN CATTELL and published every Friday by

THE SCIENCE PRESS

Lancaster, Pa.   Garrison, N. Y.

Annual Subscription, $6.00   Single Copies, 15 Cts.

SCIENCE is the official organ of the American Association for the Advancement of Science. Information regarding membership in the Association may be secured from the office of the permanent secretary in the Smithsonian Institution Building, Washington, D. C.

REGENERATION, DEVELOPMENT AND GENOTYPE[1]

By Professor CHARLES E. ALLEN

UNIVERSITY OF WISCONSIN

THE potentialities of a many-celled plant or animal were derived through the single cell from which the development of the organism can be traced. It follows that the genotype of such an organism is the genotype of its originating cell.

This statement is wholly true, to be sure, only if during the course of development the original genotype has not been modified. Environmental influences can induce changes in chromosome number, in chromosome constitution or in genes, and hence modifications of the genotype of the affected cells. The commonest visible type of such change in plants is a doubling of the chromosome number in some or many cells. Tetraploidy, resulting from a doubling of the typical diploid number, is of common occurrence. Ordinarily the "spontaneous" appearance of tetraploid cells must be assumed to result from an unrecognized stimulus. But in some species, including hemp, melons and a number of Chenopodiaceae, tetraploidy and octoploidy are regularly characteristic of certain regions. Here the change seems pretty clearly not to result from external stimuli. It is in a real sense itself an expression of the plant's genotype.

The extent to which a doubling of the chromosome number constitutes a genotypic modification can for the present be tested only by the examination of deliberately induced polyploids. From these it appears that the distinguishing characters of a tetra-

[1] Abridged version of a paper presented at the Fiftieth Anniversary Celebration of the University of Chicago, September 22, 1941.

sults of nineteen different exposures are shown in Fig. 1. The graph represents gains and losses of weight in the suit for the first six hours. Final equi-

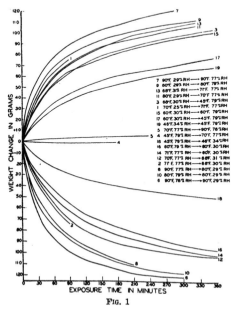

FIG. 1

librium was reached in most cases within twenty-four hours. The legend referring to each curve indicates the condition at which the suit was in hygroscopic equilibrium when exposure started, and the exposure condition which resulted in a given weight gain curve. For example, the legend for Curve No. 7 reads 90° F, 28 per cent. R.H. → 90° F, 77 per cent. R.H. This means that when the suit was in equilibrium at 90° F and 28 per cent. relative humidity and was then exposed to a condition of 90° F and 77 per cent. relative humidity, it gained weight as described by this time curve.

The significant effect of garment moisture gain or loss on skin temperature and heat balance may be illustrated from the magnitude of the weight changes in the first hour of exposure. For example, in Curve No. 7 again: In the first hour the garment picked up 76 grams of moisture which has a heat gain equivalent of about 44 calories.[1] This value is 50 to 60 per cent. of the resting hourly heat production of an adult man. If one started with a heavy garment of 3 to 4 kilos dry at moderate temperatures, the total heat evolution in the first 2 or 3 hours would obviously be at least equal to the physiological heat production at rest. All

[1] The calorie equivalent of a 10-gram change in weight is about 5.8 calories.

curves indicate that more than half the total change in weight takes place in the first two hours of exposure. Another conclusion to be drawn from the figure is that relative humidity influences the weight change far more than temperature, although the effect of 10° rises in temperature is observable for comparable relative humidities. Finally, it may be of some interest to note a hysteresis effect. At a fixed temperature, in varying relative humidity from a given low to a given high value and back to the original low again, the garment gained more moisture before reaching equilibrium at the high humidity than it lost in returning to equilibrium at the original low humidity.

A thorough knowledge of the hygroscopic properties of different materials as well as the thermodynamic implications inherent in the body-clothing system is of considerable importance in designing protective garments for optimum comfort under extreme conditions.

JEAN H. NELBACH
L. P. HERRINGTON

JOHN B. PIERCE LABORATORY OF HYGIENE,
NEW HAVEN, CONN.

TREATMENT OF RENAL OSTEODYSTROPHY WITH DIHYDROTACHYSTEROL (A.T.10) AND IRON

RENAL osteodystrophy is a generic name for osseous disorders simulating rickets, osteomalacia or osteitis fibrosa cystica, but originating from chronic renal insufficiency. The most important metabolic defect is poor calcium absorption due to large phosphorus excretion by the bowel as a result of renal insufficiency. Yet vitamin D, specific in promoting calcium absorption in rickets and osteomalacia, is singularly ineffective in renal osteodystrophy. This is true in a series of 5 cases in which detailed metabolic studies are made in this clinic. Vitamin D in ordinary therapeutic doses for prolonged periods orally or intramuscularly or in single massive dose by mouth failed to elicit any significant clinical or metabolic response.

This led us to the use of dihydrotachysterol (A.T.10), an irradiation product of ergosterol, first introduced by Holtz[1] in the treatment of hypoparathyroid tetany. Our experience with A.T.10 in 3 cases of osteomalacia[2] indicates that this compound promotes calcium and phosphorus absorption by the intestine and deposition in the bones, contrary to the earlier view[3] that A.T.10 was not anti-rachitic. In

[1] F. Holtz, H. Gissel and E. Rossmann, *Deutsche Ztschr. f. Chir.*, 242: 521, 1934.
[2] H. I. Chu, S. H. Liu, H. C. Hsu and H. C. Chao, ''Calcium and Phosphorus Metabolism in Osteomalacia.'' XII. A Comparison of the Effects of A.T.10 (Dihydrotachysterol) and Vitamin D. To be published.
[3] F. Albright, *et al., Jour. Clin. Invest.,* 17: 317, 1938; 18: 165, 1939.

view of the favorable effects on osteomalacia, two of our patients with renal osteodystrophy received by mouth A.T.10 in 3 cc daily doses for 5 four-day metabolic periods while on a high calcium and moderate phosphorus intake. In both cases there was an immediate and progressive decrease of fecal calcium. While calcium appeared in significant amounts in the urine in one case, it remained absent in the other. The net retention of calcium at the height of A.T.10 action during the last period of its administration or the following period amounted to 50 per cent. of the intake. This was followed by a corresponding phosphorus gain due to a diminution of phosphorus elimination both in the stool and in the urine. The serum calcium, low initially in both cases, was raised to normal; and the inorganic phosphorus, high to start with, was reduced to normal during the A.T.10 therapy. Thus in remedying the basic metabolic defect underlying the bone disease in renal osteodystrophy, dihydrotachysterol appears to be highly efficacious, similar to vitamin D in rickets and osteomalacia. However, the effect of A.T.10 lasts for 7 or 8 four-day periods after the therapy is discontinued, in contrast to the long-sustained aftereffect of vitamin D in rickets and osteomalacia. Therefore, to secure substantial remineralization of the skeleton in renal osteodystrophy it would be necessary to administer A.T.10 for a prolonged period of time.

Another mode of therapy which we believe to be of interest in renal osteodystrophy is the oral administration of iron salts. It is well known in elementary chemistry that iron combines with phosphate to form insoluble ferric phosphate. That similar reaction takes place in the intestine is indicated by the experimental work[4] showing that iron added to a non-rachitogenic diet of rats produces rickets. Thus iron in large doses is contraindicated in rickets and osteomalacia. However, in renal osteodystrophy with hyperphosphatemia and high concentration of phosphate in the intestine interfering with the assimilation of calcium, the phosphate-precipitating action of iron may be utilized to advantage. Accordingly, the two patients wtih renal osteodystrophy referred to above were given ferric ammonium citrate 6 gm daily for from 5 to 14 metabolic periods. The most consistent changes were a decline of the serum inorganic phosphorus and an ascending tendency of the serum calcium. The phosphorus balance showed a decline due to an increase of stool excretion of phosphorus. The fecal elimination of calcium was usually diminished, giving rise to favorable calcium balance. This increase of calcium retention is most probably the result of the calcium-sparing action of iron in combining with phosphorus in the intestine. Thus from the standpoint of combating phosphate retention and promoting calcium gain in renal osteodystrophy, iron therapy proves effective.

In view of the present unsatisfactory state of affairs in the therapy of renal osteodystrophy, dihydrotachysterol (A.T.10) and iron seem to be rational and useful items in the treatment of such condition. As far as we are aware, the use of A.T.10 or iron in osseous disorder due to renal insufficiency has not been recorded in the literature. This is a preliminary report, and the detailed data will be published elsewhere.[5]

S. H. LIU
H. I. CHU

DEPARTMENT OF MEDICINE,
 PEIPING UNION MEDICAL COLLEGE,
 PEIPING, CHINA

SCIENTIFIC APPARATUS AND LABORATORY METHODS

CONCERNING THE NATURE OF TYPE C BOTULINUS TOXIN FRACTIONS

THE first portions of condensate obtained by use of the standard lyophil apparatus in the dehydration of type C botulinus toxin consist of a high concentration of the thermo-stable fraction of this toxin. Recognition of this fraction in botulinus toxin was announced by Bronfenbrenner and Schlesinger in SCIENCE in 1921, though they gave no method of obtaining it in pure form in quantities sufficient for our study purposes.

This fraction, which for convenience may be designated as A, consists of ammonia salts. It is thermostable, and may be obtained in high concentration in almost pure aqueous solution by the method named. No antigenic property has been demonstrated for this fraction and it, therefore, has no specific antibody. Neutralization by type C antitoxin does not occur. Fraction A is a neuro-toxin which acts without delay. Sub-lethal intraperitoneal doses in mice result in nervous irritability for about 30 seconds, followed by what appears to be a complete anesthesia for four to six hours and eventual complete recovery. Thirty intraperitoneal, 18 gram mouse, mld's, administered orally to a three-pound mallard duck, result in a typi-

---

[4] J. F. Brock and L. K. Diamond, *Jour. Pediat.*, 4: 442, 1934.

[5] S. H. Liu and H. I. Chu, "Renal Osteodystrophy: Studies of Calcium and Phosphorus Metabolism with Special Reference to Pathogenesis and Effects of Dihydrotachysterol (A.T.10) and Iron." To be published.

STUDIES OF CALCIUM AND PHOSPHORUS METABOLISM WITH SPECIAL REFERENCE TO PATHOGENESIS AND EFFECTS OF DIHYDROTACHYSTEROL (A.T.10) AND IRON

S. H. LIU, M.D., AND H. I. CHU, M.D.

Department of Medicine, Peiping Union Medical College, Peiping, China

CONTENTS

NOSOGRAPHY

The purpose of this presentation is to record the metabolic observations on five cases of renal osteodystrophy in the hope that they may contribute to the understanding of the pathogenesis of this osseous disorder and add to its therapy. The term renal osteodystrophy is chosen advisedly, because while chronic renal insufficiency is fundamentally responsible for the skeletal changes in all the cases, the type of resulting osseous disorder is not uniform and may be difficult to determine without complete histological examination.   Moreover in the literature the nosography of the disease is a subject of much controversy.   The term "renal rickets", though used extensively, is objectionable because it identifies the disease of the skeleton with rickets which it is not in many cases, especially those in more recent reports, although the radiological appearance and the gross deformities of the bones resemble those seen in rickets.   The term "renal dwarfism" emphasizes only one feature of the disease which is not present in many cases especially when growth is complete and fails to indicate the osseous affection.   Objection to the term "renal infantilism" may be made on the same basis.   In view of the finding of osteitis or osteoporosis fibrosa cystica in many cases in which the pathologic study was clearly presented, Park and Eliot (1) inclined to consider osteofibrosis as the essential pathological lesion in the skeleton and agreed to the propriety of the term "renal osteitis fibrosa cystica" adopted by Albright, Drake and Sulkowitch (2).   How generally applicable this term may be will have to await the pathological studies of further cases.   The term "renal osteodystrophy" seems to be a suitable generic name to include cases of

103

osseous disorder associated with renal insufficiency, while the exact nature of the pathological process in the skeleton is still undetermined.

HISTORICAL

The association of albuminuria and late rickets was noted as early as 1883 by Lucas (3), but it was not until 1911 that Fletcher (4) clearly recognized the etiologic relationship between chronic renal disease and bone deformities. Barber (5) reported 10 additional cases under the term renal dwarfism. Parsons (6) and Teall (7) are early workers to define the roentgenologic picture of renal rickets. Brockman (8) gave the first clear histological distinction between renal rickets and infantile rickets. Recent reports by Langmead and Orr (9), Smyth and Goldman (10), Shelling and Remsen (11), Albright, Drake and Sulkowitch (2), and others (12–14) served to emphasize the frequent occurrence of diffuse parathyroid hyperplasia in renal osteodystrophy and raise the question of its possible etiologic importance in the genesis of the osseous disorder. Comprehensive reviews of the subject of renal osteodystrophy are available by Mitchell (15), Hamperl and Wallis (16) and Park and Eliot (1).

CLINICAL MATERIAL

The present study includes 5 Chinese patients with various grades of skeletal decalcification with or without other osseous changes occurring in association with moderate to advanced renal insufficiency. The clinical abstracts of these patients are to be found in the appendix. Here the salient features of each case may be briefly summarized.

Case 1 concerns a girl of 8 who had scarlet fever and acute glomerulonephritis 2 years previously. This was followed by polyuria, pain in legs and stunted growth. Examination showed dwarfism, knock-knee, enlarged wrists and ankles. X-ray revealed marked rarefaction of the skeleton with rachitis-like changes in the epiphyses. There was slight albuminuria with moderate reduction of renal function.

Case 2 is that of a girl of 19 who developed knock-knee, pain in the legs, pelvis and spine and great debility in the course of 4 years. The skeleton showed general osteoporosis and marked deformities. The pelvis exhibited cystic absorption and a triradiate deformity of the type seen in osteomalacia. The epiphyses had already been fused. Moderate anemia, slight albuminuria and very poor renal function were present. Pyelogram showed very small kidney shadows.

Case 3, a married woman of 34, was admitted in 1938 during her sixth pregnancy for edema, bone pains and spasm of hands. She had similar, but milder, symptoms in her fourth and fifth pregnancies 4 and 2 years previously. Bleeding from hemorrhoids had been present for 7 years. Examination showed severe anemia, moderate cardiac enlargement and slight peripheral edema. Signs of tetany were present. There was bone tenderness, but no deformities. X-ray showed slight rarefaction of all the bones with biconcave reabsorption of the lumbar vertebrae. Renal functional impairment was severe, and pyelography revealed very small kidneys. Slight albuminuria was present.

Case 4. This is a girl of 20 who had generalized bone aching for over a year. There was slight or moderate tenderness over the bones of the lower extremities, pelvis and chest, but no deformities. Generalized moderate osteoporosis was demonstrated on x-ray examination. There were moderately severe anemia and slight albuminuria. The renal function was markedly impaired and the kidneys appeared to be very small on the pyelogram.

Case 5 is that of a boy of 20 with pain and swelling of knees, progressive deformity of lower limbs and backache for 8 years. Examination showed emaciation, dwarfism and infantilism. Both knees were swollen and tender with effusion. The bones showed extreme rarefaction. The left femur presented an old fracture. The diaphyseal ends of both radii showed marked cupping and irregularity. The skull presented a mottled appearance and the vault was thinner than normal. The urine contained albumin and the renal function was very poor. Moderate anemia was present.

The bones of all the five patients were involved to a varying extent. Slight or moderate osteoporosis without skeletal deformity was present in Cases 3 and 4, and marked osteoporosis in the rest of the cases. In addition, Case 2 showed deformities of the pelvis and knees with cystic absorption of some of the bones. Cases 1 and 5 presented rachitis-like changes in the epiphyses. In the last case rheumatoid arthritis might also be present. The nature of the kidney disease was not determined in any of the cases. In Case 1, the history of acute nephritis following scarlet fever suggested chronic glomerulonephritis (16a). In the remaining cases there was no history referable to renal disease, and the advanced renal insufficiency was discovered on renal function tests. The small kidneys demonstrated on the pyelograms could be the result of chronic glomerulonephritis or pyelonephritis, or they were congenitally hypoplastic with interstitial nephritis.

METABOLIC PROCEDURE

All the patients were observed for prolonged periods in the metabolism ward where the procedure for making and serving constant diets and quantitative collection of excreta has been established and described previously (17). The diets for these patients were usually low in calcium and phosphorus (Table 6, Appendix). The desired high level of calcium intake was made up by the administration of a 7.7% calcium lactate solution. Higher phosphorus intake was brought about either by inclusion in the diet of phosphorus-rich food or by the administration of a mixture of monosodium and disodium phosphate of pH 7.40, disodium or trisodium phosphate solution. The diets were quantitatively consumed except in a few instances where the refused food or vomitus were saved and analysed. Complete balances in calcium, phosphorus and nitrogen were obtained in 4-day periods. Serum calcium, phosphorus and phosphatase (18) were determined at the beginning of each period. The massed data on the 5 patients are shown in Tables 7–12 in the Appendix.

Serum acid-base balance from venous blood obtained with anaërobic technic was studied occasionally in each patient and more frequently when the influence of ingestion of sodium bicarbonate or ammonium chloride was investigated. The acid-base studies included serum pH (19), bicarbonate (20), chloride (21), inorganic phosphate (22), proteins (23), total base (24) sodium (25), potassium (26), calcium (27) and magnesium (28).

Vitamin D given orally was an oily solution of irradiated ergosterol marketed as Vigantol containing 0.3 mg. or 12,000 international units per cc. or 30 drops. For intramuscular injection Vigantol was sterilized by autoclaving at 15 pounds of pressure for half an hour. A concentrated solution of irradiated ergosterol in corn oil[1] containing 1,000,000 international units per gm. was given orally for the single massive dose therapy. A.T.10, given by mouth was a 0.5% solution in oil of dihydrotachysterol (Bayer). For the oral administration of iron, a 20% solution of ferric ammonium citrate was used.

ALTERED PHOSPHORUS METABOLISM IN RENAL OSTEODYSTROPHY

The fundamental cause of renal osteodystrophy must be sought in the renal insufficiency of long standing. The duration of the renal disease in our cases can not be accurately ascertained, but probably it ranged between 2 and 8 years. The severity of the renal failure must also play a part, for in 4 of the cases in this series, the phenolsulphonephthalein output was only 6% or less, and the urea clearance varied around 10 per cent of normal, and the azotemia was pronounced. However, advanced renal insufficiency is not an invariable accompaniment of renal osteodystrophy. Case 1 showed only moderate renal insufficiency, although the osseous involvement was severe. While it is generally agreed that renal insufficiency is causally related to the development of osseous disorder, much remains to be elucidated as to the mechanism by which the osseous disorder is brought about by the renal insufficiency. Several theories have been proposed.

Mitchell's concept (15) is that in renal insufficiency a shift of phosphorus excretion from the kidneys to the intestine occurs, and "the concentration of phosphorus in the intestine thus increased so blocks the absorption of calcium from food that the child suffers a true calcium starvation." Although the theory has been accepted generally and received support from Albright, Drake and Sulkowitch (2), the experimental data demonstrating the shift of phosphorus excretion and impairment of intestinal absorption of calcium in renal osteodystrophy remain meager. The presence of chronic acidosis in renal insufficiency has been thought by many to be an important factor in the skeletal decalcification in renal osteodystrophy. In normal individuals (29) and in patients with osteomalacia (30) the production of moderate acidosis by the ingestion of ammonium chloride results in excessive calcium wastage through the urinary tract. Jaffe, Bodansky and Chandler (31) produced in animals a bone disorder similar to osteitis fibrosa by feeding them a low calcium diet and ammonium chloride. Shohl (32) found rickets in the rat fed a non-rachitogenic diet with added ammonium chloride and ammonium carbonate mixture. While acidosis does exert a deleterious effect on the calcium and phosphorus metabo-

---

[1] Supplied through the kindness of Dr. Charles E. Bills of the Research Laboratory, Mead Johnson and Company, Evansville, Ind.

lism, how important it is in the pathogenesis of renal osteodystrophy remains to be determined. Recently a third theory has been put forward, namely, that hyperparathyroidism secondary to renal insufficiency occurs and is the cause of the osseous changes. While this concept is propounded in detail by Park and Eliot (1) and Anderson (33), it has been objected to by others, notably Albright, Drake and Sulkowitch (2).

The data from the present series of cases concerning the disturbances in phosphorus metabolism may be of value in evaluating the various theories of pathogenesis of renal osteodystrophy.

(a) Serum inorganic phosphorus

In most of the reported cases of renal rickets the serum inorganic phosphorus was very much elevated. In fact, phosphate retention in the blood has been regarded by many as the *sine qua non* of renal rickets. In our series Cases 2, 3 and 4 showed initial values averaging 5.90, 6.89 and 4.76 mg.% respectively indicating definite phosphate retention (Table 1). Cases 1 and 5 had values around 4 mg.%, that is, within normal limits. As the renal functional impairment in Case 1 was only moderately severe, definite elevation of serum inorganic phosphorus may not be expected. However, we have no explanation to offer for the lack of phosphate retention in Case 5. The renal insufficiency of this patient was just as severe as that of the other patients in this series with definite elevation of serum inorganic phosphorus. We suspect that the relatively low phosphorus diet might have lowered the serum inorganic phosphorus. In fact, when these patients were examined in the outpatient clinic, their serum phosphorus was frequently lower than after admission, suggesting that the diet at home had been lower in phosphorus content or contained largely cereal phosphorus which could not be absorbed. Then there is the possibility of variations in the response of the parathyroids to renal insufficiency. An active response of the parathyroids may depress an otherwise elevated serum inorganic phosphorus to normal, while a relative inactivity of the parathyroids favors the development of hyperphosphatemia. Thus, while hyperphosphatemia is the rule in advanced renal insufficiency, exceptions do occur in view of certain modifying factors such as low phosphorus diet and activity of the parathyroids.

(b) The ratio of urine to stool excretion of phosphorus

Mitchell (15) rearranged the data of Boyd, Courtney and MacLachlan (34) on 7 cases of chronic nephritis and those of Schoenthal (35) on 1 case of renal rickets and 2 cases of chronic nephritis for comparison with the data on 4 normal children as controls. The ratio of urinary to fecal phosphorus in the controls varied from 1.02 to 2.01, while that in the nephritic children was below 1 in 6 out of 10 cases, and above 1 in the remainder. This was interpreted to indicate a shift of phosphorus excretion from the kidneys to the intestine in renal insufficiency. However, the partition of phosphorus excretion depends to a large extent on the relative proportion of calcium and phosphorus in the diet. When more calcium is ingested in relation to phosphorus (high Ca/P intake), more

S. H. LIU AND H. I. CHU

phosphorus is excreted in the feces than in the urine; and when the diet contains less calcium in proportion to phosphorus (low Ca/P intake), phosphorus excretion takes place more in the urine than in the stool. This is strikingly shown in osteomalacia undergoing repair through the action of vitamin D (36, 37). The same phenomenon to a lesser degree is also observed in normal individuals (38). Therefore the urinary and stool phosphorus data need to be interpreted in conjunction with the ratio of calcium to phosphorus intake. In the collected cases of Mitchell, the diet Ca/P ratio was high, ranging from 0.87 to 2.32, favoring high phosphorus output in the stool. Therefore, in those cases in which the ratio of urinary to fecal phosphorus was below 1, such effects could not be entirely attributed to renal insufficiency.

In Table 1 are set forth the percentage of phosphorus excretion in the urine in terms of total output in the present series of cases when the diet Ca/P intake was low, namely 0.27–0.44. In case 1, the urinary phosphorus amounted to 76% of the total output, a figure at the upper limit of normal, evidently due to the fact that her renal function was not sufficiently impaired to influence the partition of phosphorus excretion. In the remaining 4 cases where the renal insufficiency was advanced the urinary phosphorus varied from 40 to 54%, all below the average of 63% for normal individuals on similar ratio of calcium to phosphorus intake. This indicates considerable difficulty on the part of the kidneys to eliminate phosphorus under the strain of a low Ca/P intake. When the phosphorus intake remained about the same, but with the calcium intake raised so as to increase the diet ratio of Ca/P to 1.80–2.63, all showed a definite decrease in the percentage of phosphorus excretion in the urine, demonstrating the influence of a high calcium intake in diverting phosphorus excretion from the kidneys to the intestine. In general the decrease in urinary phosphorus percentage was more pronounced in advanced renal insufficiency than in normal persons and in the case of milder renal disease, suggesting that in the former the strain on the kidneys of a low Ca/P intake had been greater.

(c) Effect of increasing the phosphorus intake

Attempt was made in examining further the metabolic behavior of these patients when the phosphorus intake was raised. Under the stress of a high phosphorus intake, one expects to find phosphorus retention manifested not only by an elevation of serum inorganic phosphorus but also by a positive balance or an increase of such. The large amount of ingested phosphorus should give rise to greater increase of phosphorus output in the stool than in the urine, thus reducing still further the percentage of phosphorus output in the urine. If the stool phosphorus is sufficiently augmented, the stool calcium may be expected to increase, thus diminishing calcium retention or rendering a positive calcium balance negative. All these expectations come true to a varying extent in the four cases so studied.

Case 2. As shown in Fig. 1, periods 6 and 7 were control periods on an intake of 1207 mg. calcium and 675 mg. phosphorus. On this regime the serum phosphorus was coming down from 6.85 to 5.96 mg.%, and the serum calcium was essentially constant at 5.54–5.91 mg.%. Urinary phosphorus averaged 314 mg. per day, amounting to 43% of the total output; and the balance was on the average −56 mg. per day. The average daily calcium balance was 63 mg., the large output being all by way of the intestine. During the next two periods (periods 8 and 9), the phosphorus intake was increased to 1075 mg. per day by the administration of a solution of disodium phosphate. This was followed by a rise of serum inorganic phosphorus from 5.96 to 7.25 mg.% and by a fall of serum calcium from 5.54 to 4.86 mg.%. Clinically the patient felt worse and exhibited active tetany. The urine phosphorus increased to 418 mg. daily, namely, 44% of the total output, and the balance was changed to a positive one, namely, 117 mg. per day. With this phosphorus gain there was a slight improvement of calcium balance to 114 mg. per day. The next two periods (periods 10

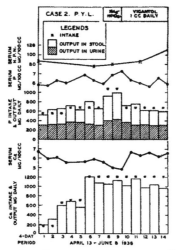

FIG. 1. CASE 2. EFFECT OF HIGH PHOSPHORUS INTAKE AND VIGANTOL ON CALCIUM AND PHOSPHORUS METABOLISM

and 11) saw a reversion of most of the alterations to the control state. It is noteworthy that during these two periods the phosphorus balance was a little more negative than in the control periods suggesting that the retained phosphorus during the high phosphorus periods was now being slowly eliminated.

Case 3. While on a daily calcium intake of 989 mg. this patient had her phosphorus intake raised from 612 mg. (periods 16–17) to 1105 mg. (period 18) and 1055 mg. (period 19) by the addition of a phosphate solution. Such a change resulted in a marked increase of the serum-inorganic phosphorus from 5.58 to 9.26 mg.% and a decrease of the serum calcium from 5.46 to 4.14 mg.% (Fig. 2). The daily urine phosphorus excretion increased from 218 to 323 mg. but the proportion in the urine increased but little (from 33 to 36%). The phosphorus balance shifted from −40 to 176 mg. per day, while the calcium balance changed from 31 to −12 indicating that an increase of stool phosphorus also increased

110   S. H. LIU AND H. I. CHU

stool calcium, leading to an adverse calcium balance. The figures for the following period (period 20) are most instructive. Although the diet phosphorus
was lowered to only 585 mg. per day, the stool phosphorus of 684 mg. was in
excess of the intake and this, together with the urine output of 257 mg., resulted
in a negative balance of 356 mg., showing that the phosphorus retained during
the 2 high phosphorus intake periods was eventually all excreted in the following
low phosphorus period. With the large increase of stool phosphorus in an attempt to excrete the retained phosphorus, there was a corresponding increase
of stool calcium, giving rise to a negative balance of 295 mg. per day. This set

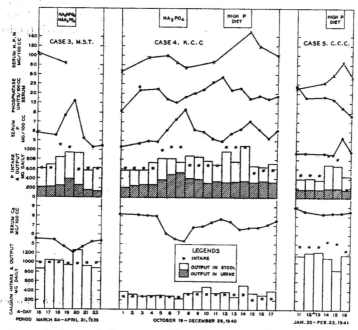

FIG. 2. CASES 3, 4 AND 5. EFFECT OF HIGH PHOSPHORUS INTAKE ON CALCIUM AND
PHOSPHORUS METABOLISM

of data affords direct evidence to the supposition that phosphorus elimination
by the bowel in large amounts does lead to a loss of calcium, and this loss con-
tinues for sometime after the phosphorus intake is reduced.

Case 4. In this patient the effect of increasing phosphorus intake was studied
while on low calcium diets (215–336 mg. per day), and the phosphorus intake was
raised by the addition of trisodium phosphate in the first series (periods 5–7)
and by the inclusion in the diet of high phosphorus-containing foods such as
millet, peanut and pork liver in the second series (periods 12–14). Periods 1–4
served as control on a diet containing 271 mg. calcium and 618 mg. phosphorus
(Fig. 2). On this diet the calcium balance was slightly negative, averaging 52
mg. per day and the phosphorus balance was barely positive, averaging 11 mg.

per day. The output of calcium was practically all in the stool, and the partition of phosphorus excretion was 40% in the urine. The serum calcium tended to lower, while inorganic phosphorus tended to rise. When the phosphorus intake was raised to 1059 mg. per day by the addition of trisodium phosphate, there was a marked phosphorus retention, averaging 256 mg. per day, and the serum inorganic phosphorus rose from 4.95 to 8.33 mg.%, with a lowering of the serum calcium from 8.04 to 5.38 mg.%. However, in this patient the increase of phosphorus intake by the addition of trisodium phosphate did not increase the stool phosphorus, showing that the phosphate in this form was easily absorbed. The urinary phosphorus increased, amounting to 58% of the total output, indicating that the kidneys were still capable of bearing most of the burden of phosphorus excretion. With the absorption of relatively large amounts of phosphate, the calcium balance showed a slightly favorable turn, the negative balance now averaging only 9 mg. per day. The post-control periods (periods 8–11) without the added phosphate witnessed an increase of stool phosphorus excretion over the pre-control periods (periods 1–4) with a persistently negative balance averaging 122 mg. per day. The serum inorganic phosphorus steadily returned to 5.00 mg.%, and the serum calcium to 7.73 mg.%. The calcium balance became less favorable, averaging −60 mg. per day.

During periods 12–14 the diet was changed to contain 1073 mg. of phosphorus. On this relatively high phosphorus intake of exclusively dietary origin, there was likewise a retention of phosphorus, averaging 124 mg. per day, and an increase of the serum inorganic phosphorus from 5.00 to 7.11 mg.% with a decrease of the serum calcium from 7.73 to 6.80 mg.%. These changes were not as marked as those of periods 5–7 when a similarly high phosphorus intake was brought about by the administration of sodium phosphate. The explanation for the difference probably lies in the poorer absorbability of the dietary phosphorus, particularly cereal and nut phosphorus. Thus the stool phorphorus during periods 12–14 showed a marked increase averaging 610 mg. per day and the urinary phosphorus came up to only 37% of the total output. The calcium balance remained negative to about the same extent as previously, namely, −62 mg. daily. In the three post-control periods (periods 15–17) with the diet changed back to a low phosphorus one, the reverse train of events followed: a decrease of the serum inorganic phosphorus and an increase of the serum calcium, a persistence of relatively large stool phosphorus excretion in spite of decreased intake, resulting in a negative phosphorus balance, and a large stool calcium excretion leading to a calcium loss.

Comparing the effects of increasing phosphorus intake by means of the soluble salt of phosphate with those of high phosphorus containing diet one finds that the former was more easily absorbed giving rise to greater retention and, in the serum, greater changes in the levels of inorganic phosphorus and calcium, but the partition of phosphate excretion was more in favor of the urinary tract leading to less phosphorus, therefore less calcium, drainage through the bowel. Clinically the patient tolerated the soluble phosphate salt better than the organic dietary phosphorus, not from the slightly greater drainage of calcium in the latter case, but from the concomitant increase of dietary protein leading to greater nitrogen retention and azotemia (blood non-protein nitrogen was raised from 86 to 150 mg.% as the result of increased protein intake).

Case 5. During the control periods (periods 11–13) on a calcium intake of 1356 mg. and a phosphorus intake of 488 mg. per day, both the daily calcium and phorphorus balances were slightly positive, averaging 149 and 92 mg. respectively (Fig. 2). While the calcium output was entirely in the stool, the phosphorus excretion was 44% in the urine. The serum calcium was 8.31 and inorganic phosphorus 3.70 mg.%. Periods 14 and 15 were test periods in which the phosphorus intake was increased to 907 and 819 mg. per day respectively by the inclusion of millet, peanut and more milk in the diet. The stool phosphorus showed a marked increase, while the urinary phosphorus was not much changed in quantity so that it amounted to only 30% of the total output. The phosphorus balance increased to 221 mg. per day, and the serum inorganic phosphorus came up to 5.36 mg.%. There was practically no change in the level of serum calcium, but the calcium balance showed a distinct improvement, averaging 460 mg. per day. In the post-control period (period 16), the serum inorganic phosphorus promptly returned to the precontrol level, the phosphorus balance became markedly negative and there was a corresponding decrease of calcium balance. In this patient the chemical alterations following the increase of diet phosphorus were not as marked as in the previous cases. This is partly due to the poorer general condition of the patient. He tolerated the high phosphorus diet so poorly that he succeeded in finishing the prescribed diet only for the first period (period 14), and the food intake during the subsequent two periods was considerably reduced. The blood non-protein nitrogen increased from 43 to 86 mg.% after two periods of increased nitrogen intake incident to the increase of diet phosphorus.

Summary. As summarized in Table 2, the most marked and consistent changes following an increase of phosphorus intake in these cases of advanced renal insufficiency consisted of a rise of the serum inorganic phosphorus and a retention of phosphorus. This increased intake also led to larger phosphorus output in the stool and somewhat larger excretion in the urine except in Case 4 during the soluble phosphate administration. Here with a ratio of calcium to phosphorus intake as low as 0.26, the kidneys were forced to bear most of the burden of increased phosphate elimination. The serum calcium usually bore an inverse relationship to the serum inorganic phosphorus. Marked lowering of the serum calcium to the tetany level occurred when there was considerable elevation of the serum inorganic phosphorus. The calcium balance was at times improved during the high phosphorus intake periods on account of increased phosphorus retention, but when the stool phosphorus was markedly increased by such a regimen, the calcium balance was usually adversely affected. After the high phosphorus intake was removed during the post-control periods there occurred a rapid elimination of the retained phosphorus largely by way of the bowel, resulting in marked negative phosphorus balance and reversion of the serum inorganic phosphorus and calcium to the control level. The large stool phosphorus elimination then gave rise to a considerable negative calcium balance in most instances. This calcium loss brought about by the necessity of large stool elimination of phosphorus sheds an important light on the mechanism of skeletal decalcification in renal insufficiency.

This is in contrast to the studies on Farquharson and Salter and their co-workers (39, 40) on individuals with normal kidneys. The ingestion of large amounts of soluble phosphates was followed by prompt elimination. Three-fourths of the excess phosphorus excretion was urinary. The calcium balance was not influenced by the administration of phosphates.

IMPORTANCE OF CALCIUM INTAKE

The usual Chinese dietary is low in calcium and various estimates place the calcium intake at 200–400 mg. per day. Such a level of intake may be sufficient for a normal person when the calcium-conserving action of vitamin D brought about by an adequate exposure to sunlight is operative, and when extra demands for the mineral such as during pregnancy and lactation are not present. However, as soon as sunlight exposure is curtailed by prolonged indoor life and repeated reproductive cycles set in, the prevailing low calcium intake is no longer adequate to prevent the mineral drainage from the skeleton. These circumstances afford an explanation for the prevalence of osteomalacia in Chinese women in the northern parts of China (41, 42). It would be of interest to examine cases of renal insufficiency to see if a low calcium diet can be a factor in the development of the osseous decalcification. In Table 3, are set forth the average daily calcium and phosphorus balances, together with serum calcium and inorganic phosphorus observed after from 2 to 4 periods on low calcium diets. These diets contained from 96 to 415 mg. of calcium per day or from 6.4 to 10.9 mg. per kg. of body weight per day. Such levels of calcium intake were most probably not less than what these patients used to take at home especially in view of their poor appetite. Normal Chinese on similar calcium intake (38) may be expected to maintain themselves in balance especially toward the end of several metabolic periods, where physiological adjustment comes into play. On the contrary these patients showed persistently negative calcium balance, averaging from 18 to 87 mg. per day. Such calcium loss, when prolonged for months or years, as it was most likely so in these cases, would inevitably lead to sufficient skeletal decalcification to be evident clinically. Therefore the prevailing low calcium intake in the Chinese diet is an important factor in the pathogenesis of the osseous disorder in renal insufficiency.

One would, then, expect a high calcium intake to be beneficial in such cases. From Table 3, it may be seen that when the calcium intake was raised approximately from 800 mg. in Case 1 to 1900 mg. in Case 3, all the calcium balances became positive. The average daily gain of calcium varied from 63 to 346 mg. It is true that some of these gains were small, but the maintenance of a positive balance for prolonged periods would add substantially to the skeletal store and alleviate the osseous changes.

The favorable influence of a high calcium intake did not stop at the improve-

ment of the calcium balance.   The effect on phosphorus balance of a high calcium intake was not uniform, because, on one hand, the increased stool calcium
would favor the elimination of phosphorus by the bowel, tending to decrease
phosphorus retention, and, on the other hand, better calcium retention might
lead to better phosphorus retention for deposition in the bones.   The resulting
phosphorus balance would, then, be the algebraic sum of the two processes which
went on at varying rates in various cases.   Thus one finds that the phosphorus
balance was improved by high calcium intake in Cases 1 and 4, impoverished in
Cases 2 and 3 and unchanged in Case 5.

However varied were the effects of high calcium intake on the phosphorus
balance, the response of the serum inorganic phosphorus was most uniform.
In all the cases there was a fall of the serum inorganic phosphorus after the high
calcium diet.   The decrease was most marked in Case 3 (from 7.60 to 4.90 mg.%)
and least in Case 2 (from 6.25 to 5.96 mg.%).   Even in Cases 1 and 5 where the
serum inorganic phosphorus was within normal limits (4.06 and 4.07 mg.% respectively) there was a distinct decrease (to 3.26 mg.% in both cases).

Serum calcium, however, behaved irregularly.   There was a distinct increase
in 2 instances (Cases 3 and 5), slight decrease in 2 (Cases 1 and 2) and no change in
1 (Case 4).

THE FACTOR OF CHRONIC ACIDOSIS

In renal insufficiency acidosis arises on two scores.   First, the retention of
phosphate, sulphate and other undetermined acid metabolites takes up base.
Second, the conversion of urea into ammonia by the kidneys for the purpose of
eliminating acid metabolites as ammonium salts becomes deficient.   Thus more
fixed base (sodium or potassium) is drawn upon in excreting acid end-products.
Both of these processes reduce the amount of fixed base available for the bicarbonate.   A decrease of the bicarbonate content tends to decrease the pH of the
serum giving rise to acidosis.   Chronic acidosis as shown by a decrease of alkali
reserve in renal rickets was first noted by Green (43) and confirmed by Lathrop
(44), Faxen (45), Elliott (46), Salvesen (47), and almost all recent authors on
the subject.   Complete serum electrolyte studies are available in some of the
reported cases (2, 35, 47).   In view of the decalcifying effects of acidosis experimentally produced in man and animals (29–32), it is generally assumed that
acidosis is an important factor in the genesis of the osseous disorder in renal
insufficiency.   The data on the acid-base equilibrium of the serum in the
present series of cases and the results of administering alkali and acid to one of
the cases lend support to this opinion.

(a) Serum acid-base balance and electrolytes

In table 4 are compiled data on serum pH and electrolytes of the cases in this
series.   The pH was around 7.25–7.30 indicating the presence of a slight or
moderate degree of acidosis.   The lowest figure of 7.10 was obtained in Case 5
when the patient was in a very poor condition with nausea and vomiting.   The
lowering of bicarbonate was, as a whole, more marked.   Very rarely did it

exceed 20 milli-equivalents per liter, and the usual level was between 15 and 19. The chloride tended to be higher than normal in Cases 2 and 4. The phosphate showed some increase in most instances, but quantitatively the increase could only account for a small part of the loss of bicarbonate. The serum albumin was within the lower limits of normal in Cases 2 and 4, but definitely lower than normal in the rest, while the serum globulin was either normal or higher than normal. As a whole the sum of base-binding values of serum proteins was within normal limits. The sum of the anions fell short of the total base by a relatively wide margin. In Cases 3, 4 and 5, the undetermined anions varied from 6.5 to 13.2 milli-equivalents per liter. Sulphates may account for 1 or 2 m.-eq., but the rest are of unknown nature.

The total base was normal in Cases 3 and 4, but tended to be subnormal in Cases 2 and 5, especially the latter. In Case 5, the decrease of sodium was mainly responsible for the marked lowering of the total base. This patient was in poor condition with marked anorexia and vomiting during the latter part of the studies.

From the above observations, acidosis, as shown by the slight or moderate lowering of pH and marked decrease of bicarbonate, was present in all the cases. The decrease of bicarbonate was due not so much to an increase of phosphate as to an increase of undetermined anions. In Cases 2 and 4, the increase of chloride seemed to be a factor in the lowering of the bicarbonate. The presence of a chloride acidosis was found by Albright et al. (48) in a case of nephrocalcinosis with rickets and dwarfism and thought to be important in the causation of the bone disease. The loss of base contributing to the acidosis occurred only when intercurrent episodes of anorexia and vomiting, or terminal events had su er-vened. It seems that in renal osteodystrophy, chronic acidosis is a constant feature and it is comparable in extent to that produced in experimental decalcification. However, in experimental acidosis in individuals with intact kidneys, an important phenomenon is the excessive urinary calcium loss, which is absent in renal osteodystrophy. In our cases the urine calcium remained small or absent. Therefore in renal osteodystrophy if acidosis has a decalcifying effect, the resorbed calcium is not drained through the kidneys. That it may be drained through the intestine is possible in view of the augmented calcium output in the stool in 2 cases of late rickets receiving ammonium chloride (30).

(b) *The effect of alkali and acid salt on calcium and phosphorus metabolism and serum electrolytes*

Experimental data of this type were available only from Case 2 (Fig. 3 and Table 5). The study was carried through 16 four-day periods with determinations of the serum electrolytes extended for some time before and after the metabolic observations. The diet contained 919 mg. calcium, 604 mg. phosphorus and 7.58 gm. nitrogen. Periods 21–24 served as control during which the positive calcium balance averaged 210 mg. per day and the positive phosphorus balance 214 mg. per day. The serum calcium tended to decrease from 5.11 to 4.57 mg.%, while the inorganic phosphorus rose from 6.25 to 7.54 mg.%. The

serum non-protein nitrogen came up from 127 to 168 mg.%. Acidosis increased
in that the pH was 7.22 and bicarbonate was only 11.6 milli-equivalents per
liter. The patient felt definitely worse so that she could not finish the diet in
Period 24. During the next period the patient was given sodium bicarbonate,
80 cc. of molar solution (6.72 gm.) daily. This brought the serum pH up to 7.35
and bicarbonate up to 22.0 m.-eq. per liter. The serum N.P.N. went down to
131 mg.%, and continued to decrease during the subsequent periods. The serum
inorganic phosphorus tended to decrease during the period of alkali administration, and the fall became more marked in the subsequent 3 periods when it
reached 5.91 mg.%. Although the serum calcium level was somewhat depressed
while the alkali was being given, it rose to its previous value immediately after

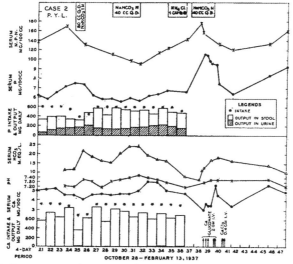

FIG. 3. CASE 2. INFLUENCE OF ALKALI AND ACID ON CALCIUM AND PHOSPHORUS METABOLISM
AND ACID-BASE EQUILIBRIUM OF SERUM

the alkali was discontinued. While the food intake during the alkali period and
the period after it was lower and irregular precluding conclusion as to the effect
of the alkali on the calcium and phosphorus balance, the clinical improvement
was so gratifying that further trial with the alkali was indicated.

By Period 27, the appetite of the patient had returned so that a quantitative
consumption of the prescribed diet was again possible. After the control observations in Periods 27 and 28, sodium bicarbonate, 40 cc. of molar solution
per day, was given in the 3 subsequent periods. In looking over the results on
the calcium and phosphorus metabolism during Periods 29–33 (Fig. 3), one notices
a progressive downward trend of the stool calcium giving rise to increasing
calcium gain, as the alkali was being administered and for some periods after
it was stopped. Although the average daily positive calcium balance of Periods
29–34 was not greater than that of the two preceding periods, the steady de-

crease of the stool calcium after alkali suggested that with the amelioration of the existing acidosis so that the pH and bicarbonate content approached normal (pH 7.40 and HCO_3 24.8 m.-eq. per liter), intestinal absorption of calcium improved, leading to better calcium balance. This improvement confirms the suggestion made before that acidosis may be associated with increased calcium loss in the stool. The increase of the serum calcium up to 6.09 mg.% was an additional evidence of improved calcium exchange. The phosphorus balance was not distinctly influenced by the alkali therapy except for a noticeable ascending trend in the urinary phosphorus elimination. The serum inorganic phosphorus was maintained below the 6 mg.% level during the alkali therapy, but it began to rise after the alkali was discontinued. Likewise after the N.P.N. decreased to a minimum of 91 mg.% at the end of alkali administration, it began to increase promptly.

Ammonium chloride in 1 gm. daily doses was given during Periods 35 and 36. The pH went down to 7.20 and bicarbonate to 8.3 milli-equivalents per liter. Thus the acidosis deepened considerably in spite of the small doses of the acid producing salt used. The serum N.P.N. rose to 142 mg.%. Clinically she felt worse again and could not finish the diet of the last period. The serum calcium and phosphorus were not much altered nor were the calcium and phosphorus balance significantly changed during the acid salt periods. However, the subsequent periods witnessed a dramatic rise of serum inorganic phosphorus and N.P.N., marked decrease of serum calcium and slight further depletion of serum bicarbonate. The patient had severe tetany with convulsions which were controlled by intravenous injections of calcium gluconate or chloride. The sodium bicarbonate solution given at this time might have aggravated the tetany, but it was responsible for correcting the acidosis and improving the renal function.

In this patient, although we were unable to witness a direct aggravating effect of ammonium chloride on the calcium and phosphorus balances, the deleterious influence on the renal function, the unfavorable changes in the serum levels of calcium and phosphorus and the systemic disturbance were impressive. The appetite was so much curtailed that adequate intake of all nutrients became impossible. Calcium intake would be especially short in view of the low calcium content of the Chinese diet. In this way chronic acidosis becomes a serious disturbing factor for the bone metabolism, not only by increasing the calcium loss through the intestine, but by curtailing the intake of all nutrients, especially calcium, through the appetite impairing influence of acidosis. The demonstration that the correction of the acidosis by alkali therapy led to an improvement of appetite and of calcium metabolism serves to emphasize the deleterious effect of chronic acidosis.

LACK OF RESPONSE TO VITAMIN D

Vitamin D, while specific in correcting the fundamental metabolic defects of rickets and osteomalacia and in rectifying the osseous changes, is without effect in cases of renal osteodystrophy. In fact, the lack of response to vitamin D has been taken as one of the important criteria for the diagnosis of the renal origin

118   S. H. LIU AND H. I. CHU

of the bone disorder. Exceptional cases have been reported by György (49), Duken (50), and Karelitz and Kolomoyzeff (51) in which the improvement in the bone condition was attributed to vitamin D. But in view of the possible spontaneous remission of the renal insufficiency in certain types of kidney disease and the lack of metabolic data, it would be difficult to appraise the value of vitamin D in these cases.

In all the 5 cases of this series, vitamin D in the usual therapeutically effective doses was thoroughly tried, and the clinical and metabolic responses were uniformly absent. In two of the cases larger doses for longer periods were also tried without effect. In two other cases of the series, the single massive dosage (1,000,000 international units of vitamin D_2) was given. One of the patients exhibited an equivocal improvement in the calcium and phosphorus metabolism,

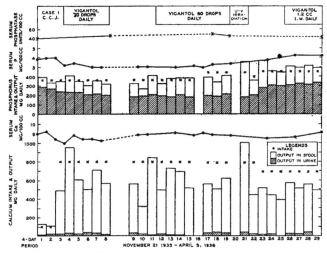

FIG. 4. CASE 1. EFFECT OF VITAMIN D ORALLY AND INTRAMUSCULARLY ON CALCIUM
AND PHOSPHORUS METABOLISM

but the other patient's response was practically negative. In view of the different experimental set-up under which the observations on the vitamin D therapy were made in the various patients, it is necessary to comment on the results individually.

Case 1. After one control period (period 3) on a constant diet with 796 mg. of calcium and 358 mg. of phosphorus per day, Vigantol in 30-drop daily doses was given by mouth for 5 consecutive periods (Fig. 4). The daily calcium balance was 312 mg. during the control period and it averaged 131 mg. for the 5 therapy periods. The daily phosphorus balance, which was 13 mg. in the control period, averaged 10 mg. for the subsequent 5 periods. The serum calcium fluctuated irregularly between 8.03 and 8.85 mg.%, although the serum inorganic phosphorus decreased from 4.06 to 3.01 mg.% through the 6 periods of observation

After a lapse of 3 weeks during which tonsillectomy was performed, meta-

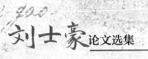
bolic studies were resumed.   Periods 9–11 served as control during which an average of 334 mg. of calcium and 24 mg. of phosphorus was retained per day. Vigantol in 60-drop daily doses was given orally during Periods 12–19.   This is equivalent to a total of 768,000 international units of vitamin D within 32 days.   Ultraviolet irradiation was given during Periods 20–21.   This massive dose of vitamin D, even with the addition of ultraviolet irradiation, did not bring about any improvement in the mineral metabolism.   In fact, the calcium balance fluctuated irregularly and averaged 191 mg. per day for Periods 12–22; likewise the phosphorus balance was irregular, averaging 9 mg. per day for the same periods.   The serum calcium remained relatively constant (8.82–9.12 mg.%), as well as the serum inorganic phosphorus (3.02–3.42 mg.%).

It was thought at the time that poor intestinal absorption might be responsible for the ineffectual oral dosage of vitamin D.   Therefore, after 3 control periods (Periods 23–25) on a new diet containing 690 mg. calcium and 454 mg. phosphorus, Vigantol in 1.2 cc. daily doses was given intramuscularly for the next 5 periods. The intramuscular route of administration of vitamin D did not prove superior to the oral dosage.   The daily calcium balance averaged 239 mg. in the control and 158 mg. during the intramuscular administration of vitamin D; and the daily phosphorus balance was 41 mg. before and −49 mg. during the therapy. There was but a slight increase of both serum calcium and inorganic phosphorus.

In contrast to ordinary rickets and osteomalacia in which the oral administration of 12,000 international units of vitamin D daily for 4 or 5 four-day periods was invariably followed by improved calcium and phosphorus absorption with large retention of these minerals (17, 52), this patient failed to respond to the same treatment.   It has been demonstrated previously (53) that a patient with osteomalacia, having received vitamin D sometime previously and still showing good mineral balance, may respond only slightly or not at all to further dosage.

This was evidently not the case in this patient as she had had no prior vitamin D therapy in the history, and the relatively small extent of calcium retention and the practical absence of phosphorus retention during the first control period were not what one would expect in a patient who had responded to previous vitamin D therapy.   Therefore one has to conclude that this patient was incapable of responding to vitamin D therapy.   The subsequent results with the second series with rather massive dosage by mouth and the third series by the intramuscular route add to the strength of this conclusion.

Case 2.   Vigantol 1 cc. daily was given for 20 days (Periods 10–14), while the patient was on a diet with 1207 mg. calcium and 675 mg. phosphorus per day (Fig. 1).   The average daily calcium balance was 173 mg. and the average phosphorus balance 8 mg.   As the vitamin D periods followed the administration of sodium phosphate (Periods 8–9) which accounted for the negative phosphorus balance during the subsequent two periods, only Periods 12–14 should be taken in computing the average phosphorus balance which then came up to 61 mg. per day.   These figures represent very slight, if any, improvement over those during Periods 6–7 which may be taken as control, namely 63 mg. of calcium and −56 mg. of phosphorus per day.   Likewise the changes in the serum calcium (from 5.91 to 6.54 mg.%) and inorganic phosphorus (from 6.29 to 5.96 mg.%) were of doubtful significance.

Case 3. After a control observation for 5 periods (Periods 1–5) on a calcium intake varying from 620 to 856 mg. and a phosphorus intake from 486 to 613 mg. per day, during which the daily calcium balance averaged 105 mg. and phosphorus balance 73 mg., Vigantol 1 cc. daily was given for 5 periods and 5 cc. daily for the next 2 periods. Thus a total of 720,000 international units of vitamin D was administered within 28 days. This constitutes a massive dose. Metabolic observations (Fig. 5) were made only during the last 4 periods (Periods 10–13). The calcium balance averaged 63 mg. and phosphorus balance −9 mg. per day.

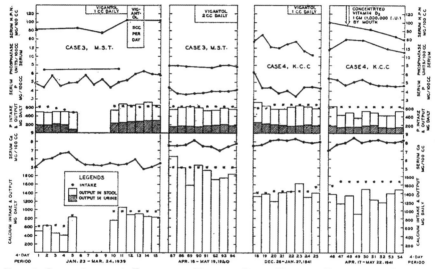

Fig. 5. CASES 3 AND 4. EFFECT OF VITAMIN D OF VARIOUS DOSAGE ON CALCIUM AND PHOSPHORUS METABOLISM

Thus the daily balances were even less favorable than during the control periods. This is all the more significant when it is noted that both the calcium and phosphorus intake were higher during the vitamin D periods than during the control. The serum calcium and inorganic phosphorus remained practically constant throughout.

Vigantol was given again a year later in 2 cc. daily doses for 5 periods (Periods 90–94) on a diet with 2009 mg. calcium and 626 mg. phosphorus. The daily calcium balance on this regimen averaged 146 mg. and phosphorus balance averaged 65 mg. These were not significantly different from those of the 3 preceding control periods. Nor were there clearcut changes in the serum calcium and inorganic phosphorus (Fig. 5).

Case 4. In this patient vitamin D was tried both in ordinary therapeutic doses and in a single massive dose (Fig. 5). Control observations were made during Periods 20 and 21 on a diet with 1451 mg. calcium and 678 mg. phosphorus per day. The patient retained on the average 136 mg. calcium and 113 mg. phosphorus daily, with the serum calcium slightly above 8 mg.% and inorganic phosphorus slightly above 4 mg.%. Vigantol 1 cc. daily was exhibited for Periods 22–25 inclusive, during which the calcium balance averaged 29 mg. and phosphorus balance averaged 60 mg. per day. The serum calcium and inorganic phosphorus showed no significant change. The observations for the next 3 periods, in which the vitamin D administration had been discontinued, likewise showed no substantial improvement in the calcium and phosphorus metabolism (See Fig. 7, Periods 26–28).

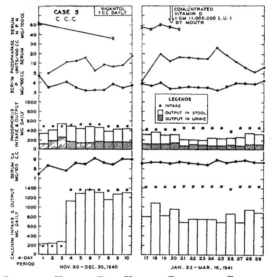

FIG. 6. CASE 5. EFFECT OF VITAMIN D OF VARIOUS DOSAGE ON CALCIUM AND PHOSPHORUS METABOLISM

On the first day of Period 48 the patient received by mouth 1 gm. of a concentrated solution of irradiated ergosterol containing 1,000,000 international units of vitamin D. The calcium intake was high (1572–1677 mg.) and phosphorus intake relatively low (624 mg.). During the control (Periods 46–47) the calcium retention was 358 mg. and phosphorus retention was 88 mg. per day; while during the next 7 periods (Periods 48–54) following the ingestion of the massive dose of vitamin D, these figures were respectively 382 and 163 mg. The serum calcium (7.91–8.15 mg.%) and inorganic phosphorus (4.63–4.60 mg.%) remained essentially constant. The response, then, even to a massive dose of vitamin D was negligible.

Case 5. This patient like the preceding one, received vitamin D at two dosage levels (Fig. 6). During Periods 7–10, Vignatol in 1 cc. daily doses was given. The average calcium balance was 96 mg. and phosphorus balance was 66 mg.

per day. These figures were not different from those of the control periods
(Periods 4–6), which were 96 and 53 mg. respectively. The serum calcium
remained at approximately 9.0 mg.%, while the inorganic phosphorus increased
slightly from 3.26 to 3.74 mg.%. Thus the response to ordinary therapeutic
doses of vitamin D was practically negative.

The single massive dose of vitamin D (1,000,000 i.u.) was given orally on the
first day of Period 20. The observations of the 3 preceding periods (Periods
17–19) served as control in which the retention of calcium amounted to 515
and that of phosphorus to 79 mg. per day. Following the massive dose of vitamin
D, the average calcium balance for the subsequent 10 periods (Periods 20–29)

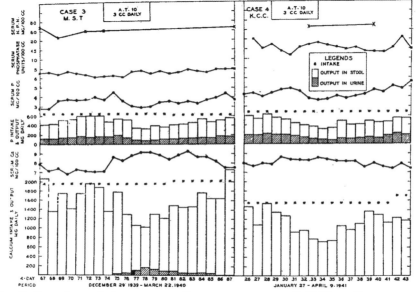

FIG. 7. CASES 3 AND 4. INFLUENCE OF DIHYDROTACHYSTEROL (A.T.10) ON CALCIUM AND
PHOSPHORUS METABOLISM

was 629 and the corresponding phosphorus balance was 193 mg. per day. While
both the calcium and phosphorus balances were somewhat improved, the improvement was slight or equivocal in comparison with the remarkable results on osteomalacia from similar dosage (54). The serum calcium remained constant, being
8.53 mg.% on the day of the massive dose and 8.61 mg.% at the end of the 10
periods. The serum inorganic phosphorus rose during the same period of time
from 3.33 to 4.18 mg.%.

Summary. All the patients were given ordinary therapeutic doses of vitamin
D and none showed any improvement in the calcium and phosphorus metabolism. Two of the patients (Cases 1 and 3) received also much larger dosage for
longer periods (respectively 768,000 and 720,000 i.u. in toto) likewise without
appreciable improvement. Of the two patients receiving the single massive

dose (1,000,000 i.u.), one (Case 4) showed practically no response and the other (Case 5) a very slight response from the standpoint of mineral metabolism. Vitamin D in ordinary therapeutic doses was given intramuscularly in Case 1, and no favorable response was elicited.

The lack of response to vitamin D may be taken to mean that renal osteodystrophy bears no etiological relationship to vitamin D. If so, one would not expect improvement in renal osteodystrophy from vitamin D therapy any more than hyperparathyroidism or osteogenesis imperfecta would be improved by the same treatment. However the anatomical changes in the bones associated with renal insufficiency may at times be indistinguishable from rickets and osteomalacia (55, 56). And both types of bone disease have certain metabolic defects in common, namely poor absorption of calcium through the intestine with large quantities of calcium in the stool, absence or negligible amounts of calcium in the urine, and hypocalcemia. Thus there is still room for the consideration that renal osteodystrophy is related to vitamin D not from any deficiency in the intake of the vitamin or in the exposure to sunlight as in osteomalacia and rickets, but from an interference with the action of the vitamin conditioned by renal insufficiency. With advanced renal impairment phosphate is retained in the blood and tissue fluids, leading to a high concentration in the intestine. The presence of large amounts of phosphate in the bowel precipitates calcium, rendering the latter difficult of absorption. While vitamin D improves the absorption of calcium in conditions where poor absorption is due to vitamin D deficiency, it may not be able to remedy a similar difficulty arising from the calcium being diverted to enable phosphorus elimination by the intestine. Such a viewpoint may hold true in advanced renal insufficiency such as Cases 2–5, where high concentration of inorganic phosphorus in the serum, large stool phosphorus and small urinary phosphorus excretion did exist. But in Case 1 where the renal impairment was only moderately severe, and consequently the urinary tract still constituted the main route of phosphorus elimination, and the serum inorganic phosphorus remained at normal level, the ineffectiveness of vitamin D in promoting calcium absorption could not be due to an interference by the high stream of phosphorus going from the blood to the intestine. We have seen cases of osteomalacia with only a slight impairment of renal function, but already showing poorer, slower or less well-sustained improvement in mineral metabolism after vitamin D therapy (53, Case 1). An alternative explanation which will take into consideration those milder cases of renal damage showing poor or no response to vitamin D would be that in renal insufficiency a certain factor is produced or retained which inactivates vitamin D, rendering it ineffectual. Such a hypothesis is difficult to investigate. But as shown in the following section, A.T.10 is effective in promoting calcium and phosphorus absorption and deposition in the bones in renal osteodystrophy just as in ordinary osteomalacia. This lends support to the hypothesis of vitamin D inactivation, and further suggests that such an inactivation, if it exists, is chemically specific for vitamin D and not generally applicable to other calcium absorption promoting compounds like A.T.10.

124   S. H. LIU AND H. I. CHU

FAVORABLE EFFECT OF DIHYDROTACHYSTEROL (A.T.10)

Dihydrotachysterol (A.T.10) is one of the products of irradiation of ergosterol, first used by Holtz in 1933–34 (57, 58) for the treatment of hypoparathyroid tetany with prompt rise of serum calcium and relief of symptoms. The efficacy of A.T.10 in the therapy of various forms of tetany has been confirmed by a host of observers (59–65). Metabolic observations by Albright and co-workers (66) on hypoparathyroidism showed that A.T.10 promotes calcium absorption by the intestine and increases phosphorus elimination by the kidneys. In rickets they (67) observed that while calcium is absorbed and retained after A.T.10 therapy, very little phosphorus is retained, thus concluding that this compound is not antirachitic. However Shohl and co-workers (68, 69) demonstrated antiricketic effect of A.T.10 in experimental rickets in the rat. Our own observations on 3 cases of osteomalacia (70) show that A.T.10, like vitamin D, promotes calcium absorption by the intestine followed by increased phosphorus absorption. The absorbed elements are retained for the replenishment of the depleted bone store and for the elevation of the serum calcium and phosphorus levels when these are low. While these favorable effects on osteomalacia from A.T.10 wear off quickly after its discontinuation in contrast to the prolonged after-effect of vitamin D, they are striking while the therapy is being given. It is therefore of interest and importance to ascertain the effect of A.T.10 in renal osteodystrophy where the difficulty of intestinal absorption cannot be rectified by vitamin D administration. Metabolic observations on A.T.10 are available in 2 cases of renal osteodystrophy in this series.

Case 3. The control observations were made during Periods 67–73 on a constant diet with 1952 mg. of calcium and 642 mg. of phosphorus per day (Fig. 7). The calcium output was all in the stool, and the average daily positive balance was 217 mg. The phosphorus excretion was 27% in the urine and the daily average positive balance was 170 mg. Throughout the 7 control periods the serum calcium fell from 7.87 to 7.08 mg.%, while the serum inorganic phosphorus rose from 2.77 to 3.72 mg.%. These changes in the serum levels of calcium and phosphorus were due to the discontinuation of ferric ammonium citrate therapy (see Section on Effect of Iron and Fig. 8). A.T.10 was given by mouth in 3 cc. daily doses for 5 periods (Periods 74–78). One notices immediately a decrease of both stool calcium and phosphorus with improved balances. As the therapy was continued, calcium began to appear in the urine in significant amount and by the 5th period of the treatment it amounted to 163 mg. per day—a remarkable figure considering the fact that in this as well as in other patients with renal osteodystrophy, absence or presence of a trace only of urinary calcium was a constant finding. The stool calcium continued to diminish so that during the last period of A.T.10 treatment, in spite of the large urinary calcium, the daily balance amounted to 927 mg. or 47% of the intake. The average daily calcium balance for the 5 periods together was 652 mg. or 33% of the intake. The phosphorus excretion in the stool, as well as in the urine, also steadily diminished so that the daily phosphorus retention during the last A.T.10 period came up to 318 mg. or 50% of the intake. The average daily phosphorous balance was

207 mg. or 33% of the intake. The serum calcium rose from 7.08 to 9.18 mg.% through the 5 periods of A.T.10 administration, while the serum inorganic phosphorus showed a diminution from 3.72 to 3.04 mg.%.

After A.T.10 therapy was discontinued from Period 79 the stool calcium began to increase and urinary calcium began to decrease so that in the course of 8 or 9 periods the pre-A.T.10 state was reached. Likewise the stool phosphorus, as well as the urinary phosphorus gradually increased to approach the previous values in the same period of time. The serum calcium decreased from 9.18 to 7.52 mg.% and phosphorus increased from 3.04 to 4.39 mg.% at the end of Period 86.

Case 4. Periods 26–28 served as control with a calcium intake of 1550 mg. and a phosphorus intake of 678 mg. per day (Fig. 7). The output of calcium was all in the stool leaving an average daily balance of 153 mg.; while the phosphorus elimination was 34% in the urine with an average daily balance of 86 mg. The serum calcium remained at 8 mg.% and the serum inorganic phosphorus at a little over 4 mg.%. A.T.10 was given by mouth during Periods 29–33 in 3 cc. daily doses. Like the preceding case, both the calcium and the phosphorus in the stool began to decrease during the first therapy period and continued to to do so throughout the following periods. Unlike the previous patient the urinary calcium remained absent or in negligible amount, although the urinary phosphorus diminished steadily. The maximum retention of calcium was 815 mg. and that of phosphorus was 359 mg. per day; both amounted to 53% of their respective intake and occurred during Period 34, the period just after the discontinuation of the A.T.10 administration. The serum calcium rose from 7.92 to 8.55 mg.% and the serum inorganic phosphorus fell from 4.41 to 3.68 mg.%.

The post-control observations showed a gradual reversal of the above described changes. From Period 35 onward, the stool calcium and phosphorus, as well as the urinary phosphorus, steadily increased so that the calcium balance approached the pre-A.T.10 level in Period 39, the 6th period after the withdrawal of the therapy, and the phosphorus balance behaved similarly 3 or 4 periods later. The serum calcium decreased from 8.55 to 7.40 mg.% and the serum inorganic phosphorus rose from 3.68 to 5.14 mg.% in the course of 8 periods (from Period 34 to 41).

Summary. The favorable influence of dihydrotachysterol on the calcium and phosphorus metabolism in renal osteodystrophy is remarkable. The primary action of this drug seems to be the improvement of the intestinal absorption of calcium and also of phosphorus, thus reducing both the stool calcium and phosphorus. A small part of the absorbed calcium was eliminated by the kidneys in Case 3 and none appeared in the urine in Case 4. The maximal retained calcium amounted to 47% and 53% of the intake respectively. The conservation of phosphorus, on the other hand, was brought about by a diminution of both stool and urine elimination. The maximum daily phosphorus retention recorded for the two patients was respectively 50 and 53% of the intake. While a minute part of the retained calcium went to increase the serum level, the major portion must be deposited, together with the retained phosphorus, in the tissues, presumably the bones. The phosphorus deposited in the tissues is contributed to also by that present in the serum, as there was a fall in the level of serum inorganic phosphorus in both cases during the therapy.

The above described metabolic results in renal osteodystrophy from A.T.10 therapy are somewhat superior to those in ordinary osteomalacia from the same treatment (70) and the favorable after-effects of the therapy appear to last somewhat longer in the former than in the latter condition. Compared with the results of the specific vitamin D therapy in rickets and osteomalacia, the maximum mineral retention brought about by A.T.10 in renal osteodystrophy is just as excellent. In fact the improvement of calcium and phosphorus metabolism in renal osteodystrophy with the administration of A.T.10 appeared so encouraging that we venture to suggest that if it were possible to maintain the therapy for a sufficiently long period of time, the skeletal decalcification would be rectified and the general well being of the patient would be improved.

That dihydrotachysterol promotes absorption and retention of calcium and phosphorus in osteomalacia with normal kidneys as well as in renal osteodystrophy indicates that renal insufficiency makes no difference to its action. In contrast to A.T.10, vitamin D is incapable of exerting similar effect as soon as renal insufficiency supervenes. The fact that this is true of milder grades of renal functional impairment without retention of phosphate and shift of phosphate excretion from the kidneys to the intestine suggests that it is not so much the peculiar type of difficulty of intestinal absorption in renal insufficiency that can not be surmounted by vitamin D as a nullification of its action inherent in renal insufficiency. Specific inactivation of vitamin D as the result of a factor retained or produced in renal functional impairment is a distinct possibility, although no direct proof is available.

EFFECT OF IRON

In the course of a study of a case of osteomalacia in pregnancy the coexisting anemia indicated the use of iron. Large doses of ferric ammonium citrate were then given. While the anemia did not improve, it was accidentally discovered that the serum inorganic phosphorus decreased and calcium slightly increased, associated with a marked increase of the stool phosphorus and a slight decrease of the phosphorus balance (71). In view of the well known fact in elementary chemistry that a soluble ferric salt precipitates phosphate from a solution by forming insoluble ferric phosphate, similar chemical reaction probably happens in the intestinal canal. Such a precipitation would limit the absorption of phosphorus and thus lower the serum inorganic phosphorus. The serum calcium would rise partly in response to the fall of the inorganic phosphorus and partly due to the calcium-sparing action of iron in precipitating phosphate in the intestinal tract. Such a procedure should remedy the situation encountered in renal osteodystrophy where the phosphate retention leads to a high concentration of phosphate in the intestine which, in turn, precipitates calcium and limits its absorption. Ferric ammonium citrate was accordingly tried on two patients of this series, and the metabolic observations are as follows:

Case 3. On a constant diet with 1978 mg. of calcium and 707 mg. of phosphorus, the control observations during Periods 30–32 showed that the average daily retention of calcium was only 67 mg. and that of phosphorus −22 mg. (Fig. 8). The serum calcium tended to increase (from 5.14 to 5.82 mg.%) and inorganic phosphorus to lower (from 4.19 to 3.72 mg.%). Ferric ammonium citrate 6 gm. daily was started from Period 33 and continued through Period 45 (altogether 52 days) after which the patient was discharged (July, 1939). The metabolic observations were made only during the first two periods of iron therapy in which the stool calcium was definitely decreased giving rise to an average daily gain of 410 mg. of calcium, and the phosphorus balance also showed slight improvement, averaging 32 mg. per day. The serum calcium and inorganic phosphorus were followed up throughout the periods of iron therapy when

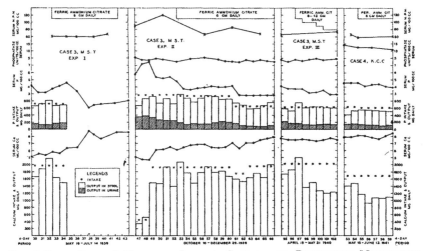

FIG. 8. CASES 3 AND 4. EFFECT OF IRON ON CALCIUM AND PHOSPHORUS METABOLISM

the high calcium intake was also maintained. The serum calcium gradually rose from 5.82 to a maximum of 9.00 mg.% during Period 38; from then on it fell somewhat but maintained a little over 8 mg.%. The serum inorganic phosphorus level initially tended to rise from 3.72 to 4.60 mg.%, but later it fell rather precipitously to a minimal value of 1 mg.% during Period 38. After this minimum had been reached, it gradually increased to and maintained itself at 2 mg.%.

The patient was readmitted in October 1939 and metabolic observations were repeated. From Period 49 to 52 the control observations on a diet with 1915 mg. of calcium and 962 mg. of phosphorus revealed an average daily balance of 346 mg. of calcium and 146 mg. of phosphorus (Fig. 8, Exp. II). The serum calcium rose from 4.74 to 6.14 mg.% and the serum inorganic phosphorus fell from 7.60 to 4.90 mg.%, apparently from an increase of the calcium intake as discussed under the Section on Importance of Calcium Intake. But the figures for the last of the 4 control periods may be taken as the base line for subsequent comparison. Ferric ammonium citrate 6 gm. daily was given from Period 53 to 66. During these 14 periods of iron therapy the calcium balance fluctuated irregularly but on the average it was less than during the control periods, namely, 157 mg. per day. The phosphorus balance was also less than the control, being 39 mg. per day for Periods 53–60, and −41 mg. per day for Periods 61–66 when a lower phosphorus containing diet was used. The serum calcium increased from 6.14 to 7.87 mg.% in the course of the 14 periods of iron therapy, while the serum inorganic phosphorus decreased from 4.90 to 2.77 mg.%, the rate of decrease being accelerated during the last 6 periods of lower phosphorus intake. These changes could be properly attributed to the iron administration because during the next 4 periods (Periods 67–70, Fig. 7) without iron, both the calcium and phosphorus balances increased to 310 and 170 mg. per day respectively with a fall of the serum calcium and a rise of the serum inorganic phosphorus.

In April-May 1940, the patient was observed for the third time in regard to the effect of iron therapy (Fig. 8, Exp. III). The control periods (Periods 95–96) followed the cessation of Vigantol administration which apparently had no effect on the mineral metabolism. During these periods the average daily retention consisted of 216 mg. of calcium and 76 mg. of phosphorus. Ferric ammonium citrate was then administered in the following daily doses: 6 gm. in Period 97, 8 gm. in Periods 98–99, 10 gm. in Period 100 and 12 gm. in Periods 101–102. The patient tolerated well the gradual increase of the dosage. The calcium balance showed marked improvement, averaging 564 mg. daily, while the phosphorus balance a slight but definite decrease, amounting to −16 mg. per day. The serum calcium, however, remained almost unchanged at the level of 7.50 mg.%, while the serum inorganic phosphorus decreased from 3.70 to 2.96 mg.%.

Case 4. This patient received iron towards the end of a long series of metabolic studies. The control observations during Periods 53–54 showed an average daily retention of 238 mg. of calcium and 149 mg. of phosphorus. The serum calcium (7.91–8.15 mg.%) and inorganic phosphorus (4.55–4.60 mg.%) were fairly constant. Ferric ammonium citrate in 6 mg. daily doses was given from Period 55 to 59, during which the calcium balance improved markedly, averaging 604 mg. per day, while the phosphorus showed a slight but definite decline, the average being 74 mg. daily. The serum calcium rose slightly from 8.15 to 8.43 mg.%, while the serum inorganic phosphorus fell from 4.60 to 3.94 mg.% through the periods of iron administration (Fig. 8).

Summary. The data on the administration of iron in the two cases are summarized in Table 6. The results are on the whole favorable. The most consistent change was a decline of the serum inorganic phosphorus level. The decline was definite in all the four trials, and most pronounced in the first trial in Case 3. As a rule the serum calcium tended to rise. This tendency was marked in the first and second trials in Case 3, slight in Case 4 and absent in the third trial in Case 3. It is to be noted that in the latter two instances the initial values of 7.50 and 8.15 mg.% were much higher than those in the former, sug-

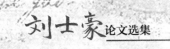

gesting that the initial height of the serum calcium level bore an inverse relationship to the extent of improvement attainable through the administration of iron.

The phosphorus balance showed a decline in all instances except the first trial in Case 3 in which the increase of phosphorus retention was relatively slight and the results obtained were from only two metabolic periods. When a decline in phosphorus balance occurred, it was invariably brought about by an increase in the stool excretion of phosphorus, thus compatible with the hypothesis that iron precipitates phosphate in the intestine and limits its absorption.

In the second trial in Case 3, the calcium balance decreased slightly following iron therapy, but it registered a substantial increase in all the rest. It was difficult to explain the decrease of calcium balance in that particular instance except that iron sometimes gives diarrhea and calcium may not be absorbed because of hurried bowel motility. Although there was no actual diarrhea during the second trial of iron therapy, the stool weight and nitrogen were higher than in the rest, suggesting increased intestinal activity. However the majority of instances were associated with an improvement in the calcium balance and the improvement was considerable. This indicates that iron does, as a rule, increase calcium absorption probably through its calcium-sparing action in combining with phosphate in the intestine.

The influence of iron on the calcium and phosphorus metabolism has received considerable attention experimentally. Cox, Dodds, Wigman and Murphy (72) demonstrated that aluminum or ferric iron added to the ration of guinea pigs and rabbits caused marked lowering of the bone ash and serum phosphorus. Using rats and adding ferric chloride to a non-rachitogenic ration, Brock and Diamond (73) produced severe rickets. Deobald and Elvehjem (74) found that chicks placed on a normal ration to which was added large amounts of soluble iron or aluminum salts developed severe rickets in 1 or 2 weeks. These authors warned against the possible danger of using large doses of iron in the treatment of hypochromic anemia. Rhem and Winters (75) found that the addition of ferric chloride to combine with one-half of the phosphorus of the diet of the rat resulted in a considerable reduction in the ash, calcium and phosphorus contents of the bodies of the animals. The influence of high phosphorus on iron metabolism has also been studied (76–78).

From the standpoint of human nutrition, Barer and Fowler (79) found that in a series of 19 patients with anemia or arthritis, the administration of ferric ammonium citrate up to 3 gm. per day failed to give rise to significant or consistent alteration in the calcium, phosphorus or nitrogen balance. Iron therapy in renal osteodystrophy with the view to facilitating the excretion of phosphate by the intestine and thereby to lower the serum phosphate has not been reported in the literature, as far as we are aware. The fact that such results could be accomplished in two cases reported above justifies further trial with this form of medication in other cases of renal osteodystrophy. The calcium balance is usually improved, but at times adversely affected by the ingestion of large doses of ferric salts in instances where diarrhea or increased bowel activity is induced. The presence of anemia in renal osteodystrophy seems to be an additional in-

130　　　　　　　S. H. LIU AND H. I. CHU

dication for the iron therapy, but this is doubtful because the anemia usually does not respond to such treatment.

PATHOGENESIS

The foregoing observations demonstrate that in advanced renal insufficiency the excretion of phosphorus by the kidneys is hampered, resulting in an elevation of serum phosphorus and appearance in the stool of larger amounts of phosphorus than normal under similar levels and ratios of calcium to phosphorus intake. The increased stool phosphorus elimination is accompanied by a negative calcium balance when the dietary calcium is low or moderate and by a relatively small calcium retention when the calcium intake is high. Thus the necessity of intestinal excretion of phosphorus hinders calcium absorption, supporting the theory of Mitchell that a shift of phosphorus excretion from the kidneys to the intestine results in calcium starvation and thereby osseous disorder. A more striking demonstration of the same train of events is afforded by increasing the phosphorus intake. Under increased strain, the serum phosphorus shows further elevation and the intestinal excretion of phosphorus assumes greater prominence. The excessive intestinal excretion of phosphorus tends to last for some time after the increased phosphorus feeding is discontinued. The calcium loss becomes evident during these post-phosphorus feeding periods when negative phosphorus balance prevails on account of the excess phosphorus being slowly eliminated by the intestine.

While the excessive intestinal excretion of phosphorus by reason of renal insufficiency plays an important role in the genesis of the osseous disorder, we believe that chronic acidosis usually present in such cases is also a serious factor. It is true that when acidosis induced in individuals with normal kidneys drains the skeletal store, it is evidenced by an excessive calcium and phosphorus output in the urine; and that this is absent in renal osteodystrophy. But in the latter condition, failing excretion by the kidneys, the minerals resorbed from the bones may be disposed of through other channels. The possibility that part of the excess calcium and phosphorus present in the intestine is derived from the skeleton on account of the decalcifying effects of acidosis cannot be excluded. Apart from its possible direct effect on the skeleton, acidosis aggravates the general condition of the patient, leading to impairment of appetite, thus curtailing the intake of all nutrients, including calcium. Chronic calcium starvation would be of serious import to the bone metabolism.

This leads to the consideration of a third factor in the genesis of the skeletal disorder in renal osteodystrophy which is especially important in China. The prevailing low calcium intake in the usual Chinese dietary is incapable of maintaining patients with advanced renal insufficiency in calcium balance. These patients require greater amount of calcium than normal in order to offset the augmented intestinal output of calcium. Therefore subsistence on a low calcium diet would render the osseous disease manifest earlier or more acutely than on a high calcium intake when renal insufficiency exists.

All the three factors enumerated above contribute to produce a lack or deficiency in the absorption or assimilation of calcium, which must have an important bearing on the skeletal decalcification in renal osteodystrophy. Such a defective mechanism of absorption and assimilation is not susceptible to rectification by the administration of vitamin D which is specific in remedying a similar defect in rickets and osteomalacia. One might suppose that the defective absorptive state in renal insufficiency, being brought about by the necessity of large intestinal excretion of phosphorus, differs fundamentally from that in rickets or osteomalacia, and is therefore not expected to improve by vitamin D. This supposition may hold true in advanced renal insufficiency in which phosphate retention and large phosphate excretion by the intestine have been demonstrated to be present, but it can not be applied to cases of milder renal functional impairment where such phenomena are not yet evident. The fact that milder cases of renal insufficiency with associated osteodystrophy are also incapable of being improved by vitamin D speaks for some alternative hypothesis to explain its inefficacy. It is possible that renal functional impairment even before it is advanced results in a condition by which vitamin D is inactivated or otherwise nullified in its action of promoting calcium absorption. The fact that A.T.10 promotes calcium absorption equally as well in renal osteodystrophy as in osteomalacia and rickets suggests that the difficulty in calcium absorption in the former condition can be surmounted. The efficacy of A.T.10 in this respect cannot be attributed to its stronger action in promoting calcium absorption, compared with vitamin D, for this is not found to be the case in comparative studies of the two drugs in hypoparathyroidism (66) and in osteomalacia (70). It seems as if A.T.10 is able to exert its full effect irrespective of the status of renal function, while vitamin D is hampered in its action as soon as renal function is interfered with. In other words, there seems to be a specific inactivation of vitamin D conditioned by renal insufficiency.

If the above hypothesis is correct, renal osteodystrophy may be regarded as a result of vitamin D deficiency, not from a lack of its intake, but from its inactivation peculiar to renal insufficiency. In this sense, terms like renal rickets and renal osteomalacia may find their full justification. The clinical and pathological picture of these conditions need not be identical with that of rickets and osteomalacia in view of such modifying factors as chronic acidosis and hyperparathyroidism secondary to renal disease.

The data on the present series of cases do not help to decide whether secondary hyperparathyroidism is an important factor in the causation of the bone disease in renal osteodystrophy. While this hypothesis has been advocated in view of the frequent occurrence of diffuse parathyroid hyperplasia and of osteitis fibrosa cystica in cases of renal osteodystrophy, it has not been generally accepted. The presence of rickets-like changes in the epiphysis which are absent in primary hyperparathyroidism in children, as pointed out by Albright et al. (2), is a serious objection, among others, to the theory of secondary hyperparathyroidism being responsible for the bone changes in renal osteodystrophy.

TREATMENT

The ultimate prognosis in renal osteodystrophy is bad in view of the irreparable kidney damage in these cases, but we feel that certain procedures may be instituted to improve the general condition of the patient, to alleviate the acidosis and to promote calcium and phosphorus assimilation. In this way the general well being of the patient will be enchanced and the bone condition will be ameliorated.

1. Diet

In view of the renal functional impairment, a diet, limited in protein and phosphorus contents but optimal in all other respects, should be given. The daily intake of phosphorus should not exceed 500–600 mg. A large intake of calcium is also necessary to offset the drain on the skeletal store. A minimum of 1 gm. of calcium a day should be taken. If this intake can not be attained by dietary means, it should be supplemented by calcium lactate or calcium gluconate. The improvement reported by Salvesen (47) in his case of renal rickets was attributed to a large calcium intake.

2. Alkali

In view of the deleterious effects of acidosis, this should be corrected. The administration of sodium bicarbonate or a sodium citrate—citric acid mixture as used by Albright et al. (48) in a case of nephrocalcinosis is indicated. The dosage is so adjusted as to maintain a normal pH and bicarbonate content of the serum. Schoenthal and Burpee (35) and Graham and Oakley (80) have stressed the value of alkali administration in renal rickets. They find that correction of acidosis results in improvement in renal function. With this our observations agree; and in addition a normal acid-base status seems to favor calcium assimilation. The only drawback of alkali administration is the tendency to produce tetany. In such cases either the dosage of alkali must be reduced or intravenous calcium gluconate be given.

3. Dihydrotachysterol

Since one of the fundamental defects of renal osteodystrophy is poor intestinal absorption of calcium, therapy should be directed to the circumvention of this difficulty. Vitamin D is ineffective in this regard. Dihydrotachysterol (A.T.10) was found to promote calcium absorption in 2 of our cases in which this treatment was tried. The increased calcium absorption led to increased phosphorus absorption and to deposition in the bones of both of these elements. This form of therapy appears to be so gratifying that it should be tried in other cases. In view of its after-effect being not long sustained following its discontinuation, A.T.10 ingestion should be maintained for prolonged periods in order to secure substantial replenishment of the skeletal store.

4. Iron

Ferric ammonium citrate facilitates the intestinal excretion of phosphorus by the formation of insoluble ferric phosphate. This spares the amount of calcium necessary for combining with phosphate to enable the excretion of the latter by the intestine. Hyperphophatemia, an evidence of strain on the kidneys, is usually promptly relieved by the ingestion of iron. Therefore such therapy is indicated in cases of renal osteodystrophy with marked elevation of serum inorganic phosphorus. Occasionally iron, in large doses, causes diarrhea, and in such cases it should be discontinued.

SUMMARY AND CONCLUSIONS

1. Metabolic observations on 5 cases of renal osteodystrophy are presented. The bone lesions varied from slight or moderate osteoporosis with no deformities to marked rarefaction with gross deformities. In two cases rachitis-like changes were also present in the epiphyses. The nature of the kidney disease in these cases was not determined; the renal insufficiency was moderate in one case and far advanced in the rest.

2. In the cases of advanced renal insufficiency difficulty in renal excretion of phosphate was evidenced by a relatively small percentage of urinary phosphorus, and by hyperphosphatemia. Such evidence could be brought out more clearly by increasing the phosphorus intake. Calcium balance was negative on low or moderate calcium intake and slightly positive on high calcium intake. Large stool excretion of phosphorus after increased phosphorus intake was usually followed by calcium loss even on high calcium intake.

3. Chronic acidosis of moderate degree was present in all the cases. Alkali administration alleviated the acidosis with improvement of renal function and favorable effect on the calcium metabolism.

4. The response to ordinary therapeutic doses of vitamin D was absent in all the cases, and it was meager even to massive doses. In contrast to vitamin D, dihydrotachysterol (A.T.10) was found to be remarkably effective in promoting calcium and phosphorus absorption and their deposition in the skeletal store. Iron was found to be efficacious in relieving hyperphosphatemia and in sparing calcium in the intestinal elimination of phosphorus.

5. In the pathogenesis of renal osteodystrophy the lack of response to vitamin D even in cases of mild degree of renal insufficiency was thought to be significant and to suggest the possibility of inactivation of vitamin D as a result of renal functional impairment. This was considered to be of primary importance in the genesis of the bone disease. A shift of phosphate excretion from the kidneys to the intestine and marked acidosis, only present in advanced renal insufficiency, were important aggravating factors.

6. For treatment, a low phosphorus, low protein and high calcium diet, alkali, dihydrotachysterol and iron were indicated. The results with dihydrotachysterol were particularly recommendable.

Acknowledgment. The authors are indebted to Drs. T. F. Yu, H. C. Chao and H. C. Hsu and a large number of housestaff and nurses who served on the metabolism ward during the last six years during which the data on the patients herein reported were accumulated.

APPENDIX

Case 1. C. C. J., a Chinese girl of 8 was admitted on November 11, 1935, for underdevelopment since birth and polyuria, polydipsia and pain in the lower extremities since 1933. The parents were both 40 years of age, living and well. The patient was the eldest child. Three younger sisters were healthy. The patient was born spontaneously at full term. She was breast fed until the end of the first year when a diet of cereals, vegetables, fish and chicken was substituted. She disliked pork and eggs, and no cod liver oil was received. She began to walk and to talk after her first birthday. Her first tooth erupted in her 13th month. She was considered to be small and inactive.

She had three attacks of "convulsions" together with fever in her 3rd year of life. In the spring of 1933 she was sick with scarlet fever which was complicated by otitis media and later by acute glomerulonephritis. She had general edema for some time. Her urine was always pale. After the attack of scarlet fever, urination became more frequent, 4–5 times in the day time and 1–2 times at night and each voiding was large. She began to drink more than usual. Pain in the legs and feet was frequently complained of. No apparent deformities were observed by the parents. The child failed to gain in height and weight. She was in school for a year in 1934. She had measles in the spring of 1935 and she stopped schooling since.

Physical examination. The patient was markedly underdeveloped and undernourished, 10.9 kg. in weight and 95.8 cm. in height. She was intelligent and suffered from no apparent distress. The skin was dry and scaly. The skull was of normal contour, fontanelles and sutures being closed. The ocular fundi were normal. The right ear canal was filled with mucoid discharge and the drum perforated. The left ear was normal. The tonsils were enlarged. There was no general lymphadenopathy. The neck organs were normal. The chest was slightly prominent on the left side. No rosaries or Harrison's grooves were demonstrated. The lungs were clear. The heart was not enlarged, the left border of dullness being 6 cm. from the midline in the 4th space. There was a systolic thrill at the apex which later disappeared. A loud systolic murmur was heard over the whole precordium. The blood pressure measured 100/60. The abdomen was soft, the tip of the spleen and the edge of the liver being just palpable. The extremities showed knock-knee, enlarged wrists and ankles. The spine was normal. There was no edema of legs. Tendon reflexes were normal.

Roentgenological examination showed normal findings in the skull except for a delay in dental development corresponding to that of a child of about five years. Both the deciduous and permanent teeth were well calcified. The bones of the extremities showed marked general osteoporosis with coarse trabeculation. The spaces between the epiphyses and the diaphyseal ends of the long bones at the wrists, ankles and knees were increased, particularly at the wrists. The diaphyseal ends of the radii and ulnae were flared and irregular, with a zone of marked rarefaction, about 5 mm. in width, adjacent to the margin. The radii and ulnae were so decalcified that no definite cortex could be made out in most portions. The ribs, clavicles and pelvic bones were likewise markedly osteoporotic with coarse and irregular trabeculation. Plain film of the abdomen showed no calcified shadows in the kidney regions.

Laboratory findings. The blood counts gave R.B.C. 4,680,000, Hgb. 13.5 gm., W.B.C. 11,350 and normal differential formula. The urine specific gravity was low. One plus albumin and variable amounts of glucose were constantly present. Acetone bodies were present on two occasions. The average of two Addis' urine sediment counts showed a specific gravity of 1.014 and a protein content of 0.224 gm., granular casts 261,000, hyaline casts 16,000, W.B.C. 417,000 and R.B.C. 65,000 in 12 hours. P.S.P. renal function test showed 23% excretion in 2 hours. Urea clearance was 24.3% of normal. Fasting blood sugar was 83 mg. %, N.P.N. 50 mg. % and CO_2 combining power 30 volumes %. The glucose tolerance curve was essentially normal. The plasma proteins were 3.17% albumin, and 1.92% globulin. The serum calcium was 9.02 and inorganic phosphorus 3.86 mg. %. The plasma chloride was 106 M. eq. per liter. The plasma cholesterol was 139 mg. %. The blood Wassermann test was negative. The stool contained ova of ascaris. The basal metabolic rate was +20.7% (oral temperature 37.7°C.). The electrocardiogram showed normal mechanism except for a P-R interval of 0.20 second. Intelligence test showed an I.Q. of 100.

Course in Hospital. Through the courtesy of Dr. Charles McKhann and F. T. Chu, the patient was transferred to the metabolic ward for study on November 20. After a preliminary observation on the low and the high calcium regimes the effect of Vigantol was determined. Since the calcium and phosphorus balances failed to improve under the influence of vitamin D, an interfering focus of infection was suspected. Tonsillectomy was done on January 3, 1936. Metabolic observation was repeated after the operation. Ultraviolet irradiation, in addition to vitamin D, was employed, again without any effect. The patient complained of anorexia and vomited several times. Finally Vigantol was administered intramuscularly from March 21 to April 10. The results were likewise negative. Throughout the patient's stay in the hospital from November 11, 1935 to April 15, 1936, she made only very slight gain in weight and no gain in height. Her skeletal condition remained unchanged. Her kidney function also remained low on repeated examinations. The patient was discharged on April 15. She failed to return to the clinic for follow-up.

Case 2. P. Y. L., a Chinese Mohammedan girl of 17 first came to the orthopedic clinic in August 1934, complaining of pain in the lower extremities and knock-knee for more than 2 years. She was born spontaneously but prematurely at 7th month in a poor family. She was breast fed during the first year with supplementary feedings with rice porridge and other starchy food. She never received cod liver oil. Her diet after the first year consisted of cereals and vegetables. Animal food was lacking. Her general health was delicate, but no important illnesses in her childhood were recalled. She had one attack of febrile illness at 11 which was not accompanied by sore throat or skin eruption and which subsided in 10 days. Both parents were living and well. Her mother had altogether 7 pregnancies. The first two pregnancies ended in early abortion. The patient was her first child. The subsequent 4 children all died in infancy from diarrhea, convulsion or smallpox. There was no family history of tuberculosis.

For more than two years the patient had noticed slight vague pain in both knees, particularly noticeable on standing or walking. She also noticed that her feet failed to meet each other when her knees were in contact. She could walk only slowly and her gait became awkward and unsteady. Examination in the orthopedic clinic showed that the girl was pale, underdeveloped and poorly nourished. Both knees turned inward especially the left. The leg and the thigh made an angle of about 150–160° on the lateral aspect of the knees. The knee joints were not red, swollen or limited in motion. There was no bowing of the legs. The hips and spine were normal. The serum calcium was 7.3, and inorganic phosphorus 4.0 mg. %. The patient disappeared from the clinic before examination was complete.

On April 1, 1936 the patient returned in much worse condition and was admitted to the orthopedic service. During the interval of two years she gradually had more pain in the lower extremities. In the last year a heavy sensation and then pain in the lumbar region and pelvis set in. In the course of time walking and even standing became difficult. She could only sit in bed and kept indoors most of the time. In the last six months pain appeared in the shoulder joints and the upper extremities became weak. Finally she was completely bed-ridden and could not even sit up. Frequently she had severe twitchings of the muscles of the lower extremities, particularly at night. She had no disturbance of urination, never puffiness of face or edema of legs. There was no visual disturbance. Her menstruation started at 13 with regular cycles. The flow became less in the last two periods.

Physical examination showed an underdeveloped and poorly nourished girl weighing 25.6 kg. and lying in bed helplessly with her lower extremities flexed at the hips and knees. Her skin and mucous membranes were pale. There were slightly to moderately enlarged lymph glands in the neck, submaxillary regions and axillae. The eye-grounds showed only slight retinal edema and anemia. The neck was normal and the thyroid was not enlarged. The thorax was asymmetrical, left upper being fuller with slight bulging of

S. H. LIU AND H. I. CHU

the upper part of the sternum. The breasts were poorly developed. The lungs were clear. The heart was normal in size. There was a loud blowing systolic murmur at the pulmonic area. No thrill or diastolic murmur was made out. The blood pressure was 90/56. The abdomen was soft and no organs were palpable. The external genitalia were normal, but pubic hair was scanty. The upper extremities presented no deformities. The lower extremities showed marked muscular atrophy with coxa vara, knock-knee and inverted feet. Active motion of the hip and knee joints was greatly impaired. Passive motions were possible except abduction and adduction at the hip and extension at the knees, which were accompanied by muscle pain. The pelvis showed marked rostration of the symphysis pubis. The sacrum was bent backward. Pelvic measurement showed a transverse outlet of 6 cm. There was no demonstrable bone tenderness. Tendon reflexes were all active. Chvostek and Trousseau signs were negative.

Radiological examination of the skeletal system showed that the pelvis was markedly deformed, with forward protrusion of the acetabulae, folding of the iliac blades, beaking of the symphysis pubis and forward protrusion of the lumbosacral prominence. Both ilia and ischia showed cystic bone absorption. Same changes were also seen in the heads and the greater trochanters of both femora. The spine showed marked lordosis of the lumbo-sacral region, slight biconcave deformity of the vertebral bodies with increased intervertebral spaces. The thoracic cage was flattened antero-posteriorly and assumed a slanting fashion. The ribs were osteoporotic. The long bones were moderately osteoporotic throughout. The apiphyses were fused and the joints were normal.

Laboratory examination. The urine had a low and fixed specific gravity and one plus albumin reaction. The sediments were normal. Addis' count showed a urine specific gravity of 1.010, 0.19 gm. of protein, 2,000 hyaline casts, 72,000 R.B.C. and 6,786,000 W.B.C. and epithelial cells in 12 hours. P.S.P. test showed 6% excretion in 2 hours and urea clearance averaged 12.4% of normal. Stool contained cysts of E. coli and ova of trichocephalus. The blood count gave R.B.C. 2,610,000 and Hgb. 8.7 gm. W.B.C. and differential counts were normal. The blood Wassermann test was negative. The serum calcium was 7.3 mg.%, inorganic phosphorus 4.2 mg.%, and phosphatase 29.1 units. The blood N.P.N. was 86 mg. per cent and CO_2 combining power 51.0 volumes %. Plasma proteins consisted of 3.97% albumen and 3.03% globulin. The B.M.R. was -13.4%. Cystoscopy showed normal findings. Retrograde pyelogram revealed that the kidney shadows were very small, approximately 3 x 5 cm., the right slightly larger than the left. The pelves and calices were proportionally small. The ureters were normal. No stone was seen. The urine culture was sterile.

The patient's general condition and the contracture of the lower extremities were considerably improved following admission. She cooperated very well during the period of metabolic observation. She developed symptoms and signs of tetany when she received disodium phosphate solution from May 11 to 18. They disappeared as soon as the phosphate medication was discontinued. Vigantol administration failed to influence her calcium and phosphorus metabolism. The patient was discharged on June 13, 1936, in fairly good condition but with the blood picture and kidney function unimproved.

The patient remained fairly well after discharge for only two weeks and then general aching returned. She had one attack of twitching of the lower extremities in the evening July 14, 1936. She could not walk and was confined indoors throughout the summer. She was readmitted on October 1, 1936 for further study. Physical findings remained essentially the same as during the previous admission. Her eyegrounds remained negative and blood pressure measured 104/70. Skeletal deformities showed no changes. Signs of tetany were absent. Urinalysis and blood counts were the same as before. P.S.P. excretion amounted to 3.5% in 2 hours and urea clearance averaged 9.0% of normal. The blood N.P.N. was 86 mg. per cent, CO_2 combining power 30.0 volumes per cent. Plasma albumin was 2.88% and globulin 3.42%. The serum calcium was 7.24 mg.%, inorganic phosphorus 4.82 mg.% and phosphatase 28.4 units.

During the second admission, the influence of alkali and acid on her calcium and phosphorus metabolism and serum electrolyte balance was studied. The patient had tetany and anorexia. Frequent nausea and vomiting made quantitative studies difficult. The administration of sodium bicarbonate, while aggravating the tetany, was followed by a decrease in the acidosis and azotemia with improvement of the appetite. Ammonium chloride in small doses relieved the tetany to some extent, but aggravated the bone ache, acidosis, azotemia and anorexia. Frequent intravenous injections of calcium gluconate resulted in temporary improvement. However, the kidney function became progressively worse, azotemia and acidosis becoming more marked. Convulsions were noted frequently. The patient became drowsy and finally unconscious on February 23, 1937. She was discharged in critical condition at the request of her mother for religious reasons on February 25, 1937. She died at home 5 days later. No autopsy was obtained.

Case 3. M. S. T., a Chinese married woman of 34 was first admitted to the obstetrical service on May 19, 1938, for pregnancy of 5 months, repeated bleeding from the rectum and general bone aching. The patient was apparently healthy in her childhood and before marriage. She was married in 1924 and went through two full term pregnancies in 1925 and 1928 respectively without any complication. Both children were living and well. Her third pregnancy ended in abortion at the third month in 1931. She began to have bleeding after bowel movement shortly afterwards. Bleeding continued at frequent intervals and the amount of blood loss was considerable. Gradually pallor, palpitation of heart and shortness of breath developed. In 1934 she had her fourth pregnancy and in the 6th month of gestation she developed marked anasarca. Her urine was scanty. She had palpitation of heart and shortness of breath on exertion. General bone aching and spasm of hands were also noticed. The pregnancy continued to full term and a living child was delivered spontaneously. The infant died of convulsions two days after birth. Edema, palpitation, dyspnea, bone aching and spasm of hands all subsided gradually after the parturition. The same symptoms recurred in the third month of her fifth pregnancy in 1936 and persisted till one month after a full term spontaneous delivery. The child again died but 6 days after birth. Her sixth pregnancy began in December 1937 and in February 1938 general bone aching returned and gradually became more marked so that she could not walk in the last 4 months prior to admission. Bleeding per rectum persisted and became worse, large blood clots being passed with each movement. Pallor, palpitation of heart and dyspnea on exertion also became worse. Puffiness of face and edema of legs and feet were noticed. Muscular aching and numbness of extremities were also complained of. Her diet consisted of cereals, vegetables, soybean products and occasionally meat. She took one egg every day during the second half of each of her pregnancies. Her husband was healthy and denied venereal disease.

Physical examination on admission showed that the patient was very pale and weak. Her face was puffy with a "butterfly" pigmentation. Slight pitting edema was present over the legs and dorsum of feet. Chvostek and Trousseau signs were both positive. The right cervical, both axillary and left inguinal lymph nodes were palpably enlarged. No lenticular opacities were noticed and ocular fundi showed only anemic changes. The ears, nose and throat were normal. The thyroid was not enlarged. The chest was normal in contour and free from rib tenderness. The lungs were clear. The heart was considerably enlarged with a blowing systolic murmur all over the precordium. No diastolic murmur was heard. The rhythm was regular. The blood pressure was 106/64. The abdomen was distended by the gravid uterus, the fundus of which was 1 finger breadth below the umbilicus. The liver was enlarged, the edge being 2 cm. below costal margin. The spleen was not palpable. Spine and extremities were free from deformities. There was no adductor muscle spasm. The joints were free. All ,tendon reflexes were present but low. No sensory disturbance was found. The pelvis was symmetrical and not contracted and its measurements were normal.

Laboratory examination. The blood count showed severe anemia, Hgb. 2.7 gm. and R.B.C. 1,420,000. W.B.C. count was 7,800 and differential formula included 84% neutrophils. Reticulocyte count was 1.8%. Hematocrit was 11.3%, giving a mean corpuscular volume of 80 cubic micra, mean corpuscular hemoglobin 19 micro-micro-grams and mean corpuscular hemoglobin concentration 24%. The urine contained one plus albumin with a low specific gravity 1.007. Urinary sediments contained variable number of white blood cells, occasionally in small clumps. There were no red blood cells or casts. Renal function test showed 15% excretion of P.S.P. in two hours and the urea clearance averaged 16.4% of normal. Urinary sediment count by Addis' technique gave granular casts 6,600, R.B.C. 600,000, W.B.C. 50,700,000 in 12 hours. The stool was negative for ova and parasites. The blood Wassermann test was negative. Blood chemical findings were: N.P.N. 50 mg.%, CO_2 combining power 33.8 volumes %, serum calcium 4.2 mg.%, inorganic phosphorus 3.0 mg.%, plasma albumin 3.60% and globulin 3.98%. Gastric analysis showed achlorhydria before and after histamine injection. X-ray of the pelvis and spine showed slight degree of rarefaction of all the bones and slight biconcave deformity of the lumbar vertebrae. Proctoscopic examination revealed external and internal hemorrhoids.

On account of the severe renal insufficiency and marked anemia it was considered undesirable to allow the pregnancy to go on. Termination of pregnancy by vaginal hysterotomy was done on June 2, 1938. The rectal bleeding stopped on bed rest. Calcium lactate, iron, cod liver oil and ultraviolet irradiation improved her anemia and stopped the tetany. When she was discharged on June 17, 1938, her R.B.C. count was 2,040,000, Hgb. 7.0 gm., serum calcium 6.7 mg. and inorganic phosphorus 3.5 mg.%. Her kidney function did not show any improvement.

Second admission. Throughout the summer, 1938, the patient could barely walk with a stick. She preferred to stay in bed most of the time. Pain in the lower extremities and back gradually returned and became worse with the onset of the winter. She was readmitted on January 17, 1939, to the metabolism ward where the first course of study was made. Physical examination on readmission showed that the patient weighed 40.8 kg. She had mild bone tenderness all over, with pain in the lumbar region on moving in bed. No deformities were found in the skeleton but the right shoulder was limited in abduction. Chvostek and Trousseau signs were negative. The eyegrounds showed slight arteriosclerotic changes. The right cervical lymph node was larger. Otherwise, the physical findings were essentially the same as on the first admission.

X-ray of the pelvis, spine and long bones showed only slight osteoporosis. The lungs were clear but the cardiac area measured 57% oversized. The skull was somewhat small and the inner and outer tables were moderately thickened.

The blood picture was that of moderate anemia, Hgb. 7.5 gm. and R.B.C. 2,260,000 and slight leucocytosis, W.B.C. 11,550. The urine findings were the same as before. P.S.P. excretion decreased to 2.5% in 2 hours and urea clearance averaged only 9.8% of normal. The blood N.P.N. increased to 96 mg.% and CO_2 combining power decreased to 22 volumes %. The serum calcium was 5.56 and inorganic phosphorus 3.46 mg.%. Gastric analysis showed persistent achlorhydria. The electrocardiogram showed normal findings. The basal metabolic rate was +12.7%.

Plain x-ray film of the abdomen showed small kidney shadows and retrograde pyelogram revealed normally filled calices and pelvis. They were small but proportional to the size of the kidney.

Ever since readmission in January 1939 the patient ran an irregular fever, sometimes as high as over 40°C. The cause of the fever was never well understood. Repeated blood and urine cultures were negative. Blood smears were free from parasites. Blood agglutination tests were negative. The enlarged gland on the right side of neck became softened and finally ruptured in April. A discharging sinus was formed and was slow in healing. Biopsy of the sinus tissue showed tuberculosis. The patient continued to have bleeding per rectum and hemorrhoidectomy was done on June 8, 1939. With large doses of calcium and iron the patient finally was much improved and the fever subsided in July. She was discharged on July 22, 1939, with a serum calcium of 8.68 and inorganic phosphorus of 1.67 mg.%. Anemia and kidney function remained unchanged.

Third admission. The patient remained fairly well throughout the summer and she was admitted for the third time for further metabolic observation on October 2, 1939. Physical findings were the same as on discharge in last July. She remained pale and weak. The discharging sinus on the right side of neck had healed. Few glands remained palpable beneath. The heart was still somewhat enlarged. The blood pressure measured 92/60. Slight pitting edema of the legs was present. Slight tenderness over the lumbar spine, iliac regions and lower ribs was demonstrated. Chvostek, Trousseau and Erb's signs were negative. X-ray of the long bones, pelvis and spine gave no new findings besides slight general osteoporosis. The urine contained traces of albumin, some W.B.C. and occasional granular casts but no R.B.C. Only a trace of P.S.P. was excreted in 2 hours. Urea clearance averaged 8.4% of normal. The blood count reported R.B.C. 1,670,000 and Hgb. 5.4 gm. The blood N.P.N. was 68 mg.% and CO_2 combining power 23.5 volumes %. The serum calcium was 5.22 mg.%, inorganic phosphorus 6.56 mg.% and phosphatase 6.77 Bodansky units. The plasma proteins contained 3.86% albumin and 2.82% globulin. Sternal bone marrow smear showed slightly active normocytic erythropoiesis and moderately active granulopoiesis. Gastric achlorhydria remained unchanged.

The patient remained afebrile throughout her stay in the hospital from October 1939 to May 1940. She cooperated very well in the study and consumed a 1,500 calorie diet quantitatively. After two periods of low calcium intake her serum calcium dropped to 4.67 mg.% and inorganic phosphorus increased to 7.25 mg.%. Signs of tetany were elicited but disappeared promptly after the calcium intake was raised. The serum calcium was raised by the high calcium intake and further raised by the administration of iron. Mild degree of bone pain and backache persisted. Slight bleeding from her external hemorrhoid also continued off and on. With the administration of A.T.10 her serum calcium was raised to 9.18 mg.% and she had the best calcium retention. Her bone pain and backache also definitely improved and almost entirely disappeared. After the effect of A.T.10 on the calcium and phosphorus metabolism was over, Vigantol was given another trial but without apparent benefit. Lastly she was given large doses of iron again and she was discharged in good condition on May 25, 1940.

The patient was regularly followed up since discharge and her general condition remained more or less stationary. She has been on large doses of calcium and iron most of the time. When she was seen last on June 19, 1941, she complained of more backache. X-ray of her skeleton revealed slightly more general rarefaction. The serum calcium was 6.46 mg.%, inorganic phosphorus 5.03 mg.% and phosphatase 5.67 Bodansky units. Blood N.P.N. remained high, 86 mg. per cent, and CO_2 combining power was 31.9 volumes per cent. There were no signs of tetany.

Case 4. K. C. C., a Chinese unmarried woman of 20 was admitted on May 14, 1940, with the chief complaint of generalized bone pain of 13 months' duration. The patient was born and brought up in Shansi province. She had measles in early childhood and otorrhea on the left side for one month at 15. Frequent dull headache was complained of since early childhood. There was no history of scarlet fever or tonsillitis. She never had urinary disturbance or edema. She completed primary school at 16 and then she stayed home learning household duties. Her diet was fairly adequate and sun exposure was available. In September 1938, on account of war she became a refugee living for several months in crowded quarters and on insufficient food. In November 1938 she began to experience a cold sensation in both thighs at night. In January, 1939, she developed pain in the ribs, noticeable on deep breathing and on pressure. Then pain was noticed in the ankles on walking. Tinnitus in both ears was noticed and her vision became impaired particularly at night. In March 1939 pain was also present in the popliteal space, trochanteric region and back. She had difficulty in walking and in straightening her back, obliging her to stay in bed. Her appetite was impaired. She became thin and pale. In August 1939 she developed moderate pitting edema of feet which subsided in October. Occasionally she had evening fever and night sweat. She never had muscle spasm, twitching or cramps. Her menstruation which started at the age of 16 with regular cycles became irregular and scanty in the last few months. Her family history was negative.

Physical examination revealed a well developed and fairly well nourished girl. She looked pale, and could hardly sit up in bed. The skin was dry with fairly marked follicular hyperkeratosis over both arms, less marked over both thighs, abdomen and back. There was no general lymphadenopathy. Her head organs were normal except for anemia of optic discs and chronic chorioretinitis. Neck organs were normal but the thyroid appeared full. The chest was symmetrical with well-developed breasts. Some tenderness was present in the lower ribs. The lungs were clear. The heart was normal and the blood pressure measured 106/74. The liver was not palpable and the spleen was barely felt. The spinal column was straight and the pelvis was not deformed. The upper and lower extremities were free from deformities and the joints were normal. Slight to moderate tenderness was present over all the bones. Tendon reflexes were normal. Chvostek and Trousseau signs were absent. There was some tenderness in the calves and thigh muscles.

Roentgenological examination showed that the pelvis was not deformed. The sacrum was slightly anteriorly angulated and the pelvic opening was slightly narrowed anteriorly. The pelvic bones showed osteoporosis with coarse striations. A pseudo fracture was present in the superior ramus of left pubic bone. The spine showed general osteoporosis and coarse striation without any deformity. The long bones of the upper and lower extremities were also osteoporotic with coarse trabeculae. There was no gross deformity. The epiphyseal lines of both radii and ulnae were still visible.

Laboratory examination. Urinalysis showed trace to one plus albumin and a normal sediment. Urine concentration test revealed a maximal specific gravity of 1.015. Phenolsulphonephthalein test showed 7.5% excretion in 2 hours. Blood count reported R.B.C. 2,510,000, Hgb. 6.0 gm. and W.B.C. 5,000 with normal differential formula and smear. Hematocrit studies showed microcytic normochromic anemia. The platelet count was 277,000. The stool was normal. The blood Wassermann test was negative. The blood N.P.N. was 67 mg.%, CO_2 combining power 29 volumes %. The serum calcium was 8.9 mg.%, inorganic phosphorus 4.4 mg.% and phosphatase 11.6 units. The plasma proteins consisted of 3.81% albumin and 2.51% globulin. The serum vitamin A was 12 international units and carotinoid 71 gamma per 100 cc. The basal metabolic rate was −12.4%. Gastric analysis showed no free acid in the fasting specimen and 22 units of free acid after histamine. Cystoscopy showed normal urinary bladder and the catheterized urine was sterile on culture. Retrograde pyelogram showed small kidney shadows and the pelves and calices were small but well outlined. X-ray of the chest showed normal lungs with a dense calcified nodule in the left middle area. After a short period of preliminary metabolic observation on the metabolism ward she was discharged improved on June 16, 1940.

After discharge the patient was seen regularly in the out-patient department throughout the summer 1940. Although backache and pain in the legs were still present she was able to get up and walk around for a few steps. She complained of palpitation and dyspnea. Her hemoglobin decreased to 4.4 gm. and the heart was slightly enlarged. She developed fever again in August, with poor appetite, constipation and amenorrhea. She was readmitted on October 12, 1940.

The patient presented essentially the same physical findings as on discharge except that her heart was slightly enlarged. The eyegrounds showed no new findings apart from the chronic chorioretinitis. The blood pressure remained normal (110/70). No skeletal deformities were demonstrated. Roentgenological survey of the skeleton revealed no new findings. Urine contained one plus albumin and normal sediment. Phenolsulphonephthalein excretion was only 3% in two hours and maximum urea clearance measured 9.6% of normal. The blood contained only 3.5 gm. of hemoglobin and 1,270,000 R.B.C. Blood N.P.N. was 86 mg.% and CO_2 combining power was 28.2 volumes %. The serum calcium was 8.52 mg.%, inorganic phosphorus 4.10 mg.% and phosphatase 10.76 units. Plasma proteins consisted of 4.59% albumin and 2.60% globulin.

On account of the severe anemia and an unexplained fever two blood transfusions of

400 cc. each were given shortly after readmission. Fever subsided within one week and the anemia gradually improved and continued to improve afterwards so that by the end of May 1941 the blood hemoglobin was 9.3 gm. and R.B.C. 3,700,000. However, the kidney function remained poor throughout. Regular metabolic study commenced on October 19. When the phosphorus intake was raised by the administration of trisodium phosphate the patient complained of numbness of face and extremities and her bone pain was aggravated. Chvostek and Erb signs became positive. All symptoms of tetany promptly disappeared on discontinuation of the phosphate. When a high phosphorus diet, which was also high in protein, was given, not only tetany and exacerbation of bone pain, but headache and anorexia were also present. She failed to finish her diet. The blood N.P.N. increased to a maximum of 150 mg.% and the CO_2 decreased to only 13.5 volumes per cent. All the symptoms gradually disappeared after the high phosphorus diet was stopped. Vitamin D in the form of Vigantol did not affect the patient appreciably. Although A.T.10 exerted a favorable influence on the calcium and phosphorus metabolism, there was relatively little subjective improvement. A bone biopsy done on the left tibia on April 8, 1941, showed typical changes of osteomalacia. Her appetite was impaired after the operation. On April 25 the patient was given 1,000,000 i.u. of vitamin D_2 by mouth and very slight, if any, improvement was obtained. Since May 23 iron ammonium citrate was administered with slight subjective improvement. Throughout the entire period of hospitalization the patient continued to put on weight. This increased from 42 to 52 kg. in the course of 8 months. The patient was discharged improved on June 14, 1941. She remained in fairly good condition when seen in the outpatient department in September.

Case 5. C. C. C., a Chinese Mohammedan boy of 20 was admitted to the orthopedic service on October 29, 1940, with the chief complaint of pain and swelling of the knees, progressive deformity of the lower extremities and backache of 8 years' standing. The patient was born into a poor family. His diet was poor, lacking in fresh vegetables and animal food. He was always thin in early childhood but his development was normal up to 1932. In the spring of 1932 his right knee was hurt during a fall. Apart from pain, the knee showed no external wound or impaired motion. Two weeks later it became swollen and painful on walking. The patient continued to have a limping gait for one year. Gradually pain in the lumbar spine was noticed, particularly on walking. This persisted till 1935 when the patient began to experience weakness in his lower extremities and back. Walking became difficult and he tumbled easily. In 1936 weakness became more marked and he could walk only with the help of a stick. Gradually he had difficulty in straightening his back and his lower extremities. Pitting edema was noticed in both feet and ankles. This would disappear on rest. He never noticed puffiness of face. There was frequent dizziness. He had no urinary disturbance. In July, 1940, the patient fell down again, injuring his left knee. Immediately he could not move his left lower limb and the left knee was swollen and painful. A dislocation was suspected and after manipulation by a native bone-setter the whole left thigh became swollen. Walking was impossible. Ever since his first accident in 1932 the patient's appetite had always been poor and he failed to grow any more. On the contrary, he became emaciated. He had diarrhea for one month in 1937. In 1938 he had night blindness which was cured by taking sheep liver. He had measles in early childhood. There was no history of scarlet fever or tonsillitis.

Physical examination revealed that the patient was much underdeveloped and markedly emaciated, weighing only 26 kg., and having slight fever. He was completely bedridden, unable even to sit up on account of pain in the back, hips and knees together with contractures of the lower limbs. The skin was dry and rough. The submaxillary lymphglands were enlarged. The skull was of normal contour. The ocular fundi were normal. The conjunctivae were free from xerosis and the cornea was clear. The chest showed prominent costochondral junctions of the lower ribs on both sides. There was no deformity of the sternum or Harrison's groove. The lungs were clear. The cardiac findings were normal. The blood pressure measured 84/64. The abdomen was normal. The external genitalia were underdeveloped. The spine showed left-sided scoliosis of the lower dorsal and lumbar segments. The lumbar spine was fixed, no lateral or antero-posterior motion being possible. Paravertebral muscles were spastic. The upper extremities showed marked muscular atrophy and the bones were slender with enlargement at the wrists. The fingers were slender and could be hyperextended to an unusual degree at the metacarpo-phalangeal and interphalangeal joints. The lower extremities were held in flexion deformity at the hip and knees. There was genu valgum. Both knees were moderately swollen with floating patella. A fracture was present at the lower third of the left femur, the upper segment overriding the lower giving rise to a prominence in the suprapatellar region. Tenderness and grating sensation were present. The ankles were enlarged but there was no limitation of motion. The pelvis was tilted, the right side being higher than the left. Tendon reflexes were normal. Chvostek sign was not obtained. Trousseau and Erb signs were positive.

Roentgenological examination of the skeleton showed very extensive osteoporosis in all the bones of the spine and pelvis. The trabeculae were coarse and irregular. The secondary trabeculae disappeared, resulting in a "washed out" appearance of the bones. The articulating facets were cloudy. The heads of both femora were flattened. Similar osteoporosis was present in the bones of both knees. The joint surface was intact. There was an old fracture of the lower end of the left femur. Marked patchy osteoporosis was present in the humeri, radii and ulnae. Irregularity and cupping were seen in the diaphyseal ends of the radii at the wrists. The skull showed mottling in the parietal region and thinning of the vault. X-ray of the chest showed no important changes in the lungs but a substernal shadow was present. Plain film of the abdomen showed no radiopaque stones in the kidney regions.

Laboratory examination showed that the urine contained one plus albumin but no abnormal sediment. The maximal specific gravity during a concentration test was only 1.013. Phenolsulphonephthalein excretion was 7% in two hours and maximum urea clearance averaged 13.2% of normal. The blood contained 9.2 gm. of hemoglobin, 3,410,000 R.B.C., 7,200 W.B.C. and 393,000 platelets. Hematocrit studies showed normocytic anemia. Sternal marrow smear showed normoblastic erythropoiesis. The blood Wassermann test was negative. The blood sedimentation rate was very rapid. The serum N.P.N. was 50 mg.%, CO_2 combining power, 28.2 volumes %, calcium 8.1 mg.%, inorganic phosphorus 3.6 mg.%, phosphatase 16.4 units, plasma albumin 3.63% and globulin 3.76%. The stool contained ova of ascaris. The basal metabolic rate was +1.2%. The liver function by the bromsulphthalein test and galactose tolerance test was normal. Gastric analysis showed achlorhydria. The joint fluid aspirated from the right knee was serofibrinous, containing 91,440 W.B.C. with 98.5% P.M.N. Smear and culture showed no organism. Cystoscopy showed normal urinary bladder. The catheterized urine was sterile on culture. Retrograde pyelogram revealed small and contracted kidneys. The kidney pelves and calices were well filled and showed no dilatation.

Shortly after admission the patient developed a relapse of his dysentery which subsided promptly. Stool examination revealed no amoeba or B. dysenteriae on culture. The patient was, through the courtesy of Drs. C. M. Meng and H. C. Fang, transferred to the metabolism ward for study. Except for frequent dizziness and irregular appetite, the first part of the metabolic observation was satisfactorily carried out. After a high calcium regime he was given Vigantol which, however, failed to bring about any change in his calcium and phosphorus metabolism. When a high phosphorus diet was next given the patient was immediately made very sick complaining of dizziness, headache, marked anorexia, nausea and vomiting. The blood N.P.N. was raised to 86 mg.% and CO_2 decreased to 30.2 volumes %. Chvostek and Trousseau signs remained negative. All symptoms promptly improved when the diet was discontinued. Vitamin D_2, 1,000,000 i.u. was given by mouth on February 4, 1941, and the improvement of the calcium and phosphorus metabolism was only slight. The joint effusion of the knees promptly subsided in November. He had a spontaneous refracture of the lower third of the left femur in February which was immobilized by a long leg splint. He had but little pain and a transient fever. Following the fracture the left knee became swollen again and aspiration was repeated. On April 5 the patient was given A.T.10, but unfortunately before the effect was manifest the medication had to be discontinued on account of fever, headache and poor appetite. Irregular fever continued without any adequate explanation. Extreme anorexia, nausea and frequent vomiting made quantitative study impossible. Fever became higher and some chilliness was also noticed. Anemia became more marked and a leucocytosis was present. Finally on May 9, the patient presented symptoms and findings of a rectal abscess. The latter subsided before surgical intervention was attempted. Fever and leucocytosis persisted. Both knees and ankles became swollen and painful again. Headache and anorexia continued. The blood N.P.N. went up to 120 mg.% and CO_2 dropped to 15.1 volumes %. Blood transfusion, glucose infusion and calcium gluconate injections failed to improve the condition. He was discharged in very poor condition at the request of his family on May 29, 1941. He died at home few days after discharge.

144   S. H. LIU AND H. I. CHU

MASSED METABOLIC DATA

TABLE 1

Partition of phosphorus excretion in relation to the ratio of calcium to phosphorus intake and renal function

CASE	LOW Ca/P INTAKE			HIGH Ca/P INTAKE			SERUM		RENAL FUNCTION	
	Period no.	Diet Ca/P	P output in urine	Period no.	Diet Ca/P	P output in urine	Inorg. P	N.P.N.	P.S.P.	Urea clearance
			% of total output			% of total output	mg.%	mg.%	% in 2 hours	% of normal
1	1– 2	0.27	76	3	2.23	68	3.97	41	23.0	24.3
2	1– 2	0.29	54	6–7	1.80	43	5.90	85	6.0	12.4
3	47–48	0.43	47	49–52	2.00	34	6.89	90	2.5	8.4
4	1– 4	0.44	40	20–21	2.14	34	4.76	86	3.0	9.6
5	1– 3	0.39	45	4– 6	2.63	32	4.09	64	5.0	13.2
Normal*		0.38	63		1.60	57	3.99	19		

* Data from 12 normal Chinese (38) in whom the urinary phosphorus varied from 57 to 74% of the total output on low Ca/P intake and from 46 to 63% of the total output on high Ca/P intake.

TABLE 2

Effect of increasing phosphorus intake on calcium and phosphorus metabolism and serum calcium and inorganic phosphorus

	REGIMEN*	SOLUBLE PHOSPHATE ADDED			HIGH-PHOSPHORUS FOOD ADDED	
		Case 2	Case 3	Case 4	Case 4	Case 5
Period no.	Control	6– 7	16–17	1– 4	8–11	11–13
	High P	8– 9	18–19	5– 7	12–14	14–15
	Post-control	10–11	20	8–11	15–17	16
P intake, *mg. daily*	Control	675	612	618	680	488
	High P	1075	1080	1059	1073	863
	Post-control	675	585	680	569	191
Ca intake, *mg. daily*	Control	1207	989	271	336	1356
	High P	1207	980	271	329	1438
	Post-control	1207	979	336	237	1270
Ca/P intake	Control	1.89	1.62	0.45	0.49	2.98
	High P	1.12	0.91	0.26	0.31	1.67
	Post-control	1.89	1.67	0.49	0.42	6.65
P in stool, *mg. daily*	Control	412	435	370	436	221
	High P	540	582	338	610	448
	Post-control	407	684	436	350	286
P in urine, *mg. daily*	Control	314	218	251	365	175
	High P	418	323	465	339	194
	Post-control	338	257	365	334	170
P in urine, *% total output*	Control	43	33	40	46	44
	High P	44	36	58	37	30
	Post-control	45	27	46	49	37
P balance, *mg. daily*	Control	−56	−40	11	−122	92
	High P	117	176	256	124	221
	Post-control	−70	−356	−122	−115	−265
Ca balance, *mg. daily*	Control	63	31	−52	−60	149
	High P	114	−12	−9	−62	460
	Post-control	114	−295	−60	−117	82
Serum inorg. P, *mg. %*	Control	5.96	5.89	4.95	5.00	3.70
	High P	7.25	9.26	8.33	7.11	5.36
	Post-control	6.02	5.24	5.00	6.14	3.86
Serum Ca, *mg. %*	Control	5.54	5.46	8.04	7.73	8.31
	High P	4.86	4.14	5.38	6.80	8.40
	Post-control	6.31	4.70	7.73	7.54	8.56
Serum N.P.N., *mg. %*	Control	76	104	97	86	43
	High P	80	84	100	150	86
	Post-control	86		86	100	55

* Figures for intake, stool and urine are averages for the whole of each regimen, and those for serum are for the end of each regimen.

145

TABLE 3

Influence of calcium intake on calcium and phosphorus balances and serum calcium and inorganic phosphorus

CASE	PERIOD NO.	BODY WEIGHT	CALCIUM			PHOSPHORUS		SERUM	
			Intake	Intake	Balance	Intake	Balance	Ca	P
		kg.	*mg.*	*mg./kg.*	*mg.*	*mg.*	*mg.*	*mg.%*	*mg.%*
			Low calcium intake						
1	1– 2	10	96	9.6	−18	358	−5	8.45	4.06
2	1– 2	25	161	6.4	−87	554	−26	6.06	6.25
3	47–48	38	415	10.9	−25	962	242	4.74	7.60
4	1– 4	40	271	6.8	−52	618	11	8.04	4.95
5	1– 3	25	186	7.4	−72	479	49	7.84	4.07
Normal*		56	471	8.4	63	1258	96		
			High calcium intake						
1	3	10	796	79.6	321	358	13	8.03	3.26
2	6– 7	25	1207	48.3	63	675	−56	5.54	5.96
3	49–52	38	1915	50.4	346	962	146	6.14	4.90
4	20–21	40	1451	36.3	136	678	113	8.14	4.02
5	4– 6	25	1353	54.1	96	515	53	9.11	3.26
Normal*		56	1205	21.5	211	760	3		

* Data from 12 normal Chinese (38) in whom the average serum calcium was 10.07 ± 0.037 mg. %, and inorganic phosphorus 3.99 ± 0.033 mg. % without significant variations in relation to the different levels of calcium and phosphorus intake.

TABLE 4

Serum electrolytes unassociated with acid or alkali administration

CASE		pH	HCO$_3^-$	Cl	HPO$_4^-$	ALB.	GLOB.	SUM OF ANIONS	UNDET. ANIONS	TOTAL BASE	Na$^+$	K$^+$	Ca^{++}	Mg^{++}	N.P.N.
1	Nov. 14, '35		13.4	106	2.3	7.3	5.7						4.5		43
2	Apr. 9, '36	7.33	22.8	103.9	4.1	9.7	5.6	146.1	4.9	151.0	141.2	3.6	2.8	2.9	85
	June 12, '36	7.35	18.6	112.0	3.0	9.7	4.9	148.2	1.7	149.9	138.3	3.6	3.1	2.6	77
	Oct. 7, '36	7.28	16.0	106.0	3.8	10.0	5.4	141.2	2.9	144.1	137.2	3.4	2.7	2.7	
3	Jan. 23, '39	7.25	19.0	104.0	2.8	7.5	7.0	141.3	13.2	154.5			2.5		82
4	Nov. 1, '40	7.24	14.1	110.4	2.9	10.3	5.1	142.8	8.6	151.4	134.9	5.6	4.0	4.0	97
	May 23, '41	7.32	19.8	112.4	2.7	9.9	4.4	150.2	6.5	156.7	135.5	4.5	4.1	3.6	59
5	Nov. 18, '40	7.25	16.5	103.7	2.7	8.7	6.8	138.2	8.9	147.1	138.0	2.9	3.7	2.8	64
	Apr. 17, '41	7.25	12.9	105.3	1.9	8.0	6.7	134.6	12.8	147.4	131.5	4.0	4.7	2.7	68
	May 8, '41	7.10	15.6	101.4	2.2	7.7	4.8	134.2	10.9	145.1					72
	May 22, '41	7.18	12.7	97.2	2.9	5.1	7.0	124.9	13.1	138.0	118.0	3.9	4.2	2.6	131
N*	Average	7.38	28.2	100.4	2.6	10.8	4.8	148.6	3.2	150.0	138.0	3.9	4.9	2.3	27
	Lowest	7.35	25.8	95.5	2.2	9.4	3.8	142.6	0	146.1	135.5	3.3	4.4	1.9	22
	Highest	7.40	31.0	104.6	3.4	12.0	5.9	151.1	7.7	154.7	140.0	4.2	5.5	2.6	34

* 12 normal controls. Figures are expressed in milli-equivalents per liter of serum except pH and N.P.N. which are in mg. per 100 cc. of serum.

TABLE 5

Serum electrolytes after alkali and acid administration

Case 2

	pH	HCO$_3^-$	Cl$^-$	HPO$_4^-$	ALB.	GLOB.	SUM OF ANIONS	UNDET. ANIONS	TOTAL BASE	Na$^+$	K$^+$	Ca^{++}	Mg^{++}	N.P.N.	REMARKS
Nov. 9, '36	7.22	11.6	107.0	4.2	8.8	4.4	136.0	9.3	145.3	135.5	3.6	2.3	2.5	168	Control
Nov. 17, '36	7.35	22.0	96.1	4.3	9.7	5.3	137.4	5.8	143.2	137.0	2.8	2.0	1.7	131	80 cc. M NaHCO$_3$ daily Nov. 13–16
Nov. 29, '36	7.32	16.1	101.2	3.5	9.4	5.6	135.8	7.8	143.6	135.4	3.4	2.3	2.1	110	
Dec. 7, '36	7.40	24.8	96.6	3.5	9.9	5.2	140.0	5.4	145.4	139.4	4.0	2.3	2.4	97	40 cc. M NaHCO$_3$ daily Nov. 29–Dec. 10
Dec. 23, '36	7.30	16.8	103.6	4.0	11.6	4.1	140.1	6.7	146.8	137.4	4.2	2.6	2.6	124	
Dec. 31, '36	7.20	8.3	106.7	3.8	9.5	4.9	133.2	6.9	140.1	132.0	3.5	2.4	2.5	142	1 gm. NH$_4$Cl daily Dec. 23–30
Feb. 22, '37	7.28	14.9	99.9	4.8	6.8	6.1	132.5	12.0	144.5	135.8	2.9	1.8	2.0	148	

Figures are expressed in milli-equivalents per liter of serum except pH and N.P.N. which are in mg. per 100 cc. of serum.

TABLE 6

Summary of results of iron therapy

	CASE 3			CASE 4
	Trial 1	Trial 2	Trial 3	Trial 1
Ferric amm. citrate, *gm. daily*....	6	6	6–12	6
Duration of iron therapy, *days*...	52	56	24	20
Serum inorganic phosphorus, *mg.* %................................	3.70 to 1.00	4.9 to 2.77	3.70 to 2.96	4.60 to 3.94
Serum calcium, *mg.* %............	5.82 to 9.00	6.14 to 7.87	7.50 to 7.49	8.15 to 8.43
Phosphorus balance, *mg. daily*....	22 to 32	146 to 5	76 to 16	149 to 74
Calcium balance, *mg. daily*.......	67 to 410	346 to 157	216 to 564	238 to 604
Phosphorus intake, *mg. daily*.....	707	929–640	626	602
Calcium intake, *mg. daily*........	1978	1919	2009	1671
Nitrogen intake, *gm. daily*.......	7.11	8.90–7.97	7.62–7.90	6.61
Nitrogen in stool, *gm. daily*......	1.70	2.10	1.67	1.36

TABLE 7

Composition of diets in gram per day

FOOD ARTICLES	CASE 1. C. C. J.			CASE 2. P. Y. L.			CASE 3. M. S. T.									CASE 4. K. C. C.										CASE 5. C. C. C.						
	1	2	3	1	2	2a	1	2	3	4	5	A	B	C	D	1a	1b	1c	2	3a	3b	3c	4	5	6	1	2	3a	3b	4a	4b	5
Wheat flour	50			150	160	150	150	150	100	100	100	100	100	100	100	150	150	150	250	250	75	150	200	150	150	150	200	150		150	200	150
Rice	80	60		40	48	50	100	100	60	60	60	100	100	100	100	100	100	100		75	75	75	75	75	50	60	60			60	60	60
Millet			20	30	24						60																					
Kau mien							30									60	60	60	120	60	60	60	60	60	60			100	100			
Kan fen														10	10	10	10	10					30			40						
Ou fen														10	10				10	20	20	20	20									
Graham bread		50																														
Pork	50																															
Beef	40																															
Chicken			40																										65			
Liver, pork			50	40	32	30						30	30	30	30	10	10	10	20	30	30	30										
Liver, beef		50																														
Liver, sheep																																
Egg white				60	40	30	30	30	30	30	30	60	60	50	50	20	20	20						30	30		100	30	30	30	30	30
Milk			30		48		200	200	200	200	200	200	200	50	50	100	100	100	100	100	100	100	100	200	200	100		200	200	100	100	100
Klim														150	100					50												
Bean curd	50			50	64	50	50	50		50		25	25	50	50	200	200	200	200	200	200	200	200			200						
Cabbage, large		30					50	50				60	110	150	100																	
Cabbage, small						50					50													150	150							
Mung bean sprout	50					30				50	100															100						
Spinach							50									100						100		100	100							
Raddish																							100									
Turnip												50			50				40													
Wosun	40													50																		
Cucumber																											200					
White potato		40	20					100	100	100	100	100	100	100	150	50	50	50	50	50	50	50	50	50	50	200	200					
Sweet potato																150	150	150	150	150	150	150	150	150	150	200	50	50	50	50	60	30
Salted turnip				10	8			25	25	25	25	30	30	10	10												200	50	50			30
Peanut		30				10						10	20	20	20																	
Chestnut			50	100	80	100																										
Apple	50											100	200	200																		
Pear	50											100	100	200																		
Persimmon															200											200	200	200	200	200	200	200

Orange							100	200	200	200	200			10																100	100	100
Banana		100																															
Butter		10																															
Peanut butter		20		20	24													40	10					30	30							
Sesame oil	30					30					5	6	8	10	10	30	30	30	30	30	30	30	30	10	5			5	5			
Soy bean sauce			20				30	15	30	10	5	10	15	20	10	10	10	30	30	30	30	30	30	30	30	30		10	10			
Vinegar													5																			
Sugar	2	2	2	2	2	40	20	20	20	20	20	20	20	20	20	20	20	10	3	3	3	3	3	10	20		10	10	10	10	20	20
NaCl	2	2	2	2	2	2	4	3	3	2	4	2	2	2	2	3	3	3	3	3	3	3	3	1	1	5						
Calories*	901	1092	819	1157	1221	1354	1564	1529	1349	1271	1274	1527	1590	1565	1546	1413	1649	1769	2394	2259	1567	1832	1996	1847	1612	1489	1568	1504	1071	1027	1273	1220
Calcium† mg.	96	92	290	161	207	119	376	333	367	389	458	415	419	252	309	271	336	336	329	210	220	248	294	548	527	186	199	302	287	165	175	228
Phosphorus† mg.	358	440	454	554	675	604	659	602	629	612	653	962	929	642	626	618	680	680	1073	578	482	588	678	691	624	479	488	907	874	415	451	515
Nitrogen†	5.06	5.54	5.42	6.57	7.62	7.57	7.00	6.70	7.29	6.27	6.19	9.79	8.62	7.69	7.34	6.84	7.14	7.14	11.89	8.94	5.46	7.29	7.80	7.42	6.75	7.63	5.74	8.58	7.38	4.73	5.49	6.91

* Calculated from "Outlines of Diets of the Peiping Union Medical College Hospital," 3rd ed., 1937.
† Analyzed values.

TABLE 8

Case 1. C. C. J. Effect of vitamin D and ultraviolet irradiation on Ca, P and N₂ metabolism

DATE 1935–36	PERIODS 4 DAY	Calcium, mg., daily — Intake	Urine	Stool	Balance	Phosphorus, mg. daily — Intake	Urine	Stool	Balance	Nitrogen, gm. daily — Intake	Urine	Stool	Balance	Serum mg. % Ca	Serum mg. % P	Remarks
Nov. 21–24	1	96	12	112	−28	358	286	109	−37	5.06	4.19	0.54	+0.33	9.02	3.86	diet 1
25–28	2	96	18	86	−8	358	265	66	+27	5.06	4.04	0.36	+0.66	9.27	4.00	diet 1
29–2	3	796	18	466	+312	358	236	109	+13	5.06	4.17	0.44	−0.45	8.45	4.06	diet 1
Dec. 3–6	4	796	30	922	−156	358	227	184	−53	5.06	4.23	0.65	−0.18	8.03	3.26	diet 1 Vigantol 30 drops daily
7–10	5	796	20	586	+190	358	229	119	+10	5.06	4.36	0.37	+0.33	8.85	3.40	diet 1 Vigantol 30 drops daily
11–14	6	796	34	462	+300	358	204	101	+53	5.06	4.23	0.34	+0.49	8.45		diet 1 Vigantol 30 drops daily
15–18	7	796	30	677	+89	358	211	145	+2	5.06	4.18	0.53	−0.25	8.48	3.01	diet 1 Vigantol 30 drops daily
19–22	8	796	17	549	+230	358	200	120	+38	5.06	4.15	0.45	+0.46	8.26	3.02	diet 1 Vigantol 30 drops daily
Jan. 12–15	9	796	29	532	+235	358	184	142	+32	5.06	3.92	0.47	+0.67	8.88	3.04	diet 1 Vigantol 30 drops daily
16–19	10	796	19	298	+479	358	190	76	+92	5.06	4.02	0.28	+0.76			diet 1
20–23	11	796	10	831	−45	358	204	206	−52	5.06	4.07	0.59	+0.40	8.90	3.04	diet 1
24–27	12	796	19	469	+308	358	192	116	+50	5.06	3.92	0.37	+0.77			diet 1 Vigantol 60 drops daily
28–31	13	796	12	715	+69	358	183	194	−19	5.06	4.28	0.57	+0.21			diet 1 Vigantol 60 drops daily
Feb. 1–4	14	796	9	685	+102	358	204	183	−29	5.06	3.61	0.56	+0.89	9.12	3.02	diet 1 Vigantol 60 drops daily
5–8	15	796	5	511	+280	358	180	207	−29	5.06	4.06	0.53	+0.47			diet 1 Vigantol 60 drops daily
9	16															diet 1 Vigantol 60 drops daily
13–16	17	792	27	534	+231	440	196	198	+46	5.54	4.62	0.54	+0.38	8.84	3.10	diet 1 Vigantol 60 drops daily
17–20	18	792	40	318	+434	440	186	158	+96	5.54	4.74	0.39	+0.41	9.10	3.02	diet 2 Vigantol 60 drops daily
21–24	19	792	33	588	+171	440	208	201	+31	5.54	4.97	0.48	+0.09	8.90	3.32	diet 2 Vigantol 60 drops daily
25–28	20															diet 2 Ultraviolet irradiation
29–3	21	792	42	963	−213	404	178	382	−120	5.54	4.16	0.98	+0.40	8.82	3.42	diet 2 Ultraviolet irradiation
March 4–7	22	784	23	416	+345	402	201	158	+43	5.13	4.52	0.42	+0.19			diet 2
8–11	23	690	16	498	+176	454	282	290	+118	5.42	4.72	0.60	+0.10			diet 3
12–15	24	690	21	418	+251	454	304	154	+4	5.42	4.46	0.35	+0.61	8.52	3.76	diet 3
16–19	25	690		399	+291	454	297	148	+9	5.42	4.82	0.39	+0.21			diet 3
20–23	26	690	24	550	+116	454	309	198	+53	5.42	4.92	0.47	+0.03			diet 3
24–27	27	690	21	487	+182	454	324	169	−39	5.42	4.93	0.49	0	8.64	4.25	diet 3 Vigantol 1.2 cc. i.m. daily
28–31	28	690	38	519	+133	454	314	203	−63	5.42	4.42	0.49	+0.51			diet 3 Vigantol 1.2 cc. i.m. daily
April 1–4	29	690	0	490	+200	454	334	161	−41	5.42	5.05	0.51	−0.14	9.19	4.20	diet 3 Vigantol 1.2 cc. i.m. daily
5	30															diet 3 Vigantol 1.2 cc. i.m. daily

TABLE 9

Case 2. P. Y. L. Effect of vitamin D, phosphate, acid and alkali on Ca, P and N_2 metabolism

DATE 1936	PERIOD 4-DAY	CALCIUM, MG. DAILY				PHOSPHORUS, MG. DAILY				NITROGEN, GM. DAILY				SERUM, MG. %			REMARKS
		Intake	Urine	Stool	Balance	Intake	Urine	Stool	Balance	Intake	Urine	Stool	Balance	Ca	P	N.P.N.	
April 13-16	1	161	0	184	-23	554	310	212	32	6.57	4.58	0.88	1.11	6.68	5.78	85	diet 1
17-20	2	161	0	312	-151	554	316	321	-83	6.57	4.78	1.09	0.70	5.94	5.68		diet 1
21-24	3	661	0	602	59	554	323	333	-102	6.57	5.18	0.96	0.43	6.06	6.25		diet 1
25-28	4	707	0	686	21	675	368	351	-44	7.62	5.70	0.84	1.08	5.56	5.99		diet 2
29-2 (May)	5	707	0	560	147	675	361	263	51	7.62	5.74	0.72	1.16				diet 2
May 3-6	6	1207	0	1212	-5	675	326	486	-137	7.62	5.33	1.00	1.29	5.63	6.85	76	diet 2
7-10	7	1207	0	1076	131	675	301	348	26	7.62	5.28	0.95	1.39	5.91	6.29		diet 2 Na_2HPO_4
11-14	8	1207	0	1055	152	1075	402	520	153	7.62	5.65	1.05	0.92	5.54	5.96	80	diet 2 Na_2HPO_4
15-18	9	1207	0	1130	77	1075	434	560	81	7.62	5.55	1.08	0.99	5.02	6.87		diet 2 Vigantol
19-22	10	1207	0	1015	192	675	369	356	-50	7.62	5.62	0.82	1.18	4.86	7.25		diet 2 Vigantol
23-26	11	1207	0	1170	37	675	307	458	-90	7.62	5.16	1.06	1.37	6.65	6.33		diet 2 Vigantol
27-30	12	1207	0	976	231	675	309	316	50	7.62	5.16	0.92	1.54	6.31	6.02	86	diet 2 Vigantol
31-3 (June)	13	1207	0	1044	163	675	296	321	58	7.62	5.16	1.15	1.31	6.60	5.62		diet 2 Vigantol
June 4-7	14	1207	0	967	240	675	307	294	74	7.62	4.95	1.00	1.67	6.20	6.54	110	diet 2 Vigantol
8	15													6.54	5.96	86	
Oct. 28-31	21	919	0	575	344	604	73	267	264	7.57	3.57	0.92	3.08	5.11	6.25	127	diet 2a
Nov. 1-4	22	919	1	736	182	604	122	276	206	7.57	4.20	0.76	2.61	5.21	5.86		diet 2a
5-8	23	919	1	636	282	604	150	264	190	7.57	5.11	0.52	1.94	5.36	6.61		diet 2a
9-12	24	874	4	849	21	552	167	178	207	7.09	5.36	0.96	0.77	4.60	7.25	168	diet 2a $NaHCO_3$
13-16	25	670	20	340	310	404	179	152	73	4.78	5.47	0.38	-1.07	4.57	7.54		diet 2a
17-20	26	690	8	616	66	453	145	271	37	5.68	5.19	0.48	0.01	4.07	7.45		diet 2a
21-24	27	919	1	864	54	604	165	424	15	7.57	4.75	0.82	2.00	4.65	6.27	131	diet 2a
25-28	28	919	6	543	370	604	149	288	167	7.57	4.50	0.70	2.37	4.75	5.91		diet 2a $NaHCO_3$
29-2 (Dec.)	29	919	0	816	103	604	148	439	17	7.57	4.62	0.92	2.03	4.57	5.97		diet 2a $NaHCO_3$
Dec. 3-6	30	919	5	766	148	604	158	392	54	7.57	5.06	0.93	1.58	4.75	5.55	110	diet 2a $NaHCO_3$
7-10	31	919	4	643	272	604	178	348	78	7.57	4.50	0.88	2.19	4.65	6.02		diet 2a
11-14	32	919	7	737	175	604	193	354	57	7.57	4.60	0.75	2.22	5.06	5.74	97	diet 2a
15-18	33	919	12	594	313	604	217	256	131	7.57	5.17	0.52	1.88	5.99	6.26	91	diet 2a
19-22	34	919	25	700	194	604	235	348	21	7.57	4.94	0.81	1.82	5.14	6.45	114	diet 2a
23-26	35	919	7	620	292	604	204	302	98	7.83	5.44	0.69	1.70		6.81	124	diet 2a NH_4Cl
27-30 31	36	904	18	676	210	528	164	314	50	6.88	4.88	0.75	1.25	4.81	6.63	142	diet 2a NH_4Cl

TABLE 10

Case 3. M. S. T. Effect of calcium, phosphate, iron, vitamin D and parathormone on Ca, P and N₂ metabolism

DATE 1939–40	PERIODS 4 DAY	CALCIUM, MG. DAILY Intake	Urine	Stool	Balance	PHOSPHORUS, MG. DAILY Intake	Urine	Stool	Balance	NITROGEN, GM. DAILY Intake	Urine	Stool	Balance	SERUM, MG. % Ca	P	Phosphatase*	N.P.N.	REMARKS
Jan. 23–26	1	620	2	507	+111	613	188	305	+120	6.40	4.31	0.94	+1.15	5.00	4.86		82	diet 1
27–30	2	629	0	628	+1	611	190	294	+127	6.25	4.16	1.07	+1.02	5.82	4.39	2.05		diet 1
31–3 (Feb.)	3	640	7	462	+171	579	222	280	+77	5.81	4.28	0.92	+0.61	6.02	5.75			diet 1
Feb. 4–7	4	624	19	392	+213	544	194	304	+46	5.40	4.64	1.08	−0.32	6.60	4.56			diet 1
8–11	5	856	0	828	+28	486	87	398	+1	5.53	4.14	1.08	+0.31	6.75	4.90			diet 2
12–15	6													5.84	4.94		86	
16–27	7–9	967	2	753	+212	629	136	405	+88	7.29	4.35	0.94	+2.00	5.28	5.82		75	Vigantol 1 cc. daily
28–3 (Mar.)	10	967	0	1069	−102	629	152	532	−55	7.29	4.99	1.16	+1.14	5.82	4.36			diet 3 Vigantol 1 cc. daily
March 4–7	11	967	0	881	+86	629	172	471	−14	7.29	4.59	1.24	+1.46	5.47	4.96	2.80	105	diet 3 Vigantol 1 cc. daily
8–11	12	964	0	908	+56	619	177	496	−54	7.29	4.85	1.08	+1.36	5.26	5.19			diet 3 Vigantol 1 cc. daily
12–15	13	967	0	944	+23	629	193	538	−102	7.29	4.95	1.45	+0.89	5.38	5.91			diet 3 Vigantol 5 cc. daily
16–19	14	967	0	932	+35	629	196	448	−15	7.29	4.97	1.50	+0.82	5.94	6.28			diet 3 Vigantol 5 cc. daily
20–23	15	989	0	866	+123	612	215	396	+1	6.27	4.66	1.15	+0.46	4.80	5.92			diet 3
24–27	16	989	0	1050	−61	612	220	474	−82	6.27	4.61	1.16	+0.50	5.06	5.89		104	diet 3
28–31	17	989	1	1037	−49	1105	252	600	+253	6.27	4.25	1.33	+0.69	5.55	5.58			diet 4
April 1–4	18	970	1	944	+25	1055	394	563	+98	6.27	2.74	1.35	+2.18	5.46	7.77	3.91		diet 4
5–8	19	979	0	1274	−295	585	257	684	−356	5.34	3.82	1.74	−0.22	4.76	9.26			diet 4 phosphate sol.
9–12	20	989	1	929	+59	612	158	411	+43	5.73	4.36	1.14	+0.23	4.14	5.24			diet 4
13–16	21	989	0	986	+3	612	135	488	−11	6.27	4.11	1.25	+0.91	4.70	4.35			diet 4
17–20	22	1058	0	1108	−51	653	160	503	−10	6.27	4.28	1.48	+0.51	5.31	4.49		84	diet 4
21–24	23	1058	3	1014	+41	653	193	440	+20	6.19	4.09	1.25	+0.85	5.09	5.08			diet 5
25–28	24	1058	0	892	+166	653	235	358	+60	6.19	3.80	1.16	+1.23	5.15	4.89			diet 5
29–2 (May)	25																	diet 5
May 3–6	26	1058	0	968	+90	653	250	382	+21	6.19	3.87	1.22	+1.10	5.50	5.39			diet 5 parathormone 40 units daily
7–10	27	1058	0	995	+63	653	255	353	+45	6.19	3.70	1.28	+1.21	5.68	5.22			diet 5 parathormone 40 units daily
11–14	28	1058	0	893	+165	653	222	345	−14	6.19	4.15	1.28	+0.76	5.69	5.01			diet 5 parathormone 40 units daily
15–18	29	1058	0	849	+209	653	174	386	+93	6.19	3.71	1.29	+1.19	5.28	4.61			diet 5
19–22	30	1978	0	1669	+309	707	160	499	+48	6.83	3.81	1.44	+1.58	5.14	4.19			diet 5
23–26	31	1978	0	1885	+93	707	130	578	−3	6.83	4.11	1.52	+1.20	5.59	3.23			diet 5
27–30	32	1978	0	2180	−202	707	130	687	−110	6.83	4.06	1.87	+0.90	5.35	3.23			diet 5
31–3 (June)	33	1978	0	1640	+338	707	168	496	+43	6.83	4.02	1.59	+1.22	5.82	3.72	3.42	60	diet 5 Fe Amm. citrate

No.	Date	(1)	(2)	(3)	(4)	(5)	(6)	(7)	(8)	(9)	(10)	(11)	(12)	(13)	(14)	Phosphatase*	Fe Amm. citrate	Diet
34	June 4–7	1978	0	1495	+483	707	180	506	+21	6.83	3.95	1.81	+1.07	6.35	4.13	5.54	60	diet 5
35	8	415	1	350	+65	962	350	317	+295.9	9.79	5.25	1.25	+3.29	5.65	4.60	3.87	90	diet A
47	Oct. 10–13	415	1	528	−114	962	378	496	+189.9	9.79	5.93	1.85	+2.01	5.07	5.82	3.27		diet A
48	14–17	1915	2	1485	+429	962	338	595	+299.9	9.79	6.73	1.87	+1.19	4.67	7.25	4.82		diet A
49	18–21	1915	3	1465	+448	962	268	475	+219.9	9.79	5.88	1.61	+2.00	4.74	7.60	4.16		diet A
50	22–25	1915	5	1927	−15	962	254	615	+93.9	9.79	6.11	1.99	+2.00	6.06	5.44			diet A
51	26–29	1915	8	1389	+521	962	249	472	+241.9	9.79	5.89	1.50	+2.18	6.24	5.28		120	diet A
52	30–2 (Nov.)	1919	0	2065	−154	929	185	809	−65	8.90	5.99	2.53	+0.48	6.52	5.52	2.46		diet B Fe Amm. citrate
53	Nov. 3–6	1919	1	1775	+144	929	130	754	+45	8.90	5.75	2.41	+0.50	6.14	4.90			diet B Fe Amm. citrate
54	7–10	1919	4	1482	+433	929	157	619	+153	8.90	6.21	1.76	+1.39	6.51	3.74			diet B Fe Amm. citrate
55	11–14	1919	1	1785	+134	929	152	729	+48	8.90	5.95	2.12	+0.57	6.90	3.57	4.43		diet B Fe Amm. citrate
56	15–18	1919	2	1940	−23	929	149	798	−18	8.90	6.03	2.12	+0.83	6.90	3.77			diet B Fe Amm. citrate
57	19–22	1919	4	1781	+134	929	187	738	+48	8.90	5.99	2.04	+0.83	6.91	3.95			diet B Fe Amm. citrate
58	23–26	1919	1	1817	+102	929	210	641	+78	8.90	6.91	1.87	+1.04	6.45	4.13	5.14	67	diet B Fe Amm. citrate
59	27–30	1919	2	1676	+241	929	204	657	+68	8.90	6.03	1.91	+0.98	6.41	4.05			diet B Fe Amm. citrate
60	Dec. 1–4	1919	4	1605	+143	929	157	592	−107	7.97	5.40	2.13	−0.19	6.48	4.19	4.10		diet C Fe Amm. citrate
61	5–8	1752	4	1533	+215	642	110	578	−46	7.97	4.32	1.98	−0.59	7.07	2.92	2.92	86	diet C Fe Amm. citrate
62	9–12	1752	4	1640	+308	642	94	490	+58	7.97	4.49	1.71	+1.94	6.32	2.83	2.64		diet C Fe Amm. citrate
63	13–16	1952	4	1682	+267	642	82	505	+55	7.97	4.58	1.90	+0.58	7.06	2.75	3.71		diet C Fe Amm. citrate
64	17–20	1952	2	1637	+313	642	94	579	−31	7.97	4.26	1.91	+1.48	7.11	2.85	2.91		diet C Fe Amm. citrate
65	21–24	1952	1	2002	−51	642	86	688	−132	7.97	4.24	2.20	+1.51	7.48	2.84	3.96	67	diet C Fe Amm. citrate
66	25–28	1952	2	2065	−116	642	112	302	+228	7.69	4.30	1.56	+1.89	7.73	2.77	3.04		diet C Fe Amm. citrate
67	29–1 (Jan.)	1952	3	1348	+602	642	116	312	+214	7.69	4.70	1.02	+2.37	7.87	2.78	2.73		diet C
68	Jan. 2–5	1952	3	1738	+211	642	136	379	+127	7.69	4.83	1.25	+1.74	7.10	3.60	3.00	46	diet C
69	6–9	1952	4	1406	+543	642	144	388	+110	7.69	4.48	1.28	+1.58	7.39	3.78	1.80		diet C
70	10–13	1952	6	1740	+208	642	171	428	+43	7.69	4.78	1.31	+1.90	6.77	3.72	3.52		diet C
71	14–17	1952	1	1954	−8	642	148	461	+33	7.69	4.48	1.51	+1.40	7.29	3.74	2.69		diet C
72	18–21	1952	1	1872	+79	642	160	449	+33	7.69	4.76	1.50	+1.71	7.11	3.98	1.82	60	diet C
73	22–25	1952	2	1349	+599	642	159	314	+169	7.69	4.95	1.17	+1.76	7.10	3.72	0.90		diet C A.T. 10 3 cc. daily
74	26–29	1952	7	1749	+176	642	187	351	+104	7.69	4.39	1.62	+2.12	7.08	4.54	1.28		diet C A.T. 10 3 cc. daily
75	30–2 (Feb.)	1952	4	1239	+664	642	139	381	+122	7.69	4.32	1.39	+1.91	8.68	3.64	1.56	60	diet C A.T. 10 3 cc. daily
76	Feb. 3–6	1952	10	953	+896	642	88	253	+301	7.69	4.52	1.15	+2.22	8.32	3.05	0.97		diet C A.T. 10 3 cc. daily
77	7–10	1952	16	862	+927	642	77	247	+318	7.69	5.08	1.21	+1.96	8.84	2.92	3.53		diet C A.T. 10 3 cc. daily
78	11–14	1952	12	1176	+652	642	85	304	+253	7.69	4.06	1.47	+1.14	9.18	3.04	3.98		diet C
79	15–18	1952	9	1116	+745	642	107	256	+279	7.69	4.65	1.16	+2.47	9.18	3.48	2.46		diet C
80	19–22	1952	9	1399	+519	642	108	303	+215	7.34	5.10	1.23	+1.46	8.88	3.57	3.66		diet D
81	23–26	2009		1399		642	108	303	+215	7.34		1.23	+1.46	8.44		2.31		diet D
82	27–1 (Mar.)	2009	5	1407	+552	626	126	296	+204	7.34	5.10	1.26	+0.98	8.89	3.36	3.31		diet D

* Phosphatase in Bodansky units per 100 cc.

S. H. LIU AND H. I. CHU

TABLE 10—*Concluded*

DATE 1939-40	PERIODS 4 DAY	CALCIUM, MG. DAILY				PHOSPHORUS, MG. DAILY				NITROGEN, GM. DAILY				SERUM, MG. %			N.P.N.	REMARKS
		Intake	Urine	Stool	Balance	Intake	Urine	Stool	Balance	Intake	Urine	Stool	Balance	Ca	P	Phosphatase*		
March 2-5	83	2009	47	1420	+542	626	128	330	+168	7.34	4.57	1.27	+1.50	9.28	3.55	4.45		diet D
6-9	84	2009	54	1710	+245	626	139	401	+86	7.34	4.50	1.43	+1.41	8.68	3.32	3.58		diet D
10-13	85	2009	46	1597	+366	626	140	326	+160	7.34	4.25	1.33	+1.76	8.66	3.70	3.00		diet D
14-17	86	2009	13	1630	+366	626	174	335	+117	7.34	4.50	1.38	+1.46	8.18	3.92	4.70		diet D
18-21	87	2009	15	2245	-251	626	161	492	-27	7.34	4.50	1.61	+1.23	7.52	4.39	4.70		diet D
22-25	88	2009	7	1986	+16	626	171	433	+22	7.34	4.63	1.56	+1.15	7.54	3.70	4.63		diet D
26-29	89	2009	1	1580	+428	626	166	356	+104	7.34	5.08	1.16	+1.10	7.61	3.57	4.12		diet D
30-2 (Apr.)	90	2009	5	2049	-45	626	152	441	+33	7.34	5.20	1.36	+0.78	8.14	3.69		67	diet D Vig. 2 cc. daily
April 3-6	91	2009	1	1937	+71	626	175	350	+101	7.34	5.13	1.23	+0.98	7.48	3.75	3.70		diet D Vig. 2 cc. daily
7-10	92	2009	5	1712	+292	626	182	356	+88	7.34	4.89	1.13	+1.32	7.43	3.94	4.78		diet D Vig. 2 cc. daily
11-14	93	2009	9	1745	+255	626	206	384	+36	7.34	4.73	1.20	+1.41	6.98	3.92	4.90		diet D Vig. 2 cc. daily
15-18	94	2009	3	1848	+158	626	177	384	+65	7.34	4.85	1.19	+1.30	7.45	3.95	4.00		diet D Vig. 2 cc. daily
19-22	95	2009	2	1736	+271	626	222	355	+49	7.34	4.50	1.16	+1.68	7.78	4.13	2.44		diet D
23-26	96	2009	0	1848	+161	626	158	366	+102	7.34	5.05	1.20	+1.09	7.53	3.77	4.05		diet D
27-30	97	2009	0	2100	-91	626	160	597	-131	7.62	4.98	1.86	+0.78	7.50	3.70		67	diet D
May 1-4	98	2009	2	1360	+647	626	130	476	+207	7.72	5.10	1.53	+1.09	7.59	3.70	3.15	67	diet D Fe Amm. citrate 6 gm. daily
5-8	99	2009	4	1496	+509	626	124	514	-12	7.72	4.90	1.60	+1.22	7.48	3.13	4.12		diet D Fe Amm. citrate 8 gm. daily
9-12	100	2009	1	1275	+733	626	132	507	-13	7.82	5.20	1.67	+0.95	7.34	3.20	4.49		diet D Fe Amm. citrate 8 gm. daily
13-16	101	2009	5	1200	+804	626	146	466	+14	7.90	5.30	1.65	+0.87	7.51	3.52	3.89		diet D Fe Amm. citrate 10 gm. daily
17-20	102	2009	8	1220	+781	626	134	464	+28	7.90	5.39	1.73	+0.70	7.76	2.93			diet D Fe Amm. citrate 12 gm. daily
21														7.49	2.96	4.73	75	diet D Fe Amm. citrate 12 gm. daily

刘士豪论文选集

TABLE 11

Case 4. K. C. C. Effect of inorganic and dietary phosphorus, vitamin D, A.T.10 and iron on Ca, P and N₂ metabolism

DATE 1940-41	PERIODS 4 DAY	CALCIUM Intake	CALCIUM Urine	CALCIUM Stool	CALCIUM Balance	PHOSPHORUS Intake	PHOSPHORUS Urine	PHOSPHORUS Stool	PHOSPHORUS Balance	NITROGEN Intake	NITROGEN Urine	NITROGEN Stool	NITROGEN Balance	SERUM Ca	SERUM P	SERUM Phosphatase	SERUM N.P.N.	REMARKS
Oct. 19-22	1	271	0	384	-113	618	209	365	+44	6.84	4.23	1.32	+1.29	8.25	4.39	10.99	67	diet 1a
23-26	2	271	0	323	-52	618	250	331	+37	6.84	4.95	1.10	+0.79					diet 1a
27-30	3	271	5	277	-11	618	272	310	+36	6.84	5.92	1.09	-0.17	8.16	4.73	21.58		diet 1a
31-3	4	271	9	296	-34	618	273	472	-73	6.84	6.61	1.26	-1.03	8.06	4.99		97	diet 1a
Nov. 4-7	5	271	1	306	-36	1020	377	451	+192	6.84	6.68	1.08	-0.92	6.11	4.95	22.37		diet 1a Na₃PO₄
8-11	6	271	8	281	-28	1078	487	344	+247	6.84	6.25	0.96	-0.37	3.58	6.17	16.93	100	diet 1a Na₃PO₄
12-15	7	271	4	229	+38	1078	530	218	+330	7.14	5.84	0.68	+0.32	5.38	7.33	15.30	86	diet 1a Na₃PO₄
16-19	8	336	7	350	-21	680	412	470	-202	7.14	5.55	1.09	+0.50	6.84	8.33	18.13	75	diet 1b
20-23	9	336	3	384	-51	680	389	466	-175	7.14	5.52	1.25	+0.37	6.94	6.22	20.38		diet 1c
24-27	10	336	3	485	-149	680	314	463	-97	7.14	4.85	1.64	-0.65	7.40	6.02	22.31		diet 1c
28-1	11	336	0	354	-18	680	346	346	-12	11.89	4.53	1.32	+1.29	7.73	5.28	26.36	86	diet 1c
Dec. 2-5	12	329	2	378	-51	1073	327	652	+94	11.89	6.72	1.47	+3.70	7.49	5.00	27.80		diet 2
6-9	13	329	4	266	+59	1073	334	430	+309	11.89	7.55	1.10	+3.24	6.66	5.81	21.97		diet 2
10-13	14	329	0	522	-193	1073	356	748	-311	7.20	6.98	1.49	-4.42	6.80	5.81	23.02	150	diet 3a & b
14-17	15	215	1	350	-136	530	326	344	-140	7.29	8.73	0.87	-2.40	7.10	7.11	17.65	120	diet 3c
18-21	16	248	3	308	-60	588	349	302	-63	7.29	7.14	0.90	-0.72	7.54	6.23	18.77	100	diet 3c
22-25	17	248	0	399	-154	588	327	404	-143	7.29	6.43	1.22	-0.04	7.64	6.30	17.63		diet 3c
26-29	18	1405	0	1328	+77	588	257	476	-145	7.29	5.74	1.22	+0.33	8.11	6.14	18.86		diet 3c
30-2 (Jan.)	19	1405	0	1384	+21	588	224	415	-51	7.29	5.62	1.07	+0.60	8.27	4.35	22.68		diet 4
Jan. 3-6	20	1451	3	1208	+243	678	205	360	+113	7.80	5.51	0.97	+1.32	8.14	4.39	15.61		diet 4 Vigantol 1 cc. daily
7-10	21	1451	3	1419	+29	678	187	378	+113	7.80	4.90	1.16	+1.74	8.34	3.76	15.01		diet 4 Vigantol 1 cc. daily
11-14	22	1451	0	1440	+11	678	171	444	+63	7.80	4.91	1.17	+1.72	8.00	4.02	17.27		diet 4 Vigantol 1 cc. daily
15-18	23	1451	0	1630	-179	678	181	472	+25	7.80	5.11	1.17	+1.52	7.88	3.37	18.81		diet 4 Vigantol 1 cc. daily
19-22	24	1451	4	1308	+139	678	203	422	+53	7.80	5.70	1.20	+0.90	8.00	4.42	13.04		diet 4 Vigantol 1 cc. daily
23-26	25	1550	1	1405	+144	678	180	399	+99	7.80	5.61	1.04	+1.15	7.72	4.46	10.98		diet 4 Vigantol 1 cc. daily
27-30	26	1550	0	1471	+79	678	196	406	+76	7.80	5.82	1.25	+0.73	7.99	4.29	20.36		diet 4 Vigantol 1 cc. daily
31-3 (Feb.)	27	1550	0	1180	+370	678	196	346	+136	7.80	5.42	0.98	+1.40	7.92	4.41	15.36		diet 4 Vigantol 1 cc. daily
Feb. 4-7	28	1550	0	1541	+9	678	216	417	+45	7.80	5.57	1.29	+0.94	7.99	4.04	17.19		diet 4 A.T.10 3 cc. daily
8-11	29	1550	2	1350	+198	678	202	360	+116	7.80	5.48	1.25	+1.07	7.92	4.41	13.85		diet 4 A.T.10 3 cc. daily
12-15	30	1550	1	1269	+280	678	201	324	+153	7.80	6.52	1.21	+0.07	7.08	4.75	12.00		diet 4 A.T.10 3 cc. daily
16-19	31	1550	0	926	+624	678	174	271	+233	7.80	7.72	1.38	+1.30	7.08	4.88	15.94		diet 4 A.T.10 3 cc. daily
20-23	32	1550	0	963	+587	678	145	258	+275	7.80	5.06	1.23	+1.51	8.39	4.60	16.07		diet 4 A.T.10 3 cc. daily
24-27	33	1550	0	784	+766	678	110	262	+306	7.80	4.96	1.42	+1.43	8.30	3.85	17.28	67	diet 4 A.T.10 3 cc. daily
28-3 (Mar.)	34	1560	0	735	+815	678	96	223	+359	7.80	6.37	1.23	+0.20	8.55	3.68			diet 4

156 S. H. LIU AND H. I. CHU

TABLE 11—Concluded

DATE 1940-41	PERIODS 4 DAY	CALCIUM				PHOSPHORUS				NITROGEN				SERUM				REMARKS
		Intake	Urine	Stool	Balance	Intake	Urine	Stool	Balance	Intake	Urine	Stool	Balance	Ca	P	Phosphatase	N.P.N.	
March 4-7	35	1550	2	754	+794	678	83	262	+333	7.80	6.59	1.37	−0.16	8.44	3.76	16.78		diet 4
8-11	36	1550	5	1066	+479	678	124	367	+187	7.80	6.50	1.49	−0.19	8.24	4.06	15.94		diet 4
12-15	37	1550	2	977	+566	678	114	296	+268	7.80	6.30	1.25	+0.25	8.22	3.82	14.78		diet 4
16-19	38	1550	3	1110	+437	678	132	286	+260	7.80	6.15	1.57	+0.08	8.22	4.06	15.60		diet 4
20-23	39	1550	4	1375	+171	678	145	343	+190	7.80	6.00	1.72	+0.08	8.00	4.29	13.81		diet 4
24-27	40	1550	5	1298	+247	678	128	333	+217	7.80	5.55	1.68	+0.57	7.62	4.71	13.47		diet 4
28-31	41	1550	3	1128	+420	678	188	277	+213	7.80	5.71	1.36	+0.73	7.64	4.51	13.43	75	diet 4
April 1-4	42	1700	3	1227	+470	691	226	328	+137	7.42	4.53	1.55	+1.34	7.40	5.14	15.56		diet 5a
5-8	43	1700	2	1170	+528	691	197	350	+144	7.42	4.44	1.58	+1.40	7.96	4.85	21.25		diet 5a
9-12	44														5.59			diet 5a
13-16	45	1572	0	1375	+197	624	179	462	−17	6.75	4.85	1.07	+0.83	7.45	6.18	14.89		diet 5a
17-20	46	1677	6	1153	+518	624	142	289	+193	6.75	5.71	0.85	+0.19	7.00	5.44	15.56	100	diet 6a
21-24	47	1677	2	1345	+330	624	155	334	+135	6.75	4.47	1.07	+1.21	7.70	5.28	13.94		diet 6a
25-28	48	1677	2	911	+764	624	156	208	+260	6.75	4.49	0.92	+1.34	7.91	4.63			diet 6a
29-2 (May)	49	1677	7	1486	+184	624	180	344	+100	6.75	5.15	0.88	+0.72	8.47	5.02	20.13		diet 6a Vitamin D₂ 1,000,000 i.u. oral
May 3-6	50	1677	0	1249	+428	624	198	284	+142	6.75	4.39	0.85	+1.51	7.90	5.31			diet 6a
7-10	51	1677	0	1184	+493	624	145	274	+205	6.75	3.75	1.07	+1.93	8.12	4.87	19.69		diet 6a
11-14	52	1677	0	1395	+282	624	137	283	+204	6.75	4.15	1.18	+1.42	8.25	4.61		83	diet 6a
15-18	53	1677	0	1482	+195	624	152	378	+94	6.75	3.81	1.41	+1.53	7.91	4.59			diet 6a
19-22	54	1671	2	1171	+498	602	134	416	+52	6.61	3.39	1.63	+1.59	7.94	4.55	14.43		diet 6a
23-26	55	1671	2	915	+754	602	122	417	+63	6.61	3.42	1.44	+1.75	8.15	4.60		67	diet 6a Fe amm. citrate
27-30	56	1671	6	1072	+593	602	118	412	+72	6.61	3.01	1.31	+2.29	8.12	4.10	12.48	59	diet 6a Fe amm. citrate
31-3 (June)	57	1671	8	1064	+599	602	98	419	+85	6.61	3.06	1.30	+2.25	7.87	4.30			diet 6a Fe amm. citrate
June 4-7	58	1671	5	1090	+576	602	109	393	+100	6.61	3.99	1.14	+1.48	7.64	4.39	12.30		diet 6a Fe amm. citrate
8-11	59													8.02	4.06			diet 6a Fe amm. citrate
12	60													8.43	3.94	11.16	60	diet 6a Fe amm. citrate

TABLE 12

Case 5. C. C. C. Effect of dietary phosphorus and vitamin D on Ca, and N$_2$ metabolism

DATE 1940-41	PERIODS 4-DAY	CALCIUM				PHOSPHORUS				NITROGEN				SERUM				REMARKS
		Intake	Urine	Stool	Balance	Intake	Urine	Stool	Balance	Intake	Urine	Stool	Balance	CA	P	Phosphatase	N.P.N.	
Nov. 20–23	1	186	6	231	−51	479	123	221	+135	7.63	4.26	0.86	+2.51	7.46	4.70		64	diet 1
24–27	2	186	9	242	−65	479	186	224	+69	7.63	4.41	1.06	+2.16	8.36	3.52	14.73		diet 1
Dec. 28–1	3	186	0	286	−100	479	263	273	−57	7.63	4.79	1.24	−1.60					diet 1
2–5	4	1353	2	1126	+225	515	173	306	+36	8.39	5.08	1.25	+2.06	7.84	4.07	20.45		diet 1
6–9	5	1353	0	1282	+71	515	138	294	+83	8.39	5.21	1.33	+1.85	8.61	3.50	21.20		diet 1
10–13	6	1353	0	1360	−7	515	145	330	+40	8.39	5.63	1.23	+1.48	8.49	3.23	22.96		diet 1 Vigantol 1 cc. daily
14–17	7	1353	0	1305	+48	515	169	294	+52	8.39	6.01	1.42	+0.96	9.11	3.26	16.19		diet 1 Vigantol 1 cc. daily
18–21	8	1340	0	1151	+189	475	160	224	+91	7.44	4.69	1.18	+1.57	8.64	3.23	19.19		diet 2 Vigantol 1 cc. daily
22–25	9	1356	0	1271	+85	488	163	262	+63	5.74	3.63	1.55	+0.56	8.48	3.89	18.29	32	diet 2 Vigantol 1 cc. daily
26–29	10	1356	0	1295	+61	488	155	273	+60	5.74	3.64	1.45	+0.65	9.05	3.49	18.70		diet 2
30–2 (Jan.)	11	1356	0	1158	+198	488	176	232	+80	5.74	3.91	1.28	+0.55	8.97	3.74	23.96		diet 2
Jan. 3–6	12	1356	1	1220	+136	488	172	209	+107	5.74	4.16	1.34	−0.24	8.56	3.72	18.07		diet 2
7–10	13	1356	1	1242	+113	907	194	508	+205	5.74	3.57	1.33	−0.84	8.31	3.70	18.52	43	diet 3a
11–14	14	1459	0	1108	+351	819	194	388	+237	8.58	4.69	1.50	+2.39	8.38	3.55	17.36	60	diet 3a and b
15–18	15	1416	0	846	+570	191	170	286	−265	7.35	5.24	1.22	−0.89	8.40	5.36	12.86	86	diet 4a
19–22	16	1270	0	1188	+82	415	122	206	+87	4.73	4.19	1.27	−2.05	8.56	3.86	8.72	55	diet 4a
23–26	17	1421	0	804	+617	415	120	248	+47	4.73	3.48	0.94	+0.31	8.68	3.72		50	diet 4a
27–30	18	1421	2	1092	+327	415	120	191	+104	4.73	3.46	1.39	−0.12	8.71	3.97	24.77	60	diet 4a
31–3 (Feb.)	19	1421	1	820	+600	415	143	178	+94	4.73	3.96	1.04	−0.27	8.53	3.33	21.07	55	diet 4a Vitamin D$_2$ 1,000,000 i.u. oral
Feb. 4–7	20	1421	0	965	+456	451				4.73	3.47	1.12	+0.14					diet 4b
8–11	21	1431	0	684	+747	451	84	123	+244	5.49	3.37	1.00	+1.12	8.73	3.48	23.18	50	diet 4b
12–15	22	1431	0	748	+683	451	108	97	+246	5.49	3.78	1.02	+0.69	8.60	3.55	22.79		diet 4b
16–19	23	1431	0	750	+681	451	96	99	+256	5.49	4.21	1.10	+0.18	8.52	3.53	22.31		diet 4b
20–23	24	1431	0	754	+677	451	86	151	+214	5.49	4.00	1.08	+0.41	8.43	3.50	22.34		diet 4b
24–27	25	1431	0	682	+749	451	79	151	+221	5.49	3.95	0.98	+0.56	8.89	3.21	27.95		diet 4b
28–3 (Mar.)	26	1371	0	866	+505	376	98	154	+124	4.25	4.66	1.04	−1.45	8.60	3.62	24.14		diet 4b
March 4–7	27	1431	1	675	+755	451	83	167	+201	5.49	4.94	1.03	−0.48	8.80	3.96	20.64		diet 4b
8–11	28	1431	2	940	+489	451	111	240	+100	5.49	4.75	1.33	−0.59	8.90	3.92	17.58		diet 4b
12–15	29	1431	1	885	+545	451	101	220	+130	5.49	4.94	1.37	−0.82	8.72	3.84	15.42		diet 4b

S. H. LIU AND H. I. CHU

REFERENCES

1. PARK, E. A., AND ELIOT, M. M.: Renal hyperparathyroidism with osteoporosis (osteitis) fibrosa cystica. Brennemann's Practice of Pediatrics, vol. 3, chap. 29, 1936.
2. ALBRIGHT, F., DRAKE, T. G., AND SULKOWITCH, H. W.: Renal osteitis fibrosa cystica: Report of a case with discussion of metabolic aspects. Bull. Johns Hopkins Hosp., **60**: 377, 1937.
3. LUCAS, R. C.: Form of late rickets associated with albuminuria, rickets of adolescents. Lancet, **1**: 993, 1883.
4. FLETCHER, H. M.: Case of infantilism with polyuria and chronic renal disease. Proc. Roy. Soc. Med., **4**: 95, 1911.
5. BARBER, H.: Renal dwarfism. Quart. J. Med., **14**: 205, 1920–21.
6. PARSONS, L. G.: The bone changes occurring in renal and coeliac infantilism, and their relation to rickets. I. Renal rickets. Arch. Dis. Child., **2**: 1, 1927.
7. TEALL, C. G.: A radiological study of the bone changes in renal infantilism. Brit. J. Radiol., **1**: 49, 1928.
8. BROCKMAN, E. P.: Some observations on the bone changes in renal rickets. Brit. J. Surg., **14**: 634, 1926–27.
9. LANGMEAD, F. S., AND ORR, J. W.: Renal rickets associated with parathyroid hyperplasia. Arch. Dis. Child., **8**: 265, 1933.
10. SMYTH, F. S., AND GOLDMAN, L.: Renal rickets with metastatic calcification and parathyroid dysfunction. Am. J. Dis. Child., **48**: 597, 1934.
11. SHELLING, D. H., AND REMSEN, D.: Renal rickets: Report of a case showing four enlarged parathyroids and evidence of parathyroid hypersecretion. Bull. Johns Hopkins Hosp., **57**: 158, 1935.
12. PRICE, N. L., AND DAVIE, T. B.: Renal rickets. Brit. J. Surg., **24**: 548, 1936–37.
13. DEROW, H. A., AND BRODNY, M. L.: Congenital posterior urethral valve causing renal rickets. New England J. Med., **221**: 685, 1939.
14. MAGNUS, H. A., AND SCOTT, R. B.: Chronic renal destruction and parathyroid hyperplasia. J. Path. and Bact., **42**: 665, 1936.
15. MITCHELL, A. G.: Nephrosclerosis (chronic interstitial nephritis) in childhood with special reference to renal rickets. Am. J. Dis. Child., **40**: 101, 345, 1930.
16. HAMPERL, H., UND WALLIS, K.: Ueber renalen Zwergwuchs ohne und mit (renaler) Rachitis. Ergebn. d. inn. Med. u. Kinderh. **45**: 389, 1933. Ueber renale Rachitis und renalen Zwergwuchs. Virch. Arch., **288**: 119, 1933.
16a. BENNETT, T. I.: The clinical manifestations of hypocalcemia in renal failure. Lancet, **2**: 694, 1933.
17. HANNON, R. R., LIU, S. H., CHU, H. I., WANG, S. H., CHEN, K. C., AND CHOU, S. K.: Calcium and phosphorus metabolism in osteomalacia. I. The effect of vitamin D and its apparent duration. Chinese Med. J., **48**: 623, 1934.
18. BODANSKY, A.: Phosphatase studies: determination of serum phosphatase. Factors influencing accuracy of determination. J. Biol. Chem., **101**: 93, 1933.
19. HASTINGS, A. B., AND SENDROY, J.: The colorimetric determination of blood pH at body temperature without buffer standards. J. Biol. Chem., **61**: 695, 1924.
20. VAN SLYKE, D. D., AND NEILL, J. M.: The determination of gases in blood and other fluids by vacuum extraction and manometric measurement. J. Biol. Chem., **61**: 523 1924.
21. VAN SLYKE, D. D., AND SENDROY, J.: The determination of chloride in blood and tissues. J. Biol. Chem., **58**: 523, 1923.
22. FISKE, C. H., AND SUBBAROW, Y.: The colorimetric determination of phosphorus. J. Biol. Chem., **66**: 375, 1927.
23. VAN SLYKE, D. D.: Gasometric micro-Kjeldahl determination of nitrogen. J. Biol. Chem., **71**: 235, 1927.
24. STADIE, W. C., AND ROSS, E. C.: A micromethod for the determination of base in blood and serum and other biological material. J. Biol. Chem., **65**: 735, 1925.

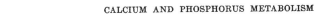
25. BUTLER, A. M., AND TUTHILL, E.: An application of the uranyl zinc acetate method for determination of sodium in biological material. J. Biol. Chem., 93: 171, 1931.

26. KRAMER, B., AND GITTLEMAN, I.: Gasometric determination of potassium. Proc. Soc. Exp. Biol. and Med., 24: 241, 1926.

27. CLARK, E. P., AND COLLIP, J. B.: A study of Tisdall method for the determination of blood serum calcium with a suggested modification. J. Biol. Chem., 63: 461, 1925.

28. BRIGGS, A. P.: Some applications of the colorimetric phosphate method. J. Biol. Chem., 59: 255, 1924.

29. FARQUHARSON, R. F., SALTER, W. T., TIBBETTS, D. M., AND AUB, J. C.: Studies of calcium and phosphorus metabolism. XII. The effect of ingestion of acid-producing substances. J. Clin. Invest., 10: 221, 1931.

30. CHU, H. I., YU, T. F., AND LIU, W. T.: Calcium and phosphorus metabolism in osteomalacia. VIII. The effects of ingestion of acid and alkali in patients with and without chronic nephritis. Chinese J. Physiol., 14: 117, 1939.

31. JAFFE, H. L., BODANSKY, A. AND CHANDLER, J. P.: Ammonium chloride decalcification as modified by calcium intake: the relation between generalized osteoporosis and osteitis fibrosa. J. Exp. Med., 56: 823, 1932.

32. SHOHL, A.: Effect of acid-base content of diets upon production and cure of rickets with special reference to citrates. J. Nutrition, 14: 69, 1937.

33. ANDERSON, W. A. D.: Hyperparathyroidism and renal disease. Arch. Path., 27: 753, 1939.

34. BOYD, G. L., COURTNEY, A. M., AND MacLACHLAN, I. F.: The metabolism of salts in nephritis. I. Calcium and phosphorus. Arch. Int. Med., 32: 29, 1926.

35. SCHOENTHAL, L., AND BURPEE, C.: Renal rickets, Am. J. Dis. Child., 39: 517, 1930.

36. LIU, S. H., HANNON, R. R., CHOU, S. K., CHEN, K. C., CHU, H. I., AND WANG, S. H.: Calcium and phosphorus metabolism in osteomalacia. III. The effects of varying levels and ratios of intake of calcium to phosphorus on their serum levels, paths of excretion and balances. Chinese J. Physiol., 9: 101, 1935.

37. LIU, S. H., SU, C. C., CHOU, S. K., CHU, H. I., WANG, C. W., AND CHANG, K. P.: Calcium and phosphorus metabolism in osteomalacia. V. The effect of varying levels and ratios of calcium to phosphorus intake on their serum levels, paths of excretion and balances, in the presence of continuous vitamin D therapy. J. Clin. Invest., 16: 603, 1937.

38. CHU, H. I., LIU, S. H., HSU, H. C., CHAO, H. C., AND CHEU, S. H.: Calcium, phosphorus, nitrogen and magnesium metabolism in normal young Chinese adults. Chinese Med. J., 59: 1, 1941.

39. FARQUHARSON, R. F., SALTER, W. T., AND AUB, J. C.: Studies of calcium and phosphorus metabolism. XIII. The effect of ingestion of phosphates on the excretion of calcium. J. Clin. Invest., 10: 251, 1931.

40. SALTER, W. T., FARQUHARSON, R. F., AND TIBBETTS, D. M.: Studies of calcium and phosphorus metabolism. XIV. The relation of acid-base balance to phosphate balance following ingestion of phosphates. J. Clin. Invest., 11: 391, 1932.

41. LIU, S. H.: The role of vitamin D in the calcium metabolism in osteomalacia. Chinese Med. J., 57: 101, 1940.

42. LIU, S. H.: Osteomalacia as a nutritional disease. Chinese J. Physiol. Nutrition Notes, No. 11, 1941 (January).

43. GREEN, C. H.: Bilateral hypoplastic cystic kidneys. Report of a case simulating chronic diffuse nephritis in a girl three years of age. Am. J. Dis. Chil., 24: 1, 1922.

44. LATHROP, F. W.: Renal dwarfism: report of a case. Arch. Int. Med., 38: 612, 1926.

45. FAXEN, N.: A case of renal rachitis. Acta Paediat., 14: 251, 1932.

46. ELLIOTT, A. R.: Renal rickets: report of a case. J. A. M. A., 100: 724, 1933.

47. SALVESEN, H. A.: Renal rickets: Report on a case with complete acid-base balance studies. Acta med. Scandin., 83: 485, 1934.

48. ALBRIGHT, F., CONSOLAZIO, W. V., COOMBS, F. S., SULKOWITCH, H. W., AND TALBOTT,

160   S. H. LIU AND H. I. CHU

J. H.: Metabolic studies and therapy in a case of nephrocalcinosis with rickets and dwarfism. Bull. Johns Hopkins Hosp., **66:** 7, 1940.

49. GYORGY, P.: Ueber renale Rachitis und Zwergwuchs. Jahrb. Kinderh., **120:** 266, 1928.

50. DUKEN, J.: Beitrag zur Kenntnis der Malacischen Erkrankungen des kindlichen Skelettsystems. II. Spätrachitis, Tetanie und chronische Schrumpfniere. Ztschr. Kinderh., **46:** 137, 1928.

51. KARELITZ, S., AND KOLOMOYZEFF, H.: Renal dwarfism and rickets. Am. J. Dis. Child., **44:** 542, 1932.

52. CHU, H. I., LIU, S. H., YU, T. F., HSU, H. C., CHENG, T. Y., AND CHAO, H. C.: Calcium and phosphorus metabolism in osteomalacia. X. Further studies on the action of vitamin D: early signs of depletion and effect of minimal doses. J. Clin. Invest., **19:** 349, 1940.

53. LIU, S. H., HANNON, R. R., CHU, H. I., CHEN, K. C., CHOU, S. K., AND WANG, S. H.: Calcium and phosphorus metabolism in osteomalacia. II. Further studies on the response of vitamin D of patients with osteomalacia. Chinese Med. J., **49:** 1, 1935.

54. LIU, S. H. ET AL.: Unpublished observation on single massive dose of vitamin D in osteomalacia.

55. TURNBULL, H. M., CITED BY HUNTER, D.: The significance to clinical medicine of studies in calcium and phosphorus metabolism. Lancet, **1:** 999, 1930.

56. KLUGE, E.: Neue Beiträge zur Kenntnis des renalen Zwergwuches und der renalen Rachitis. Virch. Arch., **298:** 406, 1938.

57. HOLTZ, F.: Die Behandlung der postoperativen Tetanie. Arch. f. klin. Chir. (Proc.), **177:** 32, 1933.

58. HOLTZ, F., GISSEL, H., AND ROSSMANN, E.: Experimentalle und klinische Studien zur Behandlung der postoperativen Tetanie mit A.T.10. Deut. Ztschr. f. Chir., **242:** 521, 1934.

59. SNAPPER, I.: The treatment of tetany. Lancet, **1:** 728, 1934.

60. HARNAPP, G. O.: Zur Pathogenese der Spasmophilie: Behandlungsversuche mit A.T.10. Monatschr. f. Kinderh., **63:** 262, 1935.

61. McBRYDE, C. M.: Treatment of parathyroid tetany with dihydrotachysterol. J. A. M. A., **111:** 304, 1938.

62. PICKHART, O. C., AND BERNHARD, A.: Treatment of post-operative tetany with dihydrotachysterol. Ann. Surg., **108:** 362, 1938.

63. MARGOLIS, H. M., AND KRAUSE, G.: Post-operative tetany: complete control of manifestation by means of dihydrotachysterol. J. A. M. A., **112:** 1131, 1939.

64. ROSE, E., AND SUNDERMAN, F. W.: Effect of dihydrotachysterol in treatment of parathyroid deficiency. Arch. Int. Med., **64:** 217, 1939.

65. WOO, T. T., FAN, C., AND CHU, F. T.: The treatment of infantile tetany with dihydrotachysterol (A.T.10). Chinese Med. J., **60:** 99, 1941.

66. ALBRIGHT, F., BLOOMBERG, E., DRAKE, T., AND SULKOWITCH, H. W.: A comparison of the effects of A.T.10 (dihydrotachysterol) and vitamin D on calcium and phosphorus metabolsm in hypoparathyroidism. J. Clin. Invest., **17:** 317, 1938.

67. ALBRIGHT, F., SULKOWITCH, H. W., AND BLOOMBERG, E.: A comparison of the effects of vitamin D, dihydrotachysterol (A.T.10) and parathyroid extract on the disordered metabolism of rickets. J. Clin. Invest., **18:** 165, 1939.

68. SHOHL, A. T., FAN, C., AND FABER, S.: Effect of A.T.10 (dihydrotachysterol) on various types of experimental rickets in rats. Proc. Soc. Exp. Biol. and Med., **42:** 529, 1939.

69. SHOHL, A. T., AND FABER, S.: Effect of A.T.10 (dihydrotachysterol) on rickets in rats produced by high-calcium-low-phosphorus diets. J. Nutrition, **21:** 147, 1941.

70. CHU, H. I., LIU, S. H., HSU, H. C., AND CHAO, H. C.: Calcium and phosphorus metabolism in osteomalacia. XII. A comparison of the effects of A.T.10 (dihydrotachysterol) and vitamin D (to be published).

71. LIU, S. H., CHU, H. I., HSU, H. C., CHAO, H. C., AND CHEU, S. H.: Calcium and phosphorus metabolism in osteomalacia. XI. The pathogenetic role of pregnancy and relative importance of calcium and vitamin D supply. J. Clin. Invest., **20:** 255, 1941.

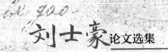
72. Cox, G. J., Dodds, M. L., Wigman, H. B., and Murphy, J. F.: The effect of high doses of aluminum and iron on phosphorus metabolism. J. Biol. Chem., 92: p. XI, 1931.

73. Brock, J. F., and Diamond, L. K.: Rickets in rats by iron feeding. J. Pediat., 4: 422, 1934.

74. Deobald, H. J., and Elvehjem, C. A.: The effect of feeding high amounts of soluble iron and aluminum salts. Am. J. Physiol., 111: 118, 1935.

75. Rehm, P., and Winters, J. C.: The effect of ferric chloride on the utilization of calcium and phosphorus in the animal body. J. Nutrition, 19: 213, 1940.

76. Day, H. G., and Stein, H. J.: The effect upon hematopoiesis of variations in the dietary level of calcium, phosphorus, iron and vitamin D. J. Nutrition, 16: 525, 1938.

77. Kletzein, S. W.: The influence of calcium and phosphorus on iron assimilation. J. Nutrition, 15: (suppl.): 16, 1938.

78. Anderson, H. D., McDonough, K. B., and Elvehjem, C. A.: Relation of the dietary calcium-phosphorus ratio to iron assimilation. J. Lab. and Clin. Med., 25: 464, 1939–40.

79. Barer, A. P., and Fowler, W. M.: Effect of iron on phosphorus, calcium and nitrogen metabolism. J. Lab. and Clin. Med., 26: 351, 1940.

80. Graham, O., and Oakley, W. G.: The treatment of renal rickets. Arch. Dis. Child., 13: 1, 1938.

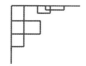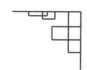

第六编　英伦进阶

　　第六编收录了1938年刘士豪教授去英国进修时发表的部分论文。他在伦敦的Middlesex医院Courtauld生物化学研究所，师从Charles E. Dodds，学习内分泌相关实验动物的研究，这在当时是非常先进的技术。其中2篇论文（《The effects of extracts of pregnant mare serum and human pregnancy urine on the reproductive system of hypophysectomized male rats》和《The effects of extracts of pregnant mare serum and human pregnancy urine on the reproductive system of hypophysectomized female rats》）是用孕马血清和人孕妇尿提取物注射去垂体的雌雄实验动物，观察它们发生的变化。这实际上和目前的内分泌功能试验是同一思路。另1篇论文（《Water balance and blood changes following posterior pituitary extract administration》是用垂体后叶提取物注射实验用兔，观察其水代谢和血容量的变化。因此，刘士豪教授的这部分研究，实际上一方面是垂体疾病研究的开端，另一方面也开了内分泌实验动物研究之先河。

124

J. Physiol. (1938) 94, 124–135   612.492.8:612.014.461.3

WATER BALANCE AND BLOOD CHANGES FOLLOWING POSTERIOR PITUITARY EXTRACT ADMINISTRATION

By E. C. DODDS, S. H. LIU,[1] AND R. L. NOBLE[2]

From the Courtauld Institute of Biochemistry, Middlesex Hospital, London

(*Received 7 July* 1938)

THE production of anaemia in rabbits after the administration of posterior pituitary extract has been previously described by Dodds & Noble [1935], Dodds *et al.* [1935]. Following a subcutaneous dose of approximately 400 pressor units of an acetone picric acid extract or standard B.P. pituitary extract a number of animals developed a severe macrocytic anaemia. This usually appeared on the fourth to fifth day, with relatively greater reduction of cell count than haemoglobin. In view of the marked reticulocytosis that accompanied the anaemia as well as increased bile elimination, the anaemia was considered to be the result of increased blood destruction. McFarlane & McPhail [1937] produced a similar anaemia in guinea-pigs, but this did not appear for 10–15 days after injection. Hypophysectomy did not result in any marked changes in the red cell and haemoglobin content of the blood, nor influence the effect of posterior pituitary extract in producing anaemia. Gilman & Goodman [1935, 1936, 1937] fully confirmed the finding of anaemia in rabbits after "pituitrin" injection. They, however, criticized the tentative suggestion put forward by Dodds & Noble that blood destruction may be controlled by the posterior pituitary gland. From their observations that the serum osmotic pressure and red blood cell count showed a parallel decrease they believed that the anaemia was a result of water retention which caused blood dilution and thereby haemolysis. In further support of their conclusions they point out that oliguria followed "pituitrin" administration, and that a dry diet of oats with water *ad lib.* prevented the production of anaemia.

From a critical consideration of the papers of Gilman & Goodman a number of conclusions may be drawn. (1) The fact that the severe

---

[1] On leave from Peiping Union Medical College, Peiping, China.
[2] Leverhulme Fellow of the Royal College of Physicians, London.

anaemia occurs only in a small percentage of rabbits has been overlooked. A large series is essential in order to determine what influence diet may have on the anaemia formation. (2) Fluid balance or blood-volume determinations were not made and therefore the implication that water retention occurs because of the oliguria is not justified. In a following paper it will be shown that the typical severe anaemia may occur in rabbits on a dry diet, and that no alteration in fluid balance or blood volume takes place.

From a physiological viewpoint the suggestion that hydraemia, so severe as to cause blood destruction, would be produced in an animal from a normal fluid intake (if this did occur) with diminished urine output, is contrary to all scientific work on the control of blood volume and concentration. The blood volume and concentration would appear to be physiological constants which are most tenaciously maintained by the body. Even after the absorption of large amounts of water it has been difficult to demonstrate any consistent blood dilution. These experiments have been reviewed in papers by Chanutin *et al.* [1924], Greene & Rowntree [1927] and Findley & White [1937]. In animals which were subjected to forced water administration, Greene & Rowntree [1927] have shown that dogs may be given by mouth 5 % of the body weight of water every 30 min. for 5–8 hr. In these animals, which exhibit the symptoms of water intoxication, the average maximal fall produced in haemoglobin was from 100 to 83 % and in serum protein to 82 %, while the increase in plasma volume was from 100 to 114 %. Similar observations have been made by Underhill & Sallick [1925]. These changes must represent the maximal alterations which can be produced by water administration, with recovery of the animal. Even so, Greene & Rowntree state that "no evidence of haemolysis or of increased destruction of erythrocytes, such as haemoglobinuria, was observed". Gilman & Goodman [1937] found that the maximal changes following "pituitrin" administration were a reduction of haemoglobin from 100 to 33 % and of red blood count from 100 to 22 % (and a loss of body weight of some 400 g.), yet concluded that this anaemia is "a result of water retention causing blood dilution".

METHODS

In the following experiments the effects of large doses of posterior pituitary extract have been observed on rabbits and guinea-pigs. In fluid-balance determinations the animals were placed in metabolism cages and the urine collected and measured at 1 or 2 day intervals. In some

126　　　*E. C. DODDS, S. H. LIU AND R. L. NOBLE*

cases a dry diet, consisting of oats, bran and chopped hay, has been used together with water *ad lib.* In order to obtain a rough idea of fluid intake, where a diet of high water content has been used, the animals were fed solely on carrots or swedes. Urine examination of specific gravity, albumin, sugar, blood, urobilin and microscopic findings was recorded. Blood examination consisted of red blood cell count, reticulocyte percentage and haemoglobin determination. The blood volume was measured using the vital red method [Peters & van Slyke, 1932]. A Leitz three-stage colorimeter was used for colour comparison, and serum taken previous to the dye administration was always used for the control. For blood volume it was found necessary to anaesthetize the rabbits with sodium amytal (75 mg. per kg. intraperitoneally), as preliminary observations without anaesthesia gave inconsistent results. B.P. pituitary extract has been administered by subcutaneous injection. In some cases the extracts used were prepared by the Kamm [1928] process, or by the acetone picric acid process [Dodds *et al.* 1934].

Results

Susceptibility. In rabbits the severe anaemia, as first described by Dodds & Noble [1935], has been produced in a relatively small number of animals. In all the experiments some sixty rabbits have received a dose of a pituitary preparation adequate to cause the severe anaemia. This, however, has occurred in only seven animals, or roughly in 11·5 % of cases. Some of these rabbits were receiving a wet diet, and one, the dry diet previously described. The anaemia has occurred in animals of both sexes and no particular strain or breed of rabbit has been used.

Slight or moderate anaemia (red cell count and haemoglobin more than 50 % of the original level) has been found to occur in nearly all the animals injected. A control extract (picrate) of anterior pituitary lobes was given in comparable doses to ten rabbits. Also, fourteen rabbits received injections of an extract (picrate) made from liver, kidney, and muscle. In these experiments there was no associated anaemia, and it is suggestive that the slight anaemia which follows posterior lobe extracts may be of significance. Liu & Noble [1938] have found that this type of anaemia also occurred after the injection of posterior lobe extracts directly into the renal artery. Under these conditions gastric haemorrhage could not be a factor in the anaemia.

Variations in extract administration. It was thought that the refractory animals might develop anaemia if the route of administration or the number of doses of the extract were altered. Pituitary extract has been administered intravenously to rabbits which failed to exhibit a severe anaemia after subcutaneous injection. Although doses as large as those used subcutaneously have been given over a short time it has not been found possible to produce anaemia in these animals. Other observations indicate that the intravenous route of injection does not materially increase the response to extracts. Thus, two rabbits of 3·3 and 2·8 kg. were injected through the ear vein with 100 and 130 pressor units of extract respectively. This was divided into three equal doses and given slowly at hourly intervals. No severe anaemia developed following this treatment or when somewhat larger doses were repeated 2 weeks later. Acute gastric ulceration has been shown to follow the administration of "pituitrin" by mouth in rabbits [Dodds *et al.* 1937]. In a few experiments it was found that no anaemia was associated with lesions produced in this manner.

Alterations in the spacing and size of dose given subcutaneously have been studied. Two animals which developed the severe anaemia from a single subcutaneous dose were allowed to return to normal and the injection then repeated. This was followed by a second period of severe anaemia. In another experiment two normal animals received 10 units, and two others 50 units three times a day for from 10 to 18 days without severe anaemia resulting. One of these animals at autopsy had a typical gastric ulcer. Large doses of 400 pressor units were injected subcutaneously into five rabbits at weekly intervals from 5 to 10 weeks. In no case did severe anaemia ensue. The effect of small doses of pituitary extract on the blood and fluid balance will be reported later in this paper.

Water balance with wet diet

In order to measure roughly the fluid intake rabbits were given 1 kg. of swedes daily as their only food. Urine was measured daily. Following the subcutaneous injection of 200 units of extract the urine excretion was markedly reduced usually for 5–6 days. During this time, however, the animals consumed very little food, and any positive water balance, if present, was not enough to be reflected in body weight. After such large injections nearly all animals developed severe diarrhoea which increased fluid loss. In Table I the alterations in fluid balance and body weight are shown in a typical experiment. The fall in urine output and food intake were maintained for 6 days, and then a rapid return to normal occurred. The blood showed a mild anaemia while the body weight remained unaltered. After a month's interval this animal received 200 units of extract given by mouth. In contrast to the previous antidiuretic action,

E. C. DODDS, S. H. LIU AND R. L. NOBLE

TABLE I. Effect of pituitary extract on fluid balance and blood of a rabbit

| Days | Urine output c.c. | Swedes eaten g. | Blood | | Body weight kg. |
			R.B.C. million/c.mm.	H.B. g./100 c.c.	
1–7 (control)	304·2	698·5	5·63	11·5	2·06

200 units B.P. pituitary extract subcutaneously

Days	Urine output c.c.	Swedes eaten g.	R.B.C. million/c.mm.	H.B. g./100 c.c.	Body weight kg.
8	65	380	—	—	—
9	14	100	—	—	—
10	14	140	6·5	—	—
11	5	300	—	—	—
12	20	300	5·4	—	—
13	0	420	—	—	2·06
14	34	320	5·3	10·7	—
15	300	800	—	—	—
16	275	560	5·0	—	—
17	240	600	—	—	—
18	355	640	—	—	—
19	345	720	5·15	—	2·06

pituitary extract administered by mouth had no effect. For 4 days previous to the extract administration the food intake was 748 g. and urine output 354 c.c. The next two 4-day periods following the extract showed food intake 750 and 728 g. and urine output 331 and 331 c.c. respectively. In another experiment an attempt was made to decrease the urine excretion, but to maintain the animal's food intake. In a previous report [Dodds et al. 1937] it was shown that the antidiuretic activity of pituitary extract could be prolonged by the addition of zinc salts. A rabbit, therefore, was given small doses (5 units) twice daily of an extract in a 5 % zinc acetate solution. With this treatment it was found that the urine output was materially reduced, but the cabbage intake was only slightly lowered. A slight anaemia developed in this case and also a lowering of the body weight. Terminally anuria occurred and the food intake dropped without any increase, however, in the anaemia. These findings are recorded in Table II.

TABLE II. Effect of small doses of zinc pituitary extract on fluid balance and blood of a rabbit

Days	Urine output average c.c.	Cabbage eaten average g.	R.B.C. million/c.mm.	Body weight kg.
Control	245·0	500·0	5·6	2·18

5 units twice daily pituitary extract in 5 % zinc acetate

Days	Urine output average c.c.	Cabbage eaten average g.	R.B.C. million/c.mm.	Body weight kg.
1–4	14·5	202·5	5·5	2·18
5–8	61·7	265·0	5·25	2·10
9–12	71·2	377·5	4·05	2·10
13–16	40·0	286·5	3·70	2·08
17–19	0·0	78·3	4·00	2·06

A series of adult guinea-pigs were injected with 30 units subcutaneously. In Table III it is seen that the effect of this on urine output and food intake (carrots) was slight. None of these animals showed the

TABLE III. Effect of pituitary extract on fluid balance and blood of guinea-pigs

	G. 71			G. 72		
Days	Urine average c.c.	Carrots average g.	R.B.C. millions/ c.mm.	Urine average c.c.	Carrots average g.	R.B.C. millions/ c.mm.
Control	120	200	6·3	65	145	6·35
	30 units B.P. pituitary extract subcutaneously					
1	25	61	—	35	128	—
2	44	172	—	43	140	—
3	110	200	—	62	152	—
4–6	109	198	5·1	55	148	6·85
7–9	50	107	4·4	31	152	6·05
10–12	72	189	5·35	64	170	5·15
13–15	79	194	5·45	34	165	5·00

	G. 73			G. 75		
Days	Urine average c.c.	Carrots average g.	R.B.C. millions/ c.mm.	Urine average c.c.	Carrots average g.	R.B.C. millions/ c.mm.
Control	65	130	5·6	83	161	6·15
	30 units B.P. pituitary extract subcutaneously					
1	31	140	—	48	120	—
2	54	180	—	53	144	—
3	72	200	—	48	157	—
4–6	68	200	5·1	80	185	6·3
7–9	68	200	5·7	86	200	5·75
10–12	84	195	6·5	60	193	5·35
13–15	99	200	4·5	65	184	5·25

typical severe anaemia, and it is apparent that a variation in the susceptibility of guinea-pigs occurs as well as in rabbits. These experiments made it appear unlikely that any increase in body fluid could account for anaemia production. Although the urine excretion was reduced there was an accompanying lowered fluid intake. Even when the food intake was maintained at as high a level as possible there was no evidence of increased blood destruction. In a further study blood volume has been measured as well as fluid balance.

Water balance and blood volume with a dry diet

In this series twelve rabbits have been given a dry diet, but with water *ad lib*. The fluid balance and the blood volume have been estimated as previously described. Four of these animals died shortly after the subcutaneous injection of 200 pressor units of extract, but the blood findings in the remaining eight are shown in Table IV. Rabbit 743 in this series

E. C. DODDS, S. H. LIU AND R. L. NOBLE

TABLE IV. Blood findings before and after 20 c.c. of posterior pituitary extract subcutaneously

Rabbit no.	Haemoglobin Before g./ 100 c.c.	Haemoglobin After g./ 100 c.c.	R.B.C. Before millions/ mm.³	R.B.C. After millions/ mm.³	Reticulocytes Before %	Reticulocytes After %	Minimum haemo-globin noted on day	Remark
742	9·7	9·4	5·04	3·80	1·0	2·0	3	Survived
743	9·9	6·0	5·01	1·98	0·8	30·0	4	Death on 4th day
744	12·4	10·6	5·63	5·50	4·8	5·0	14	Survived
745	10·9	9·1	5·02	4·12	0·2	2·8	4	Death on 18th day of uræmia
1	9·9	9·7	5·06	4·50	5·2	4·6	3	Survived
3	10·9	8·3	5·20	3·45	1·4	8·0	7	,,
4	9·5	8·9	5·10	3·56	6·4	7·0	3	,,
10	11·4	8·5	5·50	4·88	1·0	6·0	13	Death on 13th day amytal anaesthesia
Average	10·7	8·8	5·20	3·97	2·6	8·2		

developed the typical severe anaemia and showed a reduction in haemoglobin from 9·9 to 6·0 g. and in red cell count from 5·01 to 1·98 millions on the fourth day after the injection. The other animals showed slight anaemia from the third to fourteenth day after the posterior pituitary extract administration. The average reduction of haemoglobin was from 10·7 to 8·8 g. and red cell count from 5·20 to 3·93 millions. Proportionally there seemed to be a slightly greater reduction in red cell count than in haemoglobin content. Reticulocytosis accompanied the anaemia. The water balance and the blood volume of these rabbits may be seen in Table V. For 10 days prior to injection, the daily average water intake for the series was 95 c.c. and the daily average urine output was 46 c.c.,

TABLE V. Data on water metabolism and blood volume before and after posterior pituitary extract injection

Rabbit no.	Water metabolism, average per day* Water intake Before c.c.	Water intake After c.c.	Urine output Before c.c.	Urine output After c.c.	Balance Before c.c.	Balance After c.c.	Blood volume per kg. Before c.c.	Blood volume per kg. After c.c.	Body weight† Before kg.	Body weight† After kg.
742	82	73	60	24	22	49	58·6	66·5	2·44	2·54
743	132	34	71	76	61	− 42	67·9	34·5	2·71	2·12
744	133	48	66	35	67	13	—	71·4	3·36	3·12
745	54	25	22	45	32	− 20	—	82·8	2·60	2·12
1	102	103	47	41	55	62	78·5	77·6	2·80	2·86
3	94	86	38	66	56	20	89·4	79·6	2·60	2·08
4	74	78	34	32	40	46	84·2	69·7	3·06	2·74
10	88	49	33	25	55	24	79·7	75·0	2·32	1·96
Average	95	62	46	43	48	19				

* Average values of 10 days immediately before and after the injection.
† Body weight taken immediately before and 10 days after the injection.

leaving a positive balance of 48 c.c. As the animals remained fairly constant in weight the positive balance recorded represents largely the water lost through respiration and faecal elimination rather than an actual gain in body water content. After injection of the posterior pituitary extract the average daily water intake fell to 62 c.c. and urine output to 43 c.c. As the fall in water intake was much greater than that in urine output, the resulting balance of 19 c.c. after injection was much less than before. Two of the animals showed a negative balance. From

TABLE VI. Fluid balance and blood changes in R. 743 which developed severe anaemia

Days	Water intake average c.c.	Urine average c.c.	Haemo-globin g./100 c.c.	R.B.C. millions/ c.mm.	Reticulo-cytes %	Blood volume c.c./kg.	Body weight kg.
0–20	132	71	9·9	5·0	1·5	68	2·7
20			200 units pituitary extract subcutaneously				
20–22	60	120	—	—	—	—	2·35
22–24	10	40	6·0	1·98	30·0	35	2·10
	Animal dead						

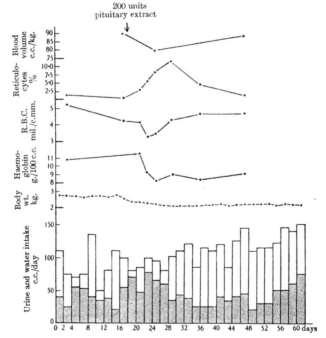

Fig. 1. Fluid balance and blood changes in R. 3 which developed moderate anaemia.

9—2

132   E. C. DODDS, S. H. LIU AND R. L. NOBLE

this it would appear that there was on the average a loss of body water after the administration of posterior pituitary extract. The loss of body water is further confirmed by the fact that most of the animals lost weight after the injection. Furthermore, the blood volume determinations (Table V) showed that most of the animals had a reduced blood volume after the injection.

From these observations it may be stated that in rabbits large subcutaneous doses of posterior pituitary extract resulted in slight to moderate anaemia in the majority of instances accompanied by loss of weight, decrease of blood volume and evidence of water loss. In R. 743 in which severe anaemia was produced, the weight loss was great, the blood volume decreased to half of its pre-injection level, and the water balance became negative. These findings are summarized in Table VI. The typical findings in an animal (R. 3) developing moderate anaemia is illustrated in Fig. 1.

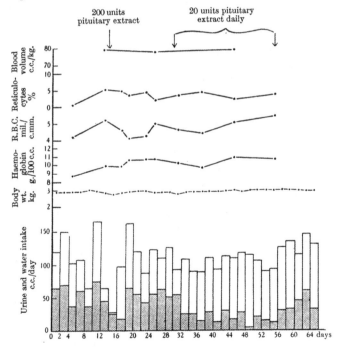

Fig. 2. Fluid balance and blood changes in R. 1 following a single and then repeated injections of pituitary extract.

Three of the rabbits (R. 742, R. 744 and R. 1), after recovery from the effects of the large subcutaneous dose of posterior pituitary extract, were given daily 2 c.c. (20 pressor units) of the extract subcutaneously for 26–39 days. No significant anaemia resulted in any of these animals. Urine output was suppressed during the period of pituitary extract administration and the water intake also decreased. The resulting water balance was not much greater than that in the control period, and the body weight remained stationary. The findings in R. 1, which is representative of the three chronically treated animals, are charted in Fig. 2.

Agglutination and haemolysis of red blood cells

In R. 743, which developed severe anaemia, it was noticed that the oxalated blood contained discrete particles which were identified under the microscope as clumps of agglutinated red cells. The plasma was intensely red, and on spectroscopic examination showed approximately 0·4 g. haemoglobin per 100 c.c. to be present. As the blood samples were taken into tubes containing isotonic sodium oxalate solution with a minimum of agitation, the agglutination and haemolysis observed were most likely intravascular. To investigate the phenomena the *in vitro* effect of posterior pituitary extract was tested. To tubes containing 0·05 c.c. of washed red blood cells 1 c.c. of normal saline, containing respectively 0, 0·05, 0·10, 0·25, 0·5 and 1·0 pressor units of the extract, were added. The mixtures were incubated at 37° C. Observations were made 3 and 20 hr. after incubation. The red blood cells of a control rabbit and those of R. 4 which had previously received 200 units of the extract subcutaneously were tested, but gave negative results. Slight haemolysis and agglutination were present in all the tubes, including the normal saline control.

Test for haemoagglutinin in serum. The technique followed was that of Donath-Landsteiner [Whitby & Britton, 1937], except that no guinea-pig complement was used. Sets of tubes were set up in the refrigerator (2° C.) and in the incubator (37° C.) and observed after 3 and 24 hr. The cells and serum of a control rabbit and those of R. 745 were examined. The latter animal had received 20 c.c. subcutaneously of posterior pituitary extract, developed slight anaemia and died of uraemia [Liu & Noble, 1938]. There was no gross agglutination of the cells in either the control or the pituitary extract injected rabbit's serum, although occasional small clumps of agglutinated cells were seen microscopically in both sera tested. The absence of clear-cut evidence of the

134   *E. C. DODDS, S. H. LIU AND R. L. NOBLE*

presence of haemoagglutinin in the serum of the slightly anaemic rabbit does not exclude the possibility of its presence in animals made severely anaemic by posterior pituitary extract administration.

DISCUSSION

The present experiments confirm the previously reported fact that posterior pituitary extract in large subcutaneous doses was capable of producing anaemia in rabbits. Although severe anaemia was only occasionally produced, slight to moderate anaemia occurred in nearly all animals. The susceptibility of individual rabbits to the anaemia-producing effect of the extract appeared to vary, and was not related to the route of administration or size of dose. Small daily subcutaneous doses for long periods, or repeated intravenous injections were no more effective in producing severe anaemia than a single large dose subcutaneously. The cause of the severe and mild anaemia would therefore appear to differ. When the relatively small percentage of rabbits which develop the severe anaemia is considered it is probable that changes in diet do not alter the susceptibility. As it was seen in R. 745, it is possible to produce anaemia in animals fed a dry diet. The occurrence of anaemia in one animal out of eight is in keeping with the frequency found in animals on a wet diet.

From the fluid balance experiments with either a wet or dry diet it may be seen that pituitary extract caused a fall in urine output. The intake of fluid, however, always fell off in a parallel fashion. Even when special means were adopted to increase fluid intake over fluid output no evidence of severe anaemia was found. The blood volume, as estimated, did not increase after pituitary extract, and in an animal which died from the typical anaemia the blood volume was materially lowered.

No evidence was found in confirmation of the contention by Gilman & Goodman [1937] that "pituitrin anaemia in rabbits is the result of water retention causing blood dilution". All the described results are incompatible with such a suggestion, and it is obvious that water retention and blood dilution do not constitute an adequate explanation of the anaemia which may follow posterior pituitary extract injection in rabbits.

As shown by *in vitro* experiments, the extract probably does not have any direct destructive effects on the red blood cells. But, on the other hand, the fact that apparently autohaemoagglutination and haemolysis were present in one of the rabbits with severe anaemia suggests the possibility that the extract acts through the production of haemo-agglutinin and haemolysin. Subsequent experiments on other rabbits failed to demonstrate conclusively the presence of such agents, but further studies along these lines would be desirable.

SUMMARY

A small percentage of rabbits develop severe anaemia following subcutaneous injections of posterior pituitary extract, but mild or moderate anaemia (probably of a different origin) is frequently produced.

Various modifications of the route or frequency of injections failed to increase the susceptibility of the animals. Diet apparently was not an important factor in anaemia production.

A reduction in urine output followed injections of extract, but the fluid intake fell correspondingly. No positive increase in water balance or blood volume could be observed even though one animal displayed the typical anaemia.

The suggestion that pituitrin anaemia is the result of water retention causing blood dilution could not be supported from the experiments described.

REFERENCES

Chanutin, A., Smith, A. H. & Mendel, L. B. (1924) *Amer. J. Physiol.* **68**, 444.
Dodds, E. C., Hills, G. M., Noble, R. L. & Williams, P. C. (1935). *Lancet*, **1**, 1099.
Dodds, E. C. & Noble, R. L. (1935). *Nature, Lond.*, **135**, 788.
Dodds, E. C., Noble, R. L., Rinderknecht, H. & Williams, P. C. (1937). *Lancet*, **2**, 309.
Dodds, E. C., Noble, R. L., Scarff, R. W. & Williams, P. C. (1937). *Proc. Roy. Soc. B*, **123**, 22.
Dodds, E. C., Noble, R. L. & Smith, E. R. (1934). *Lancet*, **2**, 918.
Findley, T. & White, H. L. (1937). *J. clin. Invest.* **16**, 197.
Gilman, A. & Goodman, L. (1935). *Proc. Soc. exp. Biol., N.Y.*, **33**, 238.
Gilman, A. & Goodman, L. (1936). *J. Pharmacol.* **57**, 123.
Gilman, A. & Goodman, L. (1937). *Amer. J. Physiol.* **118**, 241.
Greene, C. H. & Rowntree, L. G. (1927). *Ibid.* **80**, 209.
Kamm, O., Aldrich, T. B., Grote, I. W., Rowe, L. W. & Bugbee, E. P. (1928). *J. Amer. chem. Soc.* **50**, 573.
Liu, S. H. & Noble, R. L. (1938). *J. Physiol.* **93**, 13 P.
McFarlane, W. D. & McPhail, M. K. (1937). *Amer. J. med. Sci.* **193**, 385.
Peters, J. P. & van Slyke, D. D. (1932). *Quantitative Clinical Chemistry*, **2**. Baltimore.
Underhill, F. P. & Sallick, M. A. (1925). *J. biol. Chem.* **63**, 61.
Whitby, L. E. H. & Britton, C. J. C. (1937). *Diseases of the Blood*. London.

THE EFFECTS OF EXTRACTS OF PREGNANT MARE SERUM AND HUMAN PREGNANCY URINE ON THE REPRODUCTIVE SYSTEM OF HYPOPHYSECTOMIZED FEMALE RATS

BY S. H. LIU[1] AND R. L. NOBLE[2]

From the Courtauld Institute of Biochemistry, Middlesex Hospital, London, W. 1

(Received 15 February 1939)

IN a preceding paper [Liu and Noble, 1939] it has been shown that in male hypophysectomized rats, extracts of both pregnant mare serum and pregnancy urine were capable of exerting a marked effect on the testes as well as on the accessory sex organs. In the present experiments it was attempted to determine how far the results obtained on the male were comparable with those on the female hypophysectomized rats under similar experimental conditions.

METHODS

The experimental procedure was the same as previously reported [1939]. Vaginal smears were made daily to determine the oestrogenic activity. In mating experiments, normal males were placed with the hypophysectomized females at 2 weeks after the commencement of treatment.

RESULTS

Hypophysectomized controls. As shown in Table I, the rate of atrophy of ovaries and uteri of hypophysectomized rats was gradual up to 6 weeks after operation. After that time very little further decline in weight occurred. The vaginal smear showed a dioestrus condition within 3 to

Table I. *Rate of atrophy of sex organs of female rats after hypophysectomy*

Time after hypophysectomy	No. of rats	Body-weight at autopsy	Organ weights per 100 g. body-weight		
			Ovaries	Uteri	Adrenals
Weeks		g.	mg.	mg.	mg.
Unoperated	6	145–73	28·7	240	32·5
1	4	126–44	24·3	142	28·8
2	6	120–68	22·5	129	23·2
3–4	4	114–36	17·0	117	14·2
6	3	136–67	15·0	82	8·9
8	2	146–53	15·8	78	6·4
10	2	137–60	9·0	63	6·7

[1] On leave from Peiping Union Medical College, Peiping, China.
[2] Work performed during the tenure of a Leverhulme Fellowship of the Royal College of Physicians, London.

4 days after hypophysectomy; histologically the follicles rapidly degenerated and disappeared, but corpora lutea remained for relatively long periods. Even after 10 weeks, corpora lutea were still discernible, although much fibrous tissue replacement had taken place.

Pregnant Mare Serum Extract

Immediate treatment. When treatment was given immediately after hypophysectomy 0·5 m.u. of Antex daily maintained the ovarian weight and increased the uterine weight for 24 to 34 days (Table II). Vaginal oestrus continued for the duration of the experiment. However, in one animal (HRt 259), in which treatment was carried on for 42 days, the ovaries and uterus were markedly atrophied and cessation of vaginal oestrus occurred by the 27th day of treatment. Five rats treated for 12

Table II. *Results of treatment with pregnant mare serum extract (Antex) in female hypophysectomized rats*

	Treatment		Body-weight		Organ weights per 100 g.			Oestrus after treatment		
HRt no.	Daily dose m.u.	Duration Days	At operation g.	At autopsy g.	Ovaries mg.	Uterus mg.	Adrenals mg.	Onset Days	Cessation Days	Duration Days
				Immediate treatment						
172	0·5	24	200	147	30·6	246	14·3	7	no	17+
170	0·5	33	192	138	34·8	538	10·9	6	no	27+
173	0·5	34	177	120	32·5	550	11·7	6	no	28+
259	0·5	42	172	147	14·3	108	7·5	6	27	21
174	1·0	12	173	120	33·3	391	28·3	5	no	7+
260	1·0	19	160	104	31·7	435	17·3	5	no	14+
211	1·0	21	178	136	28·7	257	16·9	5	no	16+
175	1·0	23	195	113	33·6	410	15·0	5	no	18+
212	1·0	23	183	149	20·1	326	17·4	5	no	18+
				Treatment delayed 2 weeks						
161	1·0	23	180	125	22·4	267	10·4	6	no	17+
162	1·0	32	160	126	19·8	274	13·5	6	no	26+
157	1·0	47	180	138	23·2	308	11·6	6	no	41+
213	5·0	10	169	133	24·8	287	13·5	4	no	6+
135	5·0	11	182	128	47·7	365	19·5	4	no	7+
133	5·0	15	161	129	39·5	308	11·6	4	no	11+
214	5·0	34	191	136	19·9	305	8·1	4	no	30+
132	5·0	35	187	122	32·8	500	11·5	5	no	30+
				Treatment delayed 4 weeks						
109	1·0	42	177	145	9·2	157	6·9	6	no	36+
112	1·0	42	150	111	24·3	273	7·2	5	no	37+
113	1·0	42	155	109	24·8	297	7·3	5	no	37+
108	5·0	16	175	118	39·8	415	9·3	5	no	11+
107	5·0	38	184	136	21·3	280	9·6	5	no	33+

to 23 days had an approximately normal ovarian weight and distinctly heavier uterine weight than the unoperated controls (Table I). Vaginal oestrus was maintained for the entire period. The histological sections showed many large corpora lutea, with a few well developed follicles.

Delayed treatment. When Antex therapy was started 2 weeks after hypophysectomy and given in 1 m.u. daily dosage for 23 to 47 days, some regression in ovarian weight was found, but uteri were larger than normal. At a dosage of 5 m.u. per day, treatment for 10 to 15 days in three rats resulted in larger ovaries than normal, while treatment for 34 to 35 days in two other rats gave ovarian weights approaching normal, but less than those treated for the shorter period. Uteri were larger than normal in all cases, and vaginal oestrus always continued for the duration of the experiment.

When therapy was not instituted until 4 weeks after operation 1 m.u. per day of Antex for 42 days was apparently not sufficient to produce normal ovarian weight, although normal uterine weight was maintained. When the dosage was increased to 5 m.u. daily, one rat treated for 16 days gave larger ovaries and the other treated for 38 days gave somewhat smaller ovaries than normal. Uteri in both cases were large and vaginal oestrus was continuous for as long as 37 days.

Mating occurred in three animals in this series as shown by the presence of vaginal plugs, but no pregnancy followed.

Histologically the larger ovaries associated with the shorter period of treatment showed many well-formed corpora lutea with occasional fully developed follicles, but the smaller ovaries, from rats treated for the longer period, exhibited regressing corpora lutea and a few primordial follicles. Interstitial stroma appeared to be increased.

Pregnancy Urine Extract

Immediate treatment. As shown in Table III, Physex therapy started immediately after hypophysectomy in 0·5 m.u. daily doses maintained the ovarian and increased the uterine weight in the rats treated up to 22 days. One rat in the series receiving the treatment for 43 days showed marked regression in weight of both ovaries and uterus. The group receiving 1 m.u. daily consisted of nine rats treated for a period varying from 5 to 42 days. The ovarian and uterine weights showed an inverse relationship with the duration of treatment, indicating that there was an initial stimulation followed by subsequent regression. Likewise the animals exhibited continuous vaginal oestrus shortly after the commencement of treatment, but within 14 to 19 days oestrus gave place to dioestrus in spite of continued treatment. The state of anoestrus was usually associated with smaller ovaries and uteri. Histologically corpora lutea were well developed with a few atretic follicles.

c

18
S. H. LIU AND R. L. NOBLE

Table III. *Results of treatment with pregnancy urine extract (Physex) in female hypophysectomized rats*

HRt no.	Treatment Daily dose m.u.	Treatment Duration Days	Body-weight At operation g.	Body-weight At autopsy g.	Organ weights per 100 g. Ovaries mg.	Organ weights per 100 g. Uterus mg.	Organ weights per 100 g. Adrenals mg.	Oestrus after treatment Onset Days	Oestrus after treatment Cessation Days	Oestrus after treatment Duration Days
					Immediate treatment					
180	0·5	5	188	151	30·4	332	29·1	3	no	2+
182	0·5	6	199	176	33·5	372	27·8	3	no	3÷
284	0·5	18	185	129	41·1	444	19·4	7	no	11+
187	0·5	22	188	152	26·3	212	16·5	7	19	12
216	0·5	22	184	147	43·5	265	15·0	9	no	13+
179	0·5	43	200	176	8·5	990	6·8	4	19	15
183	1·0	5	191	160	29·3	356	28·1	4	no	2+
178	1·0	10	184	132	31·8	233	24·2	6	no	4+
268	1·0	11	160	126	42·8	429	33·3	6	no	5+
265	1·0	15	169	116	31·0	373	24·1	5	no	10+
266	1·0	16	154	108	25·2	282	21·3	5	14	9
185	1·0	17	169	112	26·8	433	17·0	3	no	14+
184	1·0	24	193	134	25·4	201	13·4	5	no	19+
186	1·0	25	192	140	25·7	169	15·7	5	17	12
267	1·0	42	160	135	17·3	92	11·2	2	15	13
					Treatment delayed 2 weeks					
164	1·0	20	137	102	22·5	259	11·8	4	no	16+
166	1·0	46	158	116	12·9	105	11·2	5	14	9
167	1·0	46	176	156	13·5	80	9·6	4	23	19
219	5·0	8	150	127	47·2	322	20·4	4	no	4+
136	5·0	14	164	122	29·5	285	19·7	6	no	8+
138	5·0	14	162	125	40·0	236	16·8	4	no	10+
217	5·0	15	145	98	30·6	333	17·3	5	no	10+
218	5·0	42	170	152	10·5	74	6·6	5	24	19
					Treatment delayed 4 weeks					
126	1·0	10	207	128	39·1	469	10·2	5	no	5+
127	1·0	11	223	150	26·7	230	10·7	4	no	7÷
128	1·0	42	192	161	14·9	62	11·5	4	22	18
117	5·0	20	172	120	26·7	226	9·2	4	19	15
114	5·0	42	160	150	5·3	113	6·0	5	18	13
115	5·0	42	157	116	21·5	78	7·8	5	26	21

Delayed treatment. When 2 weeks were allowed to elapse after hypophysectomy before treatment was started, 1 m.u. daily for 20 days (HRt. 164) restored ovarian and uterine weight, but when the treatment was continued for 46 days (HRt. 166 and 167), considerable regression took place. Increasing the dosage to 5 m.u. a day gave similar results, namely, a short period of treatment stimulated both ovarian and uterine growth, but a longer period of treatment failed to maintain the stimulation.

Similar observations were made on rats in which treatment was post-

GONADOTROPHIC HORMONES

poned for 4 weeks after operation. With a daily dosage of either 1 or 5 m.u. there was an initial stimulation, as shown by the greater ovarian and uterine weights in rats receiving a shorter period of treatment (10 to 20 days). This, however, was followed by regression, as evidenced by the atrophy of these organs in rats given a longer period of treatment (42 days).

Continuous vaginal oestrus was induced initially in all the rats in this series, but, like the series receiving treatment immediately after operation, dioestrus followed after a period of 9 to 21 days of continuous oestrus despite continued therapy. Similarly, dioestrus was accompanied by atrophied ovaries and uteri. The results of mating the animals in this series were negative.

Histologically corpora lutea appeared to persist in the ovaries. The larger ovaries obtained from rats receiving the shorter period of treatment showed larger corpora lutea, while the smaller ovaries obtained from rats receiving the longer period of treatment contained smaller fibrosed bodies resembling corpora albicana. Follicles were undeveloped and few in number.

DISCUSSION

From the above results it is clear that extracts of both pregnant mare serum (Antex) and pregnancy urine (Physex) were capable of maintaining and restoring ovarian weight of female hypophysectomized rats for a time, but with continued injections the ovaries began to regress. With Physex the subsequent ovarian regression was so marked that animals receiving therapy for 6 weeks showed, at autopsy, ovaries no larger than untreated operated controls for that period. With Antex, however, although some regression occurred after 6 weeks of therapy, the ovaries were usually heavier than those of untreated operated controls.

Histologically corpora lutea constituted the main part of the ovaries of animals treated with either extract. In time these decreased in size and showed degenerative changes in spite of continued treatment, corresponding to the decline in ovarian weight, especially in Physex-treated animals. In the case of the follicular apparatus, Antex-treated rats occasionally showed a well-developed antrum containing follicles early in the course of treatment; they were not seen in the later periods. With Physex follicular development was held in abeyance in all instances. Most authors agree that pregnancy urine extract possesses no follicle stimulating action. This was demonstrated in hypophysectomized rats by Leonard and Smith [1934] and Evans, Pencharz, and Simpson [1934]. On the other hand, pregnant mare serum has been shown to exert a follicle stimulating action, and Evans, Korpi, Simpson, and Pencharz [1936] have isolated from it a pure follicle stimulating fraction. The small degree of follicle stimulation in the experiments described with Antex was probably due to the predominating luteinizing action, especially in cases where treatment was prolonged.

Both extracts consistently induced continuous vaginal oestrus in hypophysectomized rats, although the duration of such differed between the two preparations. In Antex-treated animals oestrus, once initiated, was maintained in all but one for the whole of the experimental period up to 6 weeks. In Physex-treated animals, however, oestrus lasted for a period of only 9 to 21 days and did not reappear despite continued treatment. The continuous vaginal oestrus was associated with an increased uterine weight. Thus with Antex treatment, which maintained continuous vaginal oestrus up to the expiration of the experiments, uterine weights were either normal or greater than normal. With Physex treatment, which allowed the animals to pass into dioestrus within the experimental period, the uteri became atrophied. Antex, therefore, was effective in stimulating the production of sufficient oestrogen to give rise to enlarged uteri and continuous oestrus. On the other hand, the effects of Physex on the uterus and vagina were much shorter in duration. Greep [1938] under similar experimental conditions has shown that a correlation existed between the number of corpora lutea in the ovary and the duration of oestrus. The results described seem to support such an idea in that the animals which did not continue in oestrus had atrophic ovaries at autopsy, though even after the ovaries had become atrophic a month after hypophysectomy the animal still showed an oestrus response. This transitory effect of pregnancy urine extract in the female would appear to be similar to that which was found to occur in the male, and the possibility of anti-hormone formation must be considered. Mating took place occasionally in the Antex-treated animals, but in no case in the Physex-treated animals. Pregnancy did not occur in any of the treated animals; a similar failure has previously been noted by Evans, Meyer, and Simpson [1933] in the treatment of hypophysectomized female rats with a pregnant mare serum extract. The female reproductive system would appear to be so regulated that Antex or Physex, though adequate for the male under certain conditions do not constitute complete replacement therapy in the female, not at least under the experimental conditions reported.

SUMMARY

A series of female hypophysectomized rats were treated with extracts of pregnant mare serum or pregnancy urine. Treatment either immediately after hypophysectomy with small doses or delayed 2 or 4 weeks after operation with larger doses gave similar findings. With the pregnant mare serum extract the ovarian weight was maintained or restored for a time, but prolonged treatment resulted in slight regression. Uteri remained stimulated and oestrus was continuous throughout the experimental period. Mating took place, but no pregnancy followed.

Pregnancy urine extract maintained or restored ovarian weight, but regression on prolonged treatment was more marked and took place rapidly. A regression in uterine weight followed after initial stimulation. Vaginal oestrus was maintained only for a short period despite continued treatment. Mating did not occur.

REFERENCES

Evans, H. M., Meyer, K., and Simpson, M. E. 1933. *Mem. Univ. Calif.* **11**, 257.

Evans, H. M., Pencharz, R. I., and Simpson, M. E. 1934. *Endocrinology*, **18**, 601.

Evans, H. M., Korpi, K., Simpson, M. E., and Pencharz, R. I. 1936. *Univ. Calif. Publ. Anat.* **1**, 275.

Greep, R. O. 1938. *Endocrinology*, **23**, 154.

Leonard, S. L., and Smith, P. E. 1934. *Anat. Rec.* **58**, 175.

Liu, S. H., and Noble, R. L. 1939. *Journal of Endocrinology.* **1**, 7.

THE EFFECTS OF EXTRACTS OF PREGNANT MARE SERUM AND HUMAN PREGNANCY URINE ON THE REPRODUCTIVE SYSTEM OF HYPOPHYSECTOMIZED MALE RATS

BY S. H. LIU[1] AND R. L. NOBLE[2]

From the Courtauld Institute of Biochemistry, Middlesex Hospital, London, W. 1

(Received 15 February 1939)

EVANS, Meyer, and Simpson [1933] reported that in male hypophysectomized rats an extract of pregnant mare serum was capable of causing regeneration of atrophied testes and resumption of spermatogenesis and fertility. The accessory organs grew to normal size. Histologically the testes of the injected animals appeared normal. Similar results have been achieved with extracts of human pregnancy urine by Smith and Leonard [1934] and Evans, Pencharz, and Simpson [1934]. In the present experiments the relative efficiency of these two types of gonadotrophic extract have been compared in their ability to maintain and restore the reproductive system of hypophysectomized male rats.

METHODS

Male albino rats of the Wistar Institute strain, $2\frac{1}{2}$ to 3 months old, weighing 150 to 190 g. were hypophysectomized by a modified Selye technique [Collip, Selye, and Thomson, 1933]. Criteria of complete hypophysectomy were body-weight curve, adrenal weight, and examination of sella turcica at autopsy. In doubtful cases the sella was sectioned for histological study. Cases of incomplete hypophysectomy are not included in this series.

In one group of rats treatment was commenced immediately after hypophysectomy, and in the second and third series 2 weeks and 4 weeks respectively were allowed to elapse before treatment was started. The treatment was continued for 4 to 6 weeks. In another series no treatment was given, but autopsies were performed at various intervals after operation to ascertain the rate of atrophy of the reproductive organs.

The pregnant mare serum extract was Antex Leo, assayed on immature mice, one unit being described as the amount of the extract which doubles the weight of the ovaries. The pregnancy urine preparation was Physex

[1] On leave from Peiping Union Medical College, Peiping, China.

[2] Work performed during the tenure of a Leverhulme Fellowship of the Royal College of Physicians, London.

Leo, also assayed on immature mice with a unit defined as the amount causing the development of corpora lutea in 50% of the animals. The assay of these extracts has been described by Hamburger and Pedersen-Bjergaard [1937].

The extracts were dissolved in normal saline and made up in solutions containing 10 mouse units per c.c. The animals were injected subcutaneously once daily. Two dosage levels were employed in each series. In immediate treatments these were 0·5 and 1·0 m.u., and in delayed treatments 1·0 and 5·0 m.u. respectively. Each of the treated males was mated with two normal females from 4 weeks after the commencement of the injections to the 6th week.

At autopsy, the testes, prostate, seminal vesicles (with contents), and adrenals were dissected and weighed. The testes and tail and head of epididymis were examined microscopically for spermatozoa and their approximate numbers and motility. The tissues were fixed and studied histologically.

RESULTS

Hypophysectomized controls. The results on untreated hypophysectomized animals are shown in Table I.

Table I. *Rate of atrophy of reproductive system of adult male rats after hypophysectomy*

Time after operation	No. of rats	Body-weight at autopsy	Organ weights per 100 g.				Spermatozoa epididymis		
			Prostate	Seminal vesicles	Testes	Adrenals	Head	Tail	Testis
Weeks		g.	mg.	mg.	mg.	mg.			
Unoperated	11	158–80	196	149	1269	17·9	+++	+++	+++
1	4	107–40	120	52	1204	12·6	±	+	+++
2	4	112–30	109	56	854	12·6	±	±	++
3–4	5	113 56	87	42	366	8·8	0	0	0
6	2	140	54	34	273	5·7	0	0	0
10	1	109	81	40	258	7·3	0	0	0

The seminal vesicles and prostate degenerated very rapidly after operation. In 1 to 2 weeks they were approximately half the size of un-operated controls. Further degeneration occurred more slowly, and in 6 weeks it was almost complete. The decline in testicular weight was somewhat more gradual, but by 6 weeks it also reached a steady low level. Likewise there was a progressive decline in the adrenal weight until 6 weeks, when the lowest level was reached. Spermatozoa began to disappear from the head of epididymis within the 1st week, and from the tail of epididymis within the 2nd week of operation. By the 3rd to 4th week no spermatozoa could be found either in the epididymis or testis.

Pregnant Mare Serum

Immediate treatment. As shown in the first part of Table II, treatment with Antex 0·5 or 1·0 m.u. daily, maintained the testis weight for the duration of the experiment, namely, 42 days, and spermatogenesis went on unabated. Fertile mating resulted in three rats treated with 1 m.u. daily, although no litters were sired by rats receiving 0·5 m.u. daily. The substitution therapy with Antex at a dosage of 1 m.u. daily was therefore

Table II. *Results of treatment with pregnant mare serum extract (Antex) in adult male hypophysectomized rats*

| | Treatment | | Body-weight | | Organ weights per 100 g. | | | | Spermatozoa | | | |
HRt No.	Daily dose m.u.	Duration Days	At operation g.	At autopsy g.	Prostate mg.	Seminal vesicles mg.	Testes mg.	Adrenals mg.	Head epididymis	Tail epididymis	Testis	Result mating
						Immediate treatment						
332	0·5	6	169	133	287	212	1443	19·5	+++	+++	+++	—
335	0·5	7	169	132	168	56	1218	12·1	+++	+++	+++	—
331	0·5	11	149	113	225	230	1490	10·6	+++	+++	+++	—
402	0·5	14	174	120	203	85	1484	10·0	+++	+++	+++	—
336	0·5	42	188	160	80	38	1150	5·0	+++	+++	+++	0
365	0·5	42	190	150	690	948	1030	5·3	+++	+++	+++	0
401	0·5	42	187	157	436	574	1130	5·7	+++	+++	+++	0
333	1·0	11	169	130	265	253	1305	12·3	+++	+++	+++	—
334	1·0	11	154	124	292	348	1730	10·4	+++	+++	+++	—
404	1·0	18	158	119	384	504	1550	10·0	+++	+++	+++	—
337	1·0	42	167	133	262	248	1110	6·0	+++	+++	+++	+
367	1·0	42	174	132	321	355	1040	4·5	+++	+++	+++	+
403	1·0	42	196	168	510	832	1100	4·2	+++	+++	+++	+
						Treatment delayed 2 weeks						
357	1·0	28	160	128	73	30	410	5·5	0	0	0	—
358	1·0	28	168	148	115	111	426	5·4	0	0	0	—
391	1·0	28	193	158	243	253	670	6·9	0	0	0	—
390	1·0	28	172	146	336	463	638	4·8	++	++	++	—
17	5·0	28	198	130	900	980	820	4·6	++	+++	+++	—
18	5·0	42	193	140	143	74	315	4·3	0	0	0	0
200	5·0	42	183	128	677	610	860	6·2	+	+	+	0
						Treatment delayed 4 weeks						
351	1·0	28	177	151	75	49	290	6·6	0	0	0	—
352	1·0	28	178	122	105	40	219	5·7	0	0	0	—
354	1·0	28	175	138	440	427	560	4·4	0	0	+	—
406	5·0	15	172	154	394	744	556	8·4	0	0	0	—
397	5·0	21	166	139	302	1020	478	5·0	0	0	0	—
394	5·0	26	164	125	705	1250	595	5·6	0	0	0	—
400	5·0	42	185	143	1052	1023	829	4·2	++	++	++	0
78	5·0	42	198	154	493	431	860	3·9	+	++	+	0
53	5·0	42	156	119	103	69	644	5·9	0	0	0	0

Result of mating: + = normal litters sired, 0 = no pregnancy, — = not mated.

10   S. H. LIU AND R. L. NOBLE

complete as far as the spermatogenic function was concerned. The accessory organs were stimulated so that their weights at the end of 6 weeks treatment were much greater than those of normal untreated controls, the seminal vesicles being distended with secretion. Histologically the seminiferous tubules appeared to be normal with slight increase, in some cases of interstitial tissue.

Delayed treatment. When treatment was started 2 weeks after hypophysectomy when considerable degeneration had taken place, Antex 1 m.u. daily was not sufficient to bring about much repair although post-operative atrophy was somewhat slowed, especially that of the accessories. Increasing the dosage to 5 m.u. per day brought about considerably greater repair to the testes and marked stimulation to the prostate and seminal vesicles in two (HRt. No. 17 and 200) out of the three rats thus treated. Spermatozoa were present in the testes and epididymis, although mating was sterile. Histologically spermatogenesis was in evidence, but the seminiferous tubules were smaller than normal. The interstitial tissue showed marked proliferation.

The results of therapy started 4 weeks after hypophysectomy were not essentially different from those where treatment was initiated 2 weeks after operation. At the dosage level of 1 m.u. per day one rat (HRt. 354) was restored somewhat in testicular weight and stimulated in the growth of the accessories, but the other two showed no effect. However, when the dosage was increased to 5 m.u. daily, greater restoration of the reproductive organs occurred. In this group three rats were treated for 15 to 26 days, and three rats for 42 days. The latter receiving the longer period of therapy showed greater testicular weight with reappearance of spermatogenesis in the majority of instances, although the stimulation of the accessories was approximately of the same degree. Pregnancy did not occur in any of the females mated with the rats of this group. In the sections of testes from rats showing marked stimulation of the accessory sex glands, striking interstitial cell proliferation was again in evidence, as shown in Fig. 1.

Pregnancy Urine Extract

Immediate treatment. Physex at the dosage of 0·5 or 1·0 m.u. per day was ineffective in maintaining the reproductive system of hypophysectomized male rats. At the end of 42 days treatment (Table III) the testes weighed on the average but little more than those of the untreated operated controls at 3 to 4 weeks (Table I). Spermatogenesis was absent. The secondary sex organs, though somewhat heavier than those of the untreated operated controls, remained atrophic.

Delayed treatment. The data on rats receiving therapy 2 weeks after hypophysectomy were not complete (Table III). Only one animal was available, which received 1 m.u. of Physex daily for 37 days. The results showed no significant degree of restoration to the reproductive system. In the series treated with 5 m.u. daily the response of the testes was more

Table III. *Results of treatment with pregnancy urine extract (Physex) in adult male hypophysectomized rats*

HRt No.	Daily dose m.u.	Duration Days	At operation g.	At autopsy g.	Prostate mg.	Seminal vesicles mg.	Testes mg.	Adrenals mg.	Head epididymis	Tail epididymis	Testis	Result of mating
							Immediate treatment					
14	0·5	6	168	128	320	265	1280	18·7	+++	+++	+++	—
13	0·5	14	155	106	380	539	1754	11·3	+++	+++	+++	—
84	0·5	42	161	141	117	75	470	5·7	0	0	0	0
193	0·5	42	181	140	101	48	281	5·0	0	0	0	0
194	0·5	42	186	142	122	55	428	7·0	0	0	0	0
16	1·0	5	172	138	416	501	1561	20·2	+++	+++	+++	—
85	1·0	42	153	145	95	59	324	5·5	0	0	0	0
86	1·0	42	165	135	130	83	578	5·9	0	0	0	0
							Treatment delayed 2 weeks					
196	1·0	37	160	88	141	111	313	6·8	0	0	0	0
87	5·0	7	165	147	340	422	1437	8·0	+++	+++	+++	—
190	5·0	17	166	98	265	418	925	8·2	0	0	0	—
88	5·0	42	175	128	181	83	931	8·6	+	++	++	+
192	5·0	42	178	124	113	91	306	4·0	0	0	0	0
							Treatment delayed 4 weeks					
2	1·0	5	183	144	175	102	291	6·9	0	0	0	—
1	1·0	39	184	118	157	75	492	4·2	0	0	0	0
81	1·0	42	186	135	121	68	252	3·7	0	0	0	0
82	1·0	42	173	154	73	30	133	3·9	0	0	0	0
11	5·0	33	150	118	160	68	404	5·9	0	0	0	0
7	5·0	42	154	125	177	126	1126	5·6	+++	+++	+++	+
8	5·0	42	164	132	276	108	1238	3·8	+++	+++	+++	+
79	5·0	42	198	150	174	74	1008	6·7	+	+	++	0

Result of mating: + = normal litters sired, 0 = no pregnancy, — = not mated.

marked. In three instances out of four the weight was greater than that of untreated operated controls at 2 weeks, and in two instances spermatogenesis was restored; and in one case, mating was fertile. The accessories exhibited definite stimulation in the rats given a shorter period of treatment, but regression took place in those given 42 days of therapy. This suggests that Physex in adequate doses stimulates the accessory sex glands initially, but in continued administration this effect is lost, allowing regression to take place.

When therapy was delayed 4 weeks after hypophysectomy 1 m.u. a day

12　　　　　S. H. LIU AND R. L. NOBLE

was likewise ineffective in bringing about any significant repair in the atrophied testes and secondary sex glands, but a daily dose of 5 m.u. was much more efficient. In the latter group of four rats, three showed at the end of 6 weeks' treatment testicular weights approaching those of normal controls, and active spermatogenesis (Fig. 2). Fertile mating occurred in two of the rats. Of the secondary sex glands, the prostate was approximately the same in weight as the unoperated controls, while the seminal vesicles were somewhat smaller. The substitution therapy therefore was apparently complete from the viewpoint of spermatogenesis, but not so when the accessory glands were considered. An initial stimulation of the accessories followed by regression may have occurred, as shown in the group of rats treated 2 weeks after operation with 5 m.u. a day for a varying number of days.

DISCUSSION

From the above results on the rat it is clear that both the extract of pregnant mare serum and pregnancy urine have a stimulating action, but they differ in several important respects. In maintenance experiments when treatment commenced immediately after hypophysectomy, Antex in daily doses of 0·5 or 1·0 m.u. was able to sustain spermatogenesis and stimulate interstitial cell function for as long as 42 days after ablation of the pituitary while similar doses of Physex were ineffective. Thus in contrast to Antex, 1 m.u. of Physex (assayed by a different technique) does not contain sufficient gonadotrophic substance to produce significant effects on the reproductive system of hypophysectomized male rats. Higher dosage of Physex would probably be effective, as shown in reparative experiments.

In reparative treatment, Antex in 5 m.u. daily dose was more effective as an interstitial cell stimulator, but less efficient in restoring spermatogenesis than Physex in similar dosage. Thus Antex-treated rats showed greater prostate and seminal vesicle weights, but smaller testes than Physex-treated animals. While mating of Antex-treated rats did not result in any litters, it was fruitful in some of the Physex-treated animals. Increasing the dosage of Physex from 1 to 5 m.u. brought its effect on spermatogenesis from a position of relative ineffectiveness to one of marked potency; while a similar increase in the dosage of Antex failed to produce any greater effect in restoring than in maintaining spermatogenic function. This suggests that the difference between the dose required in maintenance and that in restoration is greater in the case of Antex than in Physex.

The relative lack of interstitial cell stimulating action in Physex may only be apparent rather than real, as it is possible that shorter periods of treatment produced larger prostate and seminal vesicle weights, whereas after 6 weeks treatment, regression in size had taken place. However, in the spermatogenic activity of either Physex or Antex there is no evidence of initial stimulation followed by subsequent regression in the response of the testis.

In the experiments of Evans *et al.* [1933] on the action of pregnant mare serum on hypophysectomized male rats, the interval between operation and injection varied between 29 and 41 days and the treatment was continued for 14 to 84 days. This corresponds to the delayed treatment described. The stimulation of the interstitial cells and restoration of spermatogenic function has been confirmed, but the latter was apparently not complete in that no fertile mating occurred. This failure may be related to the dosage employed. At a higher dosage level it is possible that enough enhancement of spermatogenesis may occur as to result in fertile mating. It must be pointed out, however, that the secondary effect of the androgens which are liberated in response to Antex may be an important factor in maintaining spermatogenesis. Cutuly, McCullagh, and Cutuly [1937 and 1938] showed that chemically pure androsterone and testosterone would maintain the tubules of the testes after hypophysectomy, if injection were started immediately post-operative. Once the testes were atrophied, however, the androgens would not cause repair of the tubules. The observed findings that Antex would maintain spermatogenesis if injections were started immediately after hypophysectomy, but did not restore spermatogenesis to a point where fertile matings occurred when therapy was delayed for 2 to 4 weeks, could be explained on the experimental findings of Cutuly *et al.* However, since there was definite histological evidence of spermatogenesis in some cases and a definite increase in the weight of the testes, it would seem that Antex produced a direct action on the testes in the delayed treatment experiments. The secondary liberation of androgens in the immediate experiments is probably an accessory factor in maintaining spermatogenesis.

Smith and Leonard [1934] noted that in hypophysectomized male rats, treatment with pregnancy urine extract produced an enlargement of the accessory reproductive organs and hypertrophy of the interstitial cells, but by the 30th day of treatment there was a marked regression of the accessories and the interstitial tissue. Likewise Greep and Fevold [1937] showed that in adult hypophysectomized rats partial regression of the accessory organs occurred after 30 to 40 days of treatment with luteinizing hormone of the pituitary. In the results described a similar phenomenon was apparent so that by the 42nd day of treatment with Physex the prostate and seminal vesicles were either atrophic or only slightly restored. In the experiments of Smith and Leonard they were

S. H. LIU AND R. L. NOBLE

unable to restore completely the spermatogenic function of their animals when injections of pregnancy urine extract were begun after a lapse of 20 to 75 days following operation. In the experiments described above the restoration with a similar preparation seemed complete in that fertility returned in some of the animals treated with a daily dose of 5 m.u. starting from 2 or 4 weeks after hypophysectomy.

SUMMARY

The gonadotrophic effects of extracts of pregnant mare serum and pregnancy urine were compared in adult male hypophysectomized rats. When treatment was instituted immediately after operation small doses of pregnant mare serum extract were adequate in stimulating interstitial cells with resulting enlarged accessory reproductive organs, and in maintaining spermatogenesis so that mating was fertile. Pregnancy urine extract in similar doses was ineffective. When treatment was delayed for 14 or 28 days after operation, but given in 5 or 10 times the dosage used in immediate treatment, pregnant mare serum seemed to be a more efficient interstitial cell stimulator than pregnancy urine, but the reverse was true in regard to the spermatogenic effect.

REFERENCES

Collip, J. B., Selye, H., and Thomson, D.L. 1933. *Virchows Arch.* **290**, 23.
Cutuly, E., McCullagh, D. R., and Cutuly, E. C. 1937. *Amer. J. Physiol.* **119**, 121.
Cutuly, E., McCullagh, D. R., and Cutuly, E. C. 1938. *Amer. J. Physiol.* **121**, 786.
Greep, R. O., and Fevold, H. C. 1937. *Endocrinology*, **21**, 611.
Evans, H. M., Meyer, K., and Simpson, M. E. 1933. *Mem. Univ. Calif.* **11**, 305.
Evans H. M., Pencharz, R. I., and Simpson, M. E. 1934. *Endocrinology*, **18**, 607.
Hamburger, C., and Pedersen-Bjergaard, K. 1937. *Quart. J. Pharm.* **10**, 662.
Smith, P. E., and Leonard, S. L. 1934. *Anat. Rec.* **58**, 145.

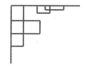
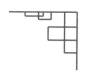

第七编　贫血探秘

　　刘士豪教授在 1938 年和 1940 年在病房收治了 2 例特殊的贫血患者，用生物化学的方法对这 2 例患者的血清进行了非常详尽的研究，其结果最终发表于 1951 年的著名血液病学期刊《血液》(*Blood*)。从这两篇论文可以管窥刘士豪教授的深厚内科功底和生物化学研究能力。

BLOOD *The Journal of Hematology*

FEBRUARY, 1951　　　　　　　　　　　　　　　　VOL. VI　NO. 2

Chronic Hemolytic Anemia with Erythrocyte Fragility to Cold and Acid

I. Clinical and Laboratory Data of Two Cases, with Special Reference to the Cell Abnormality

By S. H. Liu, M.D.

THE AIM of this paper is to report 2 cases of severe anemia which were thought to belong to the group of aplastic or "refractory" anemias, frequently seen in this locality[1] and recently restudied in the United States by Rhoads.[2] However, the history of passage of dark urine in one of the cases led to examinations for paroxysmal cold hemoglobinuria (Donath-Landsteiner) and for paroxysmal nocturnal hemoglobinuria (Marchiafava-Micheli). While the erythrocytes of this patient were found to be abnormally susceptible to hemolysis with chilling and on addition of acid, the diagnosis of either one or the other type of hemoglobinuria could not be properly made. Following the experience in this case, all the patients with peculiar or "refractory" anemia that were available at the time were similarly studied with the result that another case possessing the same abnormality of the red blood cells was found. The hemolytic nature of the anemia in these 2 patients was not evident on ordinary examination, but the demonstration of excessive hemoglobinemia in the serum and large iron excretion in the urine in both cases and finally the heavy hemosiderin deposits in the organs at autopsy in one case pointed to the presence of an abnormal in vivo hemolysis. The present report deals with the clinical data of the two patients together with the autopsy findings in one. The laboratory investigations characterizing the abnormality of the erythrocytes and the results of chilling and administering acid to the patients are included herewith. The studies concerning the serum factor necessary for hemolysis are reported in a companion paper.

Case 1

W. H. L. (74586), a Chinese farmer of 49, was admitted on November 29, 1940 for investigation of his anemia. In January 1940, the patient was noticed by his friends to be pale. However, no subjective symptoms appeared until February, when he began to experience general weakness with occasional dizziness on sudden movement of his body or abrupt assumption of an erect position. There was tinnitus with impairment of hearing. Since August the general weakness became more marked, with exertional dyspnea and palpitation. The

From the Department of Medicine, Peiping Union Medical College, Peiping, China.

The author wishes to acknowledge the valuable aid of Drs. H. I. Chu, H. C. Chao and H. K. Hsu in carrying out some of the experiments.

101

limbs were particularly weak with a tingling sensation in the hands. On inquiry as to bleeding tendency the patient admitted several attacks of dark urine. The first attack occurred in February 1940, when the urine was of the color of dilute Chinese ink; it cleared after two voidings. Similar attacks recurred at intervals of ten to fifteen days up to April. He was free from the attacks during the summer until they reappeared in September, the last attack being twenty days prior to admission. There were no chills, or other symptoms associated with the attacks. Exposure to cold did not necessarily result in attacks. The patient had had painful urination and urethral discharge eight years previously, followed twenty days later by generalized itchy skin eruption, but no penile sore was noted.

Physical examination showed pallor. The body weight was 64.8 Kg., and height 174 cm. Sclerotics were suggestively icteric. Fundi oculi were pale, especially the discs, with small hemorrhages in the retina. The tongue was normal. The lungs were clear except for a moderate degree of pulmonary emphysema. The heart was normal except for a blowing systolic murmur over the precordium. The blood pressure was 110/50. The pulse had a collapsing character, and capillary pulsation was demonstrable over the finger nails. The abdomen was relaxed and nontender. The liver, spleen and kidneys were not palpable. External genitalia were normal. No lymph nodes were palpable. There were no abnormal neurologic findings.

The urine was normal except for a few granular casts and red blood cells; the guaiac and urobilin reactions were negative. The phenolsulphonephthalein output was 40 and 49 per cent on two occasions. Blood study gave 1.54 million red blood cells, 5.1 Gm. hemoglobin, 2,700 white blood cells with 36 per cent polymorphonuclears and 54 per cent lymphocytes, 53,200 platelets and 3.4 per cent reticulocytes. Hematocrit was 16.2 per cent, mean corpuscular volume 106.5 cubic micra, mean corpuscular hemoglobin 34.2 micro-micro-grams, mean corpuscular hemoglobin concentration 32.1 per cent. Erythrocyte sedimentation rate was 75 mm. in 1 hour and 140 mm. in 2 hours (Westergren). The blood belonged to Group A. Venous pressure was 10 cm., and circulation time 13 seconds. Bleeding time was 2.5 minutes. The globulin test was negative. Icterus index was 5, and serum bilirubin 0.35 mg. per 100 cc. Fragility test showed beginning hemolysis at 0.48 per cent saline and complete hemolysis at 0.36 per cent saline, the control figures being 0.52 per cent and 0.32 per cent respectively. Sternal bone marrow showed active erythropoiesis, and normal distribution of myeloid elements. The gastric juice contained 5 cc. of 0.1 N HCl per 100 cc. on histamine stimulation. Liver function by bronsulphalein test showed no retention of the dye in 30 minutes and by hippuric acid test gave 4.16 Gm. of hippuric acid or 2.83 Gm. of benzoic acid in the urine in 4 hours.

Blood Kahn and Kline tests were repeatedly positive, and Wassermann reaction was strongly positive in three out of eight examinations, the rest being anticomplementary. Spinal fluid was normal, the mastic test and Wassermann reaction being negative. A smear of the urethral discharge contained many pus cells and gram-positive bacilli and cocci. An inguinal lymph node and blood were inoculated into rabbits on December 27, and no *T. pallidum* was isolated after two serial passages.

Donath-Landsteiner reaction was performed on December 4 and 9; on both occasions only a faint trace of hemolysis was obtained, with the patient's serum acting on his own cells but not of control cells. Titration of hemolysin titer of the patient's serum on December 14 and 16 gave equivocal results, while that on December 31 showed no hemolysis in the lowest dilution of the serum (6:10). However, the Rosenbach tests were positive on both Dec. 6 and on Dec. 17 (table 9). Chilling of both feet and legs in ice water at 5 C. for fifteen minutes gave rise to hemoglobinuria lasting for three to four hours. There were chilliness and cramps in the abdomen, but no rise of temperature.

The history of passing dark red urine in the colder months of the year and the positive Rosenbach test were strongly suggestive of the diagnosis of paroxysmal cold hemoglobinuria, but the negative Donath-Landsteiner reaction, and the persistent anemia during the paroxysm-free period were against the diagnosis. The nocturnal type of paroxysmal hemoglobinuria (Marchiafava-Micheli) was then suspected, and the acid hemolysis test devised by Ham[3] was performed. The erythrocytes of the patient were hemolyzed by small amounts of dilute acid in the presence of his own serum as well as of a control serum, in contrast to the control cells which remained intact under similar treatment. While this finding supports the diagnosis of Marchiafava-Micheli disease, certain other features of the case are not consistent with such a diagnosis. The positive Rosenbach test, together with the factor of chilling on the hemolysis of the red blood cells demonstrable in vitro in this case, has not been reported in cases of paroxysmal nocturnal hemoglobinuria in the literature. Moreover, in none of the reported cases of this condition was there historical or serologic evidence of syphilis, as in our patient. Further studies of the case, to be presented in the latter part of this paper, also failed to support the diagnosis of paroxysmal nocturnal hemoglobinuria.

Course in the hospital. For the treatment of his anemia the patient received dilute hydrochloric acid and ferrous sulfate (later ferric ammonium citrate) with no apparent benefit. Blood transfusions were given on December 19 and 23, 400 cc. of whole blood each time. This brought about an improvement in the anemia so that on January 12, 1941, the red blood cells were 2.32 million, hemoglobin 8.6 Gm., leukocytes 2,800, and reticulocytes 5.3 per cent. Liver extract 5 cc. (5 U.S.P. units) intramuscularly every day from January 21 to 27 failed to elicit any response except for a transient rise of the reticulocytes to 8 per cent. Antiluetic treatment was started on January 7, consisting of 8 weekly intravenous injections of neoarsphenamine, 0.45 Gm. each, followed by three weekly intramuscular injections of Na-K bismuth tartrate, 0.1 Gm. each. The treatment was stopped after March 18, on which date the blood Wassermann and Kahn tests remained positive as before.

From February 1 the patient began to have sharp, but transient, attacks of fever over 39 C., and continued low-grade fever in between. Except for injected throat and ragged tonsils there were no obvious foci of infection. Blood smears were negative for parasites and blood cultures were sterile. The anemia began to progress rapidly, and by the end of February, the red blood cells were 1.45 million and hemoglobin 4.9 Gm., leukocytes 2,200 and reticulocytes 2.2 per cent. The sternal and iliac crest marrow showed much fatty tissue with a few cells.

From March 1 the fever gradually rose, remaining at 39 C., and from April 1 it was around 40 C. Headache was complained of. Despite repeated blood transfusions (9 transfusions of 400 cc. each between February 21 and April 14) the anemia showed further progression. On April 10, the red blood cells were 0.86 million, hemoglobin 2.7 Gm., white blood cells 1,950, reticulocytes 1.6 per cent and platelets 20,600. Many purpuric spots appeared in the skin over the extremities and trunk and in the mucous membrane of the throat. There were numerous hemorrhages of various sizes in the retina. Singultus developed and persisted. The patient became drowsy and finally comatose. Death occurred on April 16, namely, 5 months after the patient was admitted and 16 months after he began to be ill.

Postmortem examination. This was performed by Dr. Y. Liu of the Department of Pathology, who kindly supplied the following findings. The heart was slightly enlarged, particularly the left side, weighing 400 Gm. In the arch of the aorta several longitudinal furrows were seen and above the aortic cusps there were two pale opaque rounded patches suggestive of syphilitic lesions. The lungs appeared to be voluminous, with distended air blebs along the anterior border. Caseous tubercles were present in the right upper lobe. The spleen was enlarged (245 Gm.), very soft in consistency with obliteration of the normal architecture. The liver weighed 1490 Gm., with patches of congestion in the central area. The gastrointestinal tract was normal except for several areas of erosion of the mucosa in the esophagus and a few scattered well demarcated ulcers, covered with dark blood, in the terminal ileum. Both kidneys were moderately swollen and pale, weighing 460 Gm. The surfaces appeared slightly granular, with adherent capsules. On section, the cortex was thicker than normal with blurring of the architecture. The pelvic mucosa showed a few petechial hemorrhages. The testes were normal. The marrow of the femur and ribs was yellow and that of vertebrae and iliac crest mottled yellow.

Microscopically, the aorta showed a few scars in the media with destruction of the elastic tissue and perivascular lymphocytic infiltration in the adventitia. The intima exhibited focal thickening, hyalinization, and cholesterol deposits. The lungs showed evidence of purulent bronchiolitis and emphysema. The liver presented moderate fatty change, atrophy of the liver cells in the central areas and congestion of the sinusoids. The reticulo-endothelial cells were hyperplastic, containing in their cytoplasm golden brown pigments which stained prussian blue with Turnbull's method (hemosiderin). This pigment was also seen sporadically in the liver cells. There was no evidence of thrombosis of the central veins or other vessels. The spleen showed active phagocytosis of hemosiderin, congestion of sinusoids and intimal hyalinization of the central arteries. The kidneys contained the largest amounts of the brown pigments giving Turnbull's reaction for hemosiderin. They were situated mostly in the tubular epithelium, which appeared to be autolytic. The glomeruli appeared normal except for a few sclerosed ones in the cortical layer. The interstitial spaces were edematous and the capillaries in them appeared much congested. The lymph nodes were characterized by reticulo-endothelial hyperplasia, erythrophagocytosis and hemosiderin deposits. The femur marrow was slightly hyperplastic, but the cellular elements in the ribs and verterbrae were fewer than normal. The erythropoiesis was normoblastic, with more polychromic than orthochromic erythroblasts, no megaloblasts being seen. The myeloid series was normal in distribution. Megakaryocytes were occasionally seen. There were moderate numbers of phagocytes and plasma cells, the former containing both red blood cells and hemosiderin.

Examination of the brain by Dr. Y. K. Hsu of the Neurological Service showed fresh subarachnoid hemorrhage extending over the frontal and parietal regions and over the cerebellum. There were no cerebral hemorrhages.

Comment. Anatomic diagnoses were: hemosiderosis of kidneys, liver, spleen, lymph nodes and bone marrow; slight hyperplasia of femur bone marrow and hypoplasia of rib and vertebral marrow; petechial hemorrhages in pelvic mucosa; subarachnoid hemorrhage; fatty change of liver and myocardium; syphilitic aortitis; purulent bronchiolitis; pulmonary emphysema; tubercles in lung; chronic ulcerative ileitis; scarring of kidneys.

Case 2

S. S. C. (62835), a railway workman of 43 years of age, Chinese, was first admitted on April 20, 1938, for anemia of seven years' duration. In September 1931, the patient began to notice weakness, pallor, palpitation of heart on exertion and pain along the spine on bending forward. Anemia was diagnosed and iron was given with slight improvement. The treatment was kept up for the next four or five years, but the symptoms persisted and became worse. He was first seen in the outpatient clinic in April 1936, when the blood hemoglobin was 4.3 Gm. per 100 cc.; the Wassermann reaction was moderately positive and Kahn test positive. Large doses of iron and liver by mouth were prescribed. Subsequent visits in 1936 and 1937 showed no improvement. Liver extract parenterally given for prolonged periods in 1938 was followed by no change in his symptoms. Hence he entered the hospital for further treatment.

There were no other members of his family with similar illness. His diet consisted of wheat flour, rice, millet, corn, vegetables and occasionally meat. He worked at a railway repair shop dealing with minor machinery parts, having had, to his knowledge, no contact with chemicals of any sort. He had frequent attacks of dysentery from 1915 to 1932, and of malaria in 1929–30. A penile sore developed after venereal exposures in 1923. Treatment then consisted of three injections of arsphenamine. There was no history of jaundice, skin rash or bleeding from any source except that on repeated questioning he admitted an attack of dark urine lasting for a day, without other symptoms, in April 1935.

Physical examination showed marked pallor but fairly good general nutritional status. The body weight was 53.7 Kg., and height 162.5 cm. The sclerae were clear, pupils reactive and fundi oculi normal. There were no foci of infection in the ears, nose, throat and teeth.

The arterial pulsations in the neck were prominent and radial pulse collapsing in character. The blood pressure was 132/62. The heart was not enlarged, but a loud systolic murmur was heard all over the precordium. The lungs were clear. The liver and spleen were not palpable. There was no subcutaneous edema. Neurologic survey gave normal results. No lymph gland enlargement was noticed anywhere.

Laboratory studies. Urine was normal except for the occasional presence of urobilin. The phenolsulphonephthalein output was 66 per cent in 2 hours. The stools were negative for parasites and ova. The hematologic studies showed 5.4 Gm. hemoglobin per 100 cc., 1.60 million red blood cells, 2,500 leukocytes with 42 per cent polymorphonuclears and 55 per cent lymphocytes. The hematocrit was 16 per cent, giving a mean corpuscular volume of 98.7 cu. micra, mean corpuscular hemoglobin of 34 micro-micro-grams, and mean corpuscular hemoglobin concentration of 34.4 per cent. The erythrocytes appeared normal with the reticulocytes varying between 2.6 and 5.9 per cent. The platelet count ranged between 64,000 and 214,000. The bleeding time was 2 minutes, and coagulation time 9 minutes. The erythrocyte fragility to hypotonic saline was normal, hemolysis starting at 0.44 per cent and complete at 0.28 per cent with both the patient's and the control's cells. Similar results were obtained on each of the subsequent admissions. The blood of the patient belonged to Group O. The sternal bone marrow showed increased number of primitive erythrogenic cells and decreased number of granulocytes. The bromsulphalein liver function test showed a trace of the dye in the serum in 30 minutes. The serum bilirubin was 1.0, N.P.N. 26 mg. per 100 cc., albumin 4.31 per cent and globulin 3.27 per cent. The blood Wassermann, Kahn and Kline tests this time were weakly positive, and the spinal fluid Wassermann reaction was negative. Gastric analysis showed no free hydrochloric acid in the fasting content, but 55 cc. of 0.1 N HCl per 100 cc. of gastric juice after histamine injection. Gastro-intestinal x-ray series gave no abnormal findings.

Course in the hospital. Ferric ammonium citrate 6 Gm. and whole liver 300–600 Gm. daily were started from April 27. Although the reticulocytes rose to as high as 14.8 per cent, and the white blood cells went up to 3,800, the erythrocytes and hemoglobin failed to show any increase. On May 13, the left lower extremity was swollen, and the inner aspect of the thigh was tender with enlarged inguinal lymph nodes. Thrombophlebitis of the left femoral vein was suspected. The condition, however, subsided in five or six days. A recurrence took place on May 22 and this also became better in a few days. Liver extract 5 cc. (5 U.S.P. units) a day injected intramuscularly from May 14–20 also failed to elicit any response. Blood transfusions were then given in quantities of 300 or 500 cc. at intervals of three to five days (eight transfusions from May 23 to June 19, totalling 3,000 cc.). The erythrocytes increased steadily from 1.23 to 3.78 million and hemoglobin from 4.2 to 13.0 Gm. and the leukocytes from 2,100 to 3,400 within the month of intensive blood transfusion therapy. The reticulocytes decreased from 6.2 to 2.1 per cent. There was no untoward reaction (to blood transfusion) except that for two days after a transfusion of 500 cc. of compatible blood on June 11, the urine was dark colored, giving a positive guaiac test but without red blood cells in the sediment. No symptoms were associated with the hemoglobinuria. The patient also received three intravenous injections of 0.45 Gm. of neoarsphenamine each during this admission. The blood Wassermann reaction became negative, although the Kahn test remained positive. He was discharged on June 21, 1938 in good condition except for slight residual edema of left leg.

Second admission. April 25–May 29, 1939. After the patient's discharge he continued to do well for two months, resuming light work. However, he had to stop because of weakness, palpitation, dyspnea and swelling of legs. These symptoms varied in severity with a downhill trend in the subsequent months so that on the present admission signs of congestive heart failure were present. In addition to edema of legs, the heart was definitely enlarged and liver palpable at 1 cm. below the costal margin. Teleoroentgenogram of the heart showed 75 per cent oversize, the enlargement being generalized, compatible with anemia heart. Urine contained a faint trace of albumin, disappearing a few days later (this was true also with later admissions). The anemia was more severe than during the first admis-

106   ANEMIA WITH ERYTHROCYTE FRAGILITY TO COLD AND ACID. I.

sion: Erythrocytes 0.65 million, hemoglobin 2.5 Gm., leukocytes 1,750 with 14 per cent poly-morphonuclears, 74 per cent lymphocytes and 12 per cent monocytes. The reticulocytes were 6.3 per cent and platelets 63,700. The hematocrit was 8 per cent, giving a mean corpuscular volume of 123 cu. micra, mean corpuscular hemoglobin of 38.4 micro-micro-grams, and mean corpuscular hemoglobin concentration of 31.2 per cent. Bone marrow from iliac crest again showed active erythroblastic elements. Venous pressure was 8.9 cm. of blood and circulation time (saccharine method) 17.4 seconds. Serum bilirubin was 0.6-0.8 mg. per 100 cc.

Symptoms of heart failure disappeared promptly on bed rest. The treatment consisted of blood cell transfusions which were given seven times, 200-400 cc. each time, totalling 2,150 cc. of blood cells within a month. On discharge, the red blood cells were 3.98 million, hemoglobin 9.4 Gm., white blood cells 3,800 with 49 per cent polymorphonuclears and 41 per cent lymphocytes, reticulocytes 2.4 per cent and platelets 92,000. Neoarsphenamine 0.45 Gm. intravenously at weekly intervals was given for four doses during this admission. Susbequently the Kahn test became also negative.

Third admission. June 19-September 9, 1940. After discharge the patient's condition again gradually deteriorated and two weeks before the present admission, following strenuous walking, severe dyspnea and palpitation returned together with edema of lower extremities. On admission, besides severe anemia and congestive heart failure, he ran an unexplained fever of 40 C., which subsided in two or three days. The anemia was extreme: erythrocytes 0.61 million, hemoglobin 1.7 Gm., leukocytes 2,950 with 64 per cent polymorphonuclears. Reticulocytes were 13 per cent and platelets 50,000. Sternal bone marrow study again revealed active normoblastic erythropoiesis and normal distribution of granulocytes. Blood smear was examined for the "sickling" phenomenon with negative results. Serum bilirubin was 1.6 mg. per 100 cc. The liver function was again investigated: Bromsulphalein test showed no retention of the dye in 30 minutes; ingestion of 5.9 Gm. of sodium benzoate was followed by the excretion of 4.83 Gm. of hippuric acid (or 3.28 Gm. of benzoic acid) in the urine in 4 hours. The extent of cardiac insufficiency was about the same as on the second admisson and the frontal area of the heart measured in the teleoroentgenogram was also 75 per cent oversize. In addition to the systolic murmur heard previously, there was now a rumbling diastolic murmur at the apex. This, however, disappeared as soon as improvement of the cardiac function set in. The electrocardiogram showed flat T wave in Lead I suggestive of myocardial damage.

Treatment comprised yeast and blood transfulsions. Yeast in 30-60 Gm. daily doses was given for twenty-five days without appreciable improvement in the anemia. Ten blood transfusions of 400 cc. each were given. These brought the erythrocyte count up to 2.56 million, hemoglobin to 9.1 Gm., and white blood cells to 3,150 on discharge. During this admission several bouts of fever occurred; one of these was related to a parotitis, but the rest were not explained.

Fourth admission. April 21-August 6, 1941. On admission this time, the anemia had returned to the same severity as on the third admission, although the signs of congestive heart failure were not as marked. The heart remained 75 per cent oversize, but no diastolic murmur was heard. The liver edge was 2 cm. below the costal margin, but edema of the legs was only slight. The veins in the neck were engorged; capillary pulsation and collapsing pulse were present. The blood pressure was 118/50. The urine contained a faint trace of protein, and a few hyaline and granular casts. Urobilin was also present. The urea clearance was 60 per cent of normal. The basal metabolic rate was 1,494 calories per diem (+7.7 per cent).

The erythrocyte count was 0.50 million, hemoglobin 1.8 Gm., white blood cells 1,750 with 28 per cent polymorphonuclears and 70 per cent lymphocytes, and reticulocytes 4.2 per cent. The platelets were 57,500 with a positive tourniquet test and a bleeding time of 5 minutes. Bone marrow studies again showed active erythropoiesis. Serum bilirubin was 1.04 mg. on one occasion and 3.72 mg. per 100 cc. on another. For treatment, Lederle's concentrated liver extract (15 units per cc.) 1 cc. daily was given intramuscularly for 6 days. A reticulocyte rise to 9.4 per cent was not followed by any improvement in hemoglobin. Blood transfusions had to be resorted to. Within a period of a little over three months, a total of twelve transfusions (four of 400 cc. whole blood each, and eight of 200 cc. blood cells each) was given. There were mild reactions to some of the blood transfusions in the form of chills and fever; these reactions were more liable to occur with whole blood than with blood cell transfusions. The improvement of the anemia was not so satisfactory as previously. On discharge the erythrocytes were 2.55 million, hemoglobin 7.8 Gm., white blood cells 1,700 and reticulocytes 3.2 per cent.

Comment. Diagnosis of this case presented considerable difficulty. Although the anemia was severe and macrocytic in character, there were none of the other characteristics of pernicious anemia. With the absence of response to iron, whole liver and yeast by mouth and liver extract parenterally, together with a depression of the granulocytes and thrombocytes one tends to place this case into the ill-defined group of refractory anemias. In fact, aplastic anemia had been diagnosed during the first three admissions. However, the relatively high reticulocyte percentage, the frequent increase of the serum bilirubin to above normal limits, the persistent urobilinuria in the presence of normal liver function and the active erythropoiesis in the bone marrow suggest increased blood destruction and attempts to respond to such stimulation. In view of the recent experience with Case 1, the erythrocytes were examined for abnormal susceptibility to hemolysis by chilling and by acid. Indeed they were found to possess such abnormal qualities, justifying the grouping of these 2 patients in one group. The studies of the red blood cells in vitro and in vivo are presented in the following section.

METHODS

Cold hemolysis. Blood from venipuncture was defibrinated by shaking at room temperature (24–28 C.) in a sterile flask containing glass beads. The defibrinated serum was separated from the cells by centrifuging, and the cells were washed with 0.85 per cent sodium chloride solution twice and resuspended in the saline to make a 10 per cent suspension. Portions of 0.25 cc. of this suspension were pipetted into small tubes. These were centrifuged and the supernatant saline discarded. To each of the tubes containing 0.025 cc. of cells, 0.6 cc. (sometimes 0.5 cc.) of serum was added. After the contents of the tubes were mixed, they were chilled in ice for thirty minutes and then incubated at 37 C. for two hours. The contents of the tubes were mixed once or twice during the period of incubation. At the end of two hours, the tubes were centrifuged. The degree of hemolysis in the supernatant serum in each tube was noted. The serum was then removed for the determination of hemoglobin by the photoelectric colorimeter technic of Evelyn,[1] 0.3 cc. of serum being used. The original serum served as blank. From the increment of hemoglobin in the supernatant serum and the amount of cell hemoglobin, the percentage of hemolysis, in terms of the hemoglobin originally present in the 0.025 cc. of cells, was calculated.

Acid hemolysis. The procedure was the same as above except that 0.05 cc. of N/3 hydrochloric acid was added to 1.0 cc. of the serum and 0.05 cc. of the cells, the preliminary chilling was omitted and the incubation at 37 C. was only one hour.

Serum hemoglobin. While the photoelectric technic is eminently satisfactory when only comparative values of serum hemoglobin are required, it does not give absolute values, because the serum itself, in the amount used, gives appreciable light absorption. For this purpose the benzidine method of Bing and Baker[5] was adopted without modification. To prevent hemolysis from manipulation blood obtained by smooth venipuncture was placed in paraffin-lined tubes. The blood was immediately centrifuged to throw down the cells, and the plasma was separated before clotting took place. The separated plasma was then allowed to clot and the serum was used for the hemoglobin determination. With this method normal serum contains less than 5 mg. of hemoglobin per 100 cc.

Serum bilirubin. The photoelectric technic of Malloy and Evelyn[6] was employed for the determination of total and direct reacting bilirubin of the serum.

CO$_2$ equilibration. The double tonometer method of Austin et al.[7] was used. Defibrinated venous blood, in 10 cc. portion, was placed in the small tonometer, and the large tonometer was evacuated and filled with CO$_2$ at the desired tension and then with air to atmospheric pressure through a gas manifold. The whole system was then rotated in a water bath at 37 C. for one hour. The gas and blood phases were separated without contact with outside air. The blood was centrifuged under liquid paraffin and the serum was analyzed for CO$_2$, pH and hemoglobin. The gas phase was analyzed for CO$_2$ by means of the Haldane apparatus.

Serum pH and CO$_2$. Blood was drawn by venipuncture without stasis in a syringe which contained a few cc. of sterile liquid paraffin and from which all air bubbles had been expelled. The blood was transferred to a test tube containing liquid paraffin without contact with air. The serum separated after clotting was used for the determination of pH by the colorimetric method of Hastings and Sendroy[8] and of CO$_2$ by the manometric technic of Van Slyke and Neill.[9] From these, the serum bicarbonate content and CO$_2$ tension were calculated.[10] For the frequent determination of acid-base balance of the blood in Case 1, the microtechnic of Shock and Hastings[11] was used.

Lysolecithin fragility test. The method of preparing lysolecithin extract was that of Singer.[12, 13] The dried extract from 10 cc. of serum was dissolved in 2.5 cc. of physiologic salt solution, from which 1:2, 1:4, 1:8, and 1:16 dilutions were made with saline. To each of the five tubes containing 0.025 cc. of packed washed red blood cells, 0.5 cc. of one of the dilutions of lysolecithin solution was added so as to give a series of lysolecithin concentrations equivalent to 2, 1, 0.5, 0.25 and 0.125 cc. of the original serum. The contents of the tubes were mixed, incubated at 37 C. for an hour, and centrifuged. The concentration of hemoglobin in the supernatant fluid was determined photoelectrically and percentage of hemolysis calculated.

Saponin hemolysis. The technic of Wu and Tsai[14] was followed with certain modifications. A stock solution contained 0.5 mg. or 500 gamma of saponin per cc. of physiologic salt solution, from which various dilutions were made. To test the fragility of the washed erythrocytes alone, dilutions containing 2, 4, 8, 12, 16 and 20 gamma per cc. were used. To 1 cc. of each of these dilutions, 0.8 cc. of saline and 0.2 cc. of a 10 per cent suspension of washed erythrocytes were added in that order. The mixtures were incubated at 37 C. for thirty minutes and the percentage of hemolysis in each concentration of saponin was determined. To test the protective effect of serum on the erythrocytes against saponin hemolysis, serum was mixed with the cell suspension in a ratio of 1:2 (serum: 10 per cent cell suspension). The range of saponin concentrations found useful for this purpose was from 100 to 400 gamma per cc. To 1 cc. of each of the selected concentrations of saponin, 0.7 cc. of saline and 0.3 cc. of the serum-cell suspension were added in that order. Further procedure was the same as before.

Urine iron. Urine was collected in two portions, the specimens passed from 7 A.M. to 7 P.M. constituted the day urine and those from 7 P.M. and 7 A.M. the night urine. The method of iron determination was that of Kennedy,[16] with modifications. A 5 cc. sample of the urine was digested in a pyrex test tube with 0.25 cc. concentrated sulphuric acid and 0.5 cc. of nitric acid. One or two drops of nitric acid were finally added to complete the digestion. The digest was washed into a 100 cc. separatory funnel with four or five portions of 5 cc. distilled water each. Five cc. of amyl alcohol were added, followed by 2 cc. of a 20 per cent sodium thiocyanate solution. The mixture was shaken. The alcohol layer which separated sharply, contained the colored ferric sulphocyanate and was transferred to a calibrated tube. The extraction was repeated with a second 5 cc. portion of amyl alcohol, and the alcohol layer was similarly transferred to the same tube. A reagent blank was treated the same way each time. The color measurement was made by means of the Evelyn photoelectric colorimeter, filter 520 being used. The value of K_1 determined with standard iron solutions containing 0.002–0.010 mg. of iron was 0.0395, which was used for calculation in this study.

INFLUENCE OF COLD ON IN VITRO HEMOLYSIS

The factor of cold on hemolysis in vitro in these 2 patients was ascertained in various ways. In Case 1 the washed erythrocytes resuspended in the original serum were chilled in ice for thirty minutes and then brought to room temperature. The supernatant serum showed no hemolysis immediately upon being brought to room temperature, but in half an hour gross hemolysis occurred. As shown in table 1 chilling the same serum repeatedly with fresh portions of cells produced hemolysis of 7.6–9.7 per cent of the cells each time during the first three trials, the ability of the serum to hemolyze the cells being sharply reduced on the fourth trial. Chilling the same sample of cells repeatedly with fresh por-

TABLE 1.—*Case 1. Influence of Repeated Chilling on the Hemolytic Activity of the Serum and on the Susceptibility of the Cells to Hemolysis*

A. Chilling the same serum (4 cc.) repeatedly with fresh 0.25 cc. portions of erythrocytes

Serum	Cells		Supernatent serum hemoglobin			Cell hemoglobin	Hemolysis due to each chilling
		Each mixture successively chilled in ice for 30 min. and brought up to room temp. 25°C. for centrifuging and transfer	Concentration	Δ Conc.	Δ Amount		
cc.	cc.		mg. %	mg. %	mg.	mg.	%
4.0	0.25		113	113	4.54	59	7.7
3.7	0.25		268	155	5.73	59	9.7
3.4	0.25		400	132	4.46	59	7.6
3.1	0.25		413	13	0.43	59	0.7

Total hemoglobin freed 15.16

B. Chilling the same cells (1 cc.) repeatedly with fresh 1 cc. portions of serum

1.0	1.0*	Same as in A	1314		13.14	236	5.6
1.0	1.0		69		0.69	223	0.3
1.0	1.0		40		0.40	222	0.2
1.0	1.0		64		0.64	222	0.3

Total hemoglobin freed 14.87

* 1 cc. of washed cells from a blood donor of group A suspended in 1 cc. of the patient's serum, similarly treated, showed no hemolysis.

tions of serum (table 1, B) gave rise to marked hemolysis (5.6 per cent) on the first trial, and very slight hemolysis on subsequent trials. This suggests that the cell factor necessary for hemolysis was more easily exhausted than the serum factor, or only a certain proportion of the cell population was susceptible to hemolysis. However, the total amount of hemoglobin set free in the two experiments was approximately the same. The fact that control cells suspended in the patient's serum, similarly treated, showed no hemolysis indicated that the serum factor necessary for the hemolysis of the patient's cells was not capable of acting on normal cells.

In Case 2, the effect of the duration of chilling on hemolysis of the cells in presence of the original serum was studied (table 2). Without chilling, incubation alone gave no hemolysis; with a preliminary chilling for thirty minutes, 2 per cent of the cells were hemolyzed and prolonging the time of chilling resulted in somewhat greater hemolysis. A similar experiment performed on the cells and serum of a control showed no hemolysis even after three hours' chilling indicating that the susceptibility to hemolysis on chilling was a property peculiar to the blood of the patient.

The influence of guinea pig serum will be discussed in the next paper. Suffice it here to mention that guinea pig serum added in small amounts (10 per cent of the volume of human serum) seemed to cause hemolysis of the patient's cells

TABLE 2.—*Case 2. Effect of Duration of Chillingon Hemolysis**

Time of chilling at zero degrees C. before incubation at 37° for 2 hours	Serum	Cells	Hemolysis		Hemolysis, due to g.p. serum
			N. saline 0.05 cc.	G.p. serum 0.05 cc.	
	cc.	cc.	%	%	%
0	0.6	0.025	0	5.0	5.0
30 minutes	0.6	0.025	2.0	6.4	4.4
1 hour	0.6	0.025	2.8	7.8	5.0
2 hours	0.6	0.025	3.3	8.8	5.5
3 hours	0.6	0.025	3.3	9.9	6.6

* The same set-up was run with the serum and cells of a control (Yuan) showing no hemolysis.

TABLE 3.—*Cold Hemolysis in Case 1 with Two Controls (Chi and Chang) of the same Blood Group (A)*

Untreated serum, cc.			Washed cells, cc.			Guinea pig serum	Hemolysis, %, after chilling at zero degrees C. for 30 minutes and incubation at 37°C. for 2 hours
Case 1	Chi	Chang	Case 1	Chi	Chang		
						cc.	
0.6	—	—	0.025	—	—	0.05	2.5
0.6	—	—	—	0.025	—	0.05	0
0.6	—	—	—	—	0.025	0.05	0
—	0.6	—	0.025	—	—	0.05	1.6
—	0.6	—	—	0.025	—	0.05	0
—	—	0.6	0.025	—	—	0.05	1.6
—	—	0.6	—	—	0.025	0.05	0

but not those of the control, and the extent of hemolysis so produced bore no relation to preliminary chilling.

In both cases, the cold hemolysis was studied with the technic given under "Methods" with many controls of the same blood group. In both instances (tables 3 and 4), the patient's cells were hemolyzed in his own serum as well in the control sera, while the cells of the controls were not hemolyzed in the patient's or control sera. The hemolytic activity of individual sera varied considerably; in Case 1 the patient's serum was somewhat more active than the control sera, while in Case 2, the reverse was true. In comparing tables 3 and 4, one notes greater hemolysis in Case 2 than in Case 1. However, in Case 1, the particular set of data was obtained during the later part of his hospital sojourn when he had high fever, and the earlier experiments showed a degree of cold hemolysis comparable to Case 2. It is possible that fever might have been a complicating factor in the extent of hemolysis of the erythrocytes.

In table 4 it is to be noted that without preliminary chilling, incubation alone brought about hemolysis of the patient's cells in presence of any of the sera studied. While part of the hemolysis might be attributed to the presence of guinea pig serum, it was so intense that part of it at least must be due to the activity of human sera. Preliminary chilling did play a role in that hemolysis was greater with it than without in every instance.

TABLE 4.—*Cold Hemolysis in Case 2 with Four Controls (Kuo, Liu, Chin and Pai) of the Same Blood Group (O)*

Untreated serum, cc.					Washed cells, cc.					Hemolysis, %			
Case 2	Kuo	Liu	Chin	Pai	Case 2	Kuo	Liu	Chin	Pai	G.p. serum	After chilling at zero degrees C. for 30' and incubating at 37° for 2 hours	After incubating at 37° for 2 hrs. without chilling	Serum complement
										cc			Unit/cc.
0.6	—	—	—	—	0.025	—	—	—	—	0.05	9.5	7.0	33
0.6	—	—	—	—	—	0.025	—	—	—	0.05	0	0	
0.6	—	—	—	—	—	—	0.025	—	—	0.05	0	0	
0.6	—	—	—	—	—	—	—	0.025	—	0.05	0	0	
0.6	—	—	—	—	—	—	—	—	0.025	0.05	0	0	
—	0.6	—	—	—	0.025	—	—	—	—	0.05	20.7	13.6	33
—	0.6	—	—	—	—	0.025	—	—	—	0.05	0	0	
—	0.6	—	—	—	—	—	0.025	—	—	0.05	0	0	
—	0.6	—	—	—	—	—	—	0.025	—	0.05	0	0	
—	—	0.6	—	—	0.025	—	—	—	—	0.05	37.5	32.2	29
—	—	0.6	—	—	—	0.025	—	—	—	0.05	0	0	
—	—	0.6	—	—	—	—	0.025	—	—	0.05	0	0	
—	—	—	0.6	—	0.025	—	—	—	—	0.05	19.1	10.9	50
—	—	—	0.6	—	—	0.025	—	—	—	0.05	0	0	
—	—	—	0.6	—	—	—	0.025	—	—	0.05	0	0	
—	—	—	—	0.6	0.025	—	—	—	—	0.05	16.0	13.0	
—	—	—	—	0.6	—	—	—	—	0.025	0.05	0	0	

The relationship of complement to cold hemolysis will be dealt with in the following paper, but it may be noted here that the variation in the hemolytic activity of the various sera was not correlated with the concentration of complement in the serum.

EFFECT OF ACID ON HEMOLYSIS IN VITRO

(a) *Hydrochloric acid.* The influence of acid on the hemolysis of the erythrocytes in these 2 cases was studied in view of the possibility of paroxysmal nocturnal hemoglobinuria in which Ham[16] and Dacie, Israëls and Wilkinson[17] have demonstrated a close relationship between hemolysis and acid-base equilibrum. The first patient (table 5) showed that his cells were hemolyzed to the extent of 1.1–1.8 per cent in the presence of his own serum or of the control sera when hydrochloric acid in the prescribed amounts was added, there being no hemolysis without the acid. The cells of the controls, on the other hand, exhibited no hemolysis in contact with the patient's or control sera under the same treatment, showing that the abnormality concerned the erythrocytes of the patient

TABLE 5.—*Acid Hemolysis in Case 1 with Two Controls (Chi and Chang) of the Same Blood Group (A)*

Untreated serum, cc.			Washed cells, cc.			Hemolysis, %, after incubation at 37°C. for 1 hour	
Case 1	Chi	Chang	Case 1	Chi	Chang	N/3 HCl 0.50 cc.	N. saline 0.05 cc.
1.0	—	—	0.05	—	—	1.1	0
1.0	—	—	—	0.05	—	0	0
1.0	—	—	—	—	0.05	0	0
—	1.0	—	0.05	—	—	1.8	0
—	1.0	—	—	0.05	—	0	0
—	—	1.0	0.05	—	—	1.6	0
—	—	1.0	—	—	0.05	0	0

TABLE 6.—*Acid Hemolysis in Case 2 with Four Controls (Kuo, Liu, Chin and Pai) of the Same Blood Group (O)*

Serum, cc.					Cells, cc.					Hemolysis, %, after incubation at 37°C. for 1 hour	
Sun	Kuo	Liu	Chin	Pai	Sun	Kuo	Liu	Chin	Pai	N/3 HCl 0.05 cc.	N. saline 0.05 cc.
1.0	—	—	—	—	0.05	—	—	—	—	46.1	0
1.0	—	—	—	—	—	0.05	—	—	—	0	0
1.0	—	—	—	—	—	—	0.05	—	—	0	0
1.0	—	—	—	—	—	—	—	0.05	—	0	0
1.0	—	—	—	—	—	—	—	—	0.05	0	0
—	1.0	—	—	—	0.05	—	—	—	—	44.9	3.4
—	1.0	—	—	—	—	0.05	—	—	—	0	0
—	1.0	—	—	—	—	—	0.05	—	—	0	0
—	1.0	—	—	—	—	—	—	0.05	—	0	0
—	—	1.0	—	—	0.05	—	—	—	—	78.5	20.0
—	—	1.0	—	—	—	0.05	—	—	—	0	0
—	—	1.0	—	—	—	—	0.05	—	—	0	0
—	—	—	1.0	—	0.05	—	—	—	—	67.9	0
—	—	—	1.0	—	—	0.05	—	—	—	0	0
—	—	—	1.0	—	—	—	—	0.05	—	0	0
—	—	—	—	1.0	0.05	—	—	—	—	61.2	8.0
—	—	—	—	1.0	—	—	—	—	0.05	0	0

alone. However, serum, either normal or of the patient, was necessary for the hemolysis because when the patient's cells were suspended and incubated in phosphate buffer saline solutions ranging from pH 7.8 to 6.4, no hemolysis occurred. Nor was there hemolysis when the phosphate buffer of pH 7.38 was acidified with comparable amounts of the hydrochloric acid.

The second patient (table 6) showed greater hemolysis on the addition of acid, ranging from 44.9 to 78.5 per cent. The activity of the control sera was on the whole greater than that of his own serum, and often considerable hemolysis occurred in the absence of added acid. The occurrence of hemolysis on one hour's incubation alone without acid confirms the results of table 4, showing hemolysis after two hours' incubation without preliminary chilling. Again none of the 4 controls' erythrocytes were hemolyzed under similar treatment.

In this connection it may be mentioned that the red blood cells of 2 patients with typical paroxysmal cold hemoglobinuria were examined for acid hemolysis with the same technic. No hemolysis was obtained in either case in the acidified serum of their own or of the control.

(b) *pH*. The degree of hemolysis is apparently a function of pH change. This was studied in Case 1 (table 7) by measuring the pH and percentage hemolysis

TABLE 7.—*Hemolysis by Graded Amounts of Acid Under Aerobic and Anaerobic Technic*

				March 5				March 7, Case 1			
				Case 1		Control		Anaerobic		Aerobic	
Serum	Cells	N/3 HCl	0.9% NaCl	pH	Hemolysis %	pH	Hemolysis %	pH	Hemolysis %	pH	Hemolysis %
cc.	cc.	cc.	cc.								
1.0	0.05	0	0.05	7.95	0	7.75	0	7.65	0	7.85	0
1.0	0.05	0.01	0.04	7.85	0	7.65	0	7.45	0.5	—	—
1.0	0.05	0.02	0.03	7.75	1.5	—	—	7.30	1.0	7.50	0.8
1.0	0.05	0.03	0.02	7.60	2.3	7.50	0	7.10	2.9	7.35	2.2
1.0	0.05	0.04	0.01	7.40	4.1	—	—	6.95	3.0	—	—
1.0	0.05	0.05	0	7.25	4.5	7.25	0	6.80	3.0	7.10	2.8

Note. Experiment on March 5 was done without anaerobic precaution. On March 7, the blood was withdrawn and defibrinated under liquid paraffin. The serum was separated by centrifuging, the cells washed with normal saline and the set-up incubated at 37°C. for an hour, all under liquid paraffin. This is the anaerobic technic. The other set was run without liquid paraffin—aerobic technic.

in the serum after incubation with graded amounts of hydrochloric acid. In the trial of March 5, hemolysis began at pH 7.75 and progressively increased at lower pH, being 4.5 per cent at pH 7.25. The control cells showed no hemolysis within a similar range of pH.

The absolute values of pH in this experiment could not be taken literally, because they were obtained after incubation without precaution against the loss of CO_2 which would increase the pH. Thus on March 7, with "anaerobic" technic the range of pH was on the whole lower; and hemolysis began at pH 7.45 and increased to 3.0 per cent as the pH was progressively lowered to 6.80. A similar setup incubated without "anaerobic" precaution gave higher range of pH and slightly less hemolysis. But greater hemolysis took place at higher pH in the "aerobic" set (2.2 per cent at pH 7.35) than in the anaerobic set (1.0 per cent at pH 7.30), suggesting that the pH of the former had been lower initially. On the whole the experiment showed that with the cells of Case 1 slight hemolysis occurred at normal physiologic range of pH (7.45–7.30), and lowering the pH to 7.10–7.00 brought about marked hemolysis.

(c) *CO_2 equilibration*. Hymans van den Bergh[18] was the first to demonstrate the hemolytic effect of carbon dioxide in an atypical case of hemoglobinuria, although he attributed this to a specific action of CO_2 and not to a change of pH. The effect of varying CO_2 tension and therefore of varying serum pH on the hemolysis was studied in the two patients together with two control subjects (table 8). In Case 1, equilibration of the blood at CO_2 tensions from 15 to 108.6 mm. Hg brought the pH from 7.68 to 7.18. Hemolysis began at pH 7.43 and amounted to 1.5 per cent at pH 7.18. In Case 2, the range of CO_2 tension at the end of equilibration was from 11.2 to 73.0 mm. Hg with a corresponding range

TABLE 8.—*Equilibrium of Blood under Various CO_2 Tensions at 37 Degrees C.*

CO₂ tension of gas phase			Serum CO₂		Serum pH			Increment serum hemoglobin	
Determined		Calculated mm Hg.	Total m.Eq./L.	HCO₃ m.Eq./L.	Det'd.	Calc'd.	Gross	Photoelectric mg. %	Hemolysis % of total
%	mm. Hg.								
Case 1. Blood hemoglobin 2.36 Gm./100 cc.; hematocrit 8.1%									
2.11	15.0	17.2	20.22	19.9	7.68	7.74	0	0	0
5.56	39.6	37.2	24.71	23.3	7.43	7.36	+	20.7	0.5
9.60	68.2	61.0	27.74	25.5	7.28	7.22	++	44.7	1.2
15.27	108.6	84.0	30.53	27.8	7.18	7.05	++	56.9	1.5
Case 2. Blood hemoglobin 3.49 Gm./100 cc.; hematocrit 10%									
1.58	11.2	16.1	22.27	22.1	7.75	7.90	0	7.8	0.3
4.42	31.4	30.9	25.15	23.8	7.52	7.51	+	10.4	0.4
7.98	56.8	50.2	27.42	25.3	7.35	7.30	++	39.5	1.7
11.20	73.0	73.5	29.97	27.3	7.23	7.23	+++	114.4	4.8
Control 1. Coronary occlusion. Blood hemoglobin 14 Gm./100 cc.; hematocrit 40%									
0.20	1.4	3.0	9.01	9.0	7.80	8.43	0	0	0
2.80	19.8	26.6	20.86	20.0	7.50	7.63	+	20.5	0.1
6.34	44.8	49.0	26.44	24.4	7.35	7.37	0	0	0
10.92	77.8	69.0	31.38	28.8	7.27	7.19	0	0	0
Control 2. Kala-azar. Blood hemoglobin 9.2 Gm./100 cc.									
1.18	8.3	9.0	14.85	15.1	7.80	7.76	0		
7.72	54.6	42.0	25.65	24.0	7.40	7.27	0		
14.05	99.4	68.0	28.78	26.3	7.25	7.03	0		
20.23	142.8	110.0	31.80	28.8	7.12	6.91	0		

of pH from 7.75 to 7.23. There was slight hemolysis at the high pH of 7.75 and 4.8 per cent hemolysis at the low pH of 7.23. On the other hand, the experiments on the two controls showed that while a similar range of CO_2 brought about similar change of pH, hemolysis did not occur even at the lowest pH attained.

ERYTHROCYTE FRAGILITY TO AGENTS OTHER THAN CHANGES OF TEMPERATURE AND pH

(a) *Hypotonic saline*. The fragility of the red blood cells toward hypotonic sodium chloride solutions was normal in both cases on repeated observations. The normal osmotic fragility of the cells is rather expected in view of the absence of spherocytosis and other stigmata of congenital hemolytic jaundice.

(b) *Lysolecithin.* Bergenhem and Fåhraeus[19] demonstrated that normal blood contains a hemolysin formed by an enzyme from serum lipoids. Being similar in properties to the hemolytic substance produced by the action of snake venum on lecithin, it has been called lysolecithin. Singer[12] found that the erythrocytes in congenital hemolytic anemia are more susceptible than normal to the lytic effects of lysolecithin, although the lysolecithin content of the serum in this condition is not increased, compared with normal.[13] The lysolecithin fragility of the red blood cells of Case 2 and of a control was determined. The cells of the patient were hemolyzed to the same extent as the control cells by the action of lysolecithin prepared from the patient's serum and that from the control serum. Thus, from the standpoint of erythrocyte fragility to lysolecithin, there was no difference between the patient and the control.

(c) *Saponin hemolysis.* With the technic described, the resistance of the red blood cells toward the lytic effect of saponin was studied. With the washed eryth-

TABLE 9.—*Case 1. Effect of Immersing Both Feet and Legs in Ice Water for Fifteen Minutes (Rosenbach Test)*

| | Temp. °C. | Pulse | Blood pressure | Blood | | Serum bilirubin | Urine | | Symptoms |
				WBC	Hemo-globin		Color	Hemo-globin*	
Before chilling	38.0	80	114/52	2600	—	Trace	Straw	0	No
Immediately after	38.0	106	104/60	—	—		—	—	
1 hour later	38.0	102	110/60	3300	7.0		Dark red	+++	Slight chilliness and epi-gastric dis-comfort for 2–3 hours
2 hours later	38.0	88	112/54	1900	—	Trace	Red	++	
3 hours later	38.2	84	112/50	2100	—		Pink	+	
4 hours later	38.1	94	100/50	2000	5.8	Trace	Straw	0	
17 hours later	37.5	94	102/56	2600	6.3	Trace	Straw	0	

* Oxyhemoglobin bands present spectroscopically.

roytes, approximately 50 per cent hemolysis occurred in the presence of 4–8 gamma of saponin both in Case 2 and in the control, thus showing no appreciable difference between the two in regard to erythrocyte fragility toward saponin. In the presence of their respective serum, the patient's cells were hemolyzed to the extent of approximately 50 per cent at a saponin concentration between 250 and 300 gamma, while the control cells were similarly hemolyzed at about 170 gamma, indicating greater protective power of the patient's serum than the control serum on their respective erythrocytes.

THE EFFECT OF CHILLING IN VIVO

In view of the history in Case 1 of probable hemoglobinuria in the colder months of the year, as already mentioned, paroxysmal cold hemoglobinuria was suspected. As one of the pathognomonic phenomena of the disease is a positive Rosenbach test, the effect of immersing both feet of the patient in ice water for fifteen minutes was noted. Marked hemoglobinuria followed for three hours (table 9). The test was repeated several days later with the same findings.

The Rosenbach test in Case 2 (table 10) was negative, in that no hemoglobin-uria was detected after the chilling. The serum hemoglobin showed no increase after chilling, varying between 48 and 67 mg. per 100 cc. during the test. However, the serum bilirubin showed changes which appeared to be significant. The value was 1.01 mg. per 100 cc. before chilling, went up to 1.43 immediately after chilling and to a maximum of 1.95 one hour later, the increase being more notice-able in the indirect-reacting bilirubin. There appeared to be some increase in the urinary excretion of iron after chilling.

While the Rosenbach test yielded equivocal results in Case 2, it was frankly positive in Case 1. The appearance of hemoglobin in the urine after chilling in paroxysmal cold hemoglobinuria, according to the theory of Donath and Land-steiner, is due to the presence of a hemolysin in the serum which requires a low temperature for its fixation to the erythrocytes, and hemolysis of such cells occurs when they are brought back to the body temperature in the presence of

TABLE 10.—*Case 2. Effect of Immersing Both Feet (up to Mid-Tibial Region) in Ice Water for Thirty minutes (Rosenbach Test)*

	Serum hemoglobin mg. %	Serum bilirubin			Urine		
		Direct mg. %	Indirect mg. %	Total mg. %	Iron mg./hr	Urobilin	Hemoglobin
Before chilling	66.7	0.66	0.35	1.01	0.071	+	0
Immediately after	62.8	0.66	0.77	1.43	0.149	+	0
1 hour later	47.6	0.91	1.04	1.95	0.073		
2 hours later	50.0	0.66	0.99	1.65	0.520	±	0
3 hours later	47.4	0.66	0.84	1.50	0.038	+	0
4 hours later	48.1	0.66	0.60	1.26	0.086	±	0
6 hours later	47.8	0.39	0.55	0.94	0.083	+++	0

the complement. When the concentration of free hemoglobin increase to above a certain level, it appears in the urine. Such a mechanism is not applicable to the present case, because a hemolytic factor peculiar to the patient's serum and capable of acting on normal cells has not been demonstrated, and the hemoglo-binuria in Case 1 is most likely related to the abnormal fragility of the erythro-cytes at low temperature as demonstrated in vitro.

ACIDOSIS AND HEMOLYSIS IN VIVO

In view of the in vitro demonstration of the abnormal fragility of the erythro-cytes to acid and of the in vivo production of increased hemoglobinemia and hemoglobinuria in patients with paroxysmal nocturnal hemoglobinuria by the administration of ammonium chloride by Ham,[3] it was of interest to ascertain whether acidosis so produced in our patients was associated with increased hemolysis. In Case 1 (table 11) the ingestion of ammonium chloride 3 Gm. every three hours for thirty-six hours (totalling 30 Gm.) resulted in a marked lowering of the serum bicarbonate content (from 25.5 to 15.0 m.Eq./L.), and a moderate decrease of pH (from 7.50 to 7.30). This extent of displacement of serum pH was associated with a slight increase of hemoglobinemia (from 23.9 to 31.7 mg. per 100 cc.), but no hemoglobinuria. Further evidence of increased hemoglobin breakdown was shown by the behavior of urinary iron which showed a definite increase during the period of the acid salt administration and returned to the control level within twenty-four hours after the discontinuation of the acid.

The second patient (table 12) took 4 Gm. of ammonium chloride at four-hour intervals for thirty-seven hours (totally 42 Gm.). This larger dosage brought about a greater decrease of the serum bicarbonate content (from 24.2 to 10.7 m.Eq./L.) and of the serum pH (from 7.40 to 7.22). The degree of acidosis at-

TABLE 11.—*Ammonium Chloride Experiment in Case 1*

	Date	Time	pH	HCO₃ m.Eq./L.	pCO₂ mm. Hg.	Serum Hgb. mg. %	Urine iron mg./3 hr.	NH₄Cl
1	Mar. 12	8 a.m.	7.50	25.5	35.0	---	0.184	
2	12	11 a.m.	7.45	23.0	35.0	23.9	0.334	3 Gm. at 8:10 a.m.
3	12	2 p.m.	7.49	22.0	37.7	23.9	0.583	3 Gm. at 11:10 a.m.
4	12	5 p.m.	7.38	19.3	35.0	20.6	0.225	3 Gm. at 2:10 p.m.
5	12	8 p.m.	7.35	18.7	35.3	20.6	0.349	3 Gm. at 5:10 p.m.
6	12	11 p.m.	7.30	17.2	36.5	20.6	0.437	3 Gm. at 8:10 p.m.
7	13	8 a.m.	7.30	15.7	33.0	20.6	0.536	3 Gm. at 11:10 p.m. and 8:55 a.m.
8	13	4 p.m.	7.30	15.0	31.5	22.8	0.468	3 Gm. at 8:55 a.m. and 1:00 p.m.
9	13	10 p.m.	7.30	16.5	35.0	29.5	0.444	1 Gm. at 6:45; 7:30 and 8:10 p.m.
10	14	8 a.m.	7.35	17.7	33.5	31.7	0.236	
11	14	5 p.m.	7.40	19.5	33.3	20.6	0.168	
12	15	8 a.m.	7.45	24.2	37.5	20.6	0.193	

tained was not accompanied by hemoglobinuria, nor by any increase in the extent of hemoglobinemia already present. The serum bilirubin showed a tendency to rise toward and for sometime after the end of the acid salt administration, but the tendency was not clearcut. However the rate of urinary iron excretion exhibited a more definite increase during and after the acid ingestion. A maximum excretion of 2.261 mg. in four hours was reached twelve hours after the cessation of the medication, and the rate returned to the control level forty-eight hours later.

While no hemoglobinuria was produced in either case, and a slight increase of serum hemoglobin was present in only one case, the increased urinary output of iron in both instances should be construed as evidence of enhanced hemoglobin breakdown as a result of the acidosis produced. The fact that large doses of ammonium chloride given to a normal person had no effect on the urinary excretion of iron[20] adds to the significance of the observed increase in urinary iron output in these patients.

Is There a Nocturnal Increase in the Hemolysis?

This is an important question to answer in these two patients, because in paroxysmal nocturnal hemoglobinuria, intravascular hemolysis, while present throughout the twenty-four-hour period, is more intense at night, or, as shown by Ham,[3] rather during the sleeping period. Therefore, hemoglobinuria, when present, is more liable to occur at night or on awakening in the morning. Although in one of our patients, hemoglobinuria occurred in association with exposure to cold, and in the other it followed one of several blood transfusions, spontaneous hemoglobinuria had never been observed during their long periods

TABLE 12.- *Ammonium Chloride Experiment in Case 2*

	Date	Time	pH	HCO$_3$ m.Eq./L.	pCO$_2$ mm. Hg.	Serum Hgb. mg. %	Serum bilirubin mg. %	Urine Fe mg./l hr.	NH$_4$Cl
1	May 7	8 a.m.	7.40	24.2	42.0	30.3	1.09	0.292	
2	7	12 noon	7.38	21.7	39.5	32.5	1.20	0.312	4 Gm. at 8:04 a.m.
3	7	4 p.m.	7.40	21.1	36.6	33.1	1.20	0.448	4 Gm. at 12:05 p.m.
4	7	8 p.m.	7.35	18.8	36.0	30.2	1.17	0.448	4 Gm. at 4:05 p.m. and 2 Gm. at 6:30 p.m.
5	7	12 M.	7.30	17.2	36.3	31.4	1.13	0.457	4 Gm. at 8:05 p.m.
6	8	4 a.m.	7.25	16.2	35.6	31.4	0.88	0.460	4 Gm. at 12:05 a.m.
7	8	8 a.m.	7.25	13.9	32.4	31.3	0.94	0.593	4 Gm. at 4:05 a.m.
8	8	12 noon	7.22	11.6	28.2	31.8	0.99	0.573	4 Gm. at 8:05 a.m.
9	8	4 p.m.	7.25	12.3	28.0	30.3	0.97	0.838	4 Gm. at 12:05 p.m.
10	8	8 p.m.	7.22	10.7	26.0	32.1	1.19	1.144	4 Gm. at 4:05 p.m.
11	8	12 M.	7.28	10.9	23.0	28.7	1.04	0.958	4 Gm. at 9:00 p.m.
12	9	4 a.m.	7.30	11.5	23.0	29.0	1.32	0.281	
13	9	8 a.m.	7.33	11.6	21.6	31.0	1.13	2.261	
14	9	8 p.m.	7.40	12.5	20.7	31.4	1.44	1.116	
15	10	8 a.m.	7.35	15.3	28.5	31.4	1.28	0.996	
16	10	8 p.m.	7.40	17.4	29.3	29.6	1.20	0.731	
17	11	8 a.m.	7.35	18.2	34.5	19.4	1.36	0.331	
18	12	11 a.m.	7.40	21.3	36.5	27.8	1.40	0.510	

of hospital sojourn. However, spontaneous intravascular hemolysis did occur to an abnormal degree, because the concentration of serum hemoglobin, determined on many occasions, was always high, 20–30 mg. per 100 cc. in Case 1 and 30–60 mg. per 100 cc. in Case 2. Further evidence of increased hemolysis was the frequent increase of serum bilirubin above normal in Case 2 in the presence of normal liver function.

But is there a diurnal variation in the serum hemoglobin in these cases? In Case 1, many samples taken at various times of the twenty-four-hour period on different days showed no consistent diurnal variation. More systematic studies of the serum hemoglobin and acid-base equilibrium were made during a twenty-four-hour period in both cases. In Case 1, the serum acid-base balance was determined every two hours with the micro-technic of Shock and Hastings, and there was no consistent variation of the pH (7.40–7.45), HCO_3 (21.8–24.8 m.Eq./L.) and CO_2 tension (35–41 mm. Hg.). The serum hemoglobin determined every four hours, remained within the narrow limit of 20–25 mg. per 100 cc. In Case 2, the serum was studied every four hours with the regular macro-technic for acid-base balance. Although the pH showed a progressive increase from 7.30 to 7.45 during a twenty-four-hour period starting from 8 A.M., the high pH occurred during the night. The bicarbonate content (20.5–21.2 m.Eq./L.) remained essentially constant throughout. Likewise the serum hemoglobin varied irregularly within the limits of 40–48 mg. per 100 cc. On the whole we are forced to conclude that we are unable to obtain evidence of a diurnal character for the intravascular hemolysis in these two cases.

Urinary iron. The question of the diurnal relationship was further investigated by studying the total iron in the urine passed during the night and day for many consecutive days. The method includes iron of all forms. Normally the

TABLE 13.— *Urinary Iron Day and Night*

Case	Date	No. of days of observations	Day (7 a.m.–7 p.m.) Mean ± Em mg. in 12 hr.	Night (7 p.m.–7 a.m.) Mean ± Em mg. in 12 hr.	Diff. of the Means ± Ed mg. in 12 hr.	Remarks
1	Feb.–Mar.	16	1.466 ± 0.041	1.001 ± 0.031	0.465 ± 0.051	Liver 200 Gm. daily
	Apr.	7	0.888 ± 0.079	0.592 ± 0.029	0.296 ± 0.085	Ferric Am. Cit.
2	May	29	1.798 ± 0.028	1.456 ± 0.035	0.342 ± 0.045	6 Gm. daily
	June	25	2.309 ± 0.031	2.140 ± 0.033	0.169 ± 0.034	
	July	28	3.196 ± 0.037	2.728 ± 0.027	0.468 ± 0.046	
Control	June	7	0.180 ± 0.018	0.136 ± 0.027	0.044 ± 0.032	

Em = standard error of the mean.
Ed = standard error of the difference between the means.

daily output of iron in the urine is small. Marlow and Taylor[20] reported that normally the iron content of the urine ranged from 0.03 to 0.8 mg. per twenty-four hours. In the normal subject studied by Reznikoff et al.[21] it averaged 0.35 mg. per day; in the 4 normal persons studied by Widdowson and McCance[22] the average ranged between 0.25 and 0.45 mg. per day; and in 4 normal women studied by Leverton and Roberts[23] the range was 0.17–0.29 mg. per day. This quantity was not influenced by ordinary variations in the dietary intake of iron, nor by massive doses of iron given by mouth. In cases of polycythemia undergoing treatment with phenylhydrazine,[24, 25] urinary output of iron may be increased. Any considerable increase of urinary iron output may be taken as evidence of increased hemoglobin breakdown, and indirectly of in vivo hemolysis. A nocturnal increase of such process should be evidenced by an increase or iron output in the night urine. In both cases (table 13) the daily urine iron output was large, exceeding 2 mg. in Case 1 and 3–6 mg. per day in Case 2. This is strong evidence in favor of increased blood destruction in the 2 patients. The control, a patient with probably aplastic anemia, eliminated in the urine on the average 0.3 mg. of iron per day, a value well within normal limits. As to diurnal

120 ANEMIA WITH ERYTHROCYTE FRAGILITY TO COLD AND ACID. I.

variation in the iron output, the means for the day portions were significantly greater than those for the night portions. Whether this indicates a diurnal variation in the intensity of hemolysis, it is difficult to be certain; as the urinary volume during the day was usually greater than at night.

DISCUSSION

The important features common in both patients are as follows: The anemia is severe, macrocytic and resistant to treatment with large doses of iron and liver extract. There is usually a slight or moderate reticulocytosis. The granulocytes are decreased with relative lymphocytosis. The platelets are also depressed. The bone marrow usually exhibits increased activity in erythropoiesis until the terminal state when hypoplasia or aplasia supervenes. Thus far the picture is consistent with that of "refractory" anemia described by Rhoads and often seen in this clinic. However closer examination reveals evidence of increased blood destruction or intravascular hemolysis, not ordinarily seen in aplastic anemia. Hemoglobinemia is present beyond normal limits and iron excretion in the urine is excessive. Finally the heavy deposits of hemosiderin in the various organs of Case 1 confirms the presence of excessive blood destruction. Although the repeated blood transfusions might have contributed to the formation of hemosiderin, it is unlikely that they alone could be responsible for the extensive deposits in the various organs, particularly in the kidneys. On the other hand jaundice is absent, serum bilirubin exceeds normal limits only occasionally (Case 2), and urobilinuria is not prominent. This, together with the absence of splenomegaly, spherocytosis and osmotic fragility of the erythrocytes, distinguish these cases from ordinary chronic hemolytic jaundice, acquired or congenital.

The circumstances that led to the examinations for paroxysmal hemoglobinuria é frigore and of the nocturnal type have already been mentioned. The results thus far recorded would rule out the possibility of paroxysmal hemoglobinuria é frigore.[26] Although both patients showed historical and serological evidence of syphilis (Case 1 had syphilitic aortitia) and erythrocyte fragility to chilling in vitro and in vivo (actual hemoglobinuria in Case 1 and increased bilirubinemia in Case 2), attempts to demonstrate the Donath-Landsteiner hemolysin in these cases were negative. The abnormal erythrocyte susceptibility to hemolysis by acid observed in our cases is not found in paroxysmal hemoglobinuria é frigore and the type and the refractoriness of the anemia and the fatal termination in one of the cases are very unusual for that condition.

However the question of paroxysmal nocturnal hemoglobinuria can not be dismissed so readily. This syndrome was first carefully described by Marchiafava[27] in 1928 and Micheli[28] in 1931, although similar cases had been reported previously by others. These cases were characterized by chronic anemia of the hemolytic type and hemoglobinuria occurring mostly at night, running a progressive course. Hamburger and Bernstein[29] collected 22 such cases in 1936. Subsequently one case was reported by Witts[30] in 1936, 2 cases by Scott, Robb-Smith and Scowen[31] and one case by Dacie, Israëls and Wilkinson[17] in 1938, 4 cases by Ham[3] in 1939 and one case each by Ham and Horack,[32] by Buell and

Mettier[33] in 1941, and by Pierce and Aldrich[34] and by Hoffman and Kracke[35] in 1943. Two additional cases were reported by Manchester in 1945.[36] Approximately 50 cases have been on record according to Ross.[37] The mechanism of the hemolysis remained unknown until Ham[16] demonstrated the peculiar susceptibility of the erythrocytes to hemolysis by the addition of acids in amounts which do not affect normal red blood cells, although in 1911, van den Bergh[18] found unusual fragility of the red blood cells to CO_2 in a case of probably the same disease without distinguishing it from acholuric hemolytic jaundice. The mechanism of acid hemolysis in this condition was confirmed by Dacie et al.[17] and further elaborated by Ham.[3] This led to the diagnosis of other cases with atypical clinical manifestations[31] particularly when the element of hemoglobinuria was inconspicuous.

The clinical course, the character of the anemia, the evidence of increased blood destruction (hemoglobinemia and large urinary iron output), hemosiderin deposits, and finally the abnormal fragility of the erythrocytes to acid in vitro and in vivo in our cases conform to the picture of Marchiafava-Micheli disease. However there are several features in our cases that do not agree with this syndrome. First, the erythrocyte fragility to chilling demonstrated in vitro in both cases and clinically important in one case has not been reported in the cases of paroxysmal nocturnal hemoglobinuria with one possible exception. Dacie, Israëls and Wilkinson[17] found that in an otherwise typical case the cells showed greater hemolysis after chilling apart from their susceptibility to a lowering of pH. All the rest of the cases in which the factor of chilling was recorded showed negative findings. Ham especially denied the influence of cold on hemolysis in his cases. Second, we have not been able to demonstrate any nocturnal increase in the hemoglobinemia or in the urinary iron excretion in our cases, although a nocturnal rise of serum hemoglobin with consequent appearance of hemoglobin in the urine is one of the important characteristics of the disease. Finally clinical and serologic evidence of syphilis present in our cases has not been found in cases of nocturnal hemoglobinuria in which such evidence has been sought for.

From the above considerations, one is not in a position to accept the diagnosis of Marchiafava-Micheli disease for the present cases without reservation. One is dealing either with an atypical form of Marchiafava-Micheli disease or with a special type of chronic hemolytic anemia in which the cells are fragile both to cold and to acid, without evident nocturnal intensification of the hemolytic process and in which syphilis may possibly play a role. Further study of similar cases may help to clarify the situation.

SUMMARY

Two cases previously diagnosed as aplastic anemia were found to have abnormal susceptibility of the red blood cells to hemolysis after chilling and after addition of acid in the presence of their own as well as control serum. The serum of the patients had no such effect on control erythrocytes. This erythrocyte abnormality was accompanied by a severe anemia of the macrocytic type, slight reticulocytosis, depression of granulocytes and platelets, and erythropoietic hyperactivity of the bone marrow in the early stages and hypoactivity in the late stages. Increased blood destruction was evidenced not by jaundice, but by persistent hyperhemoglobinemia in the serum and increased iron excretion in the urine, without nocturnal intensification. Chilling in vivo produced hemoglobinuria in Case 1, but only slight evidence of increased blood destruction in Case 2. Administration of large doses of ammonium chloride failed to produce hemoglobinuria in either case, although evidence of an increase in blood destruction was detectable. Both patients had historical and serologic evidence of syphilis. Autopsy of Case 1 showed, in addition to syphilitic aortitis, marked hemosiderosis of the kidneys, liver, spleen and lymph nodes.

These were clearly not cases of paroxysmal hemoglobinuria é frigore (Donath-Landsteiner). They resembled cases of chronic hemolytic anemia with nocturnal paroxysmal hemoglobinuria (Marchiafava-Micheli), but the erythrocyte fragility to chilling, the absence of nocturnal increase in the hemolytic process and the presence of syphilis rendered the acceptance of such diagnosis difficult.

REFERENCES

[1] SHEN, C. Y.: Cases of aplastic anemia in North China. National M. J. China. *14:* 389, 1928.

[2] RHOADS, C. P.: Aplastic Anemia. A Symposium on the Blood. Madison, University of Wisconsin Press, 1939. P. 31.

[3] HAM, T. H.: Studies on destruction of red blood cells. I. Chronic hemolytic anemia with paroxysmal nocturnal hemoglobinuria: An investigation of the mechanism of hemolysis with observations on five cases. Arch. Int. Med. *64:* 1271, 1939.

[4] EVELYN, K. A.: Stabilized photoelectric colorimeter with light filters. J. Biol. Chem. *115:* 63. 1936.

[5] BING, F. C., AND BAKER, R. W.: Determination of hemoglobin in minute amounts of blood by Wu's method. J. Biol. Chem. *92:* 589, 1931.

[6] MALLOY, T. H., AND EVELYN, K. A.: The determination of bilirubin. J. Biol. Chem. *119:* 481, 1937.

[7] AUSTIN, J. H., CULLEN, G. E., HASTINGS, A. B., McLEAN, F. C., PETERS, J. P., AND VAN SLYKE, D. D.: Technic for collection and analysis of blood and for its saturation with gas mixtures of known composition. J. Biol. Chem. *54:* 493, 1922.

[8] HASTINGS, A. B., AND SENDROY, J.: The colorimetric determination of blood pH at body temperature without buffer standards. J. Biol. Chem. *61:* 695, 1924.

[9] VAN SLYKE, D. D., AND NEILL, J. M.: The determination of gases in blood and other solutions by vacuum extraction and manometric measurement. J. Biol. Chem. *61:* 523, 1924.

[10] —, AND SENDROY, J.: Line charts for graphic calculation by Henderson-Hasselbalch equation and for calculating plasma carbon-dioxide content from whole blood content. J. Biol. Chem. *79:* 781, 1928.

[11] SHOCK, N. W., AND HASTINGS, A. B.: Studies of acid-base balance of blood: microtechnic for determination of acid-base balance of blood. J. Biol. Chem. *104:* 565, 1934.

[12] SINGER, K.: The lysolecithin fragility test. Am. J. M. Sc. *199:* 466, 1940.

[13] —: Lysolecithin and hemolytic anemia. The significance of lysolecithin production in the differentiation of circulating and stagnant blood. J. Clin. Investigation *20:* 153, 1941.

[14] WU, C. H., AND TSAI, C.: The antihemolytic acitvity of the normal and pathological plasma. Chinese J. Physiol. *16:* 179, 1941.

[15] KENNEDY, R. P.: The quantitative determination of iron in tissues. J. Biol. Chem. *74:* 385. 1927.

[16] HAM, T. H.: Chronic hemolytic anemia with paroxysmal nocturnal hemoglobinuria: A study of the mechanism of hemolysis in relation to acid-base equilibrium. New England J. Med. *217:* 915, 1937.

[17] DACIE, J. V., ISRAËLS, M. C. G., AND WILKINSON, J. F.: Paroxysmal nocturnal hemoglobinuria of the Marchiafava type. Lancet *1:* 479, 1938.

[18] HYMANS VAN DEN BERGH, A. A.: Ictére hèmolytique avec crises hemoglobinuriques fragilité globulaire. Rev. Med. *51:* 63, 1911.

[19] BERGENHEM, B., AND FÅHRAEUS, R. Über spontane Haemolysinbildung im Blut unter besonderer Berücksichtigung der Physiologie der Milz. Ztschr. f. d. ges. esper. Med. *97:* 555, 1936.

[20] MARLOW, A., AND TAYLOR, F. H. L.: Constancy of iron in the blood plasma and urine in health and in anemia. Arch. Int. Med. *55:* 351, 1935.

[21] RESNIKOFF, P., TOSCANI, V., AND FULLARTON, R.: Iron metabolism studies in a normal subject and in a polycythemic patient. J. Nutrition *7:* 221, 1934.

[22] WIDDOWSON, E. M., AND McCANCE, R. A.: The absorption and excretion of iron before, during and after a period of very high intake. Biochem. J. *31:* 2029, 1937.

[23] LEVERTON, R. M., AND ROBERTS, L. J.: The iron metabolism of normal young women during consecutive menstrual cycles. J. Nutrition *13:* 65, 1937.

[24] BASSETT, S. H., KILLIP, T., AND McCANN, W. S.: Mineral exchange in man. III. Mineral metabolism during treatment of a case of polycythemia vera. J. Clin. Investigation *10:* 771, 1931.

[25] McCANCE, R. A., AND WIDDOWSON, E. M.: The fate of the elements removed from the blood-stream during the treatment of polycythemia by acetyl-phenylhydrazine. Quart. J. Med. *6:* (N.S.): 277, 1937.

[26] MacKENZIE, G. M.: Paroxysmal hemoglobinuria. Medicine *8:* 159, 1929.

[27] MARCHIAFAVA, E.: Anemia emolitica con hemosiderinuria perpetua. Policlinico (sez. med.) *35:* 105, 1928; *38:* 105, 1931.

[28] MICHELI, F.: Anemia (splenomegalia) emolitica con emoglobinuriaemosiderinuria tipo Marchiafava. Haematologica (I. Arch.) *12:* 101, 1931.

[29] HAMBERGER, L. P., AND BERNSTEIN, A.: Chronic hemolytic anemia with paroxysmal nocturnal hemoglobinuria. Am. J. M. Sc. *192:* 301, 1936.

[30] WITTS, L. J.: Paroxysmal hemoglobinurias. Lancet *2:* 115, 1936.

[31] SCOTT, R. B., ROBB-SMITH, A. H. T., AND SCOWEN, E. F.: The Marchiafava-Micheli syndrome of nocturnal hemoglobinuria with hemolytic anemia. Quart. J. Med. *7:* 95, 1938.

[32] HAM, G. C., AND HORACK, H. M.: Chronic hemolytic anemia with paroxysmal nocturnal hemoglobinemia: Report of a case with only occasional hemoglobinuria and with complete autopsy. Arch. Int. Med. *67:* 735, 1941.

[33] BUELL, A., AND METTIER, S. R.: Paroxysmal nocturnal hemoglobinuria with hemolytic anemia (Marchiafava-Micheli Syndrome). J. Lab. & Clin. Med. *27:* 1934, 1941.

[34] PIERCE, P. P., AND ALDRICH, C. A.: Chronic hemolytic anemia with paroxysmal nocturnal hemoglobinuria (Marchiafava-Micheli Syndrome). J. Pediat. *22:* 30, 1943.

[35] HOFFMAN, B. G., AND KRACKE, R. R.: Chronic hemolytic anemia with paroxysmal nocturnal hemoglobinuria. J. Lab. & Clin. Med. *28:* 817, 1943.

[36] MANCHESTER, R. C.: Chronic hemolytic anemia with paroxysmal nocturnal hemoglobinuria. Am. J. M. Sc. *23:* 935, 1945.

[37] ROSS, J. F.: Hemoglobinemia and the hemoglobinurias. New England J. Med. *233:* 732, 1945.

Chronic Hemolytic Anemia with Erythrocyte Fragility to Cold and Acid

II. Serum Hemolytic Activity and Its Relation to Serum Globulins and Complement and the Role of Guinea Pig Serum

By S. H. Liu, M.D.

IN THE preceding paper,[1] the data of 2 cases of chronic anemia of the hemolytic type were presented. The erythrocytes in these cases were abnormally susceptible to hemolysis by chilling and by addition of acid in the presence of the patients' as well as control sera. Erythrocytes from control subjects, in contrast, were not hemolyzed under identical treatment. The abnormality, then, resided in the red blood cells of the patients, although a factor present in the serum of the patients as well as of normal persons was necessary for the hemolysis. These cases could be clearly distinguished from paroxysmal cold hemoglobinuria by the refractory and progressive character of the anemia, by the absence of a Donath-Landsteiner hemolysin (amboceptor) peculiar to the patient's serum capable of acting on the patient's as well as control cells, and by the presence of the erythrocyte susceptibility to hemolysis by a lowering of the pH of the serum. These findings were in favor of the diagnosis of chronic hemolytic anemia with paroxysmal nocturnal hemoglobinuria (Marchiafava-Micheli), but the demonstration of the role of chilling in aiding the hemolysis, the absence of a nocturnal increase in the hemolytic process, and the association with syphilis in our patients were not in conformity with the usual picture of that condition.

Without further speculation as to the exact orientation of our cases, it is the purpose of the present communication to report on some of the studies of the serum factor necessary for the hemolysis. In the study of an atypical case of hemoglobinuria which was most probably of the Marchiafava-Micheli type, Jordan[2] considered that in this condition the red blood cells were already sensitized spontaneously, so that contact with the normal complement-containing serum gave rise to hemolysis without preliminary chilling. The increase of hemolysis by exposure to CO_2 was attributed by Jordan to the activation of the complement under the influence of CO_2. Dacie et al.[3] concluded that in their case of nocturnal hemoglobinuria the cells had become sensitized to a potential lysin present in normal and in the patient's serum. Ham,[4] after an elaborate study of 5 cases of the disease came to the conclusion "The serum factor essential for hemolysis was closely associated with, if not indistinguishable from complement or alexin of human serum."

The study of our cases reveals findings not consistent with the theory of the human complement being the serum hemolytic substance, but suggests a separate factor, either a fraction of serum globulin or a substance having similar solubility

From the Department of Medicine, Peiping Union Medical College, Peiping, China.

124

characteristics as serum globulin, which is responsible for the serum hemolytic activity towards the red blood cells of our patients.

METHOD

Cold and acid hemolytic tests. These have already been described.[1] Defibrinated serum was used unless otherwise noted. Cold hemolysis referred to the hemolysis occurring after chilling the mixture of cells and serum for thirty minutes folllowed by incubation at 37 C. for two hours. Usually a control set was incubated for two hours without preliminary chilling. Acid hemolysis was obtained by incubating the cells with acidified serum for an hour, N/3 HCl being added in a 5 per cent by volume of the serum. Percentage of hemolysis was calculated from the increment of hemoglobin in the supernatant serum in terms of the total cell hemoglobin originally present, both determined photoelectrically.

Complement titration.[*] To 1 cc. of each of a series of saline dilutions of serum were added 0.5 cc. of a 1:8,000 dilution of anti-sheep cell rabbit serum (equivalent to 2 units of hemolysin) and 0.5 cc. of a 2 per cent suspension of washed sheep erythrocytes. The mixtures were incubated in a water bath at 37 C. for thirty minutes. The smallest amount of the serum giving complete hemolysis was considered to contain 1 unit of complement.

Separation of serum euglobulin from remaining fraction. The method of Liefmann[5] was employed. A measured amount of serum was diluted with 9 volumes of distilled water. Pure CO_2 was bubbled through the diluted serum until the precipitation was complete. This usually took one hour. The suspension was centrifuged and the supernatant fluid was saved. The sediment was washed once with CO_2-saturated distilled water, and centrifuged again to discard the supernatant. The precipitate was drained and placed in a vacuum desiccator. This constituted the euglobulin fraction. For hemolysis tests the dried precipitate was dissolved in the original volume of the serum of a M/15 phosphate buffer of pH 7.38 containing 0.5 per cent sodium chloride to maintain isotonicity (designated briefly as buffer). N/3 HCl added in a 5 per cent by volume of the buffer changed its pH to 7.00–6.80 suitable for the study of acid hemolysis. The remaining fraction (the supernatant after CO_2 precipitation) was reduced to the original volume of the serum by means of an oil pump with the suction flask kept in ice.

Cholesterol suspension. Cholesterol 20 mg. was dissolved in absolute alcohol, and 5 cc. of distilled water were added. The mixture was heated in a boiling water-bath until all the alcohol was evaporated. The remainder was made up to 5 cc. by adding distilled water.

Fractionation of serum proteins by sodium sulphate. The serum was diluted with 9 volumes of distilled water, and following the method of Howe,[6] the fractionation was started by adding anhydrous sodium sulphate to 14 per cent concentration. After standing at 37 C. for three hours, the precipitate was obtained by centrifuging. Calculated amount of sodium sulphate was added to attain the next desired concentration for the precipitation of the second portion of serum protein. The process was continued until 38 per cent sodium sulphate concentration was reached, by which most of the albumin should be precipitated. Usually the fractions obtained after 22 per cent sodium sulphate had to be separated by filtration, because the precipitate was relatively lighter than the solution and could not be thrown down by centrifuging. The various fractions were separately dissolved in the buffer and made up to the original volume of the serum, and enclosed in cellophane bags for dialysis in icebox, at first with normal saline and then with the buffer until sulphate-free. The contents of the cellophane bags were then removed for testing.

Third and fourth components of the complement. The third component was inactivated according to Strong and Culbertson[7] by zymin. Fleischmann's dried yeast 0.5 Gm. was emulsified in 5 cc. of normal saline, and centrifuged to discard the supernatant. To the

---

[*] Thanks are due to Dr. Samuel Zia of the Department of Bacteriology for the facilities afforded in carrying out complement titration.

sediment 10 cc. of absolute alcohol were added and the mixture was stirred for thirty minutes. The alcohol layer was removed after centrifuging. The same amount of ether was added and mixed with the sediment for thirty minutes. The ether layer was separated after centrifuging. Normal saline 10 cc. was then added and the mixture was boiled in water bath for thirty minutes. The supernatant was discarded. The sediment from 0.5 Gm. of yeast was mixed with 10 cc. of serum and incubated at 37 C. for seventy-five minutes. The supernatant serum was used as zymin-treated serum in which the third component of the complement had been eliminated.

The fourth component was inactivated according to Ham[4] and Gordon et al.[9] by adding 0.85 cc. N/3 NH₄OH to 10 cc. of serum. This would change the pH of the serum to 8.50–9.00. After incubation at 37 C. for seventy-five minutes, the serum was neutralized to pH 7.20–7.30 by the addition of N HCl. Usually 0.4 cc. of the acid was sufficient for the purpose. The resulting serum was used as ammonia-treated serum in which the 4th component of the complement had been inactivated.

TABLE 1.—*Heat Inactivation of Hemolytic Activity of Serum at 56 Degrees C. for Thirty Minutes*

Serum, cc.		Cells cc.	Cold hemolysis, %				Acid hemolysis, %						Serum complement, unit/cc.
			Chilling and incubation		Incubation alone		Chilling and incubation			Incubation alone			
Fresh	Heated		G.p. serum 0.05 cc.	Normal saline 0.05 cc.	G.p. serum 0.05 cc.	Normal saline 0.05 cc.	N/3 HCl 0.025 cc. G.p. serum 0.05 cc.	N/3 HCl 0.025 cc. normal saline 0.05 cc.	Normal saline 0.075 cc.	N/3 HCl 0.025 cc. G.p. serum 0.05 cc.	N/3 HCl 0.025 cc. normal saline 0.05 cc.	Normal saline 0.075 cc.	
Case 1													
0.5		0.025	5.3	5.3	0	0	6.2	7.7	4.9	2.2	2.2	0	
	0.5	0.025	0	0	0	0	0	0	0	0	0	0	
Case 2													
0.5		0.025	1.4	0	1.4	0	44.6	36.3	0	54.4	37.2	0	33
	0.5	0.025	0	0	0	0	0	0	0	0	0	0	0

BEHAVIOR OF SERUM HEMOLITIC ACTIVITY AND COMPLEMENT UNDER VARIOUS CONDITIONS

Heat inactivation. Heating the serum in a water bath at 56 C. for thirty minutes completely inactivated the serum hemolytic factor (table 1) both for cold and acid hemolysis. The addition of guinea pig serum failed to restore the activity. Heating likewise eliminated the complement of the serum. Such results confirm all the previous workers in regard to the heat inactivation of the serum factor for acid hemolysis in nocturnal hemoglobinuria.

Kaolin inactivation. Treatment of the serum with kaolin (table 2) completely eliminated the complement, and greatly reduced the serum activity for the cold and acid hemolysis in Case 2 and in a control in which such procedure was tried. The presence of guinea pig serum made no material difference to the kaolin-inactivated serum for cold hemolysis. Jordan[2] obtained no hemolysis with serum which had been shaken with kaolin in his atypical case of hemoglobinuria.

Influence of aging. It is well known that complement diminishes and disappears from the serum on standing, more rapidly at room temperature than in the ice box. The serum hemolytic activity in our cases also behaved the same way. The results set forth in table 3 were obtained with serum right after withdrawal, and after four and nine days' storage in the ice box at 8 C. After four days of storage

TABLE 2.—*Kaolin Inactivation of Serum Hemolytic Activity*

(Kaolin 2 Gm. was added to 4 cc. of serum, the mixture shaken for fifteen minutes and the serum obtained by centrifuging)

Serum, cc.		Cells, cc., from Case 2	Cold hemolysis,* %		Acid hemolysis, %		Serum complement unit/cc.
Fresh	Kaolin treated		Chilling and incubation	Incubation alone	N/3 HCl 0.025 cc.	Normal saline 0.025 cc.	
			Serum from Case 2				
0.5		0.025	8.1	4.7	44.2	0	33
	0.5	0.025	1.7	0	4.1	0	0
			Serum from control (Liu)				
0.5		0.025	23.2	19.0	37.2	0	33
	0.5	0.025	0	2.1	1.9	0	0

* Guinea pig serum 0.05 cc. was added to each of the tubes.

TABLE 3.—*The Influence of Aging and a Comparison of the Hemolytic Activity of Serum Obtained by Defibrination and that by Spontaneous Clotting (Case 2)*

Days of storage	Serum, cc.		Cells, cc. fresh	Cold hemolysis, %				Acid hemolysis, %			Serum complement, unit cc.
	Defibrinated	Clotted		Chilling and incubation		Incubation alone		N/3 HCl 0.025 cc. G.p. serum 0.05 cc.	N/3 HCl 0.025 cc. normal saline 0.05 cc.	Normal saline 0.075 cc.	
				G.p. serum 0.05 cc.	Normal saline 0.05 cc.	G.p. serum 0.05 cc.	Normal saline 0.05 cc.				
0	0.5		0.025	3.7	2.6	1.0	1.2	25.0	16.0	0	33
4	0.5		0.025	0.6	1.2	0	0	2.8	1.2	0	20
9	0.5		0.025	0	0	—	—	0.9	1.9	0	11
0		0.5	0.025	7.1	3.3	3.5	1.6	34.6	26.2	0	40
4		0.5	0.025	2.7	1.2	0.9	0.9	23.6	22.1	0	20
9		0.5	0.025	0.9	0	0	—	4.7	0.9	0	13

the defibrinated serum lost most of its activity for cold and acid hemolysis and by the ninth day the activity for cold hemolysis disappeared although a trace of the acid hemolytic activity still remained. The complement in the serum diminished more gradually and about a third of its original content still remained after nine days. The addition of guinea pig serum complement to the aged serum made no significant difference to the hemolytic activity.

Difference in serum activity between defibrination and coagulation. Serum obtained by spontaneous clotting was repeatedly found to contain greater hemolytic activity than the defibrinated serum. A sample of such data is shown in table 3. The greater activity of the clotted serum was exhibited in all phases, and the rate of deterioriation of the activity appeared to be slower. The reason for this is not clear, but the agitation involved in defibrination probably played a part in diminishing the hemolytic activity. Mechanical shaking is known to decrease complement activity.[9]

Oxalate decreased serum hemolytic activity but not complement titer. Plasma obtained by the addition of potassium oxalate was often but not always diminished in hemolytic activity. It was suspected that this depended upon the quantity of oxalate used. Therefore specimens of plasma were obtained in which graded amounts of oxalate were added, and the hemolytic and complement activities were determined. From table 4 it is to be noted that 0.1 per cent potassium

TABLE 4. *The Effect of Potassium Oxalate on Hemolytic Activity of Plasma (Case 2)*

Conc. of potassium oxalate, %	Plasma cc.	Cells cc.	Cold hemolysis, %				Acid hemolyis, %			Serum complement, Unit cc.
			Chilling and incubation		Incubation alone		N/3 HCl 0.025 cc. G. p. serum 0.05 cc.	N/3 HCl 0.025 cc. normal saline 0.05 cc.	Normal saline 0.075 cc.	
			G. p. serum 0.05 cc.	Normal saline 0.05 cc.	G. p. serum 0.05 cc.	Normal saline 0.05 cc.				
0	0.5*	0.025	11.0	5.9	9.9	6.2	31.1	22.5	0	33
0.10	0.5	0.025	15.8	4.8	11.0	4.8	19.6	5.2	0	33
0.16	0.5	0.025	5.7	0.9			29.3	11.3	0	33
0.20	0.5	0.025	3.3	4.2	2.2	2.1	3.7	3.2	0	33
0.36	0.5	0.025	0	0			2.5	0	0	33

* Serum in this instance.

oxalate had no influence on cold hemolysis, but diminished acid hemolysis; and 0.16 per cent caused a diminution of both types of hemolysis. Concentration of 0.2–0.36 per cent oxalate greatly diminished or abolished the hemolytic activity to cold and acid. On the other hand complement titration gave the same titer throughout the range of oxalate concentrations used. Guinea pig complement had no restoring action on the hemolytic activity once it was greatly reduced by the oxalate.

Cold absorption. In the paroxysmal cold hemoglobinuria, absorption of serum with red blood cells abolishes the serum activity, but renders the absorbing cells susceptible to hemolysis by normal serum at 37 C.[10] Our cases behaved differently. In Case 1 (table 5) absorption of the serum with cells at zero degrees C. for three hours was followed by some degree of hemolysis as shown by the color of the supernatant serum. The remaining cells separated and resuspended in saline, whether washed three more times with saline or not, showed no hemolysis on being tested with fresh serum for the cold hemolysis, but somewhat diminished hemolysis on the addition of acid. The cold-absorbed serum, on the other hand, retained partially its ability to hemolyze untreated cells on chilling and incubation, and almost completely its ability to hemolyze untreated as well as cold absorbed cells on the addition of acid.

For Case 2, similar cold absorption for three hours resulted in no change in the activity of the serum toward fresh cells of the patient. On prolonging the time of absorption to twenty-four hours, the serum activity for cold hemolysis

TABLE 5.—*Case 1. Influence of Cold Absorption on Hemolysis of the Cells and Activity of the Serum for Cold and Acid Hemolysis*

| Serum, cc. | | Cells, cc. | | | Cold hemolysis, % | | Acid hemolysis, % | |
Fresh	Absorbed*	Fresh	Absorbed* and un-washed	Absorbed* and washed	Chilling and incubation	Incubation alone	N/3 HCl 0.025 cc.	N. Saline 0.025 cc.
0.5		0.025			3.3	1.5	6.0	1.3
0.5			0.025		0	0	3.2	0
0.5				0.025	0	0	2.5	1.1
	0.5	0.025			1.2	0	2.4	0
	0.5		0.025		0	0	4.9	0
	0.5			0.025	0	0	1.4	0

* 10 cc. of the serum and 4 cc. of cells of Case 1 were mixed and placed in ice for three hours.

TABLE 6.—*Case 2. Influence of Cold Absorption on Hemolysis of the Cells and Activity of the Serum for Cold and Acid Hemolysis*

| Serum, cc. | | Cells, cc. | | | Cold hemolysis, % | | | | Acid hemolysis, % | | | |
| | | | | | Chilling and incubation | | Incubation alone | | N/3 HCl 0.025 cc. G. p. serum 0.05 cc. | N/3 HCl 0.025 cc. normal saline 0.05 cc. | Normal saline 0.075 cc. | Serum complement, Unit/cc. |
Fresh	Absorbed	Fresh	Absorbed and washed		G. p. serum 0.05 cc.	Normal saline 0.05 cc.	G. p. serum 0.05 cc.	Normal saline 0.05 cc.				
5 cc. serum + 2.5 cc. cells, both from the patient, in ice for 24 hours												
0.5		0.025			17.2	5.0	12.3	4.4	30.1	26.4	0	20
0.5			0.025		10.8	3.9	—	—	26.7	29.1	0	20
	0.5	0.025			1.8	1.8	—	—	26.1	27.4	0	20
	0.5		0.025		—	—	—	—	27.7	27.7	0	20
10 cc. patient's serum + 4 cc. control cells of same blood group (O) in ice for 3 hours												
0.5		0.025			7.8	4.4				28.2	0	
	0.5	0.025			6.4	3.0				45.8	0	

was greatly impaired, while that for acid hemolysis remained intact. The absorbed erythrocytes showed also lesser grade of hemolysis on chilling and incubation, but the same degree of hemolysis to acid, compared with untreated cells (table 6). As shown in the same table, cold absorption of the patient's serum with normal cells had practically no influence on the serum activity for hemolyzing susceptible cells on subsequent cold and acid tests.

On the whole, cold absorption diminished or abolished the propensity of the cells to hemolysis toward subsequent chilling, leaving the tendency to acid hemolysis uninfluenced. The serum activity after cold absorption was diminished for subsequent cold hemolysis, but unimpaired for acid hemolysis. These facts, as well as the data presented previously (table 1 in preceding article[1]) showing the exhaustion of the cold hemolysis factor in the cells on repeated chilling, suggest that only a limited portion of the cells (especially in Case 1) was susceptible to chilling and could be removed by prolonged exposure to cold, and that the remaining cells which were capable of hemolysis by acid were not susceptible to cold hemolysis. The serum, after having been chilled with the patient's cells, likewise showed reduced activity for subsequent cold hemolysis, but full activity for subsequent acid hemolysis.

CO_2 *equilibration.* It was of interest to test for cold and acid hemolysis after the blood had been subjected to the action of acid such as after CO_2 equilibration.

TABLE 7.—*Influence of CO_2 Equilibration on Subsequent Hemolytic Activity of the Serum and Susceptibility of the Erythrocytes*

Serum, cc.		Cells, cc.		Cold hemolysis, %				Acid hemolysis,		
				Chilling and incubation		Incubation alone		N/3 HCl 0.025 cc. G. p. serum 0.05 cc.	N/3 HCl 0.025 cc. normal saline 0.05 cc.	Normal saline 0.075 cc.
Fresh	CO₂ at 57–73 mm.	Fresh	CO₂ at 57–73 mm.	G. p. serum 0.05 cc.	Normal saline 0.05 cc.	G. p. serum 0.05 cc.	Normal saline 0.05 cc.			
0.5			0.025	5.3	1.0	3.6	0	29.1	18.2	0
0.5			0.025	5.4	2.3	5.2	1.0	30.7	17.0	0
	0.5	0.025		2.3	1.3	—	—	0	0	0
	0.5		0.025	3.2	1.7	—	—	0	0	0

Two portions of blood from Case 2 were equilibrated at 37 C. for one hour at CO_2 tensions of 57 and 73 mm. of Hg. respectively. The resulting hemolysis was 1.7 and 4.8 per cent. The pooled serum and cells were then tested for cold and acid hemolysis by the usual procedure. As shown in table 7, such serum exhibited no further activity for acid hemolysis, but retained most of its activity for cold hemolysis. The erythrocytes after CO_2 equilibration were capable of being hemolyzed by fresh serum to the same extent as the untreated cells in the cold as well as acid hemolysis.

Thus, in contrast to cold absorption, CO_2 equilibration did not diminish the capacity of the cells to hemolysis on subsequent chilling, and like cold absorption, it allowed further hemolysis by acidification. The behavior of the serum after CO_2 equilibration, namely, disappearance of acid hemolytic factor and persistence of the cold hemolytic factor, was just the opposite of that after cold absorption which diminished or abolished the activity for further cold hemolysis, leaving the activity for subsequent acid hemolysis intact. This may possibly speak for the nonidentity of the serum activity for cold and that for acid hemolysis, and one may be used up without affecting the other.

In summarizing the results thus far presented, one may characterize the serum hemolytic factor as heat-labile, disappearing on storage and inactivated by kaolin and probably by mechanical agitation. These properties are shared by complement.[9] Such apparent parallelism makes it tantalizing to identify complement as the serum hemolytic factor. However, several observations make this identification doubtful. For example, kaolin treatment abolishes the serum complement, but leaves some, though greatly diminished, hemolytic activity. Potassium oxalate added to the serum in sufficient amounts to eliminate the hemolytic activity does not diminish the complement titer. Aging seems to decrease the serum hemolytic activity more rapidly than the complement. The addition of guinea pig serum complement to heated, aged or kaolin-treated serum does not restore the hemolytic activity. Such facts leave room for considering the probability of a serum hemolytic factor distinct from the complement.

SEPARATION OF THE HEAT-LABILE COMPONENTS OF COMPLEMENT AND THE HEMOLYTIC ACTIVITY OF THE GLOBULIN FRACTIONS

Precipitation of serum euglobulin by CO_2 saturation. According to Liefmann,[5] complement may be resolved into two parts by CO_2 saturation. The precipitate which is usually called globulin, but in reality only euglobulin[6] contains the midpiece, while the remainder usually known as albumin fraction, contains the end piece. The two portions, when separated, have no complement action, but when recombined, show full activity. Accordingly, sera from Case 2 and a control were resolved into two components by the procedure of Liefmann and these were tested for hemolytic and complement activities separately and after their recombination.

From table 8 it is shown that neither fraction showed any complement activity, but on recombination the full complement titer was restored, thus confirming all previous work concerning this peculiar property of serum complement. However on testing for hemolytic activity for the patient's cells, only the euglobulin fraction exhibited such activity, while the residual portion was devoid of action and, when added to the euglobulin fraction, appeared to inhibit the activity of the latter. The activity of the euglobulin fraction was greater than that of the original sera, from which it was derived, both for cold and acid hemolysis. This activity was always obtained on plain incubation at 37 C., sometimes increased by preliminary chilling and frequently so by acidification. The presence of guinea pig serum had no augmentary effect on the hemolysis, and in fact inhibition was sometimes obtained. It is important to note that the euglobulin fraction had no hemolytic activity on control cells.

The hemolytic activity of the euglobulin fraction was further studied from the quantitative standpoint (table 9). An amount of euglobulin material equivalent to 0.025 cc. of the original serum was hemolytically active and the activity showed progressive increase with increasing quantity of the euglobulin material used. The inhibitory effect of the albumin fraction was confirmed by the fact that even as small an amount of it as equivalent to 0.05 cc. of the original serum

132   ANEMIA WITH ERYTHROCYTE FRAGILITY TO COLD AND ACID. II

TABLE 8.--*Hemolytic Activity of Euglobulin Fraction of Serum Precipitated by* CO_2
Saturation

Serum preparation, 0.5 cc.	Cells,* cc.	Cold hemolysis, %		Acid hemolysis, %			Complement titer Unit per cc.
		G. p. serum 0.05 cc.	Normal saline 0.05 cc.	N/3 HCl 0.025 cc. G. p. serum 0.05 cc.	N/3 HCl 0.025 cc. normal saline 0.05 cc.	Normal saline 0.075 cc.	
Serum from Case 2							
Euglobulin fraction (E)	0.025	15.2	23.8	65.6	63.5	25.1	0
Residual fraction (A)	0.025	0	0	0	0	0	0
E + A in equal parts	0.025	1.5	0	2.5	0	0	28
Original serum	0.025	8.4	3.3	33.6	25.6	0	17
Serum from Control (Kuo)							
Euglobulin fraction (E)	0.025	8.0	13.7	8.1	12.1	12.5	0
Residual fraction (A)	0.025	0	0	0	0	0	0
E + A in equal parts	0.025	1.5	0	2.0	0	0	20
Original serum	0.025	3.4	0.6	5.0	4.8	0	20

 * These erythrocytes were from Case 2. The cells from the control were also tested in a parallel series without showing significant hemolysis by any of the sera or their fractions.

TABLE 9.—*Hemolytic Activity of Various Amounts of* CO_2-*Precipitated Serum Euglobulin Fraction (E) and Inhibitory Influence of the Residual Fraction (A)*

Fraction E cc.	Fraction A cc.	Buffer cc.	Cells cc.	Cold hemolysis, %				Acid hemolysis, %		
				Chilling and incubation		Incubation alone		N/3 HCl 0.025 cc. G. p. serum 0.05 cc.	N/3 HCl 0.025 cc. normal saline 0.05 cc.	Normal saline 0.075 cc.
				G. p. serum 0.05 cc.	Normal saline 0.05 cc.	G. p. serum 0.05 cc.	Normal saline 0.05 cc.			
Euglobulin and residual fractions prepared from serum of the control (Kuo) Cells from Case 2										
0.3	0.2	0.025	7.3	9.3	9.2	5.1	14.0	19.2	7.6	
0.2	0.3	0.025	5.1	7.6	12.4	7.2	9.9	15.0	5.7	
0.1	0.4	0.025	2.4	4.8	2.7	6.9	5.7	12.9	2.5	
0.05	0.45	0.025	1.5	2.1	1.5	2.1	1.3	6.3	1.6	
0.025	0.475	0.025	1.2	1.5	0.9	0.6	1.6	4.1	0.9	
Euglobulin and residual fractions from serum of Case 2 Cells from Case 2										
0.5	—	—	0.025	5.1	5.8*	5.8	5.1*	4.7	5.4*	4.0
0.2	—	0.3	0.025	2.5	3.5	3.8	2.5	3.6	2.7	2.0
0.2	0.05	0.25	0.025	0	0	0	0	0	0	0
0.2	0.1	0.3	0.025	0	0	0	0	0	0	0
0.2	0.2	0.1	0.025	0	0	0	0	0	0	0
0.2	0.3	—	0.025	0	0	0	0	0	0	0
--	0.5	—	0.025	0	0	0	0	0	0	0

 * In these tubes heated guinea pig serum 0.05 cc. was used in place of the normal saline.

abolished the hemolytic effect of 0.2 cc. of the euglobulin fraction both for cold and acid hemolysis. Guinea pig serum complement did not restore the activity.

It was uncertain whether the inhibitory effect of the residual fraction was due to the albumin itself, for this fraction contained all that remained after the CO_2 precipitation of the euglobulin. In view of the inhibitory effect of cholesterol on hemolysis against saponin,[11] the effect of this substance was investigated. Cholesterol suspension (4 mg. per cc.) added in 11–12 per cent by volume of the original serum increased somewhat the activity for cold hemolysis, but decreased the activity for acid hemolysis. However the cholesterol suspension had practically no influence on the hemolytic activity of the euglobulin fraction both for cold and acid hemolysis. Therefore it was unlikely that cholesterol was concerned in the inhibitory effect of the albumin fraction.

Fractionation of serum proteins by sodium sulfate. As the CO_2-precipitated portion contained euglobulin, it was of interest to ascertain whether the euglobulin, as well as other protein fractions separated by various concentrations of

TABLE 10.—*Serum Protein Fractions from Various Concentrations of Sodium Sulphate and their Hemolytic Activity on Susceptible Erythrocytes*

0.5 cc. of protein solution from % Na₂SO₄	Cells cc.	Cold hemolysis, %		Acid hemolysis, %		Complement Unit/cc.
		Chilling and incubation	Incubation alone	N/3 HCl 0.05 cc.	Normal saline 0.05 cc.	
14	0.025	3.3	2.7	2.9	1.4	0
18	0.025	1.9	2.5	2.9	1.1	0
22	0.025	0	0	0	0	0
30	0.025	0	0	0	0	0
38	0.025	0	0	0	0	0
Original serum	0.025	0	0	9.7	0	20

sodium sulfate possessed hemolytic activity. The serum from Case 2 (table 10) was precipitated with 14, 18, 22, 30 and 38 per cent sodium sulfate. It was found that the fraction precipitated at 14 per cent showed hemolytic activity, corresponding to the euglobulin precipitated by CO_2. The activity was manifest on incubation alone, but after preliminary chilling or acidfication it was somewhat enhanced. In addition to the euglobulin, the fraction precipitated at 18 per cent (pseudoglobulin I) also possessed hemolytic activity, perhaps somewhat less than the euglobulin fraction. Further fractions at 22, 30 and 38 per cent sodium sulfate, however, gave no evidence of hemolytic activity.

On account of the length of time (about three days) required to complete the preparations of the various protein fractions for hemolysis test and the somewhat drastic treatment involved in the sodium sulfate fractionation, the hemolytic activity of the euglobulin from sodium sulfate appeared to be small in comparison with that obtained by CO_2 precipitation. But in comparison with the original serum which also stood for three days before testing, the hemolytic activity of the sodium sulfate-precipitated euglobulin appeared to be greater for cold hemolysis, although less for acid hemolysis.

The effect on the active globulin fractions of adding each of the other fractions was studied. The fractions at 22, 30 and 38 per cent were all inhibitory, suggesting that these fractions (pseudoglobulin II and albumin) might be responsible for the inhibitory effect of the residual serum from CO_2 precipitation on the CO_2 precipitated euglobulin. Moreover since the residual serum still contained pseudo-globulin I which was shown to be hemolytically active when isolated by precipitation with 18 per cent sodium sulfate, the absence of hemolytic activity in the residual serum was most likely due to the overwhelmingly depressant effect of the other protein fractions.

The various protein fractions were titrated for complement. No complement was detected in any of the fractions either individually or in various combinations, probably as a result of the drastic treatment involved in the sodium sulfate procedure.

The results presented in this section indicate that the euglobulin fraction from the serum of the patient and of the control precipitated by CO_2 showed great hemolytic activity for the erythrocytes of the patient but not for those of the control. The euglobulin fraction was more active than an equivalent amount of the original serum, but behaved similarly toward chilling and acidification. Fractionation of serum proteins with sodium sulfate showed that in addition to euglobulin, pseudoglobulin I also contained hemolytic activity. There seemed to be an antihemolytic factor present in the residual serum after CO_2 precipitation. It was probably not cholesterol but something in the pesudoglobulin II and albumin fractions.

The facts that the euglobulin fraction was hemolytically active without complement activity and that the reconstituted serum exhibited almost no hemolytic activity with fully restored complement titer were strong evidence that the serum hemolytic factor for our patient's cells was distinct from the serum complement. These observations were different from those of Ham[4] on his cases of paroxysmal noctural hemoglobinuria. He stated that the globulin and albumin fractions, after separation by Liefmann's technic, "showed neither complement nor hemolytic activity when employed alone, but both qualities were restored by recombination of the fractions." This would speak for a fundamental difference between Ham's cases and ours.

The Third and Fourth Components of Serum Complement

Work on complement has shown that two further components are demonstrable, namely, the so-called third and fourth components. The third component may be eliminated by yeast or zymin,[7, 12] and the fourth component may be inactivated by ammonium hydroxide or ammonium salts.[8] Both of these components are heat-stable and may therefore be reactivated by the addition of heated serum. Thus, serum was divided into four portions: portion 1 was heat inactivated, portion 2 treated with zymin, portion 3 mixed with ammonium hydroxide and portion 4 reserved for control. The treated sera, alone and combined, as well as the untreated serum, were tested for cold and acid hemolysis on the erythrocytes of the patient. The sera of the patient and 2 controls were investigated. Similar results were obtained on all three sera and the results on one of the controls, being more complete, are given in table 11. Heated, zymin-treated and ammoniated sera showed no hemolytic activity, nor did the combinations of heated with zymin-treated and with ammoniated serum give rise to any hemolysis when brought in contact with the cells of the patient in contrast to the original serum, which was active hemolytically. The guinea pig serum had no influence on the inactivated sera. The original serum had a good complement titer, but after various treatment the complement activity was lost; and combining the heated serum with zymin-treated serum did not restore the complement activity and combining with ammoniated serum gave only a trace of activity.

TABLE 11.—*Hemolytic Activity of Serum Treated to Destroy the Third and Fourth Components of Complement, and that of Euglobulin Fractions Therefrom*

Serum, 0.5 cc., after various treatment	Cells cc.	Cold hemolysis, %		Acid hemolysis, %			Complement Units/cc.
		G. p. serum 0.05 cc.	Normal saline 0.05 cc.	G. p. serum 0.05 cc. N/3 HCl 0.025 cc.	Normal saline 0.05 cc. N/3 HCl 0.025 cc.	Normal saline 0.075 cc.	
Serum treated variously							
Heated (H)	0.025	0	0	0	0	0	0
Zymin (Z)	0.025	0	0	0	0	0	0
Ammonia (N)	0.025	0	0	0	0	0	0
H + Z	0.025	0	0	0	0	0	0
H + N	0.025	0	0	0	0	0	2
Untreated	0.025	5.7	0.9	29.3	11.0	0	33
Euglobulin fraction from serum treated variously							
Heated (H)	0.025	0	0	0	0	0	
Zymin (Z)	0.025	1.8	0	3.1	0	0	
Ammonia (N)	0.025	1.8	1.5	3.1	3.3	0	
H + Z	0.025	0	0	1.6	0	0	
H + N	0.025	0	0	0	0	0	
Untreated	0.025	11.1	10.4	13.0	16.8	11.2	

The various treated sera and the various combinations of treated sera were precipitated with CO_2 so as to obtain the euglobulin fractions for hemolysis test. The euglobulin fraction from heated serum was uniformly inactive, while those from zymin- and ammonia-treated sera showed slight hemolytic activity for cold and acid hemolysis. The euglobulin fractions from combinations of heated serum with zymin-treated serum and with ammoniated serum showed practically no hemolytic activity.

The results presented do not help to decide whether the serum hemolytic activity was due to the complement, because the addition of zymin-treated or ammonia-treated serum to the heated serum did not restore the complement nor the hemolytic activity. However they show that the hemolytic activity of the euglobulin fraction was completely destroyed by heating, and only partially so by zymin and ammonia.

The Role of Guinea Pig Serum on Hemolysis

Influence of guinea pig serum in small amounts added to human serum. While the addition of guinea pig serum (diluted 1:2 with normal saline) to fresh human serum in a ratio of 1:10 by volume appeared to exert no appreciable influence on the cold and acid hemolysis of the cells of Case 1 (table 1), such procedure frequently increased the hemolytic activity of fresh human sera on the cells of Case 2 (tables 1, 3, 4, 6, 7). The data in table 12 further show the variable extent to which fresh guinea serum enhanced the hemolytic activity of sera from different individuals. Usually the hemolytic activity of human serum on incubation alone was more markedly augmented by the presence of guinea pig serum than that after incubation with preliminary chilling or after addition of acid. It is remarkable that heating the guinea pig serum in water bath at 56 C. for thirty minutes did not abolish its augmenting effect on human serum hemolytic activity.

TABLE 12.—*The Role of Small Amounts of Guinea Pig Serum in Aiding the Hemolytic Activity of Human Serum on Susceptible Erythrocytes*

Serum, cc.			Cells, cc.		Cold hemolysis, %						Acid hemolysis, %			
					Chilling and incubation			Incubation alone						
					G. p. serum 0.05 cc.		Normal saline 0.05 cc.	G. p. serum 0.05 cc.		Normal saline 0.05 cc.	Fresh G. p. serum 0.05 cc. N/3 HCl 0.025 cc.	Heated G. p. serum 0.05 cc. N3/HCl 0.025 cc.	Normal saline 0.05 cc. N/3 HCl 0.025 cc.	Normal saline 0.075 cc.
Liu*	Li* Case 2		Li*	Case 2	Fresh	Heated		Fresh	Heated					
0.5				0.025	40.4	40.8	43.6	30.2	14.8	4.2	37.8	35.5	33.9	4.5
	0.5			0.025	38.8	35.3	36.9	8.8	9.1	0	32.0	9.2	7.7	0
		0.5		0.025	9.7	7.6	0	14.5	5.6	0	33.5	32.7	26.5	0
		0.5	0.025		0	0	0	0	0	0	0	0	0	0

* Controls.

Thus heated guinea pig serum added to human sera gave greater hemolysis than saline control in all the instances of acid hemolysis and of hemolysis on incubation alone, and in one out of 3 instances of hemolysis on chilling and incubation (table 12).

However, human serum, heated (table 1), cold-absorbed (table 6), zymin-treated or ammoniated (table 11), failed to show activation in hemolysis by the addition of guinea pig serum, although serum partially inactivated by aging (table 3), by oxalate (table 4) or by CO_2-equilibration (table 7) exhibited some restoration of hemolytic activity. On the other hand the hemolytic activity of the euglobulin fraction of fresh serum was frequently suppressed by the presence of guinea pig serum (table 8). Finally it is important to point out that the effects described above for relatively small amounts of guinea pig serum added to human serum held true for the cells from the patient only, for control cells showing no propensity to hemolysis by human sera were not hemolyzed by the addition of the prescribed amounts of guinea pig serum (table 12).

Influence of guinea pig serum in large amounts without human serum. When guinea pig serum (diluted 1:2 with normal saline) was employed as the sole hemolytic agent (0.5 cc. for 0.025 cc. cells), hemolysis occurred to a slight degree, but equally with both the patient's and the control cells (table 13). In such hemolysis the addition of acid or preliminary chilling had no augmenting influence on the hemolytic activity of the serum. Absorption of the serum with human erythrocytes at zero degrees C. for three hours diminished or eliminated the hemolytic activity on chilling and incubation. Unfortunately the influence of acidification on the hemolytic activity of the absorbed serum could not be ascertained, because the addition of the usual amount of $N/3$ HCl to a dilute and under buffered guinea pig serum resulted in an excessive lowering of pH and extensive breakdown of the cells. Heat inactivation eliminated all the hemolytic activity. This experiment suggests the presence of a heterologous hemolytic factor in the guinea pig serum, which is nonspecific in regard to the

TABLE 13.—*Hemolytic Activity of Guinea Pig Serum Alone on the Erythrocytes of Case 2 and Control (Li)*

Guinea pig serum, cc.			Cells, cc.		Cold hemolysis, % of total cells		Acid hemolysis, % of total cells	
Fresh	Absorbed	Heated	Case 2	Control	Chilling and incubation	Incubation alone	$N/3$ HCl 0.025 cc.	Normal saline 0.025 cc.
0.5			0.025		5.9	8.8	4.0	4.8
0.5				0.025	4.5	9.3	23.2*	3.8
	0.5		0.025		1.2		60.6*	0
	0.5			0.025	0		15.5*	0
		0.5	0.025		0		0	0
		0.5		0.025	0		0	0

* Color of the supernatant serum was dark brown (due to hematin), indicating probably the pH was excessively lowered with the prescribed amount of acid in these particular instances.

type of human erythrocytes, and can be inactivated by cold absorption and by heating. Clearly this is different from the relatively heat-stable guinea pig serum factor that augmented the hemolytic activity of fresh human serum on the patient's red blood cells.

The guinea pig serum was further investigated by separating it into euglobulin and residual fractions by means of CO_2 precipitation. As shown in table 14, while the original serum hemolyzed both the patient's and the control cells to a slight extent on chilling and incubation and on acidification, the euglobulin and residual fractions, separately or when recombined, gave no more hemolytic activity, which was apparently destroyed by CO_2 precipitation. Complement activity was absent in the separated portions, but fully restored on recombining the fractions.

The third and fourth components of the complement were studied in the guinea pig serum (table 15) as in the human serum. Heat eliminated the hemolytic activity as shown previously. The zymin-treated serum, either alone or in combination with heat inactivated serum, showed slight hemolytic activity, but ammoniated serum was devoid of hemolytic activity even when combined with heated serum. The complement titer of zymin- and ammonia-treated serum was nil, but when heat-inactivated serum was added to either serum, the complement activity was fully restored. This result on guinea pig serum complement is to

TABLE 14.—*Guinea Pig Serum Separated into Euglobulin and Residual Fractions by CO_2 Precipitation and the Absence of Hemolytic Activity of the Fractions*

G. p. serum preparation 0.5 cc.	Cells, cc.		Cold hemolysis, % chilling and incubation	Acid hemolysis, %		Complement Units/cc.
	Case 2	Control		N/3HCl 0.025 cc.	Normal saline 0.025 cc.	
Globulin fraction (E)	0.025		0	0	0	0
Globulin fraction (E)		0.025	0	0	0	0
Residual fraction (A)	0.025		0	0	0	0
Residual fraction (A)		0.025	0	0	0	0
E + A in equal parts	0.025		0	0	0	20
E + A in equal parts		0.025	0	0	0	20
Original serum	0.025		0.8	1.8	1.0	17
Original serum		0.025	0.7	2.8	0	17

TABLE 15.—*Hemolytic Activity of Guinea Pig Serum Treated to Eliminate the Third and Fourth Components of the Complement*

G. p. serum, 0.5 cc., after various treatment*	Cells, cc.		Cold hemolysis, %	Acid hemolysis, %		Complement Unit/cc.
	Case 2	Control (Kuo)	Chilling and incubation	N/3 HCl 0.025 cc.	Normal saline 0.025 cc.	
Heated (H)	0.025		0	0	0	0
Heated (H)		0.025	0	0	0	0
Zymin (Z)	0.025		0.9	0	0	0
Zymin (Z)		0.025	0.9	1.7	0	0
Ammonia (N)	0.025		0	0	0	0
Ammonia (N)		0.025	0	0	0	0
H + Z	0.025		0	1.7	1.0	18
H + Z		0.025	0.8	2.4	1.4	18
H + N	0.025		0	0	0	20
H + N		0.025	0	0	0	20
Original serum	0.025		2.1	1.7	1.5	17
Original serum		0.025	0.8	1.2	0.6	17

* Portion of these sera were treated with CO_2 to obtain the respective euglobulin fraction, and no hemolytic activity was detected in any of the euglobulin fractions thus prepared, both the cells of Case 2 and the control being used.

be contrasted with that on human serum complement which fails to be reactivated by heated serum once it has been treated with zymin or ammonia.

The euglobulin fractions prepared by CO_2 precipitation from the variously treated sera were devoid of hemolytic activity on the patient's as well as control cells.

The present study seems to point to the existence of two separate effects of

guinea pig serum on hemolysis of human red blood cells. The first effect is specifi-
cally on the cells of the patient, evident only in conjunction with human serum,
active in relatively small amounts and not inactivated by heat. The second is
apparent when employed alone in relatively large amounts, acting on both the
patient's and the control cells to an equal extent, and inactivated by heat, by
cold absorption, by CO_2 precipitation and by ammonia, but not by zymin. Both
of these effects are distinct from the hemolytic factor of the human serum for the
hemolysis of the susceptible human cells, and from the complement present in
the guinea pig serum.

DISCUSSION

The foregoing observations afford strong evidence against complement being
the serum factor responsible for the hemolysis of the red blood cells of the two
cases of chronic hemolytic anemia with erythrocyte fragility to cold and acid.
Although the hemolytic factor resembles complement in being heat-labile and
inactivable by kaolin and storage, its inhibition by potassium oxalate is not
accompanied by any decrease of the complement titer. The serum euglobulin
fraction obtained by CO_2 precipitation, while devoid of complement activity,
was highly active in hemolyzing the patient's cells. Thus complement and hemolytic activities can be completely dissociated, making it most unlikely that complement is the hemolytic factor of the serum.

The fact that the euglobulin fraction acts on the patient's erythrocytes and
not on control cells, and shows enhanced activity with preliminary chilling and
on addition of acid, indicates that this isolated protein fraction is most probably an important factor responsible for the hemolytic activity of the serum.
Fractionation of serum proteins with sodium sulfate shows that pseudoglobulin
I also contains similar hemolytic activity. Thus the hemolytic activity resides
in serum euglobulin and pseudoglobulin I, although one can not be certain as
to whether it is the proteins themselves, or something intimately associated with
them, that possess the property of hemolyzing the susceptible cells. The wide spread
of the activity from euglobulin to pseudoglobulin I suggests the latter possibility.

It has been shown that the euglobulin fraction when separated from the
serum exhibits greater hemolytic power than the same amount of serum from
which it is derived. In fact the remainder of the serum after CO_2 precipitation
exerts a definite inhibitory influence on the euglobulin fraction. From the evidence presented cholesterol is probably not concerned in the inhibition, and pseudoglobulin II and albumin fractions seem to diminish the hemolytic activity of
the globulin fraction.

This euglobulin fraction is apparently highly labile; that prepared from heated
serum being entirely inactive, and those from zymin- and ammonia-treated sera
being much diminished in activity. It is probable that inactivation of the serum
hemolytic activity by aging, kaolin and potassium oxalate is brought about also
through an inactivation of the globulin fractions.

Prolonged cold absorption of the serum with cells diminishes its hemolytic
activity for further cold hemolysis, but not that for subsequent acid hemolysis.

On the other hand preliminary equilibration of the serum with CO_2 abolishes its hemolytic activity for further acid hemolysis without much impairment of its ability for subsequent cold hemolysis. This suggests the existence of two separate factors for the two types of hemolysis, one being used up under a given set of conditions without affecting the other. However, the phenomenon can also be interpreted as being due to two phases of activity of a single entity in view of their close association. Apart from cold absorption and CO_2 equilibration, all inactivating or inhibiting agents affect the activities for cold and acid hemolysis at the same time and to an equal extent.

Since normal serum contains the same hemolytic globulins and since only the patient's cells are susceptible to the hemolytic effects of these protein fractions, it follows that the abnormality resides in the patient's erythrocytes. How this abnormality develops can not be answered. Whether syphilis, which both patients had, is causally related to this abnormal cell fragility to cold and acid, somewhat analogous to the development of cold hemolysin in the serum of patients with paroxysmal cold hemoglobinuria, one is again not in a position to state.

The study of the role of the guinea pig serum is interesting in that it aids the human serum in the cold and acid hemolysis of the patient's cells and not of those of controls. This augmenting effect of the guinea pig serum is evident when fresh or partially inactivated human serum is used, but absent with completely inactivated (such as heated) serum. The fact that heating the guinea pig serum to 56 C. for thirty minutes does not destroy its augmenting power on the human serum hemolytic activity rules out the influence of its complement and globulin contents, for both would be destroyed by such procedure. In fact the euglobulin fraction precipitated by CO_2 from the guinea pig serum does not contain any hemolytic activity for the human cells which are susceptible to human serum euglobulin similarly prepared.

However, the whole guinea pig serum when used alone in relatively large amounts does have a slight hemolytic effect on both the abnormal and normal human erythrocytes. It is eliminated by heat, by cold absorption and by CO_2 precipitation. It appears to be a relatively labile and nonspecific (in regard to type of human cells) hemolytic factor of slight potency. It is clearly different from the augmenting factor of the guinea pig serum for human serum hemolytic activity on susceptible human cells. Nor does it bear any resemblance to the human serum hemolytic factor.

The data presented in this and preceding papers suggest a new syndrome of chronic hemolytic anemia with erythrocyte fragility to cold and acid. It is clearly distinguishable from paroxysmal cold hemoglobinuria by the presence of a primary cell abnormality and the absence of the Donath-Landsteiner hemolysin in the serum. Our cases can be differentiated from paroxysmal nocturnal hemoglobinuria by the additional cellular abnormality to the effects of cold and the absence of nocturnal intensification of the hemolytic process. Furthermore, the serum factor necessary for hemolysis, in contrast to that in paroxysmal nocturnal hemoglobinuria, does not depend on the complement, but on certain globulin fractions which are labile, yet clearly different from the former in many respects especially in being inactivable by oxalate. Another possible differential point is the behavior toward guinea pig serum which enhances the hemolytic activity of human serum toward susceptible cells. Such enhancements are brought about not by the complement nor by the englobulin but by a heat-stable factor present in the guinea pig serum.

SUMMARY

In 2 cases of chronic hemolytic anemia with erythrocyte fragility to cold and acid, although the abnormality resides in the red blood cells, serum, whether from the patients or from normal controls, is necessary for the hemolysis.

Complement is most likely not responsible for the serum hemolytic activity, because the latter, while similar to complement in certain properties, may be completely dissociated from it.

From human serum the euglobulin separated by CO_2 and sodium sulphate and the pseudoglobulin I obtained by sodium sulphate precipitation possess hemolytic activity for the cells of the patient and not those of the control. The hemolytic activity of these globulin fractions is increased by chilling and by addition of acid. It is inhibited by serum pseudoglobulin II and albumin.

Guinea pig serum aids human serum in its hemolytic activity on susceptible human cells. This augmenting effect of the guinea pig serum is not due to its complement content, nor due to its hetero-hemolysin for all human erythrocyte.

In view of the data presented in this and the preceding papers, a new syndrome is suggested which can be clearly differentiated from paroxysmal cold hemoglobinuria and from paroxysmal nocturnal hemoglobinuria.

REFERENCES

[1] LIU, S. H.: Chronic hemolytic anemia with erythrocyte fragility to cold and acid. I. Clinical data of two cases with special reference to the cell abnormality. Blood, this issue, p. 101.

[2] JORDON, F. L. J.: Studies sur l'hémoglobinurie. Acta med. Scandinav. 95: 319, 1938.

[3] DACIE, J. V., ISRAËLS, M. C. G., AND WILKINSON, J. F.: Paroxysmal nocturnal hemoglobinuria of the Marchiafava-Micheli type. Lancet 1: 479, 1938.

[4] HAM, T. H. AND DINGLE, J. H.: Studies on destruction of red blood cells. II. Chronic hemolytic anemia with paroxysmal nocturnal hemoglobinuria: Certain immunological aspects of the hemolytic mechanism with special reference to serum complement. J. Clin. Investigation 18: 657, 1939.

[5] LIEFMANN, H.: Über den Mechanismus der Seroreaktion der Lues. Müchen. med. Wchnschr. 56: 2097, 1909.

[6] HOWE, P. E.: The use of sodium sulphate as the globulin precipitant in the determination of proteins in blood. J. Biol. Chem. 49: 93, 1921.

[7] STRONG, P. S. AND CULBERTSON, J. T.: Filtrability of components of alexin. J. Hyg. 34: 522, 1934.

[8] GORDON, J. E., WHITEHEAD, H. R., AND WORMALL, A.: Action of ammonia on complement; fourth component. Biochem. J. 20: 1028, 1926.

[9] OSBORN, T. W. B.: Complement or Alexin. London, Oxford University Press, 1937.

[10] HUANG, C. H. AND SIA, R. H. P.: Paroxysmal hemoglobinuria with report of a case in a Chinese. Chinese M. J. 50: 214, 1936.

[11] TSAI, C. AND LEE, J. S.: The nature of antihemolytic substance in the plasma. Chinese J. Physiol. 16: 165, 1941.

[12] WHITEHEAD, H. R., GORDON, J. E., AND WORMALL, A.: The "third component" or heat-stable factor of complement. Biochem. J. 19: 618, 1925.

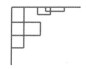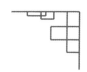

第八编　一代宗师

　　刘士豪教授在1951年出任协和生物化学系系主任，同时仍兼协和内科学教授的工作。而自1948年起，刘士豪已兼任北京同仁医院院长。1958年夏季，刘士豪卸去所有职务，创建了北京协和医院内分泌科并出任第一任科主任直至逝世。这段时间内，刘士豪对推动国内内分泌学科发展、培养内分泌和生物化学专业人才以及北京协和医院内分泌科的建设发挥了巨大作用，但多数并未以论文的形式形成成果。第八编收录了3篇论文和1篇书序，可从中初步了解这段时间刘士豪教授的工作。《甘草对阿狄森氏病的疗效》是同仁医院的工作，《微量血清碱性磷酸酶测定方法的研究》则是协和生物化学系的工作。《生物化学与临床医学的联系》在1957年问世以后影响极大，被视为与目前的转化医学思想一脉相承，而该书的序言正是刘士豪教授学术思想的重要体现。《内分泌研究发展的方向》一文则是刘士豪教授在中华医学会内分泌和肾脏病学大会上的大会报告，体现了他对内分泌学的渊博知识和深刻理解，很多观点迄今读来仍不得不佩服其高屋建瓴的学术思想。

1956年　第7号　　　　　　　　　　　　　　　· 655 ·

甘草对阿狄森氏病的疗效

四例的初步报告

刘士豪[*]　翟樹職[**]　隋樹娥[**]

阿狄森氏病，即慢性腎上腺皮質功能不全症，虽國內文献报告不多，但在臨床上並不罕見。此病之基本原因为有功能的腎上腺組織减少，而其减少的原因主要是結核，約佔68%；其次为原發性萎縮，約佔19%；其余的为淀粉样变，瘤腫，梅毒，血栓形成等，腎上腺的損坏同時影响髓質和皮質，而症狀主要是由於皮質功能不全所致。腎上腺皮質分泌多种固醇类激素，以皮質酮（Cortisone）为代表的一类与碳水化合物及蛋白質代謝有关，以醛固酮（aldosterone）[1] 为代表的一类有調節鈉、鉀及水代謝的能力，此外尚有女性激素，男性激素，孕酮等，皮質酮及醛固酮的長期缺乏是阿狄森氏病臨床表現的直接原因，故应用皮質酮及脫氧皮質酮（desoxycorticosterone，人工合成品，作用与醛固酮相似），足以使阿狄森氏病患者不致發生危象，並能恢复一部分劳动力，是一种適当的代替療法。不过，此种療法究屬昂貴，如有較簡單的治療方法，应在爭取之列。因此，甘草在这方面的应用值得研究。

甘草（glycyrrhiza uralensis, Fisch.）屬豆科植物，为多年生草，產於川陝等省[2]。中医常用其干燥根莖作为矯味剂或賦形药，有鎮咳祛痰，溫和瀉下的作用。神農本草經記載："甘草主治五臟六腑寒热邪气，堅筋骨，長肌肉，倍气力，金菪腫，解毒"。魏龍驤[3]最近介紹中医治療消化性潰瘍用甘草流浸膏有一定的療效。荷蘭人，Revers用甘草浸膏治療消化性潰瘍，認为療效很好，X-線檢查所發現的胃小弯龕影於3星期內完全消失；但应用甘草浸膏的患者每五人中有一人發生水腫。Molhuysen 等[4]的研究証明正常人每日服甘草浸膏20克可致水、鈉及氯的排泄減少，鉀的排泄增加，血紅蛋白及血清蛋白質濃度減少，以及静脉压和血压升高；因此認为甘草有类似脫氧皮質酮的作用。但是应用甘草制剂於阿狄森氏病的治療結果頗不一致。Molhuysen 等用甘草浸膏治療一例無明顯效果。Groen 等[5]先后报告兩例阿狄森氏病用甘草浸膏或甘草酸鹽治療，結果良好，認为甘草的有效成分可以代替脫氧皮質酮以控制阿狄森氏病。Cord 等[6]用甘草次酸治療一例阿狄森氏病，認为所得的效果与脫氧皮質酮和皮質酮相同。Calvert[7]报告一例本病，用甘草流浸膏起初每日60克，發生很好的療效，以后遞減至每日3克，还能使患者在良好情况下維持18个月之久，但是Borst 等[8]报告3例阿狄森氏病，其中包括Molhuysen 等曾經报告过的1例，認为甘草單独应用对腎上腺皮質功能不全者並無療效，但是与皮質酮合併应用有調節电解質代謝的作用，並能減少皮質酮的需要量。

因此，甘草对阿狄森氏病的療效在我國有研究的必要，我們曾在6例輕重不等之阿狄森氏病患者試用甘草流浸膏能，均有一定的效果，但其中4例应用时間較長，观察較詳，兹报告初步治療經过如下：

病歷摘要及治療經过

例1：住院号27860，沈姓，男，43歲，農民，於1955年5月26日入同仁医院。十年前曾發冷發热，每隔三、四日發作一次，医生認为是瘧疾，但服抗瘧药無效，並且形成持續性热，歷三、四个月之久，未治自癒，此后体力大为减退，而且皮膚逐漸变黑。近一年来腹部脹滿，食后反酸，偶尔嘔吐酸水，食慾減退，日漸消瘦，全身無力。体檢：慢性病容，全身皮膚黑褐色，唇及頰膜有紫色斑点；肝在右季肋下3厘米；胸部X線片示右上顯疑陰影。胃液分析：注射組織胺以前胃液無游离鹽酸，注射

---

　* 北京市同仁医院内科，中國协和医学院生物化学系
　** 北京市同仁医院内科
　註 中華人民共和國药典，1953，49 頁。服甘草流浸膏时，除食物所含及烹調所用的食鹽外，未加服食鹽。

后胃液每百毫升含18毫升0.1N塩酸。其他体檢及化驗(見表1及表2)。診斷:阿狄森氏病,中等度腎上腺皮質功能不全,可能与結核有关,因X線片顯示陳旧性肺結核,並有腸內鈎虫侵染。

驅虫后,即於6月14日起服甘草流浸膏,每日15毫升,分三次服(圖1)服藥后,病情好轉,食慾增加,精神較爽,体重由50增至53公斤,血壓由90/60增至110/70左右,兩手握力亦有所增加,血清鈉及氯有增加,而鉀有

表1 阿狄森氏病病例的体檢及化驗檢查

病例	体重 公斤	血壓 汞柱	手握力公斤 右	左	尿常規	糞常規	血色素	紅血球(万)	白血球	血沉 第一小時	第二小時	非蛋白氮	清蛋白	球蛋白	CO_2結合力	鈣	磷	鈉	氯	鉀	胆固醇	膽囊香草酸度	基礎代謝率	尿17-氧類固醇
1	50.0	90/60	35	15	正常	鈎虫卵	10.5	302	6000	58	70	114	27	2.9 1.9	64			132	84	5.3	190	12	-21	8.1
2	45.4	110/70	30	27	正常	正常	13.9	492	9800	14	22	70	34	4.2 2.5				140	100	5.1			-21	
3	55.0	130/90	44	46	正常	正常	12.0	371	7000	1	4	116	33	5.1 2.2	63	9.5	5.0	139	106	3.3	143	3	-2	7.9
4	43.0	91/50	6	3	正常	正常	9.0	308	3250	60	115	111	26	3.9 2.4	54	9.5	4.8	124	80	4.9	167	2	-3	8.8

* 毫当量/公升血清　　** 毫克/24小時尿

表2 阿狄森氏病病例的腎上腺皮質功能試驗(服甘草流浸膏前后的測定)

病例	甘草流浸膏治療	水試驗(Kepler, Robinson, Power) 尿量 晚小時九	次小時最一	非蛋白氮濃度 尿中	血中	氯化物濃度 尿中	血中	A值	腎上腺素(0.3毫克皮下)試驗 血中嗜酸性白血球計數 注射前	注射后	減少%	結論	垂体促腎上腺皮質激素(ACTH 25毫克肌注)試驗 血中嗜酸性白血球計數 注射前	注射后	減少%	尿中尿酸 注射前	注射后	尿中肌酐 注射前	注射后	尿酸/肌酐 注射前	注射后	比值改變%	結論
1	治療前	423	30	1170	26	600	644	0.9	414	303	27	陽性											
	治療后	890	35	280	23	473	527	0.6	423	345	19	陽性	486	411	15	38	36	43	38	0.88	0.95	-8	陽性
2	治療前	765	112	240*	19.3*	403	593	8.3					1188	9(1)2	2	38	40	75	77	0.50	0.52	3	陽性
	治療后	500	100	158*	10.5*	959	828	2.0					44	22	50	21	24	59	74	0.35	0.32	-8	陽性
3	治療前	260	110	1500	33	854	620	1.4	396	304	23	陽性	252	259	0	400	320	50	60	8.0	7.1	-11	陽性
	治療后	430	350	600	39.3	725	562	12.4	367	308	16	陽性	842	726	13	44	50	43	50	0.89	0.86	-3	陽性
4	治療前	1030	70	715	33.3	468	543	1.7					22	20	9								
	治療后	670	40	2000	34.3	527	585	3.4					176	174	1	732	800	60	50	12	16	+33	陽性

* 此例的數值是尿素氮毫克%

減少的趋势。皮膚色素沉着者於服藥后開始減退,一個月以后已減退約三分之一,一般情況大有進步,於7月15日出院。

出院后繼續服甘草流浸膏3個月,体力繼續增長,能料理家务,行走5—6公里而不覺累,色素沉着者繼續減退,11月24日追查時皮膚顏色除外耳及頸部稍黑外,与常人無异,唇及口腔粘膜的色素沉着已完全消失。11月中旬追查時,患者停用甘草流浸膏已一個半月,血壓有降低的趋势(100/70)。此后又再服,血壓開始再升。

例2;住院號112567,安姓,男,27歲,招待所服务員,於1955年7月4日入中國協和醫院。患者於一年半前發現兩頬部及前額皮膚發黑,並無其他不適,7個月前皮膚發黑逐漸進行。入院前4個月曾有高热兩次,此后常感頭昏乏力,精神差,体重減輕,性慾減退,食慾減少,並有腹瀉情况。查体:發育中等,消瘦,全身皮膚呈黑褐色,尤以顏、額、外耳、肛圍、陰囊、手背等处为著,上下肢疤痕处尤甚,唇、舌、齒齦、口腔粘膜亦呈色素沉着者。肺及腹部X線片正常。胃液分析:空腹胃液無游離塩酸,服餅干喝水(Ewald氏餐)后一小時,游離塩酸達20度,葡萄糖翻驗曲線大致正常。心电图示ST_2下降及$T_{2,3}$,aVF較低或双向。根據以上及表1—2所示,診斷为阿狄森氏病,中等度腎上腺皮質功能不全,可能

1956年　第7号

· 657 ·

由於原發性萎縮所致，因未發現体內結核病灶。

自7月23日起（圖2），每日服甘草流浸膏15毫升，分三次服，逐漸增至每日45毫升。服藥后，自覺精神較好、体力有勁、食慾較佳，体重由46增至51公斤（未見浮腫）。血壓由 $^{110}/_{70}$ 增至 $^{126}/_{80}$，血清鈉及氯顯示增加，鉀稍有降低，皮膚色素沉着亦見輕。由圖7可以看出服甘

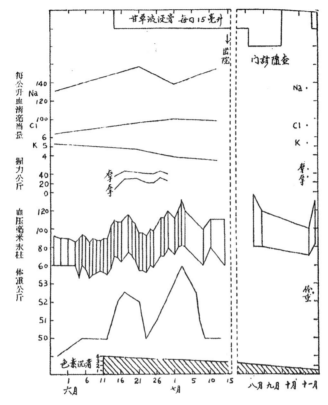

圖 1　例1的甘草流浸膏治療過程

草制剂一月余后，顏面、手背及皮膚的色素有明顯的消褪，按保守的估計，如入院时的色素沉着為4度，則出院前為2—3度之間。患者一般情况均有進步，於9月9日出院。出院后每日繼續用甘草流浸膏15毫升。休息一个月后，恢复工作（鍋爐助手）。11月12日追查时已作鍋爐助手工作一个月，不覺太累，食慾尚好。不过，此时体重已減至50公斤，血清鈉降低至120毫当量/公升，至於能否長期維持此种較重工作，須待以后随查而定。

例3：住院号28723，黄姓，男，年25歲，勘測員，因3年來呈漸進性皮膚發黑，疲倦無力，头暈。而於1955年6月28日入同仁医院。1952年夏天發覺皮膚較別人为

黑，口唇上有黑紫色斑点，以后色素沉着逐漸加深，遍及全身。体力逐漸衰弱，常有咳嗽，头昏，1953年夏症狀如前。1954年病情加重，稍累即心悸，出汗，食慾減退，2月間有惡心嘔吐，不能工作。在上海第一医學院检查認为是腎上腺皮質功能不全症，經6月29日於皮下种植脫氧皮質酮（Doca）300毫克並給皮質酮（Cortisone）每日12.5毫克口服，病情好轉。1955年1月又开始乏力，惡心，食慾減退；5月13日曾又在上海第一医學院皮下埋藏脫氧皮質酮300毫克。在上海曾服过甘草浸膏認为無效。兩三歲时患頸部淋巴腺結核，13歲时曾患慢性中耳炎。体檢：發育營養尚好，全身皮膚呈棕褐色，嘴唇呈深紫色，口腔粘膜、瞼緣、結合膜均有色素

沉著。右側頸部皮膚有以往潰糊的疤痕，皮下淋巴腺可触及。肝未摸及，脾在左季肋下一橫指，X線片檢查未發現肺部病變或腹部腎上腺部位鈣化点。結合以上病歷及表1和表2所见，認为系阿狄森氏病，中等度腎

上腺皮質功能不全（可能由結核所致），但由於5月所种植的300毫克脫氧皮質酮正在發揮代偿作用。故一般情况尚屬不坏。

入院后5个月的观察主要系在脫氧皮質酮作用的

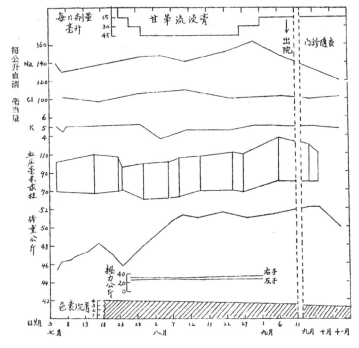

圖2　例2的甘草流浸膏治療过程

基礎上来测定甘草流浸膏的作用（圖3）。甘草流浸膏的分劑由每日15毫升增至40毫升，服藥后体重稍有增加，食慾較好，头暈头痛比以前少，体力較前稍強，血压由$^{140}/_{80}$增至$^{150}/_{90}$左右，偶有至$^{170}/_{100}$，尤其是在9月底10月初之間。自10月4日至25日停用甘草制劑，血压逐漸下降，到达25日的$^{110}/_{80}$的最低記錄，此后再給予甘草流浸膏，血压亦随之逐漸上升，虽在一个月內，尚未达到以往最高水平；皮膚色素沉著亦有減退的趋势，在4个月內估計由4度減至3度，故較其他病例色素減輕的程度为少。血清鈉，除7月13日的测定較低外，无顯著变化，血清鉀亦如是。握力無明顯的变化。本例因脫氧皮質酮的种植，症狀比其他病例較輕，故加服甘草流浸膏所得的改善，除血压增高外，比其他病例較为不明顯，可能說明甘草流浸膏的作用与脫氧皮質酮有相同之处。

例4：住院号：8225，鞠姓，男，25歲，材料員，於1955年6月2日入同仁医院，患者自謂年幼时全身皮膚較常人为黑，但無其他不適，勝任搬工工作。3年前感說体力較前为差，由搬工改为材料員。本年3月因發燒、嘔吐而入北京市立第六医院，經治痊后好轉。4月初又因同樣發作而入北京市立第六医院，此次神志模糊，經輸液后好轉。此后体力更差，不能起床，食慾減退，自覺消瘦，皮膚較前更黑。体檢：慢性病容，消瘦，不能起坐；全身皮膚呈黑褐色。手掌及足心亦發黑色，結合膜、唇、舌、口腔粘膜、齒齦均有顯著色素沉著。X線檢查發現心臟縮小，右肺第一肋間有圓形陰影，第四肋間有小片狀陰影及鈣化斑（肺結核）。相當於十二胸椎兩側有密集的鈣化斑点（腎上腺部位鈣化）。其他檢查結果見表1及表2。診断，阿狄森氏病，重度腎上腺皮質功能不全（由結核所致），右側浸潤性肺結核。

1956年 第7号

· 659 ·

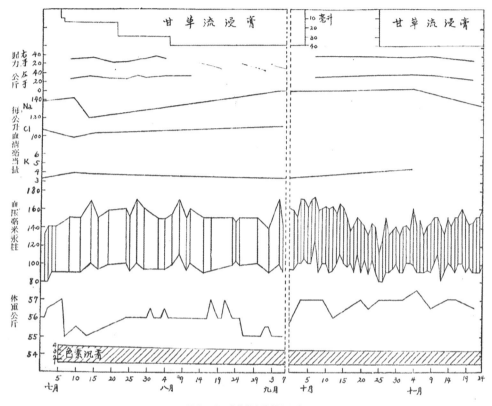

图 3 例 3 的甘草流浸膏治疗过程

入院后的第一阶段治疗经过（见图 4），自 6 月 17 日开始口服甘草流浸膏，每日 20 毫升，约一个半月以后增至 30 毫升，继而增至 45 及 60 毫升。服药后，食慾渐增，体力精神均有进步，能下地活动。体重由 43 公斤增至 46 公斤，但其中波动不定。当甘草流浸膏的分剂加至每日 30 毫升以后，血压有明显的上升，由 $^{101}/_{60}$ 升至 $^{130}/_{80}$ 毫米水柱水平。血浆钠及氯浓度亦形上升，而血钾顯示降低。皮肤色素沉着逐渐减輕，服用甘草制剂三个月后，色素沉着的程度估计由 4 度减至 2—3 度之间。

在这三个半月期间，甘草流浸膏对患者虽有上述好处，但因結核病灶的存在以及併發感染，故时常有体温升高，需要链霉素及青霉素来控制。10 月以后在服用甘草流浸膏的基础上，抗生素疗法每不易控制感染，并且發燒时常伴有昏迷的發作，發作时先有气喘，繼之以人事不省，偶有抽搐，口吐白沫，或有手足搐搦，輕 1 —5 分鐘而醒；發作时，血压並不下降，血糖及钙、磷等

測定均屬正常，發作多在体温突然上升或下降的时候。故認为体温改变的刺激对腎上腺功能重度不全者可能产生上述腦症状。为了叙述方便起見，姑且称此种發作为“危象”。單独应用甘草流浸膏已不能控制危象的發生，似有加用皮質酮（Cortisone）的必要。

第二阶段疗法，甘草流浸膏与皮質酮合併疗法見图 5。自 10 月 7 日起除甘草流浸膏每日 30—60 毫升外，合併注射皮質酮，第一天 100 毫克，第二、三天各 150 毫克，危象迅速消失，体温也降到正常，食慾恢复，精神愉快，体重由 44 增至 48 公斤，顏面有浮腫，随即将皮質酮的分剂逐渐减少至每日 10 毫克，於是浮腫消失，体重降至原来的水平，血压上升至 $^{130}/_{90}$ 左右。虽体温常有起伏，但一般情况良好。自 10 月 25 日起至 11 月 5 日停用皮質酮。單独应用甘草流浸膏，在此 12 天期間，头一星期的情况很好，但以后又有危象的發作，表示甘草流浸膏的單独使用不足控制危象，於是自 11 月 6 日起每日

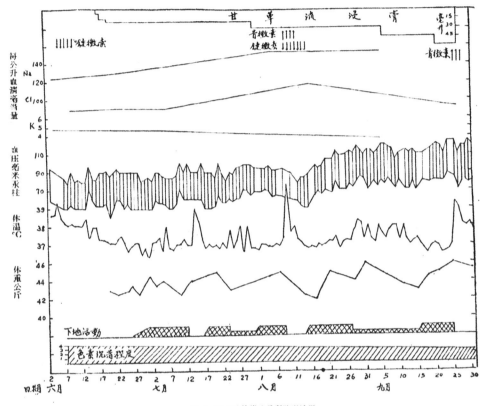

图 4 例 4 的甘草流浸膏治療过程

又注射皮質酮10毫克,没有危象產生。自11日起至17日,停止甘草流浸膏,每日只注射皮質酮10毫克,17日又有危象發生,表示單独每日使用10毫克的皮質酮不足控制危象。18日至23日恢复甘草流浸膏的併用期間又無危象的發生。因此認為甘草流浸膏与皮質酮有協助預防危象的作用,或有減少皮質酮需要量的作用。

甘草流浸膏对上述病例療效的綜述

对上述4例慢性腎上腺皮質功能不全症患者,甘草流浸膏均有一定的療效,但由於病情的輕重有所不同,甘草的療效也不一致,一般而論,甘草流浸膏对患者有促進食慾,增加体重,恢复体力的作用,例1及例2在这方面的進步較为顯著,故劳动力有所恢复,能胜任較輕的工作,例3在脱氫皮質酮的作用下已能作輕度工作,故加用甘草流浸膏对体力進一步的恢复不甚明顯。例4系重度進行性腎上腺功能不全的患者,服甘草制剂后,虽体力有所恢复,能起床下地活动,但因时常發燒而中止,以后因病情發展,甘草只能起補助作用,必須加以小量皮質酮方能有效。

对於血压,甘草流浸膏在4例中均有提高作用,收縮压及舒張压均可提升10—20毫米水銀柱。例1,2及4的血压較低,服甘草制剂后均趨正常,虽然达到正常所需的分剂可由每日15毫升(例1)至45—60毫升(例4),所需的時間可由20天(例1)至一个半月(例2)或3个月(例4),例3由於脱氫皮質酮的作用,血压比正常稍高

1956年　第7号

($^{140}/_{80}$)，經过 3 个月的甘草制剂療法，血压逐漸升至$^{170}/_{100}$，停服甘草 3 星期后血压才降至原來的水平，說明甘草对血压較高者还有加压的作用，而且此种作用在停药后需要一段時間才能消退。例4用甘草合併皮質酮療法时，血压的升高尤为顯著（圖5）。

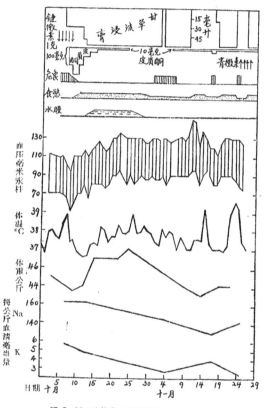

圖 5　例 4 的甘草流浸膏合併皮質酮治療过程

甘草对血清电解質的影响也很明顯，虽然我們的測定有时不够勤或及时。例1，2及4服用甘草流浸膏后，血清鈉由較正常为低的水平，如130毫当量（例1及2）或124毫当量（例4），迅速地升至150毫当量左右。例3的血清鈉原來正常（142毫当量），服甘草制剂后曾一度降低，旋即上升至150毫当量，血清氯化物經常随鈉濃度的改变而改变。血清鉀在例1，2及4均

在 5 毫当量左右，服甘草后均降低至 3 ～4 毫当量之間，例3的血清鉀可能由於脱氧皮質酮的作用，原來在 3.5 毫当量左右，服甘草制剂后未有明顯的改变。总之甘草流浸膏对血清鈉及氯的濃度确有增高的作用，而对血清鉀确有减低的作用。甘草对血清电解質的作用可能是基本的，是血压增高以及食慾和体力恢复的原因。

甘草流浸膏对皮膚及粘膜的色素沉着，在 4 例中，均有减輕的作用，例 1 的表現最为明顯，皮膚的色素沉着在三、四个月內大部消失，口腔粘膜的色素沉着完全消失，例2～4的色素沉着在三、四个月內只消退一半或三分之一。色素沉着消退的程度可能与总的病情，尤其是体力恢复的程度有关。例 1 体力恢复最好，色素沉着的消退也最多；其他病例体力的恢复均不如例1，色素沉着的消退也較慢。

上述甘草流浸膏对阿狄森氏病的影响在輕度或初期患者，甚为顯著，能恢复体力，因而恢复輕度的工作，成为適当的簡便的代替療法，不需皮質酮或脱氧皮質酮的帮助，如例1及例2所示。但是在重症或晚期患者，甘草單独的应用不能顯著地恢复患者的体力，甚至不能预防危象的發生，必須加用皮質酮才能奏效。甘草与皮質酮合併应用时，皮質酮的分剂可以大为减少，例 4 每日服 CO 毫升甘草流浸膏时，只需每日注射皮質酮10毫克，即能预防危象的發生，不然單独应用皮質酮，則所需的分剂必然大若干倍。

根据上述甘草与皮質酮似有互补或协同作用，故二者的作用必有所不同。甘草与脱氧皮質酮的作用似有相同之处。如例3所示，在脱氧皮質酮的影响下，血清电解質濃度大致正常，体力已有相当的恢复，加用甘草流浸膏后未能有更多的改变，可能表示其作用与脱氧皮質酮在这些方面是相同的，但是加用甘草后，血压繼績升高，皮膚色素沉着减退，可能說明甘草在这

些方面的作用与脱氧皮質酮不完全相同或較为优勝。总之，甘草的作用与脱氧皮質酮較为接近，与皮質酮較为不同。

4例的腎上腺皮質功能，按水試驗，腎上腺素試驗及乗体促腎上腺皮質激素試驗的結果（表2）所示，在治療前均顯著低落，符合阿狄森氏病的診断。服用甘草流浸膏一个半月至五个月之后，重复这些試驗的結果，表示腎上腺皮質功能未發生明顯的改变。除例2的促腎上腺皮質激素試驗顯示嗜酸性白血球的減少由24%增至50%，以及例3的水試驗的A值由1.4增至12.4以外，其他試驗均表示腎上腺皮質功能無進步或減低。因此可以認为甘草流浸膏对阿狄森氏病的療效不是通过腎上腺皮質功能的改進，而是一种补償作用。

討　論

甘草的主要化学成分系 5—8% 的甘草素（glycyrrhigin），甘草黄素（liquiritin），葡萄糖，甘露醇，天門冬醯胺（Asparagin），樹膠等，甘草素是甘草酸（glycyrrhizinic acid）的鉀盐及鈣盐、甘草酸經水解后，產生1分子甘草次酸（glycyrrhetinic acid）及2分子葡萄糖醛酸（glucuronic acid）：

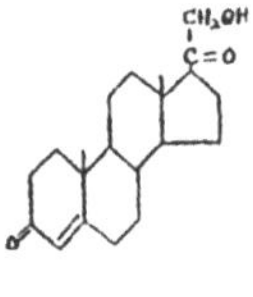

$$C_{12}H_{60}O_{16} + 2H_2O = C_{30}H_{46}O_5 + 2C_6H_{10}O_7$$
　甘草酸　　　　　甘草次酸　葡萄糖醛酸

甘草次酸系三萜类（triterpene），其構造式已由 Rugicka 等[9] 証明如式Ⅰ，甘草黄素的構造如式Ⅴ。

Card等認为甘草次酸为甘草的有效成分，因甘草次酸对正常人及阿狄森氏病患者所產生的在体重和电解質上的改变，与粗制的甘草浸膏相同。純甘草次酸的效力比含有同量甘草次酸的甘草浸膏为大，例如0.5克甘草次酸相当於20

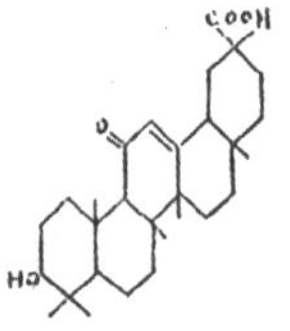

式I．甘草次酸　　　式Ⅱ．脱氧皮質酮　　式Ⅲ．醛固酮
(Glycyrrhetinic　(Desoxycortic-　(Aldosterone)
acid)　　　　　costerone)

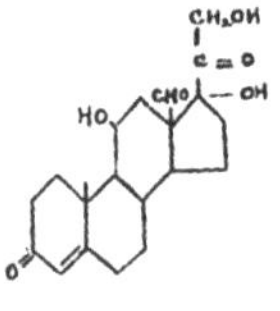

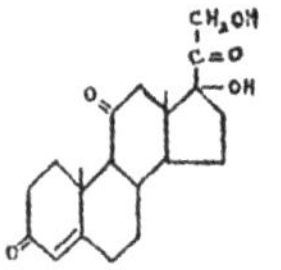

式Ⅳ．皮質酮　　　　　式Ⅴ．甘草黄素
(cortisone)　　　　　(Liquiritin)

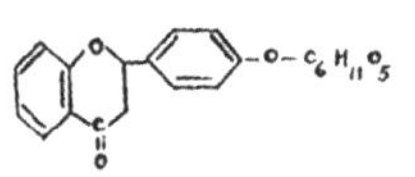

圖6　甘草次酸，腎上腺皮質激素类及甘草黄素的化学構造式

克甘草浸膏，而 20 克的甘草浸膏約含有 1 克甘草次酸。因此自由的甘草次酸的作用較大，而結合於甘草素中的甘草次酸的作用較小，因为后者在体内必須水解成自由的甘草次酸方能發生作用，而体内水解的过程可能不完全。

甘草或其有效成分甘草次酸的基本作用在於电解質代謝，即鈉和氯的存積（因而血漿及其他細胞外液的容量增加和血压升高）及鉀的排出，这样的作用正与脱氧皮質酮相同，可以矫正阿狄森氏病患者在这方面的缺陷，脱氧皮質酮因其糾正电解質代謝失常的作用，对輕度或早期阿狄森氏病患者的療效很大，使患者恢复輕度的工作；甘草流浸膏对这类患者也是如此。对重症或晚期患者，單独使用脱氧皮質酮的療效不够完全，必須加以皮質酮才能使患者恢复体力，改善患者的主观感觉；甘草流浸膏对这样患者的使用情况也是如此。因此甘草的作用与脱氧皮質酮極为相似，脱氧皮質酮主要是作用於腎曲管，使其对鈉的再吸收和鉀的排出加强以致血清鈉濃度增高，鉀濃度減低，故甘草对电解質代謝的改变，最可能也是通过对腎臟的作用。

甘草流浸膏在改進电解質代謝和恢复体力方面虽与脱氧皮質酮相似，但在升高血压和減輕皮膚色素沉着方面有所不同；在脱氧皮質酮作用基礎上，甘草流浸膏繼續使血压升高，这可能是因为甘草使血压升高的机制与脱氧皮質酮不同，或甘草在这方面的作用比脱氧皮質酮为甚。脱氧皮質酮长期应用，对阿狄森氏病患者無減輕其皮膚色素沉着的作用，而甘草在这方面的作用甚为顯著，說明甘草与脱氧皮質酮相比，有其独特之处。甘草使皮膚色素沉着減退的机制容在下面讨论。

皮質酮的作用主要在於蛋白質及醣代謝的改变，而对於电解質及水代謝的作用則远遜於脱氧皮質酮，故二者同时並用有相互补缺的效力，成为阿狄森氏病的几乎完全的代償療法，通过皮質酮的作用，体內蛋白質合成較少而分解較多，因而糖元異生作用較为旺盛。血糖較高，肝中糖元較多，这些作用，以及皮質酮的抗炎症，分解淋巴球及嗜酸性白血球等作用，对正常人有利，对重度阿狄森氏病患者必须加以补償。甘草，如脱氧皮質酮一样，似無这些作用，故对於重度腎上腺皮質功能不全者的療效不够，必须有皮質酮的补充。甘草与皮質酮並用有減少皮質酮需要量的效能，如例4的第二階段治療过程所示。甘草降低皮質酮需要量的机制是否协同作用，抑是互补作用？所謂协同作用意味着甘草加强皮質酮本身的作用。由於甘草只能对輕症阿狄森氏病有很好的療效，故Bayliss[10]認为甘草对皮質酮有协同作用，因为輕症患者可能尚有一小部分皮質功能，產生小量的皮質酮，此量本不敷体內需要，但經过甘草可能对破坏皮質酮的酶系有所抑制，小量的皮質酮可以延长其作用的时限，以应付患者所需。如果甘草有加强皮質酮的作用，則嗜酸性白血球在服藥后应較服藥前为低，但如表2所示，除例2在治療后嗜酸性白血球降低外，其他3例均無此現象，故在这方面未能肯定甘草能加强皮質酮的作用。此外，如果甘草有这样的作用，甘草应該能加强皮質酮对类風湿性关節炎的療效，或減少皮質酮的需要量，但是Hart及Leonard[11]在11例类風湿性关節炎患者的治療中，除1例給予甘草次酸每日0.5克稍減少患者对皮質酮的需要量外，其余均不顯示甘草对皮質酮有协同作用。

因此我們必须考虑甘草減少阿狄森氏患者对皮質酮的需要量是一种互补作用。阿狄森氏病患者的缺点是兩方面的，即①水和电解質代謝失常及②蛋白質和醣代謝失常。甘草只能矯正第一方面的缺点，皮質酮对第二方面的缺点有顯著的療效，如欲同时糾正第一方面的缺点，則需要大量的皮質酮方能奏效。此时如投以甘草制剂，矯正了患者在水和电解質代謝的失常，則只需小量的皮質酮以維持其蛋白質和醣代謝於正常范圍之內。故甘草降低皮質酮的需要量是一种互相补缺的作用。

甘草流浸膏对患者的皮膚色素沉着有顯著減退的作用；皮質酮长期的应用也有同样的效能。一般認为色素沉着与垂体促黑素細胞激素(Melanocyte-stinulating hormone)有关[12]，此激素作用於皮膚及粘膜的細胞，使其形成較多的黑色素，但是腎上腺皮質所產生的激素如皮質酮，对垂体有抑制作用，減少其促腎上腺皮質激素，促黑素細胞激素等的分泌，因而皮膚及粘膜的色素沉着減退。当腎上腺皮質功能不全，皮質酮產量过少时，垂体分泌促黑素細胞激素的抑制即行解除，故此激素的產量增加，皮膚及粘膜的色素沉着加重，此即阿狄森氏病色素沉着以及皮質酮減輕机制的解釋。甘草減輕色素沉着的机制可能也是通过对垂体在这方面的抑制。

綜合上述，甘草次酸与脱氧皮質酮相似，与皮質酮不同，但这只是相对地如此，因甘草与皮質酮的作用也有相同之处，例如減輕皮膚色素沉着，而甘草与脱氧皮質酮的作用也有不同之处。試看圖6的甘草次酸的化学式，可知与腎上腺皮質激素的化学式相仿，故有类似的生理作用，但由於二者的化学構造又有不同之处，故其生理作用又有所不同，說明化学結構与生理功能是緊密联系的。

結 論

1. 本文报告4例阿狄森氏病經甘草流浸膏治療后顯示体力進步，血清鈉增加，血压升高及皮膚色素沉着減退。

2. 甘草流浸膏对輕度或初期患者的療效較为顯著，單独使用可能使患者恢复較輕的工作；但对重症或晚期患者需要与皮質酮並用。

3. 甘草与皮質酮併用时，可減少皮質酮的需要量，此种作用認为是互补作用。

4. 甘草的有效成分認为是甘草次酸，其作用与脱氧皮質酮相似的地方較多。

本文的例2，承中國协和医学院内科学系主任張孝騫教授許可發表，謹此誌謝。

參考文獻

1. Gaunt, R., Renzi, A. A. and Chart, J. J.: Aldosterone—a Review. J. Clin. Endo. and Metab. 15:621, 1955.

2. 謝觀: 中國医学大辞典, 1933, 810 頁, 朱顏: 中葯的葯理与应用, 健康书店, 1955, 231 頁.
   陳諾誠: 我对甘草作用的初步探討, 上海中医葯雜誌, 1955, 11 月号, 15 頁.

3. 魏龍驤: 中医治療消化性潰瘍的介紹, 中華医学雜誌 40:613, 1954.

4. Molhuysen, J. A., Gerbrandy, de Vries, L. A., de Jong, J. C., Lenstra, J. B., Turner, K. P., Borst, J. G. G.: A licorice extract with desoxycortone—like action. Lancet 2:381 1950.

5. Groen, J., Pelser, H. E., Frenkel, M., Kamminga, C. E. and Willebrands, A. F.: Effect of glycyrrhizinic acid on the electrolyte metabolism in Addison's disease. J. Clin. Invest. 31:87, 1952.

6. Card, W. I., Mitchell, W., Strong, J. A., Taylor, N. R. W., Tompsett, S. L., and Wilson, J. M. G.: Effects of liquorice and its derivatives on salt & water metabolism. Lancet 1:663, 1953.

7. Calvert, R. J.: Licorice extract in Addison's disease, successful long term therapy. Lancet 1:805, 1954.

8. Borst, J. G. G., ten Holt, S. P., de Vries, L. A. and Molhuysen, J. A.: Synergistic action of liquorice and cortisone in Addison's and Simmonds' disease. Lancet 1:657, 1953.

9. Ruzicka, L. U. Marxer, A.: Umwandlung der glycyrrheinsäure in β-Amyrin. Helv. Chim. Act. 22:195, 1939.
   Ruzicka, L., Jeger, O. U. Jngold, W.: Neuer Beweis für die verschiedine Lage der Carboxygruppe bei der Oleanolsaure und der Glycyrrhetinsäure. Helv. Chim. Act. 26:2278, 1943.

10. Bayliss, R. I. S.: Factors influencing adrenocortical activity in health and disease. Brit. Med. J. 1:495, 1955.

11. Hart, F. D. and Leonard, J. C.: Potentiation of cortisone by glycyrrhetinic acid. Lancet 1:804, 1954.

12. Lerner, A. B., Shizume, K. and Bunding, I.: The mechanism of endocrine control of melanin pigmentation. J. Clin. Endo. & Metab. 14:1463, 1954.
   盧欣义: 黑色素代謝研究之進展, 中華医学雜誌, 41:1055, 1955.

（上接 652 頁）

拗时亦有發現（如圖 7）。

討論及結論

（1）根据以上实驗，我們認为可以証明杠柳皮含有强心性物質，其水溶性甚高，是否即为 periplocin 或类似之配糖体，尚有待化学方面之分析。

（2）根据陳克恢氏[13]測定 Periplocin，貓單位为 0.121 毫克。而我們測定國產杠柳皮的貓單位折合生葯为0.176，假定杠柳皮的有效成份为 Periplocin，則其含量近 0.07%，較 Herrmann[14] 所研究之 Periploca graeca 根皮的含量 0.03%高一倍。

（3）我們認为杠柳皮可为毒毛旋花子的代用品，有深入研究的价值。

附註：本实驗所用之生葯原料會得趙午嶠老先生之鑑定；中國葯学会中葯整理委員会代为从北京購需生葯原料；中國科学院林業土壤研究所見告杠柳產銷地点；謹此特致衷心謝忱。

參考文獻

1. 經利彬等: 南北五加皮之生理作用, 中國生理雜誌 15:361-365, 1940.

2. 趙橘黃: 五加皮与五加皮酒之中毒論 科学22卷7/8期。

3. Леман, Э. А. и Бужинский, П. В.: Врач 22:631-634, 1896. 轉自"10"。

4. Левашов, Н. М.: Известия томского университета, 16:381-390, 1900. 轉自"10"。

5. Jacobs, Walter A., and Alexander Hoffmann: Periplocymarin and Periplogenin, J. of biol. chem. 79:519-530, 1928.

6. Levi, Angelina: Periploca greca d'Italia, Boll. Soc. ital. Biol. sper. 6:111-116, 1931. 轉自 Rona's Berichte 63:544, 1932.

7. Jacobs, W. A., Elderfield, R. C.: The Correlation of Strophanthidin and Periplogenin. J. of biol. chem. 91:625-628, 1931.

8. Вершинин, Н. В.: Фармакология 250, 1952.

9. Онищев, П. И.: Сборник трудов харьковского ветеринарного института, Киев. 21:172-176, 1952 轉自 "10"。

10. Онищев, П. И.: Элиминация периплоцимарина, Фармокол. и Токсикол. 17:45-48, 1954.

11. 吳熙瑞等: 國產毒毛旋花 — 羊角拗的葯理作用, 中華医学雜誌（本期發表）。

12. Баньковский, А. И. 等: Желтушник серый 21, 1953. Медгиз.

13. Chen, K. K.: Ann. Rev. Physiol. 7:681, 1945.

14. Herrmann, G.: C. r. Soc. Biol. Paris 102:915, 1929.

营 养 学 报
第1卷 第4期 1956年12月

微量血清鹼性磷酸酶測定方法的研究

吳德昌 魏文齡 刘士豪

（中国协和医学院生物化学系, 北京）

血清鹼性磷酸酶的测定对于临床診断和营养研究都有很大的帮助[1]。血中鹼性磷酸酶的含量反映骨質的情况, 因它大部分是由成骨細胞产生的。倘佝偻病或骨質軟化症（維生素D缺乏）, 甲状旁腺机能亢进, 肾性骨質病及其他能使骨質破坏引起成骨細胞增生的疾病, 都有血清鹼性磷酸酶增加的現象。相反地, 有些骨病如老年性骨質疏松症、成骨不全等, 因为成骨細胞減少, 則血中鹼性磷酸酶正常。因此, 血清鹼性磷酸酶的测定对骨質病的鑒別診断具有重要意义[2]。

肝胆系統的疾病如阻塞性黃胆或毛細胆管胆汁性肝硬变也出現鹼性磷酸酶在血中的存积。这种存积并不反映骨質的情况, 而只反映胆道阻塞的情况;因为在这种情况下骨質及肝細胞所形成的磷酸酶不易排泄, 而潴留于血中。此时血清鹼性磷酸酶主要来自肝細胞, 因为在傳染性肝炎或严重的阻塞性黃胆中, 黃胆虽深, 但由于肝細胞坏死, 不能产生磷酸酶, 故血清磷酸酶的含量不見增加[3]。因此, 血清鹼性磷酸酶的测定也有助于黃胆的鑒別診断。

血清鹼性磷酸酶的测定也可以作为营养調查中維生素D及鈣磷代謝情况的指标。Motzok[4]發現鷄雛产生佝偻病后, 血漿鹼性磷酸酶含量与維生素D分剂的对数呈正比关系, 并应用这种关系作維生素D的生物鑒定。

根据上述, 血清鹼性磷酸酶测定的用途是很广泛的。但是一般所采用的Bodansky氏法[5]需要大量血清（2毫升）, 不适宜于小动物的研究和嬰兒幼童的檢查, 故有建立微量法的必要。Kaplan和Narahara[6]最近所建議的方法只需0.01毫升血清, 作用时間为半小时, 且操作方便。我們对此法进行了研究和試用。在試用的时候, 稍加改进, 并建立了微量血清采取法, 使这个方法能更方便地应用于小动物的研究和嬰兒的檢驗。

測 定 方 法

（一） 原理

鹼性磷酸酶作用于一苯磷酸二鈉基質, 將酚釋出, 酚与紅B鹽（Red B Salt**, 即2

---

* 1956 年 8 月 12 日收到。
** National Aniline Company, New York 的出品。

氨基5硝基苯甲醚的偶氮化合物)生成紅色化合物。紅色的深度反映所释出的酚量，亦即反映磷酸酶的含量。以标准酚溶液的不同濃度为横坐标，以其与紅B鹽所生成紅色，在光譜光度計上所得出的吸光度为縱坐标，繪出标准曲綫，由此可讀出血清醇的含量。反应式大致如下：

（二）　試剂

1. 基質 0.05M 一苯磷酸二鈉：溶解 1.09 克一苯磷酸二鈉于蒸餾水，稀釋至 100 毫升。在使用前須取 1.5 克一苯磷酸二鈉用热酒精 25 毫升处理二次，过濾，干燥后备用。

2. 硼酸鹽緩冲液 pH 9.8：秤 9.5 克 $Na_2B_4O_7 \cdot 10 H_2O$ 加 950 毫升蒸餾水，然后加入 30 至 40 毫升 N NaOH 至 pH 9.8，稀釋至 1,000 毫升。

3. 氯化鎂 20% 溶液：溶解 20 克 $MgCl_2$ 于蒸餾水，稀釋至 100 毫升。

4. 緩冲基質：取上述基質 10 毫升加 1 毫升 20% $MgCl_2$，用硼酸鹽緩冲液稀釋至100毫升。

5. 甲醛 1.5 M 溶液：取 120 毫升 HCHO(38%)，用蒸餾水稀釋至 1,000 毫升。所用甲醛需要过濾，蒸餾，沸点为 98°C。

6. 飽和硼酸鹽酒精溶液：取 150 毫升 95% 酒精加 850 毫升蒸餾水及 35 克 $Na_2B_4O_7 \cdot 10 H_2O$，搖匀，未溶解的部分保留于瓶底。

7. 紅B鹽試剂：將蒸餾水和 1.8 N H_2SO_4 冷却至 5°C，溶解 0.125 克紅B鹽于冷却的 100 毫升蒸餾水中，过濾，加 1 毫升冷的 1.8 N H_2SO_4。此溶液需保存于冰箱中，使用期限最好不超过一星期。超过二星期者不能再用。

8. 标准酚溶液：溶解 0.940 克无水酚于 100 毫升蒸馏水中，此溶液的浓度为 100 微克分子/毫升。酚在使用前需要以磨口玻璃蒸馏器蒸馏之，沸点为 182°C。

9. 应用标准酚溶液（0.05 微克分子/毫升）：将 1 毫升标准酚溶液稀释至 100 毫升，取此稀释溶液 5 毫升再稀释至 100 毫升即得。使用时需新鲜配制。

10. 校准标准酚溶液的碘滴定试剂：0.1N $KH(IO_3)_2$，0.1N $Na_2S_2O_3$，化学纯 KI，5% HCl，0.1N I_2 溶液（每升含 KI 25 克和 I_2 12.7 克），1% 淀粉溶液。

（三）步骤

1. 标准酚溶液的校准和标准曲线的制备：制备标准酚溶液时，虽可称定量的酚溶于一定量的蒸馏水中，但由于酚的纯度不易保证，所以应用以下校准方法（其原理即以标准 I_2 溶液校准酚溶液，以 0.1N $Na_2S_2O_3$ 校准 I_2 溶液，以 0.1N $KH(IO_3)_2$ 溶液校准 $Na_2S_2O_3$ 溶液）。置 3 毫升标准酚溶液于一带玻璃塞的 250 毫升容量的锥形瓶中，加 50 毫升 0.1N NaOH，在 65°C 保温 15 分钟，然后加入 25 毫升标准 I_2 溶液，用 KI 溶液封瓶口。在暗处放置 45 分钟后用标准 $Na_2S_2O_3$ 溶液滴定剩余的碘，以淀粉溶液为指示剂。同时准备空白，即以 3 毫升蒸馏水代替标准酚溶液，同样处理。空白滴定值减去酚溶液滴定值即为酚所用去的碘，代入下列公式，即可求出酚的浓度。

3 毫升所含的酚毫克数 $= 1.568 \times$（空白滴定所用 0.1N $Na_2S_2O_3$ 毫升数 — 样品滴定所用 0.1N $Na_2S_2O_3$ 毫升数）。

制备标准曲线时，取 0、0.5、1.0、2.0、3.0、4.0 毫升应用标准酚溶液，加入 1 毫升硼酸盐缓冲液，然后加蒸馏水补足为 5 毫升。加 4 毫升饱和硼酸盐酒精溶液，摇匀后再加入 1 毫升红 B 盐试剂，立即摇匀。十分钟后在 Dr. B. Lange 牌的光谱光度计上比色（波长选择为 500mμ，原作者用光电比色计），以所得透光度换算为光密度。以光密度作为纵坐标，以酚微克分子浓度×200 为横坐标，作成曲线，即得标准曲线。以酚微克分子数代表磷酸酶单位数。按此法的规定，凡 1 毫升血清在 37°C 作用 1 小时所释出的酚的量为 1 微克的时候，就等于一个单位的硷性磷酸酶。

2. 硷性磷酸酶的测定

（1）大量血清法　将 0.5 毫升血清在体积量瓶中用生理盐水稀释至 50 毫升。以稀释血清 1 毫升（即等于 0.01 毫升血清）为测定时应用的样品量。测定时需准备标准空白、样品空白和样品三个试管。原作者只用样品空白及样品两个试管，但我们认为标准空白是需要的，因为它可以使测定时的情况符合于制订标准曲线时的情况，以免去红 B 盐本身颜色所引起的误差。样品空白的作用为抵消血清本身颜色所引起的误差。

①标准空白管：1 毫升硼酸盐缓冲液加 4 毫升蒸馏水。

②样品空白管：2毫升缓冲基質加2毫升甲醛溶液及1毫升稀釋血清。

③样品管：2毫升缓冲基質在恒温水浴（37℃）中保温15分鐘后加1毫升稀釋血清，保温30分鐘后取出，加2毫升甲醛溶液。

上述三管中各加4毫升飽和硼酸鹽酒精溶液，搖匀，加紅B鹽試剂1毫升，搖匀后10分鐘比色，所求得三者的透光度按下列公式計算：

$$\log \frac{T_0}{T_1} - \log \frac{T_0}{T_2} = \log \frac{T_2}{T_1} = 血清鹼性磷酸酶濃度的光密度。$$

$T_0 =$ 标准空白的透光度，$T_1 =$ 样品的透光度，

$T_2 =$ 样品空白的透光度。

根据此光密度由标准曲綫求出每毫升血清中鹼性磷酸酶的濃度，即單位。

- (2) 微量血清法　此法的操作与大量血清法相同，不过以1毫升生理鹽水代替1毫升稀釋血清，幷以特制微量吸管（見下面）將0.01毫升血清直接加入基質中。此法可节省血清的用量。在实际操作中，样品空白管加入2毫升緩冲基質及1毫升生理鹽水后即加入2毫升甲醛溶液在室温下放置；而样品管于加入緩冲基質及生理鹽水后则置于37℃水浴中保温15分鐘，然后用0.01毫升微量吸管加入血清样品，搖匀，記录时間以便恰好保温30分鐘后即加入2毫升甲醛溶液以停止酶的活动。血清样品加入样品管后，随即用同一微量吸管加血清样品于样品空白管中以免用两个微量吸管采取同一血清样品。样品管加入甲醛停止酶活动后，对样品管和样品空白管各加入4毫升飽和硼酸鹽酒精溶液及1毫升紅B鹽試剂，立即搖匀，也利用标准空白管，在光譜光度計上比色，計算如前。

(四) 对原作者微量法的研究、改进和补充

在上面测定方法中曾提到改用光譜光度計和加用标准空白以增加比色的准确度。此外，对原作者的方法进行了以下的研究、改进和补充。

1. 紅B鹽試剂呈色反应与时间的关系。标准空白管中加入各試剂后，在光譜光度計上每隔10—15分鐘讀其透光度，在2小时內讀数的改变不超过0.6格，此种改变甚小可以不計。样品空白管和样品管加入各試剂后，透光度在5—10分鐘內稍有变动，10分鐘后趋于稳定，直至22分鐘仍保持稳定，故决定在加入紅B鹽試剂10分鐘后比色。

2. 甲醛对酶的抑制作用的情况。按原作者的操作方法，样品空白管中加入血清需在样品管中加入血清之后半小时，同一血清需用两个微量吸管，手續复杂。为了节省微量吸管的使用，我們改变为在加血清于样品管后，随即用同一吸管加血清于样品空白管中，在室温中停留半小时，待样品管在水浴中保温完畢后，一同加入試剂比色。用这种

操作程序和原作者的操作方法測定同一血清，所得結果完全一致。这表明兩種操作方法對甲醛抑制酶的能力沒有影响，樣品空白管沒有在水浴中保温或待樣品管作用完畢再加血清的必要，当樣品管保温15分鐘后需加血清时，也即时把血清加入樣品空白管中，如此可簡化手續，节省微量吸管的使用。

　　3. 紅B鹽儲存時間对于显色的影响。原作者認为紅B鹽試剂配制后可应用二星期，但在放置于冰箱內二星期过程中，其顏色由淡黄逐漸加深呈橙黄色。因此試剂可能在空气中氧化，所以用新鮮配制的和放置一定時間的試剂測定同一标本的鹼性磷酸酶以了解儲藏時間的影响。表1的結果說明紅B鹽試剂放置一星期左右后，顏色雖加深，

表1　紅B鹽試剂儲存时间对血清鹼性磷酸酶（單位数）測定的影响

血　清　樣　品	新　配　的　試　剂	儲　存　的　試　剂	儲　存　期　限
A	3.7	3?	一星期左右
B	2.3	2.4	一星期左右
C	1.?	1?	一星期左右
D	3.4	3.3	一星期左右
E	5.?	4.1	一星期左右
F	2.6	2.5	一星期左右
G	1.5	0.6	超过二星期
H	4.8	1.4	超过二星期

但有标准空白和樣品空白的校正，故一般不致产生很大的誤差，但有时也有相当的誤差，如樣品C和E。放置超过二星期者影响很大，不能使用。后来測定时为了避免紅B鹽試剂改变的影响，一般皆新鮮配制，应用时限最多不超过一星期。

　　4. 溶血对鹼性磷酸酶值的影响。血液标本需放置一段时間才能分出血清，还需要用玻璃棒刮離血塊使其易出血清，故有时产生溶血現象，可能影响結果。所以將血清与小量紅血球混合加入基質中使其破裂，产生溶血，与未溶血的血清測定鹼性磷酸酶作比較。結果見表2。

　　由以上的結果可見溶血对血清鹼性磷酸酶的測定有一定的影响，但影响不大，而且溶血的血清的数值多較不溶血者为小，故輕度溶血不足妨碍測定。但鹼性磷酸酶既是用血清測定，仍应避免溶血。

　　5. 用微量吸管代替原作者所用的0.1毫升十等分的精細吸管吸取0.01毫升血清作測定。所使用的0.1毫升十等分的精細吸管，由于管尖粗厚，容易粘附血清，不能准确量出0.01毫升，遂依照Bessey的方法[7]，制备0.01毫升微量吸管。法以一段10厘米長、4毫米直徑的玻璃管在火焰上把中間部分拉長成毛細管，最細部分的內徑约为0.2

284 营 养 学 报 1卷

表2 溶血对血清碱性磷酸酶测定結果(單位数)的影响

血 清 样 品	溶 血	不 溶 血
a	2.3	2.2
b	3.7	3.6
c	1.1	1.4
d	3.4	4.7
e	13.9	14.6
f	1.5	1.2
g	2.6	2.5
h	1.0	2.0
i	1.7	1.8
j	2.2	2.4
k	1.3	1.7

—0.3毫米。在此处切断成为兩个微量吸管。在尖端2—3毫米处弯成140—150°角度,在粗端套以橡皮管(如血球計数吸管所用者)以便使用 。刻度和校准的方法是把十等分的0.1精細吸管吸入蒸餾水后,平放于桌上,將微量吸管的尖端接触于精細吸管的开口,准确吸入0.01毫升的水,試驗几次后,划上刻度,然后在微量天秤上秤吸入的0.01毫升水的重量,由水在当时温度的比重,計算吸入的水的体积。用这个方法校准四个微量吸管所得的体积与0.01毫升分别相差为0.28, 0.89, 0.57和 —1.6%。微量吸管一般可允許1—2%的誤差,故此四支均可应用。这也証明所用的十等分0.1毫升吸管的刻度尙屬准确,以后校准微量吸管的时候可以不必在微量天秤上秤出水的重量。

6. 毛細血管取血法及微量血清分离法。由于微量吸管的应用,可以避免静脉抽血而采用皮膚毛細血管取血,所以有必要建立由毛細血管取血和由小量血液分离血清的方法。法以事先洗净而干燥的毛細玻璃管(內徑约1毫米,长約10厘米)的一端与血滴接触,血液即可进入管中。用火漆把毛細玻管的另一端封口,切勿使火漆与血液接近以免燒坏血液。在离心机中旋轉使血清与血球分离。用小鋸把血球与血清交界处鋸断,插入微量吸管即可定量取出0.01毫升血清样品。

此法的优点在于适用于嬰兒和小动物。嬰兒可由脚跟部的毛細血管取血。小动物如大鼠可將其尾巴用温水加温(較大者,可不必加温)。切去其尖端1—2毫米,按讓鼠头向上尾向下,用手指輕輕地沿着尾巴向下赶,使血流出,与毛細玻管接触,即可得到所需的血量。所需的血量最多为0.1毫升血液可分离出0.03—0.04毫升血清,足供样品空白和兩个样品测定之用。

7. 大量血清法与微量血清法的比較。用上述大量血清法(將0.5毫升血稀釋至50

毫升,取用1毫升稀释的血清)和微量血清法(以微量吸管直接取用0.01毫升血清)同时进行同一血清的碱性磷酸酶的测定以作比较。

表8 大量血清稀释后和直接用微量吸管取0.01毫升血清所得碱性
磷酸酶的结果(单位/毫升)的比较

血 清	大量血清稀释100倍取1毫升		用微量吸管直接取0.01毫升血清	
	测 定 值	平 均	测 定 值	平 均
甲	2.8, 2.8	2.8	2.3, 2.4, 2.4	2.4
乙	2.2, 2.0	2.1	2.8, 2.9	2.9
丙	1.1, 1.2	1.2	1.3, 1.4, 1.4	1.4
丁	1.3, 1.4	1.4	1.5, 1.4, 1.4	1.4
戊	0.6, 0.6	0.6	0.7, 0.7, 0.7	0.7

由表8的五个样品的结果可见两个方法的重复性都很满意,二者的平均值也很接近。因此,以后一般的测定均采用微量血清法。

結果与討論

(一) 人血清碱性磷酸酶的正常值

为了用微量法得出正常人血清碱性磷酸酶的数值,我们检查了55名在本院工作的人员。这些人的健康是无问题的,年龄由20岁到50岁,绝大多数在25—35岁范围之内。其中有39名男性,16名女性。如表4所示,男性血清碱性磷酸酶的范围为0.4—3.0单位,平均数为1.78单位,其标准差(S.D.或σ)为±0.66单位,平均数的标准误为±0.11单位。女性血清碱性磷酸酶的范围是0.7—3.0单位,平均数是1.36单位,其标准差是±0.49单位,平均数的标准误是±0.12单位。男女性别的平均数的差别,即1.78—1.36=0.42,是否显著可由平均数差别的标准误来决定。

$$平均数差别的标准误=\sqrt{男性平均数标准误^2+女性平均数标准误^2}$$
$$=\sqrt{0.11^2+0.12^2}=±0.16$$

平均数的差别为平均数差别的标准误的0.42/0.16=2.6倍。按统计学的规定,两个平均数相差凡大于差别的标准误2.5倍者,则认为显著,故两性血清碱性磷酸酶平均数的差别应当是有一定意义的。不过女性样本很少,远少于男性样本,可能发生偏差,应待以后较多女性的测定来证实血清磷酸酶在性别上的差别。因此,两性的数值目前暂可以混合计算,所得的混合平均数为1.68单位,其标准差为±0.63单位,平均数的标准误为±0.09单位。

(二) Bodansky 法与微量法的比值

表4　用微量法测得的正常人血清硷性磷酸酶值

（单位/毫升血清）

号　数	酶　值	号　数	酶　值	号　数	酶　值
男性		男性		女性	
1	2.2	24	0.8	40	0.9
2	2.5	25	1.0	41	1.5
3	2.0	26	1.6	42	1.7
4	2.0	27	2.2	43	1.0
5	1.8	28	2.4	44	1.3
6	2.3	29	2.3	45	0.9
7	1.1	30	2.3	46	1.1
8	2.6	31	2.5	47	1.1
9	1.4	32	2.5	48	0.9
10	0.6	33	2.1	49	1.8
11	1.1	34	2.4	50	3.0
12	1.4	35	2.9	51	1.8
13	1.4	36	1.8	52	1.4
14	0.4	37	1.9	53	1.3
15	3.0	38	0.9	54	1.4
16	1.9	39	1.4	55	0.7
17	1.9				
18	1.1	均　　数	1.78	均　　数	1.35
19	0.9	标　准　差	±0.66	标　准　差	±0.45
20	2.3	均数标准误	±0.11	均数标准误	±0.12
21	1.4				
22	1.9		男女总均数＝　1.68 单位		
23	1.7		标　准　差＝±0.63 单位		
			平均数标准误＝±0.09 单位		

　　临床通用以测定血清硷性磷酸酶的方法之一是 Bodansky 法。此法以磷酸甘油为磷酸酶的作用基质，经1毫升血清所含的酶的水解作用1小时所释出的无机磷毫克数为单位数，以100毫升血清计算。此法虽需要较大量的血清，但沿用较久，临床上对于此法的正常和不正常的数值均较熟悉，故引用新方法时，似应与此法比较，求得二法的比值，可能以新方法的数值来推算 Bodansky 法的数值。为此，我们检查了38名职业供血者，6名实验室工作人员和2名非骨质病或黄胆病患者，共46名。年龄由20至50岁，其中12名为女性，其余为男性。每人由静脉取血，分离血清，同时按 Bodansky 法和微量法作硷性磷酸酶的测定。结果列于表5。在这一系列的受检者中，血清硷性磷酸酶的范围按 Bodansky 法为1.7—8.8单位/100毫升血清，而按微量法为0.7—4.8单位/毫升血清。两法的比值的范围为1.3—3.5，平均数为2.1，其标准差为±0.55，平均数的标准误为±0.08。因此，微量法所得的单位数字比 Bodansky 法为小，平均约为一半。

表5　Bodansky 法与微量法測定血清鹼性磷酸酶的數值和比值

号　數	Bodansky法 單位/100毫升	微量法 單位/毫升	Bodansky法 微量法	号　數	Bodansky法 單位/100毫升	微量法 單位/毫升	Bodansky法 微量法
1	4.4	2.5	1.8	27	2.7	0.9	3.0
2	8.8	4.5	2.0	28	1.7	0.7	2.4
3	5.6	3.2	1.8	29	3.6	2.2	1.6
4	5.1	3.2	1.6	30	3.1	1.7	1.8
5	2.9	1.4	2.1	31	5.5	1.9	2.8
6	2.5	1.6	1.6	32	3.8	2.5	1.5
7	3.6	1.8	2.0	33	6.8	3.2	2.1
8	5.7	3.0	1.9	34	7.6	4.1	1.9
9	5.2	3.1	1.7	35	2.6	2.0	1.3
10	4.1	2.5	1.6	36	3.8	2.6	1.7
11	3.6	1.1	3.2	37	6.2	3.9	1.6
12	6.4	3.5	1.8	38	5.8	3.9	1.5
13	6.6	3.6	1.8	39	5.2	2.9	1.8
14	4.7	1.9	2.4	40	3.9	1.4	2.8
15	2.5	0.8	3.0	41	2.7	1.4	1.9
16	3.0	1.4	2.1	42	2.4	0.7	3.3
17	6.0	3.1	1.9	43	4.0	1.8	2.2
18	5.8	3.2	1.8	44	6.0	1.8	3.3
19	8.0	4.5	1.8	45	3.7	1.9	2.0
20	5.4	2.9	1.8	46	4.2	2.1	2.0
21	3.7	2.3	1.6				
22	7.0	4.8	1.5		卜氏法/微量法的比值:		
23	3.2	2.3	1.4		平均數 　= 2.1		
24	3.5	1.0	3.5		標准差 　= ±0.55		
25	6.2	4.2	1.5		平均數標准誤 = ±0.08		
26	3.0	1.4	2.1				

〈三〉　大鼠血清鹼性磷酸酶

我們曾用微量法測定 7 只体重約 160 克的正常大白鼠的血清鹼性磷酸酶, 其范圍為9.3 至 24.1 單位, 平均數为 15.2 單位, 标准差为±4.5 單位, 平均數的标准誤为±1.7 單位。

我們也初步檢查过兩只体重約 60 克的大鼠用正常飼料、致佝僂病膳食和維生素 D₂ 治疗以后的血清鹼性磷酸酶的变化。如表 6 所示, 兩只大鼠用致佝僂病膳食 10 天后, 血清鹼性磷酸酶顯著增加, 但持續喂这样的膳食十几天以后, 磷酸酶值不但不继續升高, 反而下降, 隨后給以治疗剂量的維生素 D₂ 10 天之后, 磷酸酶值也不下降。此系探討式的試驗, 可能有一些因素未能控制, 故引用大鼠血清鹼性磷酸酶值作为維生素 D 生物鑒定的指标是否可行, 尚待进一步的研究。

表 6　致佝偻病膳食和維生素 D_2 对大鼠血清鹼性磷酸酶的影响

日　期	鼠 188	鼠 189	附　　　　注
II，23	10.8	15.3	正常撮食
III，5	60.5	53.5	致佝偻病膳食 10 天
III，14	40.8	30.0	致佝偻病膳食 19 天
III，15	28.1	22.8	致佝偻病膳食 20 天
III，16	27.6	28.4	致佝偻病膳食 21 天
III，28	29.5	24.7	維生素 D_2 治疗 10 天

总　结

利用一苯磷酸二鈉为作用基質，用紅 B 鹽試剂以測定所釋出的酚的量，Keplan 和 Narahara 設計了一种敏感的微量血清鹼性磷酸酶測定方法。我們对这个方法进行了研究，加以改进，認为是一个簡便而准确的方法。本法的优点在于只需要 0.01 毫升的血清样品和半小时的作用时間，而且整个操作可在一只試管中完成。为了使这个方法适用于婴兒和小实驗动物的检查，我們运用了毛細玻璃管从皮下毛細血管采血和分离小量血清的方法，而且自制了微量吸管以便定量加入 0.01 毫升血清。按照这个方法的測定結果，55 名正常成年男女的血清鹼性磷酸酶的范圍为 0.4—3.0 單位/毫升，平均数为 1.68 單位，其标准差为 ±0.63 單位，平均数的标准誤为 ±0.09 單位。用 Bodansky 法和本法同时測定 46 人的血清鹼性磷酸酶，Bodansky 法对本法所得的單位数值的比例平均約为 2。正常大鼠 7 只的血清鹼性磷酸酶平均为 15.3 單位。初步試驗两只大鼠給以致佝偻病膳食，繼之以維生素 L 治疗以观察血清鹼性磷酸酶的变化，結果未能令人滿意，须待进一步的研討。

参 考 文 献

[1]　Roche, J. in: Sumner and Myrback: The Enzymes, New York, Academic Press, 1950, Vol. I, Part I, pp. 473-510.

[2]　Bodansky, O.: Biochemistry of Disease, New York, The MacMillan Company, 1952, p. 756-804.

[3]　Hoffman, W. S.: The Biochemistry of Clinical Medicine, Chicago, The Year Book Publishers, 1954, pp. 324-325.

[4]　Motzok, I.: Studies on the plasma phosphatase of normal and rachitic chicks. 3. The assay of antirachitic preparations by a method based on the determination of plasma phosphatase activity. *Biochem. J.* 1950, 47: 196.

[5]　Bodansky, A.: Determination of serum inorganic phosphate and of serum phosphatase. *Am. J. Clin. Path. Tech. Suppl.* 1937, 1: 51.

[6] Kaplan, A. and Narahara, A.: The determination of serum alkaline phosphatase activity. *J. Lab. and Clin. Med.* 1953, **41**: 819.

[7] Bessey, O. A.: Microchemical Methods in: Gyorgy, P.: Vitamin Methods, New York, Academic Press, 1950, Vol. I. pp. 293-295.

A STUDY OF THE MICRO METHOD FOR THE DETERMINATION OF SERUM ALKALINE PHOSPHATASE

Wu Teh-chang, Wei Wen-ling and Liu Shih-hao

Department of Biochemistry, Chinese Union Medical College, Peking

Utilizing disodium phenylphosphate as substrate and determining the amount of phenol set free by its reaction with red B salt, Keplan and Narahara devised a sensitive micro method for the determination of serum alkaline phosphatase. We have studied the method and found it, with a few modifications, convenient and accurate. The chief advantages of this method lie in the fact that it requires serum samples of only 0.01 ml. and a reaction time of only 30 minutes, and that the whole procedure can be completed in one test tube. In order to make the method applicable to the examination of infants and small laboratory animals, we have introduced a glass capillary method for collecting cutaneous blood and separating small amounts of serum, and a micro pipet to deliver 0.01 ml. accurately. With this method, the serum alkaline phosphatase of 55 normal adult Chinese of both sexes ranged from 0.4 to 3.0 units per cc. and averaged 1.68 units with a standard deviation of ± 0.63 units and standard error of the mean of ± 0.09 units. Parallel determinations with Bodansky's method and this method were done on a series of 46 individuals, the ratio of the unitage of serum alkaline phosphatase by Bodansky's method to that by present method was found to be on the average, approximately 2. The serum alkaline phosphatase of a small series of normal rats was found to average 15.2 units per cc. A preliminary trial with rats to ascertain the effect on serum alkaline phosphatase of rachitogenic diet and vitamin D failed to give consistent results. This aspect of the work requires further studies.

《生物化学与临床医学的联系》序言

本書是根据历年給生物化学进修学生和临床医师講授"生物化学与临床医学的联系"的講稿修改补充而成的。

生物化学在医学院校是基础学科之一，旨在給予医学生及医师們一部分理論基础，作为更好地了解發病机制、診断及治疗疾病的依据。同时，临床上所發现的問題也时常需要帶到生化实驗室进行研究和解决，这样也就丰富了生物化学的理論和内容。因此，生物化学与临床医学的發展和成长有相互依賴的关系，故二者有密切联系的必要。为了这个目的，著者自1952年會于四班生化进修生的学習中选擇了一部分个人比較熟悉的而又与生化有关的临床問題，如糖尿病、肝功能、腎炎、矿物質代谢、内分泌病等进行编写，作为生物化学与临床医学的联系的内容。据一般的反映，認为这样可以使生物化学工作者进一步了解临床上的問題，和临床工作者进一步利用生物化学上的知識。

但是，生物化学是一門新兴的科学，發展极为迅速，领域日益广闊；现代临床医学發展虽較慢，但历史較长，从事研究者較多，故领域更屬辽闊；如欲作二者全面的、深入的而又系统的联系，是极为繁重艰巨的工作，必需發动多数人和多方面的力量才能完成。故本书的编写只能代表个人在联系生物化学和临床医学的初步嘗試，具有局限性和片断性，缺乏系统性和全面性。如果能引起生化工作者深入临床，临床工作者深入生化，使二者更密切地结合起来向医学进軍，则本书抛磚引玉的目的卽已达到。

同时，就本书现有的内容而言，由于个人水平和时间的限制，缺点和错誤必然很多，欢迎讀者予以批評和指正。

　　在修訂过程中，承我院譚壯教育長的鼓励和我系全体同志的帮助，尤其是池芝盛教授的修改，曹苹子同志的校閱，張学全同志的繪圖和吴春华同志的抄写，謹此志谢。

刘士豪

中国协和医学院生物化学系

1957 年 4 月

內 分 泌 研 究 发 展 的 方 向

刘 士 豪

（北京协和医院）

　　本文就內分泌的調节与控制，激素的生物合成，激素的轉运机制，激素的化学結構与功能的关系，內分泌的免疫学、激素的作用机制等六个在內分泌学中的重要問題，評述目前的認識和今后研究的方向。內分泌的調节分为代謝物对內分泌的反饋調节、激素对內分泌的調节及反饋控制和神經的調节等三重机制，以保证內分泌腺的分泌活动受到精确的切合实际的控制。甲状腺激素和类固醇激素生物合成的途径和有关的酶系已知端倪，但蛋白质激素的生物合成尚属无知，因为一般蛋白质的結構至为复杂，其在体內合成的机制尚未闡明，它的闡明将有助于蛋白质激素生物合成問題的解决。激素在血液循环中的轉运，以甲状腺激素为例，依靠血浆中的特殊的具有携帶能力的蛋白质，如甲状腺素結合球蛋白（TBG）、清前蛋白（TBPA）等。腎上腺皮质激素的轉运也有蛋白质載体。这些載体的重要性在于調节激素进入細胞的速度，从而控制其作用和代謝的速度。激素化学結構的闡明在于改造其結構以突出某种为治疗所需的作用而降低其它不必要的作用，例如类固醇激素的人工改造制成的类似物中有作用强而副作用少的抗炎皮质激素，促进蛋白质合成的类固醇以及口服避孕药等。蛋白质激素，如促腎上腺皮质激素的結構弄清以后，即有合成較簡单而有效的激素的嘗試。免疫学在內分泌学的发展沿着两个方向，其一是內分泌腺的自身免疫作为某些內分泌病的发病机制，其二是寻找免疫学方法以测定体液中微量的蛋白质激素以助診断和研究。最后，激素的作用机制这个中心問題的了解目前尚属片断，有的激素可能影响細胞外膜或內膜，使代謝物的进入加速、或者改变酶的活性，作为輔酶或誘导酶的生成。总之，以上問題近年来研究較广泛、較深入，但也提出許多問題，值得继續研究，是今后发展的方向。

一、內分泌的調节与控制

　　內分泌系統的主要功能是調节体內代謝过程，它与神經系統配合，时常是在神經系統的主导下，成为高度整合而又密切相互关联的神經体液調节系統，控制机体的全部活动和行为以达到整体統一和机体与环境的互相平衡。內分泌腺旣是这个調节的重要組成部分，則有必要弄清它們的分泌活动是如何受到調节和控制的。近二十余年来生理和生化学家在这方面做了許多工作，把內分泌的調节和控制的知識推进一大步，但因还存在不少問題，也是內分泌今后发展的一个重要方向。临床工作者也試图利用这方面的知識和技术以加强对疾病的認識、診断和治疗。內分泌的調节和控制机制，归納起来，可分为代謝物对內分泌的反饋調节，激素对內分泌的調节及反饋控制和神經的調节

　　內分泌学是一比較新兴的学科，近年来发展极为迅速。在生物学和医学的广闊領域中，从組織胚胎，生理，生化，药理，病理直到临床各科都涉及到內分泌問題，都需要进行对內分泌的研究，并累积了丰富的經驗和知識。把散在各科門的有关內分泌的經驗和知識集中化和系統化以便为生产服务，为人民健康服务是內分泌学的任务，是近年来成立和发展內分泌专业学科的动力。因此，这門学科的內容是高度綜合性的，旣有基础理論部分，也有实际应用部分，旣有实驗內分泌学，也有临床內分泌学。因为工作性质和特点有所不同，实驗与临床分工是必要的，但为了更好地完成研究任务解决問題，二者相互沟通、配合、協調更屬重要。內分泌学的发展是多方面的，現謹择其几个重要者，略指出其目前水平和动向，供同志們参考。

三种。

(一) 代謝对内分泌的反饋的調节作用

最明显的例子是胰岛素产生低血糖，血糖这个代謝产物浓度的降低对胰岛的分泌有抑制作用；相反，血糖浓度的升高则促进胰岛素的分泌；因此，胰岛素影响物質代謝所产生的血糖浓度的差异成为調节和控制胰岛素分泌的重要因素，虽然血糖对胰岛 β 細胞的詳細作用机制尚不明了。同时，胰岛 α 細胞产生致糖素 (glucagon)，有升高血糖的作用，血糖浓度的升高却有抑制 α 細胞的分泌作用，而低血糖相反则有促进致糖素分泌的作用，保証飢餓时血糖不致过低。这說明从胰岛就有两种作用相反的激素来維持血糖的稳定性，它們的分泌也都受血糖浓度的調节，只是两种細胞的反应则完全相反。

甲状旁腺的分泌也是受代謝产物控制的。低血清鈣增强甲状旁腺的分泌，高血清鈣使之减弱。最近，Copp 等发現甲状旁腺分泌另一种控制血清鈣的因素，称为鈣控制素 (calcitonin)，其作用与甲状旁腺素相反，是降低血清鈣，对高血鈣有增强其分泌的反应以防止高血鈣症的发生。因此，鈣控制素与甲状腺素的分泌，分别于血清鈣的起伏而增加，从而双重地、相互地保証血清鈣水平的稳定性，故在一般情况下鈣进量和吸收虽有波动，但血清鈣仍能保持相当恒定。

垂体后叶抗利尿激素的释放，因細胞外液渗透压的波动而有所增减，腎上腺皮质醛固酮的分泌因体液鈉或/和鉀含量的改变而有所消长[2]也都是代謝物調节内分泌活动的范例。当鈉入量增加时，細胞外液渗透当量升高，高渗当量导致抗利尿激素的释出，后者加强远端腎小管对水的回吸收以降低細胞外液渗透压，这样細胞外液渗透压得以保持正常，但势必引起容量扩大。不过，細胞外液容量的扩大或其鈉含量的增加抑制了醛固酮的分泌。从而腎小管 $K^+ \leftrightarrow Na^+$ 和 $H^+ \leftrightarrow Na^+$ 两种离子交换机制的活动减弱，以致鈉的排出增加，并伴有水的排出，这样扩大了的細胞外液容量得以恢复原状。因此，抗利尿激素改变水的排量以影响体液的渗透压，而醛固酮则改变鈉的排量以影响体液的容量；二者的互相配合旣維持了体液的渗透压，也保存了体液的容量。

(二) 激素对内分泌的調节及反饋控制

激素具有調节内分泌腺活动的作用的认識是从垂体功能的发現开始的。垂体前叶所分泌的多种激素中，除了生长激素具有普遍作用以外，其余均有各自的靶腺作为調节其分泌的对象。即促腎上腺皮质激素 (ACTH) 調节腎上腺皮质，促甲状腺激素 (TSH) 調节

甲状腺，促性腺激素調节性腺的分泌活动。这些激素有其靶腺以外的作用，但維持靶腺的形态与功能以及促进其内分泌的形成和释出是主要的，使垂体成为内分泌腺中的主导腺体。这种认識的发展使垂体前叶分泌活动的調节問题提到議事日程。前叶的分泌活动，除了接受中枢神經系統的調节，这个問題将要在下面談到以外，也被相应的靶腺所分泌的激素，如皮质激素，甲状腺素，性腺激素等所制約。这些激素反过来对垂体分泌活动的制約称为反饋控制，是内分泌学中目前研究得最热烈的方面之一，也是今后若干年的一个重要研究方向。

从許多作者的实驗資料看来，腎上腺皮质激素对垂体 ACTH 分泌的反饋控制的机制尚未获得一致的結論，因为有的实驗结果支持下丘脑是皮质醇的反饋作用点，有的主张垂体，也有的指出腎上腺皮质。但权衡各方面的实驗结果，似乎支持下丘脑的論据較多，垂体次之，腎上腺較少[8]。甲状腺素对 TSH 的分泌有反饋控制作用，已有大量实驗来說明。垂体和下丘脑对甲状腺素的抑制作用均很敏感，微量的、皮下注射无效的甲状腺素剂量对垂体或下丘脑注射均可使甲状腺的分泌减少；垂体内注射的抑制作用出現很快，而下丘脑内注射的作用延緩 6—9 小时后才出現，虽然二者均可持續 20 小时[4]。因此，甲状腺素对 TSH 释出的反饋抑制的作用对象主要是垂体，但下丘脑的抑制也很重要，使垂体的抑制延續下去。除了腎上腺和甲状腺的分泌以外，性腺激素对垂体和下丘脑也表現反饋控制。故反饋控制是下丘脑-垂体-靶腺这类系統自动調节分泌的特点。

(三) 神經的調节作用

中枢神經系統对内分泌活动有調节作用是公认的事实。具体到不同的腺体，则神經系統的作用方式各异。归纳起来，神經調节的方式有两种。即直接的通过神經冲动和間接的通过激素传递。腎上腺髓质的腎上腺素和去甲基腎上腺素是直接由交感神經的冲动而释放的。胰岛的分泌，除了受血糖浓度的控制以外，还受中枢神經系統的直接影响；假飼、咀嚼动作和条件反射均可增强胰岛素的分泌，說明这种分泌活动必然来自中枢神經系統的神經冲动，可能是通过迷走神經的传递而到达胰岛的[6-7]。垂体后叶释放抗利尿激素和催产素，也是与直接的神經冲动有关。

垂体前叶的分泌活动与中枢神經系統，尤其是下丘脑的神經活动有密切联系。但由于垂体前叶具有解剖上的特点，即前叶沒有明显的神經纤維，而从下丘脑的中隆到前叶却有无数的毛細血管网形成的垂体門

脉系统，因此中枢神經系統对垂体前叶分泌机能的控制只有間接地通过液递的化学物質，或称神經介质，或称神經分泌[7]。下丘脑可以认为是中枢神經系統与垂体之間的总联絡站。利用局部切除或損伤或电刺激等实驗技术，已能将下丘脑与垂体的不同促激素有关的部位加以大致定位。例如控制 ACTH 释放的区域位于下丘脑中隆的中部，"促甲状腺区"位于中隆的前部，而控制黃体形成激素释放的地点是在灰白結节。这些区域的神經細胞影响垂体机能的方式是通过分泌各自的神經分泌对而对垂体相应的激素起到释放作用。促肾上腺皮质激素释放因子(CRF)、促甲状腺激素释放因子(TRF)和黃体形成激素释放因子(LRF)均可从下丘脑提取[8]。上述各种释放因子是特异地针对着垂体所分泌的相应的激素而发挥作用的，动物切除垂体后无效。CRF 可以从血中检出[9]，TRF 可由尿中排出[10]。虽然这些因子的化学性質属于多肽，与后叶激素有相似之处，但其化学結构尚不清楚。估計今后在这方面将会开展許多研究工作。不过，根据现有的资料，足以说明中枢神經系統，通过下丘脑各部所分泌的神經分泌能够液递到垂体前叶，使其分别释出不同的促激素，后者作用于各自的靶腺，以实现神經系統对内分泌系統的控制。

虽然CRF不是垂体后叶激素，但抗利尿素(ADH)的分泌在某些应激时却增加，一定量的 ADH 有发动前叶分泌 ACTH 的作用，从而增加肾上腺皮质激素的分泌，临床上应用ADH的注射观察血中和尿中 17 羟皮质类固醇含量是否增加，作为鑑別肾上腺皮质功能失調是来自垂体或下丘脑的依据。如果注射后增加则垂体功能尚属正常，而下丘脑可能是病理的来源；如果注射后不增加，则垂体显然有病。垂体功能情况也可用地噻咪松抑制試驗加以鑑定。肾上腺皮质本身的功能状态可用 ACTH 刺激試驗和2-甲基-1，2 双吡啶丙醇 (Metopyropone, SU 4885)試驗以查了解。

二、激素的生物合成

有关激素在腺体内合成的途径和有关的酶系以及能量代謝的知識尚不完备，对不同类型激素在这方面的知識頗不平衡。甲状腺素在甲状腺上皮細胞内合成的步驟以及某些酶系缺乏所造成的甲状腺肿和机能减退症前几年已有大致的了解[11]。类固醇激素在肾上腺皮质和性腺的生物合成近年来略知端倪。而蛋白質或多肽激素在垂

体，胰島，甲状旁腺的形成方式几无所知。兹将类固醇激素的生物合成，以肾上腺皮质为代表，简单介紹如下[12]：

大多数学者认为肾上腺皮质合成类固醇激素的原始材料是胆固醇，C^{14} 标記的乙酸盐与肾上腺保温也可以产生带放射性的皮质激素，这并不意味着从乙酸可以直接合成皮质激素，因为肾上腺皮质有从乙酸合成胆固醇的能力。肾上腺組織所含的胆固醇。約占60%来自血液循环，其余是自己制造的，胆固醇合成方式概括如下图(图1)：

Acetate→Mevalonic acid→Squalene→Cholesterol
乙酸盐　3,5二羟-3甲基戊酸　　鯊烯　　胆固醇
$$\Downarrow$$
Cholesterylesters
胆固醇酯

图 1　从乙酸盐合成胆固醇和胆固醇酯

在肾上腺中，胆固醇与胆固醇酯同时存在，当人的肾上腺受 ACTH 刺激而形成皮质激素时，所消失的不是胆固醇，而是胆固醇酯。在肾上腺中与胆固醇結合成酯的脂肪酸和血液胆固醇酯有所不同，以油酸和落花生酸較多，而亚麻油酸少。人的肾上腺束状带"清亮"細胞含有大量的胆固醇酯，經 ACTH 刺激后，失去其脂質；而网状带"密致"細胞則含胆固醇酯很少。在体外保温时，清亮和密致細胞产生等量的皮质醇，只有加入 ACTH 后，清亮細胞才增加皮质醇产量。这意味着在日常生活中，两种細胞从血液中取得葡萄糖和胆固醇以合成小量皮质醇以供平时之需；而在应激时，清亮細胞从胆固醇酯合成大量皮质醇以应急需。

从胆固醇合成孕酮的途径可能如图2。这个途径

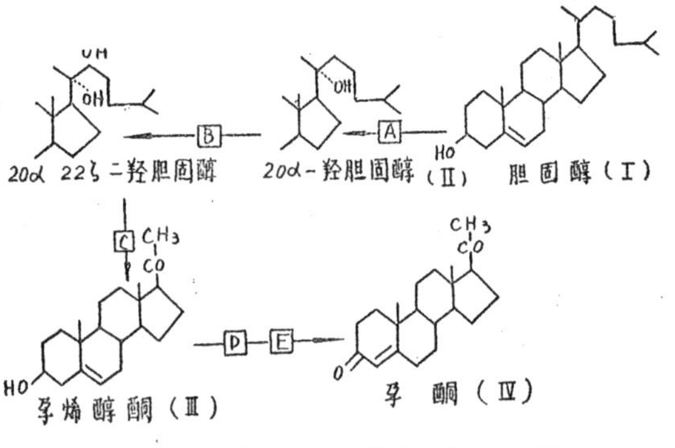

A：20 α-羟化酶；B：22-羟化酶；C：20.22 解重碳酶；D：3 β-羟类固醇脱氢酶；E：异构酶。

图 2　从胆固醇合成孕酮的途径的設想

在所有分泌类固醇激素的腺体普遍存在。所形成的孕酮是許多类固醇激素生物合成的起点。

　　孕酮在不同位置的羟化反应是合成皮质激素所必需。这些反应需要分子氧和还原型三磷酸吡啶核苷（TPNH）的存在才能进行。羟化酶在肾上腺皮质的分布大致如下：17β-羟化酶存在于束状带和网状带，18-羟化酶只存在于球状带，而11β-和21-羟化酶在各带均有。羟化反应有一定的次序，一般按17、21、11位这个顺序进行。11-脱氧皮质酮一旦形成，则不能在17位进行羟化，但可在11位羟化以产生皮质酮，进而合成醛固酮（图3）。从孕酮形成皮质醇，羟化反应的顺序可按17、21、11位，也可按11、17、21位这个次序进行（图3）。

　　肾上腺皮质合成雄激素的途径与睾丸間质细胞相仿，但睾丸酮的产量很少，去氢异雄酮是主要的雄激素，雄烯二酮次之，而且 $C_{19}O_3$ 化合物如11β-羟雄烯二酮是肾上腺产生的特异的雄激素（图4）。肾上腺皮质产生雌激素的途径与卵巢似，C-19 位必须先进行羟化才能轉变为雌酮（图4）。不过，在正常情况下，肾上腺雌激素产量极微。

　　了解腺上腺皮质激素生物合成的途径及其有关的酶系，不仅对肾上腺的正常生理有所闡明，而且对垂体肾上腺系统的一些疾病的发病机制和治疗也很有帮助。例如，先天性肾上腺增生症是由于皮质从17-羟孕酮合成皮质醇所需要的酶缺乏，故皮质醇较少，从而垂体 ACTH 的分泌增强，使皮质增生，产生大量的不正常的代謝产物所致[18]。最常見的缺陷是21-羟化反应发生障碍，这样就使17-羟孕酮的产量增加，17-羟孕酮的主要代謝产物是孕三醇（pregnanetriol）和17-羟孕醇酮（17-hydroxypregnanolone）故这两种化合物在尿中的排量

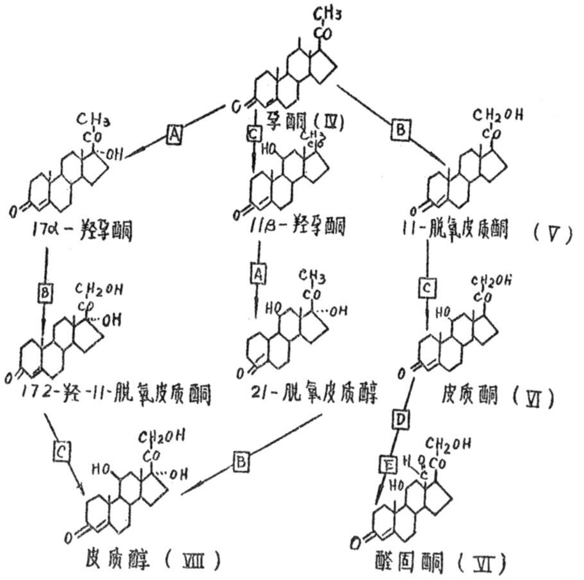

A：17α-羟化酶；B：21-羟化酶 C：11β-羟化酶；D：18-羟化酶；E：18-羟类固醇脱氢酶
　　[注]图中醛固酮（Ⅶ）应改为（Ⅶ）
图 3　C_{21} 皮质类固醇生物合成中孕酮的羟化

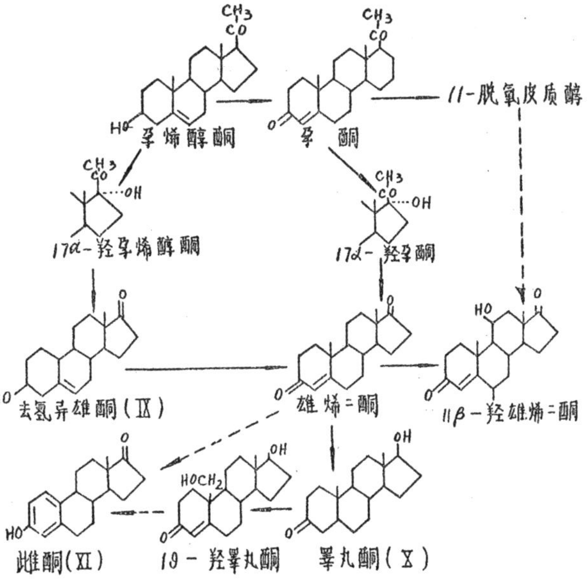

图 4　肾上腺雄激素和雌激素的生物合成途径

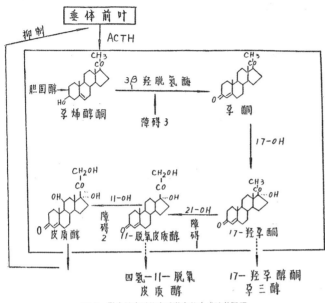

图 5　肾上腺皮质的皮质醇生物合成及其障碍

远比正常为多（图5）。同时，由于患者肾上腺11-羟化酶并不缺乏。故有一部分17-羟孕酮在11位上羟化，形成21-脱氧皮质醇，后者的代谢产物为11-酮孕三醇和11-羟孕三醇。这两种化合物在尿中出现对先天性肾上腺增生症也有诊断意义。本症的主要临床表现为性器官异常发育，在女性婴幼儿为假两性畸形，其外生殖器类似男性。在男性儿童此症表现为巨生殖器体和性早熟症。

第二种生物合成障碍在于缺乏11-羟化酶系。由于11-羟化酶缺乏，故11-脱氧皮质醇（11-deoxycortisol）的产量增加，11-脱氧皮质酮（DOC）的产量也增加（图5）。在尿中这两种类固醇激素的代谢产物，即四氢11-脱氧皮质醇、孕三醇、四氢11-脱氧皮质酮、孕二醇的排量增加，作为本症的诊断指标。这类病人除了外生殖器发育异常以外，常伴有高血压。高血压是由于11-脱氧皮质酮所致。

第三种生物合成的缺陷在于3β-羟类固醇脱氢酶系障碍。这类病人不能将Δ⁵类固醇转变为Δ⁴类固醇，故尿中出现Δ⁵孕烯三醇、Δ⁵孕烯二醇、去氢异雄酮等化合物（图5）。这些患儿，除了先天性肾上腺增生症的一般表现以外，还从尿中丢失大量的钠，呈低血钠症。其他类型先天性肾上腺增生症患者有时也表现失钠现象。失钠的原因尚在争论之中，但最近的

意见是17-羟孕酮大量的存在有排钠的作用，抵消了醛固酮的存钠效应；同时21-羟化酶的缺乏对醛固酮的合成也不利，在17-羟孕酮排钠的情况下不能相应地增加醛固酮的产量而进行代偿。

这几种类型的先天性肾上腺增生症患者对于皮质醇或皮质素疗法均有良好反应。

三、激素的转运机制

激素从腺体分泌出来进入血液之后，它在循环中转运或携带的方式与其代谢和作用有密切关系；转运方式失常可以产生病理状态；因而激素的转运机制在内分泌学中占有一个重要的领域。在这方面，甲状腺素（T₄）和三碘甲腺原氨酸（T₃）在血液循环中的转运形式研究得比较深入，取得不少成绩[14]。利用电泳法研究血浆蛋白质，发现有四种蛋白质，具有与甲状腺激素结合的能力。首先发现的是甲状腺素结合球蛋白（TBG），它泳动于α₁和α₂球蛋白之间，为量虽微，但与甲状腺素结合的能力甚强，也能与三碘甲腺原氨酸较松弛地结合，并不受常用作电泳的巴比妥缓冲液的影响（图6）。其次是甲状腺素结合清前蛋白（TBPA），在电泳中走在清（白）蛋白之前，在巴比妥缓冲液中只能与四碘甲腺乙酸（TA₄）和三碘甲腺乙

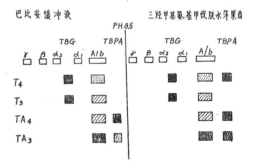

图 6　放射性甲状腺素（T₄）、三碘甲腺原氨酸（T₃）、四碘甲腺乙酸（TA₄）、三碘甲腺乙酸（TA₃）在人血清蛋白质低电泳上的分布。放射性分布：<15%，15—30%，>30%。

酸(TA_3)結合，但在其他緩冲液中也是特异地結合 T_4 的蛋白质。第三种是清蛋白，有小量的 T_4，較大量的 T_3 和 TA_4，以及大量的 TA_3 与之結合。最后还有蓝蛋白（含銅的 Ceruloplamin)，它也能和甲状腺素結合，但在激素的生理浓度下不易检出。因此，TBG 是 T_4 和 T_3 的主要載体，而 TBPA 是 T_4 的第二載体。

甲状腺激素与这些載体蛋白质相互作用，按质量作用定律形成自由激素与結合激素之間的平衡；平衡时，絕大部分是結合的，只有小量是自由的。只有自由型甲状腺激素才能进入細胞，这就使激素的轉运机制成为調节激素被利用、发生作用以及降解代謝的速度的重要因素。結合甲状腺激素的蛋白质在传染性肝炎或妊娠中毒症时增加，而某些血浆蛋白低減症或代謝障碍可使此种蛋白质減少，造成甲状腺素的作用不足而形成甲状腺功能低下。甲状腺激素結合型的存在使激素不易在肝脏破坏，不易經过腎小球濾过而被丢失。脂质性腎病或慢性腎炎腎病期在尿中漏出大量蛋白质，因而失去許多結合型甲状腺激素，这可能是这类病人基础代謝率低減的一个重要原因。

三碘甲腺原氨酸是甲状腺产生的第二种甲状腺激素，在血液中比甲状腺素要少得多，但其作用强度为 T_4 的 3—5 倍，且作用迅速，不象 T_4 有几天的潜伏期。据此，有些学者认为甲状腺素起作用的形式是三碘甲腺原氨酸，T_4 必須脱下一个碘原子成 T_3 才起作用。这个观点被以后的工作所否定。甲状腺素并不在組織內脫碘成 T_3。如将代謝率升高为纵座标，时間为横座标，繪制 T_4 和 T_3 作用的曲綫，則基綫到曲綫所占的面积二者相等，說明二者总的效能是一致的。二者的作用强度和速度的区别在于 T_4 与 TBG 結合較紧，且与 TBPA 結合，故自由型 T_4 进入組織較慢，作用高峰較低，但作用时間延长；而 T_3 与 TBG 結合較松，且不与 TBPA 結合，故进入組織較快，作用高峰較高，但时間較短。故 T_4 和 T_3 总的作用不相上下，T_3 并不比 T_4 更强。

类固醇激素如皮质醇的轉运机制亦有不少的研究[15]。用 C^{14} 标記的皮质醇加入血浆，进行平衡电泳，发現放射性高峰位于 α-球蛋白地带。加入的皮质醇約有90%与这个 α-球蛋白結合，故称之为皮质激素結合球蛋白（CBG）或称皮质激素載体（transcortin)。血浆清蛋白也与皮质醇結合，但亲和力很弱，只有小量皮质醇与之結合。皮质醇分别与这两种結合蛋白质同时进行两种反应，即結合与解离。平衡时，两种反应的速度相等，可計算平衡常数。正常血浆对皮质醇的結合力为 100 微克/100 毫升。孕妇或接受雌激素注射的正常人的血浆对皮质醇的結合力显著增强，这是由于皮质激素載体增加所致。故妊娠或注射雌激素使血浆皮质醇含量增加时，主要是結合型皮质醇增加，自由的皮质醇含量几无改变。新生儿血浆 CBG 的浓度很低。在妊娠期間，胎儿循环对皮质醇的結合力較低，而母体循环的結合力較高可以解释 C^{14} 标記的皮质醇注入羊水后迅速进入母亲的血液。这可能是某些原发性或继发性腎上腺皮质功能不全的患者在妊娠时病情緩解的一个原因。腎病綜合征和多发性骨髓瘤患者血浆 CBG 低減，說明这类患者血浆 17羥皮质类固醇水平下降不一定反映皮质功能不全。

四、激素的化学結构与功能的关系

动物的主要內分泌可以分为三大类，即胺类及氨基酸激素、类固醇激素和蛋白质激素。神經介质、腎上腺髓质分泌的腎上腺素及去甲基腎上腺素和甲状腺的激素等比較簡单的分子属于第一类。腎上腺皮质和性腺分泌类固醇激素；而垂体、甲状旁腺和胰島的內分泌均属于多肽或蛋白质激素。类固醇激素分子水平的研究是三十年前开始的，当时睾丸和卵巢分泌的类固醇性质业已确定，睾丸酮首先于 1935 年人工合成，随之雌激素也能人工合成，40 年代是人工合成腎上腺皮质激素的开始阶段。随着这些合成工作的完成，进行了大量的化学結构与生物活性的关系的研究。这些研究不仅奠定了內分泌的生理、生化、葯理、病理等理論基础。而且为临床提供了有利治疗工具。除了腎上腺皮质和性腺原有的激素可以大量供应以作研究和补偿治疗之外，尙有它們的衍生物多种以供治疗更广泛的非內分泌疾病或达到其它目的之用。归納起来，这些类固醇衍生物可分为三个类型。第一类是抗炎激素，如去氢皮质素、去氢皮质醇、地噻咪松等。第二类是合成代謝类固醇，如甲基睾丸酮、19-去甲基睾丸酮苯丙酸脂（Durabolin)等。第三类是口服避孕类固酮，如脑罗丁(Norethisterone)、美傑司脫罗（Magestrol)、克罗美地侬（Chlormadinone)等。这些化学結构与功能的研究成果对医学是一巨大的貢献，也是今后的一个发展方向。

由于蛋白质激素的复杂性，它們的化学結构的研究进展較类固醇激素为慢，到 50 年代才进入分子水平[16]。經过多年的工作，Sanger 等于 1949 和1953年分别肯定了胰島素 B 鏈 30 个氨基酸和 A 鏈 21 个氨基酸的排列顺序。继之，1953 年 du Vigneaud 等闡明了垂体后叶激素，即催产素和加压素的八肽結构，

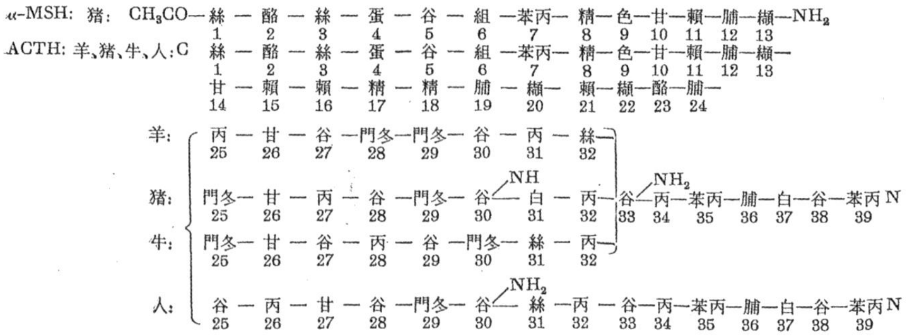

α-MSH: 猪：CH₃CO—絲—酪—絲—蛋—谷—組—苯丙—精—色—甘—賴—脯—纈—NH₂
　　　　　　　　　1　　2　　3　　4　　5　　6　　7　　8　9　10　11　12　13

ACTH: 羊、猪、牛、人：C　絲—酪—絲—蛋—谷—組—苯丙—精—色—甘—賴—脯—纈—
　　　　　　　　　　　　　1　　2　　3　　4　　5　　6　　7　　8　9　10　11　12　13
　　　　　　　　　　　　　甘—賴—賴—脯—精—纈—脯—纈—纈—酪—脯—
　　　　　　　　　　　　　14　15　16　17　18　19　20　21　22　23　24

羊：丙—甘—谷—門冬—門冬—谷—丙—絲—
　　　25　26　27　28　　29　　30　31　32

猪：門冬—甘—丙—谷—門冬—谷ᗜNH/白—丙—谷—丙—苯丙—脯—白—谷—苯丙 N
　　　25　　26　27　28　29　　30　31　32　33　34　35　36　37　38　39

牛：門冬—甘—谷—丙—谷—門冬—絲—丙—
　　　25　　26　27　28　29　30　　31　32

人：谷—丙—甘—谷—門冬—谷ᗜNH₂/絲—丙—谷—丙—苯丙—脯—白—谷—苯丙 N
　　　25　26　27　28　29　　30　31　32　33　34　35　36　37　38　39

图 7　ACTH 和 α MSH 氨基酸排列次序的比較

并加以人工合成。不同动物垂体 ACTH 的化学結构于 1953—1956 年相继由几组研究人員提出；人的 ACTH 結构是 1961 年李德勋[17]研究出来的（图7），这些 ACTH 都是由 39 个氨基酸組成，以絲氨酸为 N 末端氨基酸，以苯丙氨酸为 C 末端氨基酸。它們 N 末端第 1—24 位和 C 末端第 33—39 位氨基酸的排列次序完全一致。只是在第 25—32 位上略有不同（图7）。

同时，黑素細胞刺激素（α-MSH 和 β-MSH）的結构也逐渐阐明，α-MSH 是 13 肽，以后在实驗室能以合成。致糖素是由 29 个氨基酸組成，其排列順序是 1957 年由 Bromer 等确定的。垂体生长激素、促甲状腺激素、甲状旁腺素的制品均已达到均一的程度，其氨基酸成分和末端氨基酸种类有所了解；垂体的三种促性腺激素仍在純制的阶段；这些蛋白质激素的結构将有待今后进一步阐明。

关于 ACTH 結构与功能的关系的研究，用羧基肽酶及其他消化酶降解这个分子，使其 C 末端失去15 个氨基酸而保存共 N 末端的 24 个氨基酸，这个不完全的 ACTH 分子尚不失去活性。但是如果 N 末端的氨基酸稍有变动，则 ACTH 活性就会损失，說明这个分子的 ACTH 活性依靠 N 末端結构的完整性。根据这个观察，化学家們从 N 末端开始，合成了具有ACTH 活性的 17—23 个氨基酸的肽鏈[18]。

在 ACTH 的分离和純制的过程中，每一含有促腎上腺皮质作用的产品均有扩张黑素細胞的活性，使人搞不清楚是否 ACTH 制品混杂有 MSH，还是二者就是一个东西。一旦 ACTH 和 MSH 的結构証明 ACTH 的头 13 个氨基酸就是 α MSH 的全部組成成分，这种混乱就立刻澄清了。ACTH 的黑素細胞刺激作用是由于其分子結构具有 MSH 的氨基酸排列順序，虽然 ACTH 在这方面的活力只有 MSH 的百分之一。

上述黑素細胞刺激作用只是 ACTH的腎上腺皮质以外的作用之一，ACTH 还有許多其它全身性影响。在体内最明显的腎上腺外的影响是降低血糖（加强葡萄糖耐量）和动員脂肪，表现为血浆自由脂肪酸和酮体增加以及脂肪肝出现；在体外試驗，脂肪組織的脂肪酶对 ACTH 的激活而释出自由脂肪酸也最敏感。在不同的合成的类似 ACTH 的肽鏈中，能保持促腎上腺皮质、动員脂肪、降低血糖等作用全部活性的最短肽鏈是 20 个氨基酸残基，但短至 13 个氨基酸残基的肽鏈仍有部分活性。一但将 N 末端的絲氨酸的氨基酸氧化掉，这个分子就失去刺激腎上腺的作用，但尚能保持大部分动員脂肪和降低血糖的效能。如果将末端絲氨酸的氨基乙酰化，则促腎上腺和动員脂肪的活性明显降低，血糖升高代替了血糖降低，而且刺激黑素細胞活性加强。最后一点可以理解，因为 α MSH 的絲氨酸是乙酰化的（图7），但这样的分子改变又引入了增高血糖这一新的作用。这就提出了不正常肽分子产生病理状态的可能性。

从腺体可能分泌不正常的肽分子的观点出发，则某一腺体功能不全不一定都是分泌不足，有可能是分泌不正常肽分子，这种分子不发生作用。例如，单独一个垂体前叶激素缺乏綜合征是因为该种激素分泌的缺乏，还是所分泌的激素分子沒有活性呢？垂体嫌色細胞瘤在診断前若干年常有促性腺激素功能不全的表现，这种性功能不全是由于鞍内压增高所致，还是因为合成促性腺激素的缺陷，使下丘脑的神經分泌未受到抑制而分泌较多，以致刺激垂体嫌色細胞瘤的形成，正如先天性甲状腺合成的障碍可以引起甲状腺肿一样呢？

垂体功能亢进綜合征不一定代表正常分泌过多。例如，垂体来源的或因其它組織的肿瘤而产生的柯兴氏综合征常常伴有皮肤色素沉着，其强度远比因血中ACTH增加而增加的促黑细胞作用所带来的色素沉着为深。这里是否伴有 MSH 的分泌，还是所分泌的ACTH 不正常，具有较高的内在 MSH 活性，是值得探讨的一个问题。又如，一些促甲状腺激素(TSH)制品对豚鼠和鱼产生突眼。这种实验常出现球后组织和泪腺粘多糖代谢的改变。这些显然是甲状腺以外的影响，因为甲状腺切除的动物同样可以产生。有些作者能从 TSH 分离出一种产生突眼的物质，称为突眼素(EPS)，认为 TSH 和 EPS 是垂体分泌的两种激素。但是回忆 ACTH-MSH 争辩就可以想到在化学制备过程中，TSH 的两种活性之中的一种被取消的可能性。除此以外，也应考虑临床上的恶性突眼症可能有激素生物合成上的缺陷以致所产生的 TSH 偏重于突眼作用而缺少促甲状腺的作用。

五、内分泌的免疫学

(一) 蛋白质激素的免疫化学测定

不同种系的同一蛋白质激素的化学结构常有所差异，这种蛋白质注射给另一种动物即成为异种蛋白质，起抗原的作用，该动物对之产生抗体，可从其血清检出。这种含有抗体的血清加入抗原即可起抗体抗原反应，利用不同方法进行定量，借以获得微量激素的定量。这种方法比生物鉴定法的准确性高、敏感度强，是目前内分泌迅速发展的一个方向，具有广阔的前途。所需要的条件是高度纯制的蛋白质激素进行对动物免疫以获得高滴定度的抗体血清以及特异而敏感的抗原抗体反应系统，作为激素定量之用。

在胰岛素免疫测定法中，以 Berson 和 Yalow 的放射免疫电泳法比较成功，能测出的最低量是 10 微单位/毫升血浆[10]。血浆生长激素的免疫化学测定法多用致敏的羊红血球凝集抑制试验，其敏感度约为 10 微克/100 毫升血浆。其他垂体激素以及致糖素也有免疫测定法，但均不够稳定，须待改进。最近，Berson 和 Yalow[20] 提出的甲状旁腺素的放射免疫测定法似属敏感可靠[20]。

(二) 内分泌腺的自身免疫

关于自家免疫作为内分泌腺疾病的成因，甲状腺方面的研究比较深入，有大量文献出现[31]。自从1956年发现桥本(Hashimoto)氏甲状腺炎患者血清含有抗甲状腺抗体以来。陆续观察到甲状腺有三种蛋白质成分可以做为抗原：(1)甲状球蛋白；(2)腺泡胶状质中第二种蛋白质；(3)上皮细胞微粒体中的抗原。抗这些蛋白质的抗体都集中在血清 γ 球蛋白部分。第一种

抗体可用沉淀法或甲状球蛋白致敏的鞣酸红血球被动凝集法检出；第二种抗体用补体结合试验或鞣酸红血球法检出；第三种抗体以补体结合试验查出，并对甲状腺组织培养起细胞毒素作用。所有典型的 Hashimoto 氏甲状腺炎都有这三种抗体，且滴定度高。成人原发性粘液性水肿患者的80%和甲状腺机能亢进患者的65%也有这些抗体，但滴定度较低。胶状质甲状腺肿只有30%具有低滴定度的抗体。中年正常女性也可能有10～30%有低度的抗甲状腺抗体，但年龄越轻，抗体检出率越低。正常男性的检出率只有女性的半。这说明甲状腺自家免疫抗体的存在是一较为普遍现象，低滴定度不一定具有病理意义。

原发性肾上腺萎缩有时是阿狄森氏病的原因，肾上腺皮质显示淋巴浸润和上皮细胞增生，提示本病的发病机制与自家免疫性甲状腺炎相似。具有抗肾上腺提取物的结合补体的抗体曾在几例阿狄森氏病患者中检出。原发性粘液性水肿合并自发的肾上腺萎缩偶可见到，也提示这两种病有共同来源。

曾有不育男性血和精液中发现凝集精子的抗体。在 2015 对不育夫妇中，男性血清精子凝集素的滴定度高于 1/32 者占 4％。凝集素有抗精子头，精子尾尖部和精子尾体部三种。该作者认为输精管阻塞和精子漏入间质组织会引起自家抗体的形成。非特异性肉芽肿性睾丸炎似乎与自家免疫有关，因为在这些病人血清中可以找到精子凝集素。动物实验将同种睾丸提取液给母豚鼠注射，能降低这种动物的繁殖率。以上研究为计划生育提供线索和方向。

六、激素的作用机制

关于各种激素的作用，总的概念是调节各器官组织的物质代谢，至于它们怎样调节物质代谢，目前的认识尚属片断，颇不全面。归纳起来，激素的作用机制有两大类型，即(1)通过对细胞内外膜通透性的影响；(2)通过对酶作用的影响。在这两大类型中，又有几种不同作用方式，兹举例略加介绍如下：

(一) 通过对细胞内外膜通透性的影响

1. 加强细胞膜对有机物质的通透。胰岛素的作用机制之一是增加细胞膜的通透性，使葡萄糖，甚至氨基酸易于进入细胞以增加这些代谢物在细胞内的浓度，从而加强它们的代谢。胰岛素能够增加细胞膜对代谢物的转运这一机制是有许多实验证明的，但胰岛素怎样影响细胞膜的转运机制尚属正在探索的问题。

2. 加强细胞内微结构膜的通透性。线粒体是细胞浆内一种膜样结构，其中排列有生物氧化的酶系统，

借以传递物质氧化所脱下的氢与分子氧结合成水，这是氧化的部分，也就是耗氧的部分。同时，物质氧化所释放的能量，在正常情况下，大部分储存于无机磷酸键上。这种具有高能磷酸键的磷酸与二磷酸腺苷(ADP)结合而形成三磷酸腺苷(ATP)，这是磷酸化的部分，也就是消耗无机磷酸的部分。在正常情况下，氧化与磷酸化是偶联的，称为氧化磷酸化，即用氧与消耗无机磷酸(P:O)有一定的比值。小量或生理剂量的甲状腺素使綫粒体膨胀，說明綫粒体膜此时对水及代謝物的通透性增加；同时氧化也加强，伴有磷酸化相应地加强，故 P:O 比值正常。当甲状腺素剂量加大时，綫粒体肿胀更甚，氧化也更强，但磷酸化并不相应地增加，故 P:O 比值降低，称为氧化磷酸化脱耦联，也就是大量氧化所产生的能量不能以 ATP 的形式储存备用而以热量的形式散发消失。这就是甲状腺机能亢进的表现，故有人称甲状腺机能亢进症为綫粒体的疾病[22]。

3. 加强整个细胞对水和小分子物质的通透性。抗利尿激素(ADH)对远端肾小管细胞有加强其回吸收水的能力。根据一些实验[23]回吸收水的作用机制在于 ADH 的双硫基 (-S-S-) 与细胞受体的硫氢基 (-SH) 起反应，进行交换，形成激素与受体之间的双硫键，并在激素分子上形成一个硫氢基(图8)。这个硫氢基又可打开受体原有的双硫桥。这种激素与受体之间的 -S-S- 与 -SH 的进行性交換即可分裂细胞蛋白质中的作为扩散屏障的 -S-S- 桥，使分子构形敞开，孔道扩大以便水、尿素及其它小分子通过，有如图8所示。

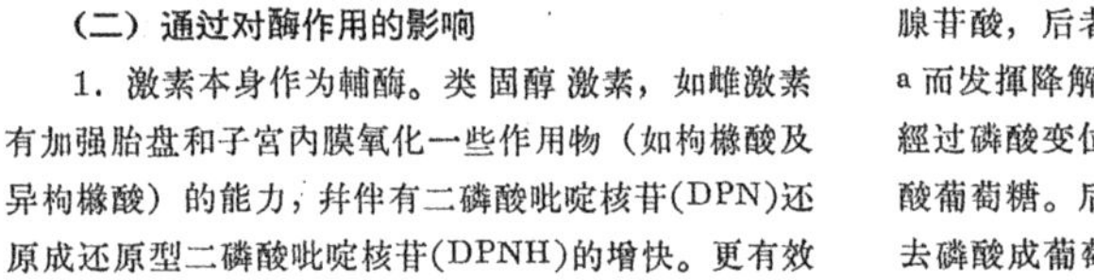

图 8 抗利尿激素与细胞受体多次进行 S-S 和 SH 交换直向前进分开蛋白质扩散屏障中的纤維成分以便利水的通透。

(二) 通过对酶作用的影响

1. 激素本身作为辅酶。类固醇激素，如雌激素有加强胎盘和子宫内膜氧化一些作用物（如构橼酸及异构橼酸）的能力，并伴有二磷酸吡啶核苷(DPN)还原成还原型二磷酸吡啶核苷(DPNH)的增快。更有效地增快 DPN 还原为 DPNH 的因素是加入少量的三磷酸吡啶核苷(TPN)。从这一观察出发，Talalay等[24]认为 TPN 促进代謝物的氧化而被还原成 TPNH，后者将氢递给雌酮，使其还原成雌二醇-17β。雌二醇

-17β 与 DPN 反应，将氢递給 DPN，形成 DPNH，而自己氢化为雌酮。实际上雌激素起着辅酶的作用，在转氢酶 (transhydrogenase) 的影响下，参与氢在 TPNH 和 DPN 之间的传递。

$$\text{雌二醇-17}\beta + \text{DPN} \rightleftharpoons \text{雌酮} + \text{DPNH}$$
$$\text{TPNH} + \text{雌酮} \rightleftharpoons \text{TPN} + \text{雌二醇-17}\beta$$
$$\overline{\text{TPNH} + \text{DPN} \rightleftharpoons \text{TPN} + \text{DPNH}}$$

图 9 雌激素作为辅酶把 TPNH 的氢转给 DPN 成 DPNH 以加强代謝的方式。

2. 激素促进酶的活性。激素通过刺激酶活性而发生作用的例子较多，如胰岛素加强己糖激酶的活性，雄激素加强转氨酶的活性等。下面重点討論 ACTH 激活肾上腺皮质磷酸化酶的机制。磷酸化酶有两型，a 型多一个磷酸，有促进糖元分解成葡萄糖的作用，b 型去掉了这个磷酸，无活性。从 b 型变为 a 型须赖 3′,5′-一磷酸腺苷(3′,5′AMP)，或称环状腺苷酸(图10)。环

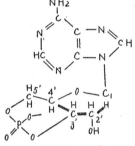

图 10 3′,5′-一磷酸腺(3′,5′AMP)或环状腺苷酸。

状腺苷酸能将 ATP 的末端磷酸加入磷酸化酶 b 的絲氨酸上而成磷酸化酶 a，是此酶的激活物。环状腺苷酸的形成需要一种环化酶 (Cyclase)，使 ATP 脱下焦磷酸，剩下的磷酸也与核糖的第 3′ 碳结合而成环状(图10)。肾上腺皮质具有环化酶，經过 ACTH 的作用而被激活，这样就形成了环状腺苷酸，后者将磷酸化酶 b 转变为有活性的磷酸化酶 a 而发挥降解皮质的糖元为 1-磷酸葡萄糖的作用。經过磷酸变位酶的催化，1-磷酸葡萄糖轉变为 6-磷酸葡萄糖。后者进一步代謝可能有三条途径，即脱去磷酸成葡萄糖或經酵解成丙酮酸或經磷酸戊糖途径而将葡萄糖第一位碳氧化而成葡萄糖酸。最后一条途径在肾上腺皮质占优势，故有较多的 TPN 还原为 TPNH。还原型 TPN 是类固醇皮质激素合成中若干步骤，尤其是羥化作用所需的氢的来源[25]。这样，

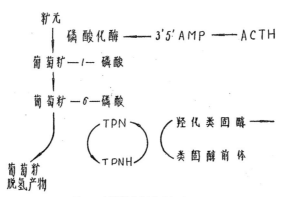

图 11 ACTH 的作用机制示意图

ACTH 加强肾上腺皮质物质代谢而促进皮质激素合成的机制有了较为满意的解释(图 11)。

肾上腺素或致糖素加强肝糖元的分解而使血糖升高的机制也与 ACTH 的作用机制相似。

3. 激素诱导酶的生物合成。机体在适应内外环境改变时，有时会出现酶的生物合成增加。例如，作用物的增加往往能诱导作用于该作用物的酶的生成。除了作用物的影响以外，激素对于酶的生成也起诱导作用。例如，皮质醇有加强葡萄糖-6-磷酸酶的活性，故血糖可因皮质醇的应用而升高。动物实验发现乙硫氨酸(ethionine)。这一蛋白质合成的抑制剂能够抑制皮质醇的这一作用，但加入乙硫氨酸的拮抗剂甲硫氨酸，则皮质醇的作用又可恢复。

又如，肾上腺皮质激素对肝脏的色氨酸吡咯酶(tryptophan pyrrolase)有诱导生成的作用。此酶的作用是裂开色氨酸的吡咯环，从而导致菸草酸(尼克酸)的合成，也是合成 DPN 和 TPN 等辅酶的首先步骤。在皮质激素的作用下，与此酶活性增加的同时，肝脏的蛋白质和核酸的量以及更新率都增高，说明蛋白质合成加强。经过提纯，色氨酸吡咯酶的含量却因皮质激素的影响而有所增加[23]。

结尾语

上面粗略地介绍了内分泌学中六个比较重要的问题和它们在国际上现代发展的情况。有关这些方面的研究虽属比较深入，但尚有许多问题须待解决，是今后努力的方向。内分泌学的发展将仍然与化学、生物化学、生物物理、生理学、免疫学、组织形态学等基础学科和临床医学各学科的发展分不开的；同时它的

发展也依靠同位素、电子显微镜、电泳、层析、逆流分布等技术的发展。

参考文献

[1] Copp, D. H., et al., Endocrinology 70: 638, 1963　[2] Blair-West J. R., et al., The Rec. Progr. Hormone Res. 19: 311, 1963　[3] 朱壬葆，生理科学进展 5: 141, 1963　[4] Yreen, L. A., et al., Ann. New York Acad. Sc. 86 (Art. 2): 669, 1960　[5] 王志均，生理科学进展 1: 13, 1957　[6] 谭得圣等，中华内科杂志 10: 92, 1962　[7] 朱鹤年，生理科学进展 6: 1, 1964　[8] Guillemin, R., et al., Endocrinology 73: 564, 1963　[9] Brodish, A., et al., Endocrinology 71: 298, 1962　[10] Abê, C., Folia Endocrinol. Japon. 35: 1651, 1961　[11] 刘士豪，中华内科杂志 10: 890, 1962　[12] Grant, J. K., Brit. Med. Bull. 18: 99, 1962　[13] Brooks, R. V., Brit. Med. Bull. 18: 148, 1962　[14] Tata, J. R., Rec. Progr. Hormone Res. 18: 221, 1962　[15] Mills, I. H., Brit. Med. Bull. 18: 127, 1962　[16] Behrens, O. K., et al., Ann. Rev. Biochem. 27: 57, 1958　[17] Lee, T. H., et al., J. Biol. Chem. 236: 2971, 1961　[18] Engel, F. L., et al., Am. J. Med. 35: 721, 1963　[19] Berson, S. A., et al., Coll. Endocrinol. 14: 182, 1962　[20] Berson, S. A., et al., Proc. Nat. Acad. Sc. 49: 613, 1963　[21] Doniach, D., et al., Ann. Rev. Med. 13: 213, 1962　[22] Hoch, F. L., New England J. Med. 266: 446, 1962　[23] Schwartz, I. L., et al., Proc. Nat. Acad. Sc. 46: 1288, 1960　[24] Talalay, P., et al., Rec. Progr. Hormone Res. 16: 1, 1960　[25] Haynes, R. C., et al., Rec. Progr. Hormone Res. 16: 121, 1960　[26] Feigelson, P., et al., Rec. Progr. Hormone Res. 18: 491, 1962.

附录一

刘士豪教授论文题录

◆ **1924**

  Liu SH. The influence of cod liver oil on the Calcium and Phosphorus metabolism in tetany. Chin Med J, 1924; 38: 793.

◆ **1925**

  Liu SH, Chang HC. Hypoglycemia, report of a case unassociated with insulin administration. Arch Int Med, 1925; 36: 146.

◆ **1926**

  Liu SH, Gault AS. Acute mercuric chloride poisoning with report of a case. Nat Med J China, 1926; 12: 927.

  Liu SH Parathyroid Hormone: A review of recent literature. Nat Med J China, 1926, 12: 349.

◆ **1927**

  Horvath AA, Liu SH. The effect of soy-bean sauce on blood sugar and phosphorus. Japan Med World, 1927, 7: 71.

  Liu SH, Mills CA.. The effect of insulin on blood cholesterol, fat and sugar in nephrosis. Proc Soc Exp Biol & Med, 1927, 24, 191.

  Liu SH. The partition of serum calcium into diffusible and non-diffusible portions. Chin J Physiol, 1927, 1: 331.

  Liu SH. The effect of thyroid medication in nephrosis. Arch Int Med, 1927, 40: 73.

◆ 1928

Hsieh CK, Liu SH. Cholecystography. Nat Med J China, 1928, 14: 382.

Liu SH. A comparative study of the effects of various treatments on the calcium and phosphorus metabolism in tetany: I. Chronic Juvenile Tetany. J Clin Invest 1928, 5: 259-76.

Liu SH. A comparative study of the effects of various treatments on the calcium and phosphorus metabolism in tetany: II. Chronic Adult Idiopathic Tetany. J Clin Invest, 1928, 5: 277-84.

Liu SH. Plasma acid-base equilibrium in malaria. Chinese J Physiol., 1928, 2, 151.

Ling SM, Liu SH. Studies on plasma lipoids. I. Fatty acids of blood plasma in diabetes and nephrosis. Chinese J Physiol, 1928, 2: 157.

Liu SH. Tissue fibrinogen in the treatment of hemorrhage. Nat Med J China, 1928; 14: 283.

◆ 1929

Liu SH. The phenoltetrachlorphthalein as an aid in the diagnosis of liver diseases. Nat Med J China, 1929; 15: 1.

Liu SH, Chu FT. Sex, age, and seasonal distribution of tetany of orphanage in Peking. Am J Med Sci, 1929;177:599.

Sendroy J, Liu SH, Van Slyke DD. The gasometric determination of the relative affinity constant for carbon monoxide and oxygen in whole blood at 38℃. Am J Physiol, 1929, 90: 511.

◆ 1930

Sendroy J, Liu SH. Gasometric determination of oxygen and carbon monoxide in blood. J Biol Chem, 1930, 89: 133.

◆ 1931

Liu SH, Hastings AB. Acid-base paths in human subjects. Proc Soc Exp Biol & Med, 1931, 28: 781.

Liu SH, Chu HI, Wang SH, et al. Nutritional edema I. The effects of level and quality of protein intake on nitrogen balance, plasma proteins and edema. Proc Soc Exp Biol & Med, 1931, 29: 250.

Liu SH, Chu HI, Wang SH et al. Nutritional edema II. The effects of alkali and acids on nitrogen balance, plasma proteins and edema. Proc Soc Exp Biol & Med 1931, 29: 252.

◆ 1932

Liu SH, Chu HI, Wang SH et al. Nutritional edema I. The effects of level and quality of protein intake on nitrogen balance, plasma proteins and edema. Chin J Physiol, 1932, 6: 73-94.

Liu SH, Chu HI, Wang SH et al. Nutritional edema II. The effects of alkali and acids on nitrogen balance, plasma proteins and edema. Chin J Physiol, 1932, 6: 95-106.

Van Slyke DD, Sendroy J, Liu SH. Manometric analysis of gas mixtures: ii. carbon dioxide by the isolation method. J Biol Chem, 1932, 95: 531-546.

Van Slyke DD, Sendroy J, Liu SH. Manometric analysis of gas mixtures: iii. manometric determination of carbon dioxide tension and phs of blood. J Biol Chem, 1932, 95: 547-568.

◆ 1933

Liu SH, Chu HI, et al. An optimal diet in promoting nitrogen gain in nephrosis. Proc Soc Exp Biol & Med, 1933, 30: 986.

Liu SH, Wang SH, Fan C. Acidocis in cholera. I. Path of displacement of serum acid base equilibrium. Proc Soc Exp Biol & Med, 1933, 30: 417.

Liu SH, Fan C, Wang SH. Acidocis in cholera. Ⅱ. Changes in serum electrolytes. Proc Soc Exp Biol & Med, 1933, 30: 419.

◆ **1934**

Hannon RR, Liu SH, Chu HI, Wang SH. Calcium and phosphorus metabolism in osteomalacia. I. The effect of vitamin D and its apparent duration. Chin Med J, 1934; 48:623-636.

◆ **1935**

Liu SH, Chu HI. An optimal diet in promoting nitrogen gain in nephrosis. J Clin Invest, 1935, 14: 293-303.

Liu SH, Hannon RR, Chu HI, Chen KC, Chou SK, Wang SH. Calcium and phosphorus metabolism in osteomalacia. II. Further studies on the response to vitamin D of patients with osteomalacia. Chin Med J, 1935, 49: 1-21.

Liu SH, Hannon RR, Chou SK, Chen KC, Chu HI, Wang SH. Calcium and phosphorus metabolism in osteomalacia. III. The effects of varying levels and ratios of intake of calcium to phosphorus on their serum levels, paths of excretion and balances. Chin J Physiol, 1935, 9: 101-118.

◆ **1936**

Chu HI, Chou SK, Chen KC, Wang SH, Liu SH, Hannon RR. Calcium and phosphorus metabolism in osteomalacia. IV. Report of an unusual case in a male with acute parathormone poisoning. Chinese Med J, 1936, 50: 1-16.

Chou SK, Chen KC, Liu SH, Fang SS. Serum electrolytes and mineral metabolism in a case of Addison's disease with observations on the use of suprarenal cortical extract (eschatin). Chin Med J, 1936, 50: 1013.

Liu SH, Loucks HH, Chou SK, Chen KC. Adenoma of pancreatic islet cells with hypoglycemia and hyperinsulinism: Report of a Case with Studies on Blood Sugar and Metabolism before and after Operative Removal of Tumor. J Clin Invest, 1936,

15: 249-60.

◆ 1937

Liu SH, Su CC, Chou SK, Chu HI, Wang CW, Chang KP. Calcium and phosphorus metabolism in osteomalacia. V. The effect of varying levels and ratios of calcium to phosphorus intake on their serum levels, paths of excretion and balances in the presence of continuous vitamin D therapy. J Clin Invest, 1937, 16: 603-611.

Liu SH, Su CC, Wang CW, Chang KP. Calcium and phosphorus metabolism in osteomalacia. VI. The added drain of lactation and beneficial action of vitamin D. Chin J Physiol, 1937, 11: 271-294.

Chou SK, Liu SH. Comparison of pituitary gonadotropic extract and prolan on ovarian and uterine response in immature rats. Proc Soc Exp Biol & Med, 1937, 34: 228–234.

◆ 1938

Dodds EC, Liu SH, Noble RL. Water balance and blood changes following posterior pituitary extract administration. J Physiol, 1938, 94: 124-35.

Liu SH, Noble RL. Renal insufficiency following intra-renal arterial injection of posterior pituitary pressor principles. J Physiol, 1938, 93: 13P.

◆ 1939

Liu SH. Pathological states produced by the administration of posterior pituitary pressor principal. Chin Med J, 1939, 55: 448.

Liu SH, Noble RL. The effects of extracts of pregnant mare serum and human pregnancy urine on the reproductive system of hypophysectomized male rats I. J Endocrinology, 1939，1: 7-14.

Liu SH, Noble RL. The effects of extracts of pregnant mare serum and human pregnancy urine on the reproductive system of hypophysectomized female rats II. J Endocrinology, 1939, 1: 15-21.

Snapper I, Liu SH, Chung HL, Yu TF. Sun HM. Hematuria, renal colic and acetyl-sulfapyridine stone formation following sulphapyridine administration. Chin Med J, 1939, 56: 1.

Snapper I, Liu SH, Chung, HL, Yu TF. Anaemia from blood donation: A hematological and clinical study of 101 professional donors. Chin Med J, 1939, 56: 403.

Snapper I, Liu SH, Ch'in KY. Liver degeneration following neo-arsphenamine and mapharsen treatment with some remarks on catarrhal jaundice and arsenioal jaundice and their relation to acute yellow atrophy. Chin Med J, 1939, 56: 501.

◆ 1940

Liu SH, Chu HI, Su CC, Yu TF, Cheng TY. Calcium and phosphorus metabolism in osteomalacia. IX. Metabolic behavior of infants fed on breast milk from mothers showing various states of vitamin D nutrition. J Clin Invest, 1940, 19:327-347.

Chu HI, Liu SH, Yu TF, Hsu HC, Cheng TY, Chao HC. Calcium and phosphorus metabolism in osteomalacia. X. Further studies on vitamin D action: Early signs of depletion and effect of minimal doses. J Clin Invest, 1940, 19:349-363.

Chu HI, Liu SH, et al. The effect of vitamin C on the calcium: phosphorus and nitrogen metabolism in scurvy and osteomalacia, Chin J Physiol, 1940, 15 : 101-118.

Liu SH, Ch'in KY, Chu HI, Pai HC. Osteamalacia: clinical, metabolic and pathologic studies of a case with parathyroid hyperplasia and right-sided cardiac hypertrophy from thoracic deformaities vitamin B1 deficiency. Chin Med J, 1940, 58: 141.

Liu SH. The role of vitamin D in the calcium and phosphorus metabolism in osteomalacia. Chin Med J, 1940, 57: 101.

Liu SH, Chu HI, et al. Osteogenesis imperfecta Ⅰ: Observation on the effect of vitamin C and D, and thyroid and pituitary preparation on the calcium, phosphorus, and nitrogen metabolism with a report on bome analysis. Chin Med J,

1940, suppl 3: 515.

Chu HI, Liu SH, Chen KC, et al. Osteogenesis imperfecta II: Observation on the effect of vitamin C and D, and thyroid and pituitary preparation on the calcium, phosphorus and nitrogen metabolism with a report on bome analysis. Chin Med J, 1940, suppl 3: 539.

Huang CH, Liu SH. Acute epidemic encephalitis of Japanese type: clinical report of six proven cases. Chin Med J, 1940, 58: 427.

◆ **1941**

Liu SH, Chu HI, Hsu HC, Chao HC, Cheu SH. Calcium and phosphorus metabolism in osteomalacia. XI. The pathogenetic role of pregnancy and relative importance of calcium and vitamin D supply. J Clin Invest, 1941, 20:255-271.

Liu SH. Osteomalacia as a nutritional disease. Nutritional Notes, 1941, 11: 1.

Chu HI, Liu SH, Hsu HC, Chao HC, Cheu SH. Calcium, phosphorus, nitrogen and magnesium metabolism in normal young Chinese adults. Chinese Med J. 1941, 59: 1-33.

Liu SH, Chu HI, Yu FT, et al. Anemia in vitamin C deficiency and its response to iron. Proc Soc Exp Biol & Med, 1941, 46: 603.

Liu SH, Chu HI, Yu FT, et al. Water and electrolytes metabolism in diabetes insipitus. Proc Soc Exp Biol & Med, 1941, 46: 682.

◆ **1942**

Liu SH, Chu HI. Treatment of renal osteodystrophy with dihydrotachysterol (A.T.10) and iron. Science. 1942, 95: 388-389.

Wang K, Liu SH, Chu HI, Yu TF, Chao HC, Hsu HC. Calcium and phosphorus metabolism in osteomalacia. XIII. The availability of inorganic phytin, and dietary phosphorus and the effect of vitamin D. Chin Med J 1942, 61:61-72 (also published in vol. 62:1-16, 1944).

◆ **1943**

Liu SH, Chu HI. Studies of calcium and phosphorus metabolism with special reference to pathogenesis and effect of dihydrotachysterol (A.T. 10) and iron. Medicine, 1943; 22:103-161.

◆ **1949**

Chu HI, Liu SH, Hsu HC, Chao HC. Calcium and phosphorus metabolism in osteomalacia. XII. A comparison of the effects of A.T. 10 (dihydrotachysterol) and vitamin D. Chin J Physiol, 1949, 17: 117-134.

◆ **1951**

Liu SH. Chronic hemolytic anemia with erythrocyte fragility to cold and acid. I. Clinical and laboratory data of two cases, with special reference to the cell abnormality. Blood, 1951, 6: 101-23.

Liu SH. Chronic hemolytic anemia with erythrocyte fragility to cold and acid. II. Serum hemolytic activity and its relation to serum globulins and complement and the role of guinea pig serum. Blood, 1951, 6: 124-41.

◆ **1956**

刘士豪，翟树职，隋树娥. 甘草对阿狄森病的疗效. 中华医学杂志，1956；42：655-664.

吴德昌，魏文龄，刘士豪. 微量血清碱性磷酸酶测定方法的研究. 营养学报，1956；1（4）：279-289.

◆ **1962**

刘士豪. 内分泌学的近代进展. 中华内科杂志，1962；10：890.

◆ **1964**

刘士豪. 内分泌研究发展的方向. 国外医学动态，1964；10：569-578.

刘士豪. 抗炎性肾上腺皮质激素的临床应用. 中级医刊，1964；1：49-52.

刘士豪. 抗炎性肾上腺皮质激素的临床应用（续）. 中级医刊，1964；2：116-119.

◆ **1984**

Zhu XY, Liu SH. The effect of a single massive dose of vitamin D (D2 or D3), on calcium, phosphorus and nitrogen metabolism in osteomalacia. Chin Med J (Engl), 1984, 97: 295-306.

协和百年忆前贤

——北京协和医院内分泌科
资深专家回忆刘士豪教授 [1]

---

[1] 2020 年 9 月 9 日与 14 日，北京协和医院内分泌科分别对资深教授白耀、周学瀛、陆召麟、吴从愿、孙梅励、邓洁英、金自孟、曾正陪就刘士豪教授的话题进行了深入访谈，采访人李乃适。孟迅吾教授提供了书面回忆录。

白耀教授访谈录

李乃适：白老师，大家都知道，您是我们科的元老，很早的时候您就已经在科里工作了；刘士豪教授是我们科的奠基人，大家想请您说一说当年您跟刘士豪教授的交往。

白耀：好。今年是刘士豪教授诞辰 120 周年，刘教授离开我们已经整整 46 年了。我在内分泌科和恩师刘教授工作过十几年，受到过他的亲切的指导和教诲。虽然已经过去几十年了，老人家的慈祥、温厚、谆谆善诱的模样，至今仍然深深地印在我的脑海里。我院内分泌科是在 1961 年成为和内科同样的独立科室。建科初期，内分泌的临床部分只有 4 个大夫，主任是刘士豪教授，副主任是池芝盛副教授，史轶蘩大夫和我都是主治医师。因为建科以后需要有人做总住院医师，就由当时年纪最轻的我来担任总住院医师。那个时候总住院医师每天早上经常有些科内的医疗或者其他的事情，要向主任请教，向刘教授汇报前 24 小时科里边所发生的一些特殊的医疗事件和其他的事。每当我去 8 楼 2 层——现在这个地方还有，8 楼 2 层的外边是我们内分泌科办公室——我进门的时候多半看到他是坐在办公室专心看书。当细心听取我的工作汇报以后，他对我提出的问题，经常中间插入提问。他要知道很详细的情况，在他了解以后总是耐心地做解答，还提出一些相关的问题，让我回去好好思考，或者查找一些答案。在我汇报工作后，他有时候还亲自去现场看看，对我提出的问题总是给予满意的答复。这种严谨的对待工作、对待医疗的治学精神对我的帮助都很大，现在印象还很深。建科之初，因为临床人员少，我连续做了一年半的病房主治医生，有幸经常聆听刘教授定时或不定时的主任查房分析。他平时不善言谈，在查房或看病人以后，话语也不多，讲话的时候语句和缓，声音较低；但言辞稳重准确，谈的一些问题都击中要害。有的时候我坐在离他不远的地方，就能更清楚地听到他对病情的讲解。在精辟的发言当中，他解决了病人存在的问题，我们也获得了一些有益的、书本上得不来的知识和经验。

刘教授善于做科研工作是有传统的。1962年，我做病房主治医生的时候，上海广慈医院报道了首例原发性醛固酮增多症，随后我院收治了全国第2个病例。这个病人我现在仍记得很清楚，她是北京地质学院的一位讲师。她的一些形象，至今印象仍然清晰。对这个病例，刘教授全面细致地进行了临床观察和研究，亲自设计科研和诊治方案，组织安排病房和实验室有关人员科学精准地采集、保存和测定病人的血、尿、大便和唾液这些标本，组织了一支精干的科研团队。同时，他详细地交代临床工作人员耐心地对各种检查从科学的角度做好病人的解释工作。做科研工作的时候，要给病人注射一种叫美蓝的显示剂；注射以后，病人皮肤黏膜都呈现蓝色，但没有任何危害。如果事先病人不知道可能出现这种现象，就会有很多顾虑。我们在事先向病人做了很周密仔细的解释，病人本人也是搞科学的，对这些问题都能够理解，因此顺利地取得了病人的主动积极配合。通过这个事例可以看出，刘士豪教授既完满地完成了临床科研工作，又培养了一批能够做好临床科研工作的团队，为今后科内开展各项临床科研工作做出了样板，奠定了坚实基础。我们现在做很多科研工作，基本上还是按照这样一个规程来做的。

刘教授在上个世纪50年代中期，根据自己多年的临床经验和基础医学知识的一些实际经验，编写了一本《生物化学与临床医学的联系》的著作，对学习临床内分泌学的人员以及其他医务工作者都是一本非常好的参考书。这本书内容很有启发价值。它不仅使读者知道了临床现象，更能够使读者进一步深入了解生物化学的基础原理和彼此之间的内在联系。这本书在上世纪50年代出版以后，曾经是医学领域的畅销书。初入临床内分泌学科的我，通过这本书的学习，在临床和科研工作方面都获得了很好的教益。

记得在上世纪60年代，我和科里几位同事在一个天气比较冷的上午，到史家胡同刘教授的家里拜访。那时候他家住在院落的南房里，房子里几面靠墙的书架都摆满了书，有很多新的专业医学杂志，有的杂志是原版的；在那个时候，在我们医科院的图书馆，这些医学杂志多半都是影印的，而且影印的书多半是在原版书出版半年之后，大约一个月以后才能看得到。刘教授他很早就能看到原版书，在书里头他夹了很多小纸条以备参考；进到他家以后就像走进图书馆，放在他桌边的都是书。我就在想，老教授在办公室里多在看书，回家以后仍然继续不顾疲倦地还在苦苦钻研。他是在面向科学的未来，面向未来的内分泌学的发展。

值此刘士豪教授诞辰 120 周年之际，我作为他的后辈和他亲自教导的学生，深深怀念我们可敬的老主任，缅怀一代内分泌宗师刘士豪教授！

李乃适：您觉得刘士豪教授当时的一些工作，对我们内分泌科临床和科研的布局有哪些是有影响的，或者说具体产生了什么影响？

白耀：刘教授对我们协和内分泌科成科后的定位，不仅只是一个临床科室，而是一个临床与科研紧密结合的内分泌科；同时，他也非常重视内分泌领域的教学和干部培养。我们科有较完整的生物化学基础及实力雄厚的实验室科研力量的支撑，使得临床工作开展得扎扎实实，使得我们的内分泌学科发展成为后来院内不少学科发展借鉴的样板。

李乃适：白大夫，您觉得刘士豪教授在人才培养上的风格是怎样的？

白耀：他对干部的培养主要是言传与身教，另外具体做的事情不仅是看在眼里，而且是实践在行动上。所以我们现在的科研工作，好多方面是按过去的传统和规程传下来的，基本上是这样一个情况。另外就是说刘教授他在很多地方对执行计划工作人员的安排，都是言传身教；比如说查房也好，或者是我做总住院医师（汇报工作也好），他都是从正面来引导你，应该怎么做，这方面印象很深，受益匪浅。

李乃适：有资料表明，刘士豪教授 1964 年参加了全国的内分泌和肾脏病学大会。您当时参会了吗？

白耀：1964 年全国内分泌和肾脏病学术会议召开时，我在病房做主治医师，当时科里人少，没有人接替我的病房医疗工作，我未能去参加会议，但协和内分泌包括临床和实验室参会的人员还是不少的。据参加会议人员回来介绍情况，我们在会上交流了多篇论文，受到与会人员的重视和好评。我虽未能到场，但带了我署名的文章 7 篇，其中有论文，也有的是工作总结分析，在会议学术汇编中是文章署名最多的。

李乃适：关于刘士豪教授生活的一些事情，您了解吗？

白耀：知道得不多，只知道刘教授的夫人是原来六楼二层代谢病房的护士长，我们去他家时，都会热情接待。另外，刘教授来医院上下班都乘定时接送的人力车。

李乃适：白老师另外想问一下，您刚才说的刘士豪教授去查房，会指出一些很关键的地方。您还记得有哪些例子吗？

白耀：刘教授看病人、问病情、做体检时，既能抓住重点，也不漏过可疑之处。譬如对糖尿病人，靠近体表的血管改变从不轻易漏过，一些关键病史也非常重视。在听取我们介绍病情后，他常会再深入检查病人存在的许多问题。那时候不像现在借助很多仪器，当时查房都很仔细，包括黏膜是否苍白、有没有贫血，都要看的，现在这方面一般都看得很少了。另外比如摸肝脾，我们有时候摸不清楚，刘教授就摸得很清楚。老医生尤其是他要想到这个病可能要排除哪些疾病的时候，他看得就很细，不忽略特殊体征，一些一般的体征都是很注意的。刘教授他虽然实验室工作做得比较多，在临床工作方面经验同样是很丰富的。

孟迅吾教授回忆录

刘士豪是我国杰出的内分泌学家、临床学家和生物化学家，是我国内分泌学的开拓者和奠基人之一，是代谢性骨病学领域的先驱。

1925 年北京协和医院创立了当时极为先进的代谢病房和代谢实验室，开创了中国佝偻病和骨软化症的研究先河。刘士豪等对中国佝偻病和骨软化症钙磷代谢的研究于 20 世纪三四十年代在《临床研究杂志》(*J. Clin. Invest.*) 等杂志上发表了 13 篇系列文章。1942 年刘士豪和朱宪彝在国际著名期刊《科学》(*Science*) 上撰文，首次提出肾性骨营养不良 (renal osteodystrophy, ROD) 的病名，并开创性地推论肾脏疾病时可能存在的维生素 D 抵抗，提出了肾脏与维生素 D 的联系。直至 30 年后 Holick MF 和 Deluca HF 等分离和证实了维生素 D 的活性代谢产物 1,25-$(OH)_2$D，随后在肾脏发现了 1α 羟化酶，证实维生素 D 需要经过肾脏 1α 羟化才能代谢为其活性形式 1,25-$(OH)_2$D。

刘士豪教授为我国第一个内分泌科（北京协和医院）的主任，作为住院医师的我切身感受到其丰富的临床经验、坚实的理论知识、有预见性的科研工作。他重视人才培养，其科学研究成果在国际上享有盛誉。

每周一次内科大查房，刘士豪教授总是第一个发言，思路清晰，临床特点与基础理论相联系。他撰写的《生物化学与临床医学的联系》是我们各级医师必备的案头参考书。他积极支持池芝盛教授倡导的把知识教给病人、发挥病人在治疗中的主观能动性。

上世纪 60 年代初，Yalow 和 Berson 成功建立了放免法测定胰岛素，刘教授敏锐地预见到这一微量的分析技术，必将带来巨大变革。1962 年他指导放射专业的研究生从事此项研究，1965 年成功建立了放免法测定胰岛素，此后生长激素、甲状旁腺素等放免法相继成功建立，大大提高了相关疾病的医疗和科研水平。

1963 年刘士豪教授主持组织了内分泌高级学习班，系统授课。参加学员有诸多进修医师和本科青年医师。经过一年严格训练，学员们受益匪浅，以后很多成为学科带头人。学员中有伍汉文、富朴云、时钟孚、潘长玉和林丽香等，潘长玉至今还保留听课笔记。

　　1981 年我以访问学者身份赴美国麻省总医院，首次见导师 Neer 教授，他知我来自北京协和医院，立马翻开手头的杂志，指出文中载有刘士豪和朱宪彝教授对钙磷代谢研究做了很大成效的研究。1985 年美国代谢性骨病学权威帕菲特（Parfitt AM）访问中国时，点名要参观北京协和医院的代谢病房和代谢实验室。史轶蘩教授带领我们接待了他。此后，他在《国际钙化组织》（*Calcified Tissue International*）载文指出，20 世纪三四十年代全球有关钙磷代谢的研究，大部分出自北京协和医院，构成了现代内分泌研究的基石，给予高度评价。

周学瀛教授访谈录

李乃适：周老师您好，大家都知道您来协和医院的时候刘士豪教授是内分泌科的主任。想请问一下您对刘士豪教授的第一印象是什么样的？

周学瀛：我是1962年刚毕业的时候就和邓洁英、吴从愿、陈智周三位同志一起分到协和来了。我是南京医学院毕业，但是最后两年是在医科院学的生物化学专业，所以毕业后分配到协和医院做基础研究。当时就是刘士豪教授领导我们四个人。当时刘士豪教授和池芝盛教授，一位是主任一位是副主任，告诉我们内分泌是临床与基础相结合的。我来到协和医院以后，我上面还有一个高年资的讲师，杨德馨，她是直接带我的。她说，刘士豪教授告诉我们，有时间的话就多去听听查房。搞实验室搞技术的为什么还要听查房呢？就是临床实践要和实验室相结合。这一点给我印象很深。因此，从那以后，杨老师、我以及其他人，要是有时间都会去听查房，特别是刘教授查房的时候。

还有一个印象是，刘教授平时话不多，但是平常说一句话可以说都是言简意赅。1963年，时任卫生部部长钱信忠到医院来视察。钱部长一个人来内分泌科视察，来到内分泌实验室时，我正在用纸层析的方法分离尿中的醛固酮。我给他们介绍之后，当时刘教授就说："很好，加油。"后来我们做的一些结果当时没有发表，但做完以后确实是发现原醛患者的醛固酮要比其他病人高。1964年在湖北召开全国第一届内分泌肾脏病会议时，刘士豪教授作了中国第2例原发性醛固酮增多症的临床和实验室的报告，引起很好的反响。

第三个给我的印象是，刘教授平时看起来很严肃的一个人，话也不多。但是对下边的人还是很关心的。他的一个研究生陈智周在结婚的时候，老主任还当了证婚人。婚礼就在现在的护士楼里办的，我们都去了。他除了工作时间以外，其他绝大部分时间都在图书馆里面。回到家他还有个小图书馆，他在家里订了很多重要的杂志，有的甚至比医院的大图书馆都早出来半年。刘教授平常非常刻苦，他很少出去，平时除了工作就是看书。还有一个印象就是，他对下面的年轻同事都很关心。当时在7楼2有一间办公室，是刘教授和池教授一间。当时我们几个年轻人看书没有地方去，当时医大的大楼还没有盖好，刘教授就说："你们晚上没地方看书，就到我这来看吧。"我们当时听了都很高兴。

　　还有我感觉呢，在咱们医院，刘士豪教授可以说是临床和基础很好结合的第一人，到现在也很少有人能超过他。这是有原因的。1941年太平洋战争爆发，协和医院被关闭了。当时有人劝刘教授，说国外有人聘请他，但他不去。当时他一边自己开诊，一边又受同仁医院聘请当院长，还去当时的华北军区医院查房。到1947年，张孝骞回来的时候，亲自到史家胡同去聘请刘士豪教授，担任协和医学院生化系主任兼协和医院的临床教授。所以他基础和临床这两方面都具有非常扎实和渊博的知识。所以，我们协和的这些老教授，包括原来眼科的胡天圣，不知在我跟前说了多少遍，"哎呀，你们这刘士豪啊，刘士豪啊，那是咱们协和的临床和基础相结合的、理论联系实际的第一大家啊。"

　　另外，刘士豪教授给我的感觉是，他善于总结。比如，原来这个肾性侏儒和肾性囊性纤维样骨炎，当时在业界已经存在了很长的时间。大家讨论但是没有统一。但是刘教授把这些统一成一种病，就是肾性骨营养不良。这是非常了不起的，国外目前也一直在沿用。当然，现在搞骨代谢的一些人，认为这个应该再改一改，他们叫作CKDMBD，把CKD（慢性肾脏疾病）和骨病联合起来这样叫，实际我自己觉得现在这个概念还是比不上刘士豪教授所提出的肾性骨病。第二，刘士豪教授敢于挑战当时权威的意见。以双氢速变固醇为例，当时认为双氢速变固醇对肾性骨病作用不大，但刘教授并不认同；刘教授发现用普通维生素D治疗效果不好，而用AT10，也就是双氢速变固醇治疗效果还不错。所以刘教授可以说是推翻了当时权威的结论，提出双氢速变固醇可以有效治疗肾性骨病。另外，刘教授勇于探索，能根据自己的经验提出自己的假说。比如他提出的肾性骨病为什么用普通维生素D治疗不起作用。就上世纪二三十年代年代末的条件来讲，他提出在这种疾病状况下，维生素D本身被灭活，而这种灭活因子在肾性骨病中具有化学专一性，所以维生素D不起作用，但是这种灭活因子对AT10不起所用，所以AT10治疗效果可以。当时没有人提出这种假说，直到1971年肾脏1α羟化酶——一种具有化学专一性的灭活因子——的发现正好证明了他当时提出的假说。当时刘教授提出这种假说，第一次把肾脏和内分泌联系起来。虽然现在看具体的这个灭活因子的提法是不对的，但是在那个年代刘教授这种思想是完全正确的。所以，他敢于提出假说，我不知道他当时这篇文章有没有被国外看到，因为直到30年以后才发现了1α羟化酶，当时有没有人是受到刘教授的思想的启发，从而联系到肾脏就不好说了。所以说，刘教授敢于提出假说，是了不起的一件事情。

另外，刘教授还会不断地探索。比如说他的研究生做胰岛素的放免测定这件事。他很快抓住放射免疫这个苗头，让自己的研究生去做，经过三年这个方法基本建成，但是可惜因为时代的原因，没有正式发表。但是它可以实际应用。也说明他当时抓住这个苗头是非常正确的。另外，在他的领导下，池芝盛教授开展了对糖尿病病人的研究。一个是糖尿病的普查（在石景山），一个是对糖尿病病人的教育。这两项研究也是我们国内近二三十年主要在做的工作。所以，刘教授不断地探索、不断地研究新的方法，是值得怀念的。

总的来讲，刘士豪教授是中国现代内分泌的奠基人。我觉得他是第一奠基人，当然对于骨矿物质代谢的研究更是他打下了基础。朱宪彝教授比他晚毕业5年，1930年毕业，后来也加入了这个队伍，立下了不少功劳。

刘士豪教授在他的业绩中，给我们留下的财富是什么？是精神财富。这个精神财富就是两个字：创新。比如在他之后，池芝盛教授开展了糖尿病教育，创建了糖尿病学会，并编辑了我们国内第一本《糖尿病学》。另外，史轶蘩大夫在垂体研究方面获得突破，孟迅吾教授在代谢性骨病、骨质疏松方面取得了令人瞩目的成绩。刘教授的创新精神，不但影响到了他的同时代人还影响到了他的后继人，对我们现在的内分泌来讲是很大的启发和传承。

最后，我想谈谈他对于人才的培养方面。在刘教授所办的学习班当中，协和自己的人就不说了；东北原来有一个富朴云，西北有一个吴伟，贵州的时钟孚，华西的梁荩忠，广州的黄葆均，福州的林丽香，山东齐鲁的教授我记不起名字了，郑州的欧阳，再加上北京的颜纯、潘长玉……刘教授培养的这些人最后都成为我们内分泌学界的顶梁柱。这方面刘教授的影响也很大。

陆召麟教授访谈录

李乃适：我们知道刘士豪教授在建科开始一直到 20 世纪 60 年代实际上做了很多开创性的事情，您觉得他哪些事情对我们科的科研布局（包括以后的发展）产生了大的影响？

陆召麟：刘士豪教授眼光远大，对世界上的内分泌发展的趋势他非常清楚。上世纪 60 年代激素测定用的是生化方法，灵敏度不高，特异性差，费时费力。后来 Yalow 提出了放射免疫法测定激素，这是一个革命性进步。刘士豪教授敏锐地抓住这个契机，就带了一个研究生陈智周，开始筹建胰岛素的放射免疫法测定。这可能是国内最早的。吴从愿大夫在 20 世纪 60 年代建立蛋白结合法测定皮质醇的测定方法。1974 年我从英国回来以后，和邓洁英教授等建了国内第一个生长激素放射免疫测定。在刘士豪教授思想的指导下，在史轶蘩教授的领导下，经过内分泌科全体同仁的共同努力，内分泌科所有激素测定都得到更新，使内分泌科的医疗、教学和研究水平有了很大的提高。

吴从愿教授口述实录

我叫吴从愿，1962 年到协和内分泌科来当研究生。1965 年毕业后一直在这个科工作到退休。退休以后还经常到科里来看看。

我感觉到协和内分泌科有很好的发展是跟刘士豪教授这位伟大的舵手分不开的。他很早就为内分泌科的发展绘制了完美的航海蓝图。既有临床内分泌，也有基础内分泌。基础内分泌当时已经有了三个组，第一个是内分泌生化，第二个是内分泌生理，第三个是内分泌组织形态。内分泌生化是杨德馨和许建生两位留美高才材生牵头；生理和组织形态分别由金孜琴讲师和倪祖梅负责。在当时，他不仅是分了组，还从医科院专业班要来了四个应届毕业生，一个是周学瀛，他当时是生化专业毕业的；还有邓洁英，她是生理专业毕业的；我和陈智周是放射专业毕业的。所以当时这个发展的蓝图是绘制好了，就是内分泌要从三个方面来发展：第一生化，第二生理，第三组织形态。当时临床内分泌最有名的就是我们的刘士豪教授了，他是 1900 年出生的；第二就是上海的邝安堃教授，他是 1902 年出生的；第三就是天津的朱宪彝教授。刘士豪教授和朱宪彝教授配合非常默契。

刘教授很重视基础研究，他指派池芝盛副主任主管生理和组织形态方面。池芝盛教授早在 1948 年就在巴黎大学从事内分泌实验研究，1952 年回国在上海军科院创立内分泌研究室，1956 年调到医科院从事内分泌病理生理的研究。他主要负责基础方面的研究比较多。当时有几位搞基础内分泌研究很有名的教授，一位是军科院的朱壬葆，他是著名动物生理学家，我国造血干细胞实验研究的创始人；一位是中国科学院动物研究所的张致一教授，他是生殖内分泌的权威；还有一位是北医的王志均教授，他是我国胃肠内分泌的创始人。当时我们搞基础研究的人有两本书必读。一本是刘教授的《生物化学与临床医学的联系》。另一本书是王志均教授 1955 年由人民卫生出版社出版的《慢性实验外科技术》。刘教授除了临床以外重点就研究生化方面。池大夫负责基础方面。我主要是搞性腺方面；通过和妇产科合作，我们研究长效口服避孕药的作用机制，促成第一个女用国产口服避孕药问世。

我觉得刘教授当时是虽有"力拔山兮气盖世"的豪气，却因"时不利兮骓不逝"无法施展其才华。如果"时利兮"能继续掌舵，协和内分泌的航船就有可能乘风破浪，排除千难万险到达彼岸。他为人非常好，是谦逊好学，很有人缘的顶尖学者，备受同行的尊敬，我们也获益匪浅。例如，我因研究课题的需要，经常请教朱壬葆，张致一和王志均教授（他们是我的院外辅导和硕士毕业论文答辩的老师），他们都因为我是刘士豪教授下面的年轻人而热情耐心教导。给我印象最深的是，他对底下工作的人非常疼爱，非常照顾。每次到外面出差回来以后，首先他会介绍一些开会的情况，然后根据这个情况我们要做一些什么工作，他都有个想法，有个交代，有个启发和布局。例如，上世纪60年代，他在莫斯科参会时，同世界上首次分离纯化9种垂体前叶激素的美籍学者李卓皓深度交流后得到启发，回国后就指示有关人员要收集和妥存垂体手术切除的标本。还有一次，他到东北开会，回来带了两箱苹果，来给所有的年轻的大夫们吃，这在1962年那个困难的时期是非常珍贵的。我最后一次见到刘教授，回想起来我就要掉眼泪了。他在八楼三病房当清洁工，擦窗户、拖地板和打扫厕所后，拖着骨瘦如柴的身体艰难地来到东门公共浴室洗澡堂。我们在澡堂里面洗澡，一边洗一边聊天，当时他的一句话对我影响很深。他说："我，是不行了，以后内分泌的发展就靠你们这些后来人了。"多么感人肺腑的嘱托！不是豪言壮语，胜过豪言壮语。大有"没有我刘士豪，自有后来人"的内分泌学术大师的自信。刘仙师，您在天之灵大可放心了，内分泌航船虽然换了几位舵手，驾驶的熟练程度有所差异，但航船一直在破浪前进，每年每站都有大的收获。如今，临床内分泌仍居榜首，基础内分泌虽暂居第二，但有望取得更大的跃进，因为我们全体后来人都在齐心协力，奋发向前！

孙梅励教授访谈录

李乃适：孙老师，大家都知道您到协和医院工作的时候，正是刘士豪教授当我们科第一任主任的时候，想请问您一下，您刚来的时候对刘士豪教授是什么印象？是他亲自来安排您工作的吗？

孙梅励：我是 1964 年 7 月底分到中国医学科学院，后因为刘士豪教授要一个北大毕业生，所以就把我又分到协和医院。当时我在人事科，刘士豪教授有一天穿着白大衣到了人事处，全体人事科的老师们都站起来欢迎他，我就觉得这人不简单，这就是刘士豪教授，内分泌科主任。当时的科长我记得是任玉珠医师，他把我介绍给刘士豪教授。刘士豪教授笑着说："欢迎你来参加我们内分泌科的工作。"然后他就把我领到了内分泌科，当时内分泌科的办公室是在 15 楼 4 层，西边的一个房间里头。到那以后，他询问了我的家庭、学业和历史。我向他介绍了以后，心里很紧张。他又问："你的论文导师是谁？"我说是沈同教授。他说："哦，他是我的朋友。"他那么和蔼可亲地跟我说，我们就很自然地聊起来了。然后他说："这样吧，我带你下楼去认识认识科里的同志。"他就领我到了当时叫 319 实验室，也就是在 10 楼 3 层的内分泌实验室。当时进去以后，里头有 4 个人，他跟我说："这个是孙老师，这个是刘老师，这个也是小刘老师。哦我说错了，（他应该是叫的先生），这是孙先生，刘先生和小刘先生。"我当时也跟着就说："老师好！"当时我就挺奇怪的，怎么会有人穿的是白大褂，有人穿的是隔离服。后来我知道了，穿隔离服的是技术员，穿白大褂的是教授。那时候穿衣服是有等级的，代表着职称的不同。从 319 实验室出来以后，我们去现在的医科大学研究所的一层的实验室叫 490 内分泌实验室，这个实验室比较大，人也比较多，里头有杨德馨讲师、许建生讲师、助理研究员倪祖梅，另外还有四五个进修大夫。金孜琴讲师当时是我们的支部书记。刘教授一一向我介绍，"这都是先生，以后都是你的老师"。他也把我介绍给吴静波进修医生，说："以后他就做你的老师，你跟着他学尿醛固酮的提取方法。"

然后又指着杨德馨讲师说：“她是这实验室的负责人，你有什么事就找她。”她以后负责辅导你们内分泌的英语。”所以从那以后，我们每星期二或星期三晚上，吃完晚饭都要到实验室来学英文。从实验室出来，他说你先回家安排安排，明天来上班。我就被安排在内分泌490实验室了，也就是现在医大一层里的实验室。

第二天刘士豪教授给我打了一个电话，让我10点钟到西门的图书馆去等他。西门是咱们的医科院图书馆。到那以后带我先认识一个管理员，那个管理员我记得姓关，非常和蔼的一个中年人。之后他又带我到了图书借书处，卡片箱里头有好多层。他就来教我怎么去查卡片，怎么找内分泌的书和杂志，然后又教我怎么去写卡片来预约。教完以后，他问我：“懂了吗？”我说：“我懂了，我在北大学过。”之后，他带我从一楼爬到三楼，看看常用的内分泌的书和杂志。一层当时都是杂志，他就告诉我第1间到第4间都有内分泌的书和杂志，以及哪些杂志是常用的、哪些杂志应该怎么去查阅。然后他又把一本杂志翻过来，里头都有插的卡片，教我怎么用卡片写预约，并说预约的时间到了，就会通知你来借。我们一直走楼梯，从一楼爬到二楼，二楼到三楼，三楼当时是医科院的馆藏的旧书，有些也是新书。然后他又教我怎么找书看，内分泌、内科或其他科的书都放在哪。他又告诉我怎么约书。那天我记着一直到11点多钟，他就一直陪着我。最后问我：“你学会了吗？你留在这再学习学习。”他就走了。我在这里过了第二天。

第三天的时候，他突然叫我去拿一个纸条。我一看是叫我借什么杂志、什么书。他还告诉我：“你去借的时候，找不着就问昨天见的管理员。”所以第三天我的主要任务就在图书馆去找杂志和借书。因为在北大学过，做学年论文和毕业论文都曾查过，虽然这个图书馆的那些规则不是特别明白，但在他的带领下我还是很快掌握了。借回来的文献我都努力把它看明白，翻译出来，第二天交给刘教授。其实我觉得来这也不轻松，在学校的时候觉得老师要求挺严的，但没想到一进内分泌科，回家的作业还是挺多的。这就是我接触到刘士豪教授的第一印象。因为他的精心安排，我就很快地熟悉了整个的工作环境，也就马上从一个学生就转变为了一个工作人员。吴静波老师也耐心地指导我，手把手地教我，使我觉得这个集体很温暖，也体会到刘教授是怎样对待一名新员工、怎样亲自培养他的学生。学生的第一课是要先学会查文献、学文献、翻译文献，然后才能去工作，而且还要不断学习。这就是我对刘士豪教授的第一深刻印象。但是当时因为我的工作没有直接的领导，就由刘士豪教授指导，所以我做的所有的工作都要直接向刘士豪教授汇报，而且听他的指示。

李乃适：孙老师您跟着刘士豪教授做了很多的学术研究，那么让您印象特别深刻的有哪些呢？这个过程当中有哪些事情让您觉得印象很深刻，也是他的风格。

孙梅励：刘士豪教授对学术要求是很严格的，也可以说非常严谨。第一次接触，我的工作是跟人家学，后来他给我的一个任务是要建立血浆和尿里的血糖试纸的测定实验。这已是 1964 年的下半年了。开展这项工作的时候，他给我的第一任务是查文献，自己去设计课题，自己去把文献先翻译出来，然后把它写出来，打算怎么做写出来流程，而且把翻译的论文和写的流程再交给他。看完以后，把我叫去跟我讨论，怎么做合适，让我试试看。他要求我必须拿一个小本。这个小本干什么呢？一边做一边记，把你看到的现象、做的步骤还有出现的意外情况都记在这小本上。你必须把这些成功的、失败的现象，都整理在科研处发的科研记录本上，内容要求写出研究目的、实验流程、出现的问题、明天准备怎么做，都必须写清楚，然后把你的草稿本和你这次实验记录本第二天必须交给刘教授。我觉得因为我在学校里受过这样训练，所以不感到陌生，做起来也还比较顺利。但是由于我边实验、边记录，所以记录都写得很潦草。刘教授批评我，字要写得工整，要让人看明白。（以后我培养我的研究生时，也是要求他们准备一个小本，随时做记录，然后课下随时把正规记录写好）。我的实验小本和记录交给他以后，他不仅要看，而且他把我的错别字都给改了，同时还要和我一起讨论，他问我实验失败的原因是什么？问题出在哪里？你要怎么改？当我回答不出来时，他就启发我。所以，我跟他讨论问题时就像我和导师讨论一样，一点都不紧张，而且愿意把做错了的地方和他说。他要求我第二天必须向他汇报前一天的工作。正好这是 1964 年的下半年了，转眼就 1965 年了。在这个过程中，我受到了严格训练并培养了精益求精的科研态度。刘士豪教授虽然很忙，但对于培养年轻一代他绝对不放松，而且也绝对不马虎。有一次我记得汇报的时候，正好赶上邢台地震，当时窗户都摇得很厉害，他仍然镇静不乱。等我汇报完，我们一起下楼。那对我真正感觉到他稳于泰山、处事不惊的精神。

李乃适：孙老师您那时候做的尿糖试纸的结果如何？后来怎样？

孙梅励：后来就和检验科合作，进行尿糖试纸实验，实验结果应用于临床，并且投给化工厂成批生产了。血糖试纸最早一次还用在临床救过一个病人。后来因为特殊时期了，就没有再做。以后我与检验科合作，把血糖和尿糖试纸与北京化工厂合作，转化成产品，广泛用于临床。

李乃适：另外一方面，您的经历当中，您觉得有什么事能特别体现刘教授的这种大医的情怀和临床的高度？

孙梅励：刘士豪教授是学识渊博的一个人，这是大家都知道的。他是协和医学院毕业生中第一个被提为教授的。此外，他从来不自傲，也不显摆，特别能够与时俱进。比如说就做放射免疫这件事，是 1964 年美国学者 Yalow 第一次发表了做 ACTH 的放射免疫试验，刘士豪教授就马上买了牛血清白蛋白，让他的研究生陈智周开展了胰岛素的放射免疫实验，同时也让我做血尿醛固酮的放射免疫试验。这就证明了刘教授很快跟上了国际科研发展形势。

另外，至今我都记忆犹新的一件事是：当时有一个妇女带着一个男孩来了我们医院，要求给她的孩子做诊断和治疗。这个孩子长得特别怪，一身的毛，鼻子和头特别大，大家都觉得像个小怪物。孩子的妈妈说她走遍了全国好多地方，都没有人诊断这是什么病、怎么治，希望咱们协和医院能够给出一个诊断治疗的方法。当时医院说请刘士豪教授去给看一看。我很深刻地记得，那时候是在院子里，刘教授很自然地走到自来水管那去洗了洗手，然后就开始坐在院子里，给孩子从头到尾做了一个体检，并问了孩子的病史和家族史。孩子的爸爸和妈妈是近亲结婚，好像我记得是表兄妹还是姑表兄妹。不到 10 分钟刘教授就检查完了。他严肃地告诉孩子的妈妈："回家吧，没什么可治的办法。这是一个黏多糖沉积病，也叫承雷病。它是一个骨营养缺乏症，是家族的一个遗传病，也是一个近亲结婚的结果。在目前情况下，没有什么好办法治。"他说："你别再跑了，也别再花钱。回家吧！真的是没有什么好的办法给孩子治。"我记得很清楚，当时那个妈妈泪流满面，给刘教授深深鞠了一躬。我看到刘教授满目惆怅，毫无办法地在那站了一会儿，转身他就走了。后来妈妈带着孩子回家了。我觉得这个病确实在当时好多人都不认得，他去了许多地方，但是只有刘教授看了 10 分钟，他就能诊断出什么病。好像我了解到这个病至今也没有什么特效的治疗办法。这体现了什么？体现了刘教授的学问，也体现了他对病人的无限同情。他是做骨代谢的一个很知名的专家，但他也无济于事。我当时看了很感动，这一时刻到现在我记忆犹新。

这就是我心中永远尊敬的导师和学者，并且是我在成长中做人做事的楷模。

李乃适：孙老师，您到协和医院之后，在您跟刘士豪教授的接触当中，您觉得他对内分泌科的这种科研布局和科研思想有什么样的影响？

孙梅励：刘大夫自己本身就是搞科研的。他又是医生，也是科研人员，他之前是从北京医院做科研调到医科院的，这是我知道的，详细不太清楚，但是好像是这样的。刘士豪教授当时跟我的北大老师，一些很有名的生化专家，比如沈同、陈同度……这些老专家都关系密切，也很友好，因为他们是搞基础研究的。我想说的就是图书馆的所有的新书卡片和杂志的卡片，第一个登记的不是刘士豪教授，就是张孝骞教授，别人都抢不过，就说明他们老是去到图书馆去看书，而且这些新书他们必须第一个看，首先看。他们紧跟国际科研发展前沿。

另外就是对内分泌的布局，当时内分泌科的布局是相当不错的，有两个留美的讲师，有一个留苏联的助理研究员，还有一个是医科大学毕业的倪祖梅助理研究员。另外还有两个老技术员，就是关炳江和刘书勤。还有一个搞生理肌电的金孜琴讲师。所以这个实验室是专门做科研的。进修大夫不仅是进修临床，他们还必须到实验室进修一年的实验室操作。所以我来的时候实验室有 4 个进修大夫，现在这 4 个进修大夫都是当地的有名的专家和建立内分泌科的主任。还有一个实验室就是 319 实验室，那个实验室是专门做临床测定的，尿 17 酮、17 羟化酶这些所有的临床测定以及血糖测定等都在这个实验室。这个实验室有两个老技术员，也有一个讲师就是刘昌河教授。同时还有一个基础代谢实验室，当时的负责人我记得姓田。田老师每天要接病人来做基础代谢。还有一个专门抽血的实验室，那个实验室是专门做完基础代谢以后要做留尿查血或其他化验的。还有一些内分泌必要的观察，如吃药后的 24 小时激素节律，也在这个实验室。所以这个实验室对于临床的配合来说，是很全面的：有搞科研的，有搞临床的，有配合临床需要观察的和需要节律性的取血的。所以我那个时候实验室的层次是上有主任（当然临床就是临床那一部分了），下有讲师，有助理研究员，有实习研究员，有技术员，而且有专门搞科研的，还有研究生，整个的内分泌科当时在协和医院是一个庞大的内分泌科，而且该实验室是当时在全国也是排第一的，别的医院都没有。可以说，那个时代相当多的全国各地的内分泌主任都是从协和内分泌科进修过的。因为他们来了不仅要进修临床，还要进实验室。正因为这样，我们协和内分泌科被美国的 Wilson 教授称为"中国的内分泌殿堂"，因为内分泌科很全面，有人有物。改革开放恢复实验室以后，我们很快建了一系列各种激素的放射免疫测定，紧跟当时世界内分泌学发展水平。

邓洁英教授口述实录

　　我，邓洁英，于 1962 年来到协和医院内分泌科，一直在那里工作到 2005 年退休。跟刘士豪教授相处大概有两年多时间。这两年里给我印象很深刻的一点就是，刘士豪教授很重视从临床出发进行基础研究，很注重对年轻人的基础理论和基本功教育和培养。刘士豪教授作为一个内分泌学专家，既是一个临床专家，又是一个生物化学专家，不但有丰富的临床经验，而且基础知识非常丰富。1961 年内分泌科刚刚恢复，1962 年我来到内分泌科，对我国来说当时科内已有较完整设备的内分泌实验室，可做 17 羟皮质类固酮、17 酮皮质类固醇和血清蛋白结合碘及基础代谢率等内分泌病的诊断常规。在研究人员的配备上也很齐全，实力雄厚，我觉得研究人员好像比临床还要强。当时除了刘士豪和池芝盛两位教授统管临床和研究以外，临床里有史轶蘩大夫、白耀大夫、孟迅吾大夫、王姮大夫、潘孝仁大夫……大概就五六个大夫；但实验室力量像更强一点，有杨德馨、许建生和金孜琴三位讲师，而且基础都很牢固。杨德馨和许建生都是留美学生化的，他们是从刘士豪教授在生化系时就已经在一起了，后来一起到内分泌科的。除有三个讲师以外，还有高年资研究人员，如倪祖梅、刘昌和。1962 年以后增加我和周学瀛两个研究人员和吴从愿、陈智周两个研究生。整个研究队伍实力雄厚。1962 年除了招收新的研究人员和研究生以外，还从全国的大医院招收一批有临床经验内分泌医生作为进修生。为了对我们这些新生力量加强基础理论的培训，从那时起，开始了"内分泌的生理和生化"的课程，每周有一次课，要求住院大夫、研究生、研究人员和进修生参加听课。这个课程从生理、生化以及病理生理对经典内分泌腺体以及内分泌激素进行一个非常详细的介绍。这个课程很多课是刘士豪教授亲自讲援的。刘士豪教授讲的课是非常有吸引力的。他讲的课很详细、很系统，而且条理非常清楚。他记忆力很好，讲课时候讲到激素的水平，可以精确到小数点后第二位都不用看讲稿的。这门课不但要求学生按时听课还要掌握并记忆激素的生物合成及代谢的每一步，牢记并能画出图表。这门课结束后还有一个严格的考试。我的印象里，这个考试是我参加那么多的考试里比较难的考试，很严格。因为要掌握的知识很多，要理解还要记住，很不容易。经过这个培养，让我们这些新入内分泌学门的人在短期里就基本上掌握了内分泌腺体以及激素的最基本的知识，为进行内分泌的临床和研究打下坚实基础。对于我们新进入实验室的研究人员，除了基本理论的学习以外，还有对基本操作进行培训。这个训练从一开始就比较严格。当时我们内分泌实验室就已经有三位讲师了，我们分别有不同的讲师带我们学习基本操作。周学瀛是杨德馨讲师带；陈智周是研究生，她由许建生带，外面还找了好多老师带；我是由金孜琴带教的。我们实验室有4个实验员，他们除了做内分泌常规以外，还带我们学习最基本的操作，包括如何清洗实验用品。我们当时的实验用品不像现在是一次性的，包括吸管试管都是玻璃的，要反复使用。如果清洗得不干净，就会影响实验结果。如打破就没得用，且要赔偿才能领新的。这些严格的培训使我们较快掌握了内分泌的基本理论和规范的生化实验操作技术，为以后的研究打下坚实的基础。对进修大夫，除了参加临床工作、查房、听课以外，也安排时间在实验室做实验，所以当时的进修大夫经过一年的全面培训，回去后都成为当地的内分泌学科骨干和带头人，带动了全国内分泌学的发展。本院的临床大夫也尽量安排做一些实验，如王姮有时间也到实验室做一些钙的测定。

另外，看到刘士豪教授亲自组织的临床基础研究也使我印象深刻。例如，当时有一例醛固酮增多症的研究，刘士豪教授就像一个作战的指挥官一样制订详细的计划。他不但制订计划，还安排和督促计划的执行，每天都要了解研究的进展情况。如当天的代谢平衡（包括留尿、尿量是否准确）要详细掌握。所以刘士豪教授的基础研究是非常严谨、严密、严格、认真的，科学性很强。

刘士豪教授结合临床进行基础研究是我们的先驱和典范。今天我们纪念他要学习他严谨的科学态度，严格的工作作风，做好我们的临床和研究工作，使我们的内分泌水平有所突破和创新。

金自孟教授访谈录

李乃适：金大夫，您能不能给我们讲一讲您跟刘士豪教授的一些接触和比较感动的事情。

金自孟：我来协和医院以后就下了医疗队和社教工作队，并且在下面待的时间比较长，一直到了 1967 年 1 月份才结束，所以正式上班已经是 1967 年 3 月份。当时特殊情况下，我在内科病房，跟方圻大夫一个病房，病房里已经取消了主治大夫，更没有主任查房。因为我当时还是一个刚参加工作的住院医师，所以实际上什么事情都要问方圻大夫，方大夫等于是我的主治医师。因为没有名义上的主治大夫了，就是每个人管一个组，所以我和刘士豪教授实际上在那时没有什么接触。那么一直到 1968 年年底和 1969 年的阶段，我轮转到了内科门诊，在门诊的工作当中，就遇到了一些内分泌的问题。当时内分泌科年资最高的是池芝盛副主任。池大夫碰到疑难的病例的时候，曾经让我偷偷地去找过他，请刘教授会诊。

我能够记得比较清楚的有两次。两例病人都牵扯到性腺和肾上腺的一些问题。当时池大夫本身是擅长性腺，但是因为病情比较复杂，所以池大夫就叫我去找刘大夫交流。两次我都是在 8 号楼地窨子厕所那里找到刘士豪教授，偷偷带到 10 号楼门诊的小屋子里。这两个病人，分别是一个年轻的男病人和一个女性病人，都是牵扯到有性行为的异常，是不是肾上腺性腺方面有问题不能确定，所以当时请刘教授会诊。我感觉刘士豪教授在学术上面确实是没有人能够代替的。因为那个时候的内分泌和现在不一样，还没有一个激素的测定，还停在一个生化的阶段，所以临床的经验、临床的判断是最最重要的。刘士豪教授在这方面是最有经验的。像池大夫有这么多的临床经验，他尤其擅长性腺方面，在女性内分泌这方面是专家，他遇到问题也要请教刘士豪教授。刘教授来了以后从临床仔细地一个一个地分析，这两个病例都是刘教授解决的。因为这两个病人都是牵涉到一些特殊情况，需要在医学方面给出一个明确的意见，不能是模棱两可的，最后都是靠刘士豪教授来了以后给拿出的主意。所以虽然我跟刘教授接触不多，但是我能在年轻的时候，听到刘士豪教授对病人的分析，我觉得他的临床经验确实是非常丰富的，而且结合他在实验方面也是很擅长的。所以他来了以后当时就给出了临床的判断，送病人来的部门也感到非常满意。

李乃适：另外，您觉得当时刘士豪教授做的一些工作对我们后来的工作有什么影响？

金自孟：影响非常非常大。内分泌的基础是他打下的，当时内分泌是不分科的，1979 年的时候开始分科，成立了垂体组，这是当时创造的，国内国外都是没有的。当时史大夫是组长，临床就是史大夫和我两个人，实验室就是邓洁英研究员和高素敏技术员，我们四个人。垂体组是怎么成立的呢？因为陆召麟原来是内科传染组的，到了 69 年的时候，开始跟国外有一些交流。当时国家选派的，我们协和医院选派了两个人，一个陆召麟，一个江永晶，要到英国去进修，陆召麟要进修实验方面，而不是临床。但是他之前没有进过实验室，当时内分泌的实验室是全医院、全中国非常好的实验室，所以史大夫带他在我们实验室训练实验技能，在我们这里训练了半年，然后出国。出国回来时候英国的老师给了他一些生长激素的标准品，但是给的量很少，按照常规方式进行动物实验不够用来打出抗体。后来大家商量用改良的方法，多点皮下注射，后来加强用的静脉的 1% 的很小剂量。大家知道如果静脉里打蛋白类的激素发生免疫反应是可能死掉的，当时没有人这样做的，但是 1% 的量静脉注射，结果成功了，兔子没有死掉，而且抗体产生得非常好。这是全中国第一个生长激素的抗体，由此建立了生长激素测定的方法、放射免疫的方法。那么为什么能那么顺利地进行，就与刘士豪教授有关。1960 年、1961 年，美国的 Yalow 创立了放射免疫的方法。刘士豪教授看到这个报道之后，马上就开始安排研究，1962 年，陈智周做的就是胰岛素的放射免疫的测定方法。陈智周于 1965 年毕业，建立了胰岛素的放射免疫测定方法，但还没有正式地在临床推广应用该方法，就碰上特殊年代了，这个工作就停顿了。但是由于过去这个工作，我们就有了技术储备，包括放射免疫方法怎么开始、选择什么样的实验动物、怎样进行免疫，等等。所以，因为建立了胰岛素的放射免疫的这个测定方法，第一代的，就有了这个技术储备；这样等我们有了一点点生长激素之后，才能很顺利地把生长激素的这个放射免疫测定完成，没有遇到那么大的困难。此外，技术上还有一点创新，就是静脉注射的加强免疫。建立以后呢我们就能进行生长激素测定了，这样我们在全中国首先应用于治疗生长激素过多的疾病，就是肢端肥大症和巨人症。这个应用比我们国内其他医院能够测定激素提前了十年多一点。这样我们在这方面领先做了很多的工作，包括各种抑制试验、兴奋试验、正常值测定，再用于临床。由于我们比国内其他医院早做了 10 年的激素测定；1979年成立了垂体专业组以后，由内分泌科牵头，我们又联合了院内的其他 8 个科室，对垂体瘤的基础与临床进行了更深入的研究。后来我们得到了国家科技进步一等奖。这个国家科技进步一等奖在协和历史上只有两个。这项工作是史大夫带领我们几十个人做的，但是这个起步，这个技术的起点，实际上是跟刘士豪教授先前的工作有着很大的关系。我们等于说是站在他的肩膀上，更上了一层。

另外，我觉得刘教授教给我们一种思想，就是临床上看到每一个病人，不仅是看病为病人解决问题，每一个病人也是一个学习的对象、研究的对象。他要求我们要把病史写好，要进行分析。所以内分泌科有个比较好的风气，就是病历书写比较完整，病历资料比较完整。内分泌科从建立开始的第一份住院病历到现在，全部的资料都完整地保存下来。这些思想都是刘教授留下来的。

李乃适：我记得史大夫说，刘士豪教授他去首钢去调查糖尿病，这个事情对后来池大夫在酒仙桥做的糖尿病，或对潘孝仁大夫，当时也去了首钢，有没有影响？

金自孟：应该有。因为老池大夫本身也是内分泌学专家，他从上海到协和医院来也是慕刘士豪教授的名，就是奔着刘士豪教授来的。现在我们做的很多工作，比如糖尿病的教育，是 1964 年从一个以色列的教授开始的，以后全世界把糖尿病教育当作糖尿病治疗的一个重要的环节。但实际上，协和医院的糖尿病教育从 1958 年就开始了。在"大跃进"的年代，我们办了学习班，把糖尿病的知识教给病人，让病人自己查尿糖、调整饮食，及时跟医生交流，实际上就是糖尿病教育。以前我们内分泌科内部有个糖尿病组，池大夫是组长，当时还有潘孝仁。那时候潘孝仁和我是两个最年轻的，就在糖尿病组。这个传统一直延续到现在。像现在我们的工作叫 MDT，实际上全世界的 MDT 就是我们 1979 年成立的垂体瘤的协作组，由内分泌科牵头，联合神经外科、耳鼻喉科、眼科、妇产科等 8 个科室，大家一起对一个专病进行研究，进行攻关。基础的、临床的，包括病理科的。然后一直到 20 世纪 90 年代的后期，MDT 开始流行了。实际上现在来看，40 年以前，我们是全世界第一个 MDT。所以垂体瘤的 MDT 是一个典范，最早的起步就是在协和医院。

曾正陪教授访谈录

李乃适：曾大夫您好。刘士豪教授是我们科的创始人，大家都知道您考上协和医大的时候，正是刘士豪教授已经创建了内分泌科并担任第一任内分泌科主任的时候；您开始工作的时候应该也有一段时间能够见到他。我们想请您谈一谈您跟刘士豪教授交往的经历，或者您当时从学生的角度听说的刘士豪教授的一些特别的事迹。

曾正陪：好的。我是 1961 年进入协和，当时我们学校叫中国医科大学，它的前身就是北京协和医学院，三年预科在北京大学。1964 年我从北大来到协和，在学校见过刘士豪教授。1974 年，我回到协和学习，现在想起来都是非常有意义的一段经历。当时我在协和内科轮转，在 8 楼 3 消化内科病房当住院医生，我们叫"回炉"学习。我记得在 1974 年 5 月份，刘士豪教授因为有神经系统的一些症状先在神经科住院，但是检查以后发现主要还是内科的问题，当时他也有发热，诊断肺炎，后来就从神经科 8 楼 1 转到了 8 楼 3。在 8 楼 3 的时候，因为当时我们在那工作嘛，我参加了当时的查房。我记得特别清楚的一次就是张孝骞主任带着我们这些年轻医生查房到了刘士豪教授的床前，刘教授看到我们这些年轻人，他就说你看张教授比我就大两岁，但是他现在还能够带你们查房，还能正常地工作；他说："我已经是一个病人躺在这儿了。"当时我就觉得非常遗憾，这是他那个时候给我们讲的话。后来到了 5 月底，他的病情就加重了。他不是我直接管的病人，但是在 6 月 2 日我值夜班，那时刘士豪教授的病情已经非常危重，我接班以后就一直和当时在场的很多大夫一起参加抢救。我记得当时他的心跳停止后，我们给他打过六次心内"三联"注射。当时我们都觉得刘教授的心脏功能还是很强大的，因为心内"三联"注射以后，心脏又复跳了。但是非常遗憾，我们还是没能把他抢救过来。最后刘教授就离开我们了，我记得当时是我和刘教授的研究生陈元方大夫，我们一起把他送到太平间去的。

李乃适：另外一个重要的问题，您认为刘士豪教授的工作，对我们后来的内分泌科产生了什么样的影响？不管是他在建内分泌科以前的工作，还是在建科以后的工作，以及刘教授对于内分泌学科整个的思路，等等。

曾正陪：刘士豪教授是内分泌科的创始人，当时在北京协和医院创建了全国第一个内分泌科，并在全国首先开创了内分泌激素的临床实验室的研究。建内分泌科以后有好几个"第一"，除了大家现在知道的在骨代谢、钙磷代谢、骨软化等方面在国内以及在国际上有很大的影响之外，其实刘教授在我们内分泌的肾上腺方面也作了非常大的贡献。

我去查过一些病例了 1939 年，当时在协和内科，刘教授与内科主任 Snapper 教授诊断了我们中国的第一例嗜铬细胞瘤，因为嗜铬细胞瘤是 1886 年在国际上首次报告，但是到了 1939 年在协和就诊断了。那个病人是一个 13 岁的男孩，他是以发热待查收住院的，但是入院以后当时的临床医生观察到他每天下午有血压的剧烈波动，后来观察到是阵发性高血压发作。然后患者接受了一系列检查。这在当时的条件下其实是很困难的，因为没有激素的测定，只是根据临床症状和通过腹膜后充气造影，发现了肾上腺肿瘤而诊断的嗜铬细胞瘤。当时是刘士豪教授和 Snapper 教授他们共同诊断的。所以在 1939 年他们就诊断了一个非常重要的内分泌高血压疾病。

1962 年，刘士豪教授诊治了国内第 2 例原发性醛固酮增多症。1955 年，美国 Conn 教授报告了全球首例原发性醛固酮增多症。1957 年，上海瑞金医院邝安堃教授报告了国内第 1 例。我们协和医院是 1962 年发现第 1 例原发性醛固酮增多症、肾上腺腺瘤的病人。在那时的条件下，没有那么多检查的手段，但是刘士豪教授带着我们内分泌科的医生，给病人做了很多关键性的检查，包括做了 ACTH 刺激试验，并且检测了病人的血容量。这个病人是容量增多的高血压，而原醛正是血容量增加的高血压。最后病理也证实是原发性醛固酮增多症。而且，这个病人在手术病理证实诊断后，一直随访到 1976 年，情况仍然很好。当时我们没有现在的 CT 等现代化的设备；我们通过临床的观察，通过一些功能试验，还有通过腹膜后充气造影，最后从临床和病理诊断了原醛症，这当时在国内也是很不容易的。所以在刘士豪教授，还有我们的其他前辈（包括池芝盛教授、史轶蘩教授）的努力下，我们协和内分泌科除了在骨代谢方面以外，在肾上腺肿瘤方面的工作也很出色。在此基础上，北京协和医院的肾上腺／高血压诊疗水平也得到了很大的发展。当时刘教授带着内分泌科同仁，制备了醛固酮抗体，而且建立了醛固酮的放射免疫测定方法。我们后来在临床上诊断治疗了越来越多的原发性醛固酮增多症和嗜铬细胞瘤患者，这些都是在刘教授创建协和内分泌科和实验室的基础上逐渐做到的。所以我们现在在内分泌科的发展是在他们建立的基础上，也就是说在巨人的肩膀上来进一步发展的。

李乃适：曾大夫您刚才说了刘士豪教授对于我们科肾上腺方面的发展起到了开创性的贡献。那么您觉得后来您受他的影响有哪些？

曾正陪：我到内分泌科以后，史大夫就给我定了内分泌高血压的研究方向。所以几十年来，我也一直就在做内分泌高血压，包括嗜铬细胞瘤和原醛的诊断治疗的工作，这其实也是在刘教授和史教授他们建立的基础上。在内分泌性高血压方面，在协和内分泌科其他医生的共同努力下，我们取得了很多成绩，包括在2003年我们诊断了国内第一例心脏的副神经节瘤，当时还叫嗜铬细胞瘤。这么多年来，我们协和内分泌科诊断的嗜铬细胞瘤也好，原发性醛固酮增多症也好，我们诊断治疗的病例数应该在国内外都是名列前茅的。特别是心脏的副神经节瘤，我们现在已经有二十几例，这个在国际上绝对是单家医院第一位的。所以在我们协和医院的肾上腺这个亚专业，特别是内分泌性高血压、原醛和嗜铬细胞瘤方面还是取得了很大的进步。最近我也刚刚完成了中华医学会内分泌学分会的嗜铬细胞瘤副神经节瘤诊断治疗的2020版专家共识。这是在我们协和医院诊治经验的基础上，总结参照了国内外其他医院在这方面做的工作。但是总的来说我们在肾上腺高血压方面还是做了很多的工作，在国内外还是有一定地位的。这些都是和我们的前辈——刘士豪教授、史轶蘩教授他们的工作分不开的。我们是在他们精神的鼓舞下，在他们打下的这个基础上，我们才能做到的。

李乃适：曾大夫，您在中华医学会内分泌学分会曾经担任了很重要的职务，请问您觉得全国的内分泌同行对刘教授的事迹了解的情况怎样呢？

曾正陪：因为协和内分泌是全国第一个成立的内分泌科，后来成为全国学术带头人的一些内分泌教授们，他们当年都是在我们协和医院进修的。那个时候在刘士豪教授、池芝盛教授和史轶蘩教授的带领和指导下，北京协和医院内分泌科给全国各地培养了很多内分泌学科带头人。中华医学会内分泌学分会对刘士豪教授给予了很高的评价。在史大夫的带领下我参与和担任学会的工作近20年，最早从当内分泌学分会的秘书开始，后来到常委、副主委、主委、前任主委、名誉主委。我记得1993年当时在南京开全国内分泌大会的时候，内分泌学会首次隆重纪念中国内分泌的主要创始人，就是刘士豪、朱宪彝、邝安堃三位教授。

我是2005年担任内分泌学分会主任委员。中华医学会内分泌学分会在2009年全国内分泌大会上隆重举行了刘士豪、朱宪彝、邝安堃三位教授的铜像揭幕典礼，并决定从2009年开始，在内分泌学会的每年年会设立以刘士豪、朱宪彝和邝安堃三位教授的冠名讲座并颁发奖牌。十余年来，每一年都选择国内在内分泌代谢领域作出了比较大的贡献的专家教授来做这三个冠名讲座的讲者。非常荣幸，我在2010年全国内分泌大会的刘士豪教授冠名讲座上做了"北京协和医院嗜铬细胞瘤和原发性醛固酮增多症的诊治"报告并获得了中华医学会内分泌学会的杰出贡献奖。这十来年，除了自己获奖以外，我也多次担任过刘士豪冠名讲座的主持人，包括邀请的外宾和国内著名教授的讲座。另外我非常高兴、也非常欣慰的是，10年后在今年，2020年，我们北京协和医院内分泌科的现任主任夏维波教授也成为刘士豪教授冠名讲座的讲者，报告了我们协和医院在骨代谢方面所做出的成绩。从刘士豪教授冠名讲座的这十年的情况看，也是体现了我们协和医院内分泌科的一个传承。所以我觉得设立了这个冠名讲座对我们协和人是一个鼓舞，更是一个鞭策。现在在学会上，大家对这三个冠名讲座还是有很高的期待的，也是给予了一个很高的荣誉。

李乃适：谢谢曾教授，我们都学到了很多。在百年协和即将到来之际，您觉得还有什么想对我们说的吗？

曾正陪：北京协和内分泌科是刘士豪教授创建的国内第一个内分泌科，我希望我们协和内分泌要不断地前进。我们现在应该有一个危机感和紧迫感，要在我们的前辈创建的基础上，把我们的协和内分泌做强做大，再创我们协和内分泌的辉煌。我觉得这是我作为曾经的科主任，也是作为协和人的一个传承吧。我觉得我的位置应该是一个承上启下的作用。我们的前辈给我们打下的基础，在我们这一代继承下去，我们也做了一些力所能及和传承的工作，我觉得我自己还是无愧的。但是这个传承下来就希望我们现在的年轻人、内分泌现在的同仁们，应该是后浪推前浪，后浪应该要体现他更强大的优势和力量。希望把我们北京协和内分泌科，在刘士豪教授、池芝盛教授、史轶蘩教授还有王姮教授他们所创建的我们内分泌科的实力和基础上，能够让我们的内分泌科更加强大起来，应该再创辉煌，让我们的内分泌科在各个方面有全面的提高。纪念刘士豪教授，让我们的年轻人应该要感到作为一个协和内分泌人的光荣和责任，同时更是一个鞭策。我们每个人都必须要为协和内分泌添砖加瓦，要贡献我们大家的力量。只有这样，我们北京协和内分泌才能更加地强大起来。这也是我对他们现在这一代人的期望。

附录三

《高山仰止——纪念刘士豪教授诞辰 120 周年》纪念片解说词

高山仰止
——纪念刘士豪教授诞辰 120 周年

李乃适

1941 年 12 月 7 日，日军突然奇袭珍珠港，继而在接下来的 1942 年席卷南洋，全世界陷入一片灰霾之中；我国的抗日战争也同时进入了最为艰难的时期。

被誉为"东方霍普金斯"的协和，这座坚持了 4 年的北平"学术孤岛"，最终也未能逃脱蹂躏于日军铁蹄之下的命运。

在协和玉碎之际，全世界为之愤懑，全世界为之痛惜。不过，阴霾的 1942 年也偶尔会透出一丝的亮色，协和人命名"肾性骨营养不良"的一篇短文于 4 月发表于《科学》(Science)，让全球医学界稍感欣慰。而这篇论文的作者，正是我国内分泌学奠基人、协和内分泌与肾脏病领域的核心人物刘士豪教授和他的师弟朱宪彝教授。

刘士豪，16 岁即考入湘雅预科的武昌天才少年，在 1918 年愉快地接受了多读一年预科并参加选拔考试的要求，考入刚满周岁的新建北京协和医学院。

这是北美医学教育改革的核心人物，威廉·韦尔奇，在洛克菲勒基金会的强力支持下，以约翰·霍普金斯医学院为蓝本，在中国建立一所符合医学教育理想的医学院，一所不亚于欧美的医学院，一所可能成为全球典范的最高水平的医学圣殿。如鱼得水的刘士豪逐渐开始了"学霸"生涯，毕业时以医本部期间总成绩第一荣获"文海奖"，并留任协和内科住院医师。

3 年住院医师工作期间，刘士豪发表了从汞中毒到甲状腺提取物治疗等一系列临床论文，继而留美师从生化巨擘范斯莱克。聪慧勤勉再加名师指点，刘士豪在临床和科研上的能力均得到了飞速提高。1930 年回国后，刘士豪正式进入内分泌和肾脏研究团队，并于 4 年后成为团队核心。

钙磷代谢领域是刘士豪的主攻方向。在前期工作的基础上，运用国外所学的最新生物化学理念，刘士豪用极为精细的代谢平衡法完成了一例又一例骨软化症的钙磷代谢研究。曾经有一个故事流传至今：一位正处于临床研究期间的住院患者进餐时，一小团米饭不慎掉落在地；刘士豪立即上前捡起了这团米饭，然后将其放置于精密天平的托盘上进行称重，并通知营养部将科研所用膳食量相应扣除。如何对待这一小团饭，体现的是老一代协和学者严谨求精的治学态度。刘士豪团队历经十余年，先后发表了 13 篇以"骨软化症的钙磷代谢"为题的系列论文，被誉为"世界钙磷代谢研究的基石"。

这一时期，先后有 5 例肾衰后的佝偻病或骨软化症患者收入代谢病房。用代谢平衡法获得基础数据以后，刘士豪和朱宪彝经过深入分析，得出了这样的结论：对于肾衰后出现的佝偻病或骨软化症，尽管用维生素 D 无效，但用双氢速变固醇治疗有显著疗效！尽管这一结论与当时的国际学术权威观点相悖，但刘士豪和朱宪彝对协和代谢病房的数据充满信心，并且为这类疾病提出了一个新的命名。他们将这一成果投稿到著名期刊《科学》（Science），从此有了中国人命名的第一个疾病名称——"肾性骨营养不良"。

20 世纪 30 年代堪称老协和的"黄金时代"。除了钙磷代谢，对我国第一例胰岛素瘤的研究、对下丘脑 - 垂体 - 性腺轴的实验研究、对垂体后叶和水代谢的研究……刘士豪的学术成就使他在 40 岁时就晋升为内科学教授，这也是协和毕业生中第一位临床学系教授。

　　然而，刘士豪在协和这座"孤岛"中的象牙塔之梦终被战火无情击碎。待到再次和平，已经是百废待兴的新中国成立之时。1951年，刘士豪出任协和生物化学系系主任。一本《生物化学与临床医学的联系》，其思想堪称开转化医学之先河。

　　知行合一，刘士豪教授在1958年8月将生物化学系的激素研究组与内科的内分泌组合并，创建了我国第一个独立于内科的内分泌科——北京协和医院内分泌科。尽管他悉心钻研的胰岛素放射免疫测定法和首钢糖尿病研究最终因时代原因未能实现"到临床中去"，但一代代协和人正是在刘士豪教授指引的道路上砥砺前行……

　　高山仰止，景行行止。虽不能至，然心向往之……